Livestock Diseases: Clinical Assessment and Treatment

Livestock Diseases: Clinical Assessment and Treatment

Edited by Salvador Barker

SYRAWOOD
PUBLISHING HOUSE
New York

Published by Syrawood Publishing House,
750 Third Avenue, 9th Floor,
New York, NY 10017, USA
www.syrawoodpublishinghouse.com

Livestock Diseases: Clinical Assessment and Treatment
Edited by Salvador Barker

International Standard Book Number: 978-1-64740-441-3 (Hardback)

Cataloging-in-publication Data

Livestock diseases : clinical assessment and treatment / edited by Salvador Barker.
p. cm.
Includes bibliographical references and index.
ISBN 978-1-64740-441-3
1. Livestock--Diseases. 2. Livestock--Diseases--Treatment. 3. Livestock--Diseases--Diagnosis. I. Barker, Salvador.
SF745 .L58 2023
636.089--dc23

TABLE OF CONTENTS

PREFACE

Livestock animals may be affected by infectious diseases caused by parasites such as tsetse flies, ticks, mosquitoes, and Culicoides midges, or by microorganisms such as viruses, fungi and bacteria. Some of the examples of infectious diseases in animals include bovine virus diarrhea (BVD), tuberculosis, Johne's disease, and brucellosis. Infectious diseases in animals are caused due to factors such as the addition of new member to a herd and contaminated water. The assessment or diagnosis of livestock diseases is essential for detecting the cause and nature of the disease, which, in turn is essential for ensuring faster treatment planning. Livestock diseases are diagnosed using techniques such as analysis of blood, tissue, urine, or stool to detect the presence of proteins, antibodies, or general indicators of overall health. The first step in the treatment of the infected livestock animals usually involves isolating the affected animal from the rest of the herd. Additionally, the infected animals are also given anti-inflammatory drugs and antibiotics. This book unravels the recent studies on the diagnosis and treatment of diseases in livestock. It is appropriate for students seeking detailed information in this area of veterinary science as well as for experts.

This book is a result of research of several months to collate the most relevant data in the field.

When I was approached with the idea of this book and the proposal to edit it, I was overwhelmed. It gave me an opportunity to reach out to all those who share a common interest with me in this field. I had 3 main parameters for editing this text:

1. Accuracy - The data and information provided in this book should be up-to-date and valuable to the readers.

2. Structure - The data must be presented in a structured format for easy understanding and better grasping of the readers.

3. Universal Approach - This book not only targets students but also experts and innovators in the field, thus my aim was to present topics which are of use to all.

Thus, it took me a couple of months to finish the editing of this book.

I would like to make a special mention of my publisher who considered me worthy of this opportunity and also supported me throughout the editing process. I would also like to thank the editing team at the back-end who extended their help whenever required.

Editor

1

Detection and Molecular Characterization of Bovine Leukemia Virus in Egyptian Dairy Cattle

Rania Hamada[1,2]*, Samy Metwally*[1,3,4]*, Meripet Polat*[5]*, Liushiqi Borjigin*[5]*, Alsagher O. Ali*[2]*, A. A. A. Abdel-Hady*[6]*, Adel E. A. Mohamed*[2]*, Satoshi Wada*[1] *and Yoko Aida*[3,5*]

[1] Photonics Control Technology Team, RIKEN Center for Advanced Photonics, Saitama, Japan, [2] Department of Animal Medicine, Faculty of Veterinary Medicine, South Valley University, Qena, Egypt, [3] Laboratory of Global Animal Resource Science, Graduate School of Agricultural and Life Sciences, The University of Tokyo, Tokyo, Japan, [4] Department of Animal Medicine, Faculty of Veterinary Medicine, Damanhour University, Damanhour, Egypt, [5] Nakamura Laboratory, Baton Zone Program, RIKEN Cluster for Science, Technology and Innovation Hub, Saitama, Japan, [6] Department of Surgery, Anaesthesiology and Radiology, Faculty of Veterinary Medicine, South Valley University, Qena, Egypt

***Correspondence:**
Yoko Aida
aida@riken.jp

Bovine leukemia virus (BLV) causes enzootic bovine leukosis (EBL), the most common neoplastic disease in cattle worldwide. The first EBL outbreak in Egypt was reported in 1997. To date, there are few studies regarding BLV diagnosis using only serological detection and no studies investigating the distribution of BLV provirus, which is the retroviral genome integrated into the host genome, in Egypt. The genetic characteristics of Egyptian BLV strains are also unknown. Therefore, we aimed to detect BLV provirus and determine BLV genetic variability among dairy cattle in Egypt. We collected 270 blood samples of dairy cattle from 24 farms located in five provinces in Egypt. Out of the 270 samples, 58 (21.5%) were positive for BLV provirus. Phylogenetic analysis based on 18 420-bp selected sequences out of 50 isolates of the BLV *env*-gp51 gene demonstrated that Egyptian BLV isolates were clustered into genotype-1 and-4, among 11 genotypes detected worldwide. Furthermore, phylogenetic analysis and alignment of the 501-bp sequence of the *env*-gp51 gene revealed that at least six genetically different strains are present in Egypt. Genotype-1 isolates comprised four different strains (G1-a, G1-b, G1-c, and G1-d) and genotype-4 isolates included two different strains (G4-x and G4-y). Moreover, in one farm with 100% infection rate, we identified three isolates of G1-a strain, 35 isolates of G4-x strain, and two isolates of G4-y strain. Overall, this study provides the new report on molecular prevalence of BLV in Egypt and records the coexistence of BLV genotype-1 and-4 in Egyptian cattle.

Keywords: bovine leukemia virus, Egypt, dairy cattle, prevalence, BLV genotype

INTRODUCTION

Bovine leukemia virus (BLV), an oncogenic member of the family *Retroviridae*, genus *Deltaretrovirus*, is closely related to the human T-cell leukemia virus types 1 and 2 (1, 2). It causes enzootic bovine leukosis (EBL), the most common neoplastic disease of cattle globally, and imposes a severe economic loss to the dairy industry (1–3). Most BLV-infected cattle are apparently healthy in the aleukemic stage and approximately one-third can enter the persistent lymphocytosis stage characterized by non-malignant polyclonal expansion of B-lymphocytes; however, only 1–5%

develop B-cell leukemia, manifesting clinical signs of lymphoma after a long latency (1, 2). BLV infection can be transmitted both vertical route and horizontal route in addition to the other iatrogenic procedures involving the transfer of infected blood between animals (i.e., dehorning, ear tattooing, rectal palpation, and needle reuse), and is responsible for disease propagation in a herd (4). BLV has spread worldwide via the continual trade of breeding cattle between several countries (3). However, vaccines and effective treatments are not yet available for practical application (1).

BLV proviral load (PVL), which represents the retroviral genome integrated into the host genome (5, 6), correlates strongly with not only BLV infection capacity as assessed by syncytium formation (7, 8), but also EBL progression (7, 9, 10). Additionally, it is a useful index for estimating transmission risk (11, 12). For example, previous reports have posited that as determined by the BLV-CoCoMo-quantitative polymerase chain reaction (qPCR)-2 method, the quantitative measurement of PVL (7, 13), BLV provirus was detected in the milk, nasal mucus, and saliva samples from dairy cattle with PVL >10,000, 14,000, and 18,000 copies/10^5 cells in blood samples, respectively (11, 12). It has been suggested that these infected cattle may increase the risk of BLV transmission via direct contact with healthy cattle. In contrast, cattle with low PVL are known to prevent natural BLV infection (14).

BLV genome consists of four structural and enzymatic regions that encode genes namely, *gag*, *pro*, *pol*, and *env*, along with the pX region that encodes two regulatory, *tax* and *rex*, and two accessory genes, *R3* and *G4*, and is flanked by two identical long terminal repeats (LTRs) at the 5′ and 3′ termini (1, 2). The BLV *env* gene is transcribed as an envelope glycoprotein (Env) protein complex that comprises the surface (gp51) and transmembrane (gp30) proteins (1), which play a major role in the virus lifecycle and entry into the host cell (15). gp51 is the target for neutralizing antibodies (16). The conformational epitopes (F, G, and H) located in the N-terminal half of gp51 are strongly involved in syncytium formation and viral infectivity (15, 16). The C-terminal half contains linear epitopes (A, B, D, and E) mapped with antipeptide antibodies (17). In contrast to gp51, gp30 is poorly immunogenic (1) and therefore, BLV *env*-gp51 sequencing is mainly used for BLV phylogenetic studies (3). At least 11 BLV genotypes have been identified worldwide based on the phylogenetic analysis of *env*-gp51 sequences of BLV after identifying BLV genotype-11 in China (3, 18). Three genotypes of BLV, namely genotype-1,-4, and-6, has been mainly detected worldwide (3).

Egypt is a transcontinental country spanning the northeast corner of Africa and southwest corner of Asia. The bovine sector in Egypt is well-integrated with cropland since there are limited natural pastures. Female cattle and buffaloes are used for milk production, while male animals and infertile females are fattened for meat (19). Native cattle in Egypt are called "Baladi," literally meaning "local" without genetic subdivisions. They are reared throughout the country, acclimatized to Egyptian conditions, and have a high tolerance to endemic diseases. Due to the low milk productivity of these animals, genetic improvement schemes have involved crossbreeding with exotic high producing cattle breeds such as Holstein, Brown Swiss, and Simmental (20–22), resulting in a large scattered population raised in small- or medium-sized herds by local farmers under the breed name "Mixed," as described and characterized by the Ministry of Agriculture and Land Reclamation. Egyptian livestock import has increased over the last 10 years, improving the dairy industry performance. Germany, Netherlands, and the United States of America remain the top suppliers of live dairy cattle to Egypt (23).

Sero-epidemiological surveys have shown that BLV infection is widespread in all continents except Europe, where the disease is present only in the eastern European countries (3). However, reports indicate that BLV infection prevalence in the Middle Eastern countries is somewhat lower than that in the other regions of the world (3). In Egypt, the first EBL outbreak occurred in 1997 in Assiut province, Upper Egypt with typical clinical signs of leukosis in a closed herd of Holstein-Friesian cattle imported from Minnesota, USA 8 years earlier (24). Thus, the authors assumed that these cattle were imported as clinically healthy BLV-infected cattle during the herd construction period and the disease progressed to lymphoma after the latent period passed (24). It was believed that this outbreak introduced BLV in Egypt (25). After completely eradicating the infected animals in the herd (24), Egypt was reported to be BLV-free (3, 26). In 2012, a seroprevalence study for BLV infection among dairy cattle in Egypt was conducted, which reported that 15.83% of the tested dairy cattle were BLV-infected (27). Recently, 20.8% BLV seropositivity was reported during the survey for BLV infection among Egyptian cattle (28). These findings indicate that BLV still infects Egyptian cattle. However, to date there has been no reports on BLV genotyping in Egypt.

In this study, we investigated BLV infection prevalence among dairy cattle in five different regions of Egypt to cover representative area of the country to include the northern (Beheira and Damietta provinces), the central (Fayoum province), and the southern (Qena and Luxor provinces) parts using CoCoMo-qPCR-2 assay. Furthermore, we demonstrated that the BLV PVL level varied among different regions of Egypt. Moreover, by conducting the phylogenetic analysis of BLV *env*-gp51 gene sequence, we investigated the six genetically distinct strains present in Egyptian cattle. Overall, this study provides a new evidence for the molecular detection of BLV in Egypt and records the coexistence of BLV genotype-1 and-4 among Egyptian cattle.

MATERIALS AND METHODS

Sample Collection and DNA Extraction

Blood samples were collected from 270 cattle of 24 different dairy farms located in five provinces in Egypt, namely Luxor, Qena, Fayoum, Beheira, and Damietta, between November 2018 and January 2019 (**Figure 1** and **Table 1**). These cattle comprised various breeds of dairy cattle, such as the Egyptian Native breed, some foreign breeds (Holstein and Simmental), and the Mixed breed, the crossbreed between foreign breeds and Native cattle, and included cattle of both sexes aged 3-months to 12-years (**Table 1**).

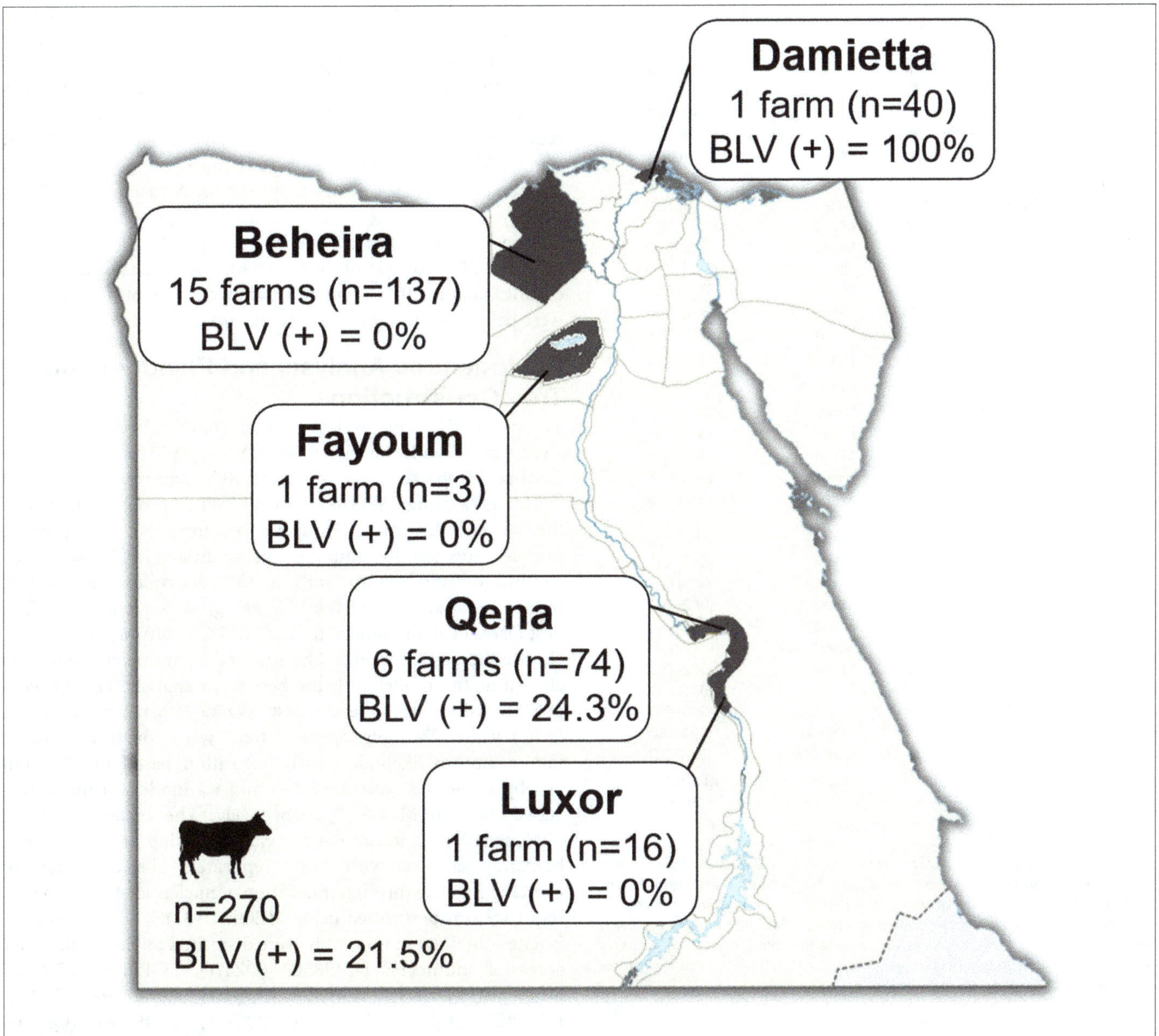

FIGURE 1 | Map of Egypt showing the location of dairy farms for sample collection. Dark gray colored area indicates the geographic location of each region in our study. The number (n; head) of cattle and number (n) of farms in each province and throughout Egypt are indicated in Square. BLV(+) % indicates the BLV prevalence rate.

Genomic DNA was extracted from 300 µl whole blood using the Wizard Genomic DNA Purification Kit (Promega; Madison, WI, USA), following manufacturer's instructions. The concentration of extracted DNA samples was measured using NanoDrop One Spectrophotometer (Thermo Fisher Scientific; Waltham, MA, USA). DNA samples were diluted in nuclease-free water to a final concentration of 30 ng/µl for PCR experiments.

Evaluation of BLV PVL Using CoCoMo-qPCR-2

BLV PVL was estimated using CoCoMo-qPCR-2 (RIKEN Genesis; Kanagawa, Japan), as described previously (7, 13). Briefly, a 183-bp sequence of the BLV LTR regions was amplified in a reaction mixture containing THUNDERBIRD Probe qPCR Mix (Toyobo; Tokyo, Japan), using the degenerate primer pairs, CoCoMo FRW and CoCoMo REV, and a 15 bp 6-carboxyfluorescein (FAM)-labeled LTR probe. To normalize the viral genomic DNA level within the host cellular genome, a 151-bp sequence of *BoLA-DRA* was amplified using the primer pairs, DRA-FW and DRA-RW, and a FAM-labeled DRA probe, as previously described (13). The PVL was calculated using the equation (number of BLV-LTR copies/number of *BoLA-DRA* copies) × 10^5 cells.

TABLE 1 | Detection of BLV infection in five provinces in Egypt as determined by CoCoMo-quantitative PCR (qPCR).

Province	Town	Farm ID[a]	Breed	(Positive no. /Tested samples no.) Positive %
Luxor	EL-Qurna	LQ1	Mixed	(0/14) 0.0
			Native	(0/ 2) 0.0
Qena	EL-Brahma	QB1	Mixed	(3/10) 30.0
		QB2	Mixed	(1/ 4) 25.0
		QB3	Mixed	(3/ 5) 60.0
		QB4	Native	(2/ 5) 40.0
			Mixed	(0/ 2) 0.0
		QB5	Native	(2/ 4) 50.0
			Mixed	(2/ 5) 40.0
	Qena-city	QC6	Holstein	(5/39) 12.8
Fayoum	Tamia	FT1	Holstein	(0/ 3) 0.0
Beheira	Abu-Elmatamir	BA1	Mixed	(0/ 9) 0.0
		BA2	Mixed	(0/ 2) 0.0
		BA3	Mixed	(0/ 7) 0.0
		BA4	Mixed	(0/ 2) 0.0
		BA5	Mixed	(0/15) 0.0
		BA6	Mixed	(0/ 4) 0.0
			Native	(0/ 1) 0.0
		BA7	Mixed	(0/ 6) 0.0
		BA8	Mixed	(0/ 3) 0.0
		BA9	Mixed	(0/ 2) 0.0
		BA10	Mixed	(0/19) 0.0
		BA11	Mixed	(0/ 6) 0.0
		BA12	Mixed	(0/ 2) 0.0
		BA13	Mixed	(0/ 7) 0.0
		BA14	Mixed	(0/ 5) 0.0
		BA15	Holstein	(0/43) 0.0
			Simmental	(0/ 4) 0.0
Damietta	El-Zarqa	DZ1	Holstein	(40/40) 100.0
Total farms		24	Total	(58/270) 21.5

[a]List of farm ID tested for BLV infection: 17 farms (QB1–QB5, BA1–BA4, BA6–BA9, and BA11–BA14) are small holder breeders, having less than 10 heads in each farm, 3 farms (LQ1, BA5, and BA10) are semi-intensive farms (over10 to 50 heads) and both of these small farms and the semi-intensive ones raring cattle of Native and Mixed breeds, and the other 4 farms (QC6, FT1, BA15, and DZ1) are intensive farms, having a cattle herd of more than 300 heads, rearing Holstein cattle except for farm BA15 that has few number of Simmental cattle rearing together with Holstein cows.

Nested PCR Amplification of BLV *env*-gp51 Gene Fragment and Nucleotide Sequencing

A 598-bp fragment of BLV *env*-gp51 gene was amplified via nested PCR using Prime STAR GXL DNA Polymerase (Takara Bio Inc.; Otsu, Japan) as described previously (29–31). The primer set External Forward (5′-ATGCCYAAAGAACGACGG-3′) and External Reverse (5′-CGACGGGACTAGGTCTGACCC-3′) resulted in the first-round amplification of the 913-bp fragment of full length BLV *env* gene corresponding to the nucleotide positions 4826 to 5738 of the whole BLV genomic sequence recorded in GenBank (accession No. EF600696) (32), and then internal ENV_{5032} (5′-TCTGTGCCAAGTCTCCCAGATA-3′) and internal ENV_{5608r} (5′-AACAACAACCTCTGGGAAGGGT-3′) resulted in the second-round amplification of the 598-bp fragment of the BLV *env*-gp51 gene corresponding to the nucleotide positions 5037 to 5634 of the whole BLV genomic sequence.

Positive second-round PCR products were purified using 5 × Exo-SAP IT (USB Corp.; Cleveland, OH, USA) and directly sequenced on an ABI3730x1 DNA Analyzer using ABI PRISM BigDye Terminator v3.1 Ready Reaction Cycle Sequencing Kit (Applied Biosystems; Foster City, CA, USA) using the primers ENV_{5032} and ENV_{5608r}. The resulting sequences included a 501-bp region of the *env* gene, corresponding to nucleotide positions 5084 to 5584 of the whole BLV genomic sequence. The editing, alignment, and identification of nucleotide sequences were performed using MEGA 7 software (33).

Phylogenetic Analysis and Phylogenetic Tree Construction

The partial BLV *env*-gp51 sequences from the Egyptian isolates were aligned with the 51 partial BLV *env*-gp51 sequences from GenBank (representative of the 11 BLV genotypes distributed worldwide) using MEGA 7 software. Phylogenetic analysis of the partial BLV *env*-gp51 sequences from 50 BLV positive samples successfully amplified using nested PCR were also conducted using MEGA 7 software (33). For robust and accurate phylogenetic analysis of the BLV *env*-gp51 sequence, the "find best DNA/Protein models" tool of MEGA 7 software was used to choose the best fit model. The Kimura-2 parameter model was chosen as the model with the best fit to analyze the BLV *env*-gp51 sequence with the smallest Akaike information criterion (AIC) value. Two phylogenetic trees were constructed using the maximum likelihood (ML) algorithm based on 420 and 501 bp sequences with the K2+I and K2 models of nucleotide substitution in MEGA 7, respectively. The reliability of the phylogenetic relationships was evaluated using non-parametric bootstrap analysis with 1,000 replicates. The deduction of protein sequence through translation of nucleotide to amino acid sequence was performed using MEGA 7 (33). The sequences of isolates obtained in this study were deposited in GenBank under accession numbers: LC498589 (DZ1.1), LC498590 (DZ1.2), LC498591 (DZ1.3), LC498592 (QB1.1), LC498593 (QB3.1), LC498594 (QB5.1), LC498595 (QC6.1), LC498596 (QB2.1), LC498597 (QB4.1), LC498580 (DZ1.4), LC498581 (DZ1.5), LC498582 (DZ1.6), LC498583 (QB1.2), LC498584 (QB3.2), LC498585 (QB5.2), LC498586 (DZ1.39), LC498587 (DZ1.40), LC498588 (QB5.3), and LC500799∼LC500830 (DZ1.7∼DZ1.38).

Statistical Analysis

The significance of PVL difference between the cattle from different geographic regions was tested using multiple comparison by Tukey's test after the analysis of variance. $P < 0.05$ was considered significant.

RESULTS

Prevalence of BLV Among Egyptian Cattle

Blood samples were collected from 270 dairy cattle of 24 farms located at five provinces of different geographic location in Egypt (**Figure 1**). Cattle samples were classified as Native Egyptian

(12 samples), Holstein (125 samples), Mixed (129 samples), and Simmental (4 samples) cattle (**Table 1**). All samples were tested for BLV infection using BLV-CoCoMo-qPCR-2 assay, which detects the two copies of BLV LTRs present per provirus. Our results showed that BLV infection rate varied among the cattle tested from farms in different regions (**Table 1**). Interestingly, BLV infection was detected only in the cattle from two provinces (Qena and Damietta), while those from the other three provinces (Beheira, Luxor, and Fayoum) tested BLV-negative. In Qena province, 74 blood samples were collected from the cattle of six farms, namely, QB1, QB2, QB3, QB4, QB5, and QC6. Five (QB1, QB2, QB3, QB4, and QB5) are small farms (<10 cattle) located at El-Brahma town, harboring either Native or Mixed breed cattle, while the sixth (QC6) is a large farm (~300 cattle) located at the provincial capital town, harboring only Holstein breed cattle. It was interesting that the cattle from all 6 farms were BLV-positive and the infection rate for each distinct breed was 0–60% (**Table 1**). In Damietta province, 40 blood samples were collected from the cattle of a large intensive farm (DZ1) located at El-Zarqa harboring ~500 cattle of Holstein breed. Surprisingly, all the tested samples were BLV-positive, thus having 100% infection rate (**Table 1**). A total of 137 samples were collected from the cattle of the 15 farms (BA1–BA15) located at Abu-Elmatamir in Beheira province, among which 14 are small or semi-intensive farms harboring Native or Mixed breeds and BA15 is a large intensive farm harboring Holstein and Simmental cattle. All the tested samples were BLV-negative, thus having 0% infection rate for each farm. In Luxor province, the 16 samples collected from Native and Mixed cattle in one small farm (LQ1) located at EL-Qurna were BLV-negative. A limited number of available samples from Holstein cattle in one large dairy farm (FT1) from Fayoum province was tested, but none of them were BLV-positive.

Our results demonstrated that 58 samples among the 270 tested samples were BLV-positive (21.5%; **Table 1** and **Figure 1**) and BLV infection was distributed only in two provinces; thus, BLV infection in Egypt may be limited to particular regions.

Phylogenetic Analysis of the 420-bp Sequence of BLV *env*-gp51 Region of the Selected 18 Typical BLV Strains in Egypt and Known Strains From Different Geographic Locations Worldwide

To analyze the genetic variability among the BLV strains in Egypt, phylogenetic characterization was carried out after sequencing the BLV *env*-gp51 gene. Out of the 58 BLV-positive samples collected from the cattle in six different farms in Qena province and one farm in Damietta province as shown in **Table 2**, 50 samples were successfully amplified by nested PCR for partial BLV *env*-gp51 gene and a 501-bp sequence corresponding to the nucleotide positions 5084 to 5584 of the full-length BLV genome of the reference strain FLK-BLV subclone pBLV913 (accession number EF600696) were obtained.

For phylogenetic analysis of BLV genotypes in Egypt, the 420-bp sequences corresponding to the nucleotide positions 5126 to 5545 of the full-length BLV genome were used in order to be shared with all the currently known 11 genotypes of BLV in the world to our references. The 18 selected BLV isolates out of the 50 PCR-amplified samples were aligned with those from BLV strains representing all known 11 different BLV genotypes (genotype-1 to-11) deposited in GenBank. An ML phylogenetic tree was constructed using the best K2+I model of nucleotide substitution (33). The results of phylogenetic analysis were similar to those published in previous studies and BLV strains were classified into 11 genotypes (3, 18, 29, 34–36), as shown in **Figure 2**. Interestingly, our phylogenetic analysis also showed that the Egyptian BLV isolates were clustered into genotype-1 or -4.

Identification of the Six Genetically Distinct Strains Present in Egyptian Cattle by Phylogenetic Analysis Based on the 501-bp Sequence of BLV *env*-gp51 Region

To gain insight into the genetic variability of BLV strains present in Egyptian cattle, we classified all the 50 BLV isolates via another

TABLE 2 | Distribution of the six genetically distinct BLV strains circulating in Egypt cattle throughout the infected dairy farms.

Province	Town	Farm ID	BLV infectivity by CoCoMo-qPCR (%)	BLV isolated strains						
				G-1				G-4		No. of detected isolates by nested PCR
				a	b	c	d	x	y	
Qena	El-Brahma	QB1	3/10 (30.0)	–	1^{m}	–	–	1^{m}	–	2
		QB2	1/4 (25.0)	–	–	1^{m}	–	–	–	1
		QB3	3/5 (60.0)	–	1^{m}	–	–	1^{m}	–	2
		QB4	2/7 (28.6)	–	–	–	1^{n}	–	–	1
		QB5	4/9 (44.4)	–	1^{m}	–	–	1^{n}	1^{m}	3
	Qena-city	QC6	5/39 (12.8)	–	1^{h}	–	–	–	–	1
Damietta	El-Zarqa	DZ1	40/40 (100.0)	3^{h}	–	–	–	35^{h}	2^{h}	40
Total				3	4	1	1	38	3	50

^{m}*Mixed breed*; ^{n}*Native breed*; ^{h}*Holstein breed.*

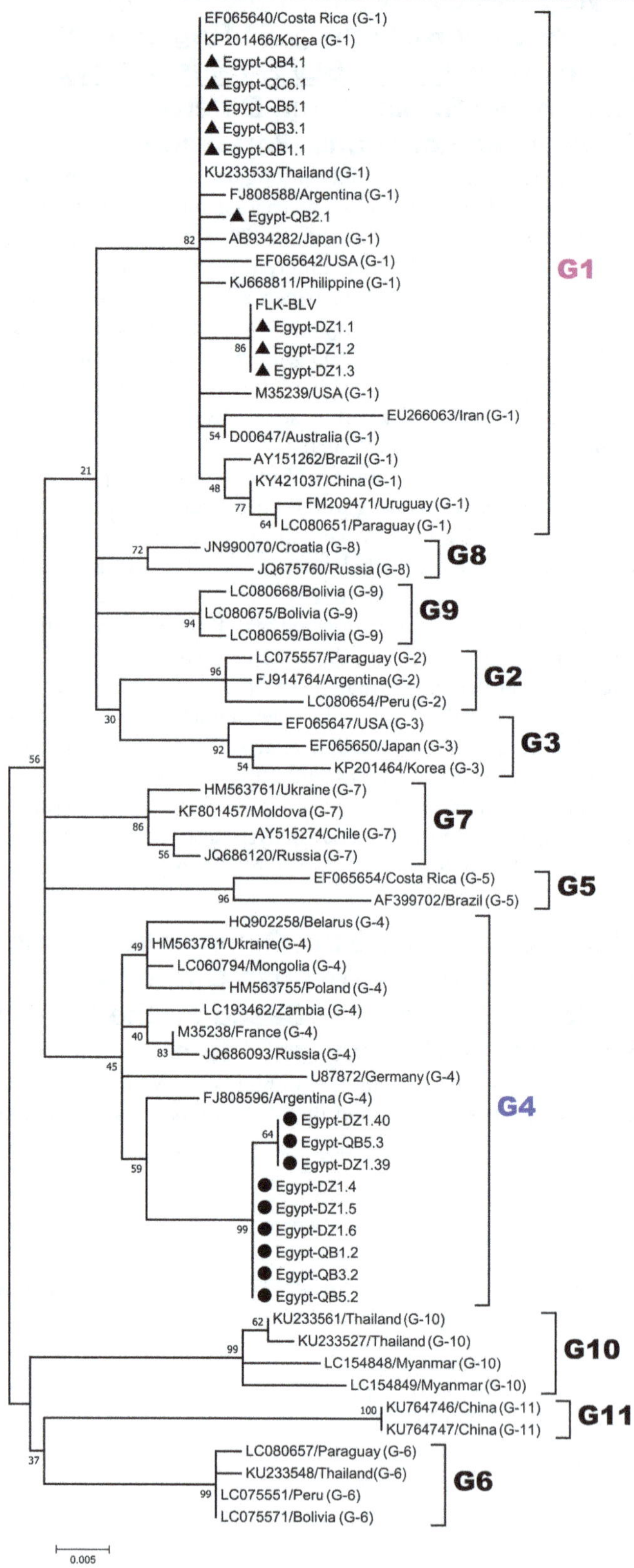

FIGURE 2 | Maximum likelihood (ML) phylogenetic tree based on 420-bp nucleotide of partial BLV *env*-gp51 gene sequences from the selected 18 typical BLV isolates in Egypt and 51 BLV isolates from other countries worldwide. The Egyptian isolates are indicated by the country name together with the sample ID and farm origin. Other isolates are indicated by the accession number and country name. Egyptian BLV isolates are aligned as shown in **Figure 4**, and those clustered into genotypes-1 and-4 are marked by filled triangles (▲) and circles (•), respectively. BLV genotypes are indicated by numbers on the right side of the tree. The bottom bar of the tree denotes distance.

(Continued)

ML phylogenetic tree based on the 501-bp sequence of BLV *env*-gp51 region (**Figure 3**). In this tree, all the 50 BLV isolates were aligned with the reference strain. It clearly showed that nine out of 50 BLV sequences belonged to genotype-1 and were further classified into four distinct strains (G1-a, G1-b, G1-c, and G1-d). In contrast, the remaining 41 BLV isolates belonged to genotype-4 and were further classified into two distinct strains (G4-x and G4-y). Thus, our results indicate that six genetically distinct BLV strains are present in Egyptian cattle.

Nucleotide and Amino Acid Sequence Analysis of the 501-bp Sequence of BLV *env*-gp51 Region of the Six Genetically Distinct Strains Present in Egyptian Cattle

The similarity of the 501-bp sequence of BLV *env*-gp51 region of all 50 Egyptian isolates ranged from 96.7 to 100% (data not shown). The sequence from the nine Egyptian BLV isolates belonging to G1-a, G1-b, G1-c, and G1-d strains exhibited the highest similarity (96.7–100%) to that from all BLV strains representing genotype-1 from various geographic locations worldwide used as references for the phylogenetic analysis (data not shown). In contrast, the sequence from the 41 Egyptian BLV isolates belonging to G4-x and G4-y strains were 97.7–99.1% similar to that from all BLV strains representing genotype-4 (data not shown).

Nucleotide sequences for the 18 typical selected BLV isolates representing the six genetically distinct strains (G1-a, G1-b, G1-c, G1-d, G4-x, and G4-y) were aligned with that of the reference strain (**Figure 4**). The three sequences for G1-a strain showed 100% similarity with that of the reference strain. The four sequences for G1-b strain exhibited two silent nucleotide substitutions: one located in the third base of residue 149 (nt 447) and the other in the third base of residue 203 (nt 609). We found only one sequence for G1-c strain, which exhibited three nucleotide substitutions: two of them were similar to those in G1-b strain sequences, while the third was located in the third base of residue 112 (nt 336); however, all of them were silent substitutions. Similarly, we detected one sequence for G1-d strain, which exhibited three nucleotide substitutions: two of them were silent and at the same positions as those in G1-b strain sequences, while the third one was a G to T substitution in the second base of residue 99 (nt 296), which changed the deduced amino acid located in the neutralizing domain (ND1) and the $CD4^+$ epitope region of gp51 protein from glycine to lysine. We found 15 nucleotide substitutions for G4-x strain. Among them, 13 were silent and included

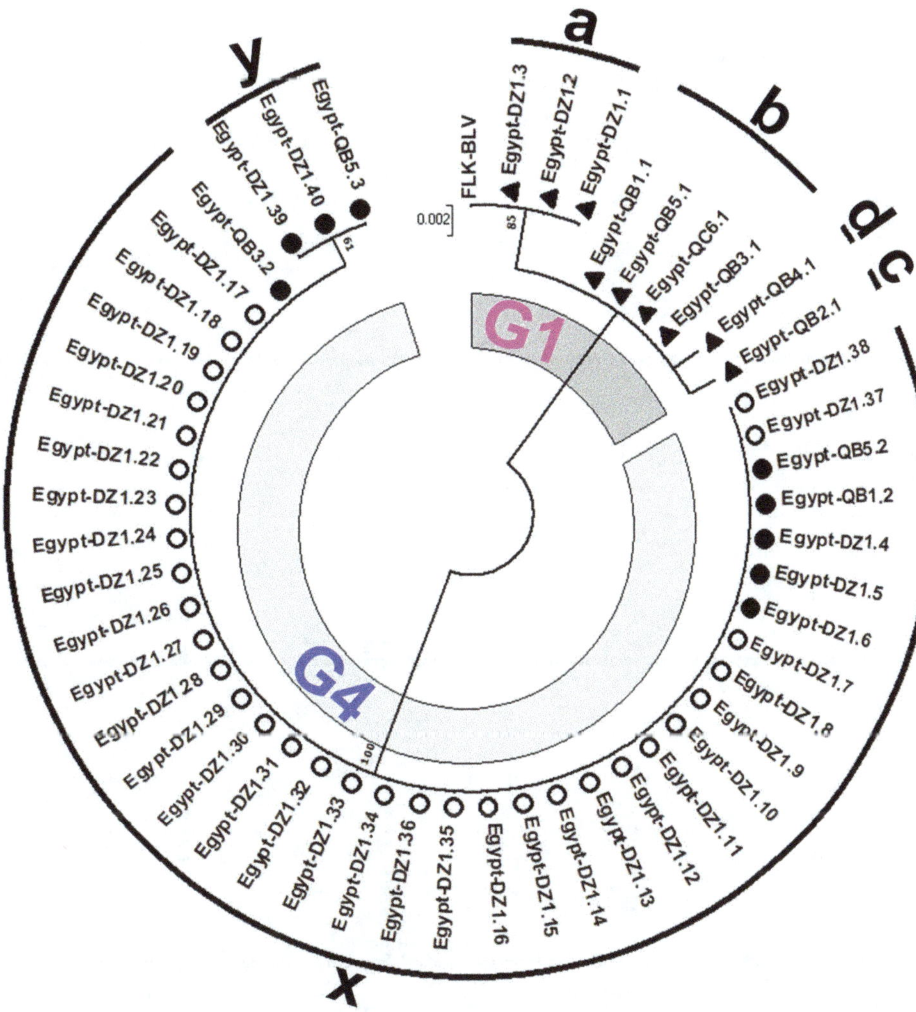

FIGURE 3 | Maximum likelihood (ML) phylogenetic tree based on 501-bp nucleotide of BLV *env*-gp51 gene from 50 BLV isolates classified into the six genetically distinct strains identified in Egyptian cattle (G1-a, G1-b, G1-c, G1-d, G4-x, and G4-y). This tree was constructed with the sequences of 50 BLV isolates detected in the cattle from different farms at two geographic locations in Egypt, including the 18 typical BLV Egyptian isolates as shown in **Figure 2** and other Egyptian isolates detected in different locations, and the reference strain FLK-BLV subclone pBLV913 (accession number EF600696). Egyptian BLV sequences on the tree are indicated by farm ID, and sample number. BLV isolates that belong to genotype-1 are indicated using filled triangles (▲), while those that belong to genotype-4 are indicated using open (○) and filled (•) circles. Sequences for each distinct BLV strain are indicated via alphabets around the circumference of the figure. The 18 typical Egyptian BLV isolates from identical samples were aligned as shown in **Figure 4** and are indicated by filled circles (•) and triangles (▲). Other isolates are indicated using open circles (○). The genotypes are shown as G1 and G4. The bar at the above portion denotes distance.

residues 90 (nt 270), 125 (nt 375), 136 (nt 408), 149 (nt 447), 161(nt 483), 175 (nt 525), 185 (nt 555), 187 (nt 559), 196 (nt 588), 197 (nt 591), 203 (nt 609), 205 (nt 615), and 239 (nt 717), but the other two substitutions were not silent. The first substitution (G to A) occurred in the second base in residue 121 (nt 362), changing the deduced amino acid located in the epitope G of gp51 protein from arginine to histidine, while the second substitution (A to G) in the first base in residue 233 (nt 697) changed the amino acid located in the B epitope region from isoleucine to valine. The substitutions for G4-y strain were identical to those for G4-x strain; however, one additional non-silent substitution (G to A) in the first base of residue 239 (nt 715) was detected, which changed the deduced amino acid from glycine to serine, which is a non-synonymous residue of gp51 protein.

Distribution of the Six Genetically Distinct Strains Throughout the Infected Farms in Egypt

We summarized the distribution of the six genetically distinct strains at different farms to specify the strain present in the cattle from each BLV-infected farm (**Table 2**). Strain G1-a was detected in three different cattle from DZ1 farm located at El-Zarqa in Damietta province. Strain G1-b was found in four different cattle: three isolates were detected as identical in the cattle from QB1,

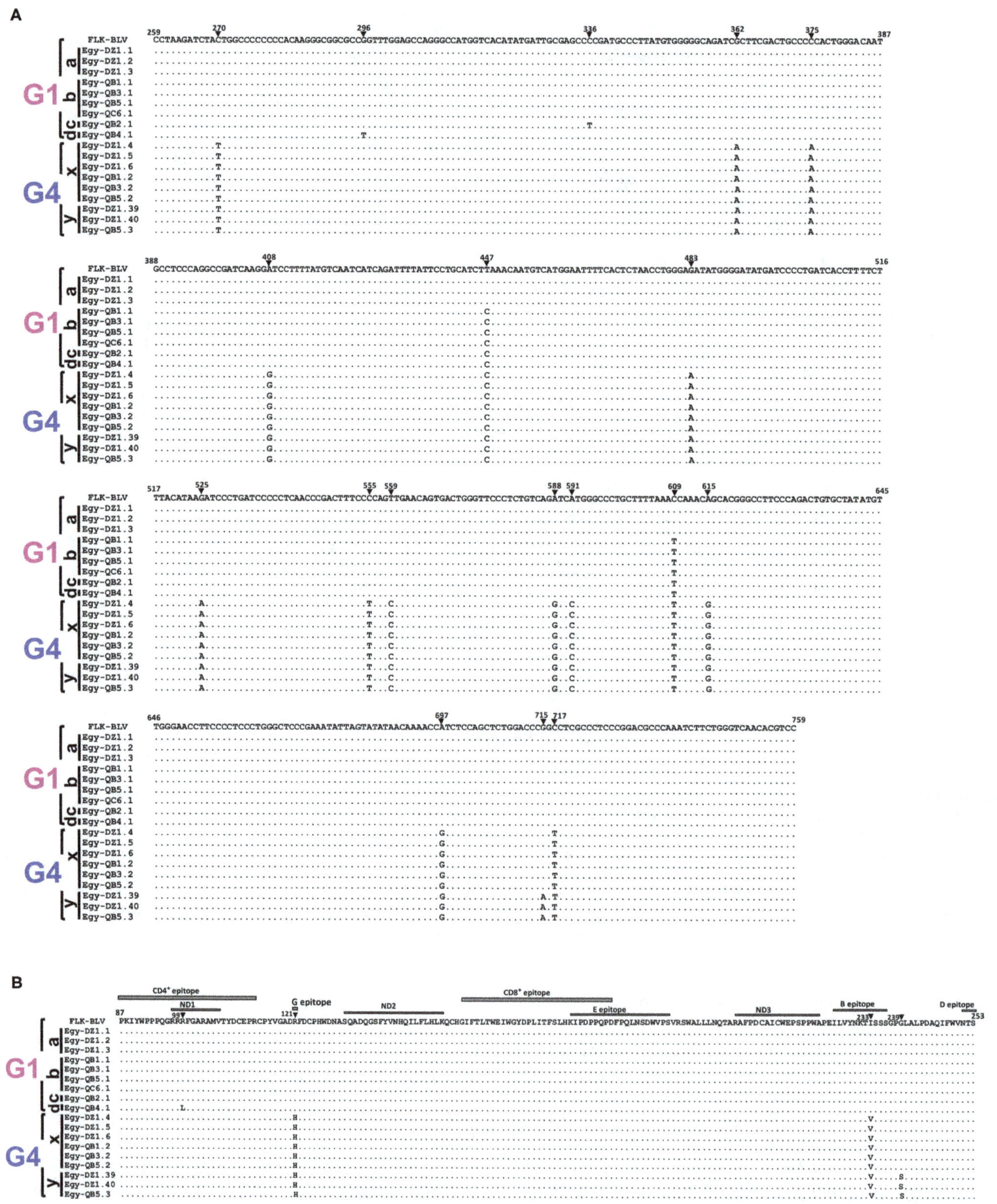

FIGURE 4 | Alignment of nucleotide sequences and deduced amino acid sequences of 501-bp nucleotide of BLV *env*-gp51 gene from the six genetically distinct strains identified in Egyptian cattle. Alignment was performed for the selected 18 typical Egyptian BLV isolates representative for the six genetically distinct strains

(Continued)

FIGURE 4 | circulating in Egyptian cattle (G1-a, G1-b, G1-c, G1-d, G4-x, and G4-y). Egyptian BLV isolates are shown by the country name abbreviation (Egy), farm ID, and sample ID. **(A)** Nucleotide sequence alignment showing the nucleotide substitutions are indicated using numbers and filled triangles above the sequences. **(B)** The deduced amino acid alignment showing the amino acid substitutions are indicated using numbers above the sequences; the labeled gray rectangles refer to coding sequences of the antigenic determinants of the gp51 protein. The black bars at the left side of the figure indicate Egyptian BLV isolates that belong to each particular strain. Genotypes (G1 and G4) are indicated using black braces at the far-left side of the figure. Dots indicate identity with FLK-BLV subclone pBLV913 (accession No. EF600696), which was used as a reference in a reference in this work.

QB3, and QB5 farms located very close to each other at El-Brahma in Qena province, while the fourth isolate was detected in the cattle from QC6 farm located in the provincial capital town. One isolate of strains G1-c and G1-d each were detected in the cattle from QB2 and those from QB4 farm, respectively, both located at El-Brahma. Among the 38 isolates classified as G4-x strain, 35 were detected in the cattle from DZ1 farm located at El-Zarqa in Damietta province and one each were detected in cattle from QB1, QB3, and QB5 farms. Among the three isolates classified as G4-y strain, two were detected in the cattle from DZ1 farm and the third was detected in those from QB5 farm.

Regarding the distribution of the six genetically distinct strains present in Egyptian cattle, our results concluded that genotype-1 and-4 strains coexisted in most BLV-infected farms.

Estimation of BLV PVL Among Egyptian Cattle

PVL is an important risk factor of BLV-associated disease progression and transmission risk (7–12). Therefore, BLV PVL was calculated by CoCoMo-qPCR2 assay and its level was summarized with BLV infection rate in each tested province of Egypt, as shown in **Figure 5**. In Qena province, 18 out of the 74 tested samples were BLV-positive, their PVL ranging from 7 to 125 copies/10^5 cells with a mean value of 41 copies/10^5 cells. In DZ1 farm from Damietta province, all 40 tested samples were BLV-positive and the PVL ranged from 45 to 98,725 copies/10^5 cells with a mean value of 22,522 copies/10^5 cells. Our previous reports (11, 12) suggest that a PVL of around 10,000 copies/10^5 cells in cow blood might be an indicator of efficient BLV spreading within the whole body, thereby easily detecting BLV proviruses into milk, nasal mucus, and saliva. Interestingly, 17 cattle from DZ1 farm (42.5%) had high PVL ($>10^4$ copies/10^5 cells) ranging from 16,985 to 98,725 copies/10^5 cells, indicating that they may be high-risk transmitters. Indeed, all tested samples from DZ1 farm were BLV-positive with infection rate of 100% (**Table 2**). In addition, 15 of these 17 cattle were infected with G4-x strain and 2 with G4-y strain, as shown in **Table 2**. In contrast, all 18 BLV-positive cattle from 5 different farms in Qena province had low PVL ($\leq 10^4$ copies/10^5 cells).

DISCUSSION

This study provides a new molecular evidence for BLV infection in Egyptian cattle. First, we successfully detected BLV provirus, which integrates into the host genome, in the blood of BLV-infected cattle with a prevalence rate of 21.5%, since the previous studies focused only on the serological detection of BLV in Egyptian cattle. BLV infection was detected in cattle from dairy farms in two of the five tested provinces, suggesting that BLV infection might exist in only particular regions. However, it is possible that the absence of BLV infection in the other three regions resulted from the small number of samples investigated. Therefore, further studies are required to accurately determine the prevalence of infection through a nation-wide survey. Second, the phylogenetical analysis and alignment of the partial BLV *env*-gp51 sequences clearly showed at least six genetically distinct strains, which belong to genotype-1 and-4 among the 11 globally detected genotypes, are present in Egyptian cattle. This is the new report of BLV genetic diversity in Egypt through molecular characterization. Third, we concluded that BLV PVL level is associated with viral horizontal transmission under field conditions in Egypt. Interestingly, in DZ1 farm, where all collected samples were BLV-positive, 35 among the 40 cattle were infected with G4-x strain and the PVL in 15 among these 35 BLV-infected cattle was $>10{,}000$ copies/10^5 cells, indicating they may be high-risk transmitters. We demonstrated that BLV-infected cattle with high PVL are a source of infection in BLV-free cattle in Egyptian dairies, which supports the results of previous studies (7–12, 37). In addition, this result supported the previous report that major strain was the source spread at the farm, which existed several BLV strains (38).

Egypt is located between the three continents of Africa, Asia, and Europe. Most of the neighboring countries of Egypt are BLV-infected, including Greece (3), Turkey (39), Jordan (40), Syria (41), and Saudi Arabia (42), however there is no information for the disease in several neighboring countries including Libya and Sudan (43). The total percentage of BLV prevalence determined in our study was 21.5%. This result is in agreement with the results of the recent seroprevalence study reporting BLV infection rate to be 20.8% among Egyptian cattle (28) and similar to the previously reported BLV infection prevalence rate of 15.83% (27). Likewise, BLV infection rate reported in some of the neighboring countries include 20.2% in Saudi Arabia (42) 7.75% in Iraq (44), despite being high (48.3% in herd level) in Turkey (39). In contrast, the BLV infection rate among cattle of Egypt reported in this study was close to or lower than that in India (27.9%) (45). However, the BLV infection rate reported here compared with that reported in some other Asian countries was being higher than that reported in Philippines (4.8–9.7%) (29) and markedly lower that in Japan (40.9%) (46), Korea (42.16%) (47), and Myanmar (37.04) (36). The Egyptian livestock import has increased over the last 10 years and the Egyptian dairy industry is completely dependent on imported cattle for herd construction. Germany, Netherlands, and the United States of America represent the major cattle

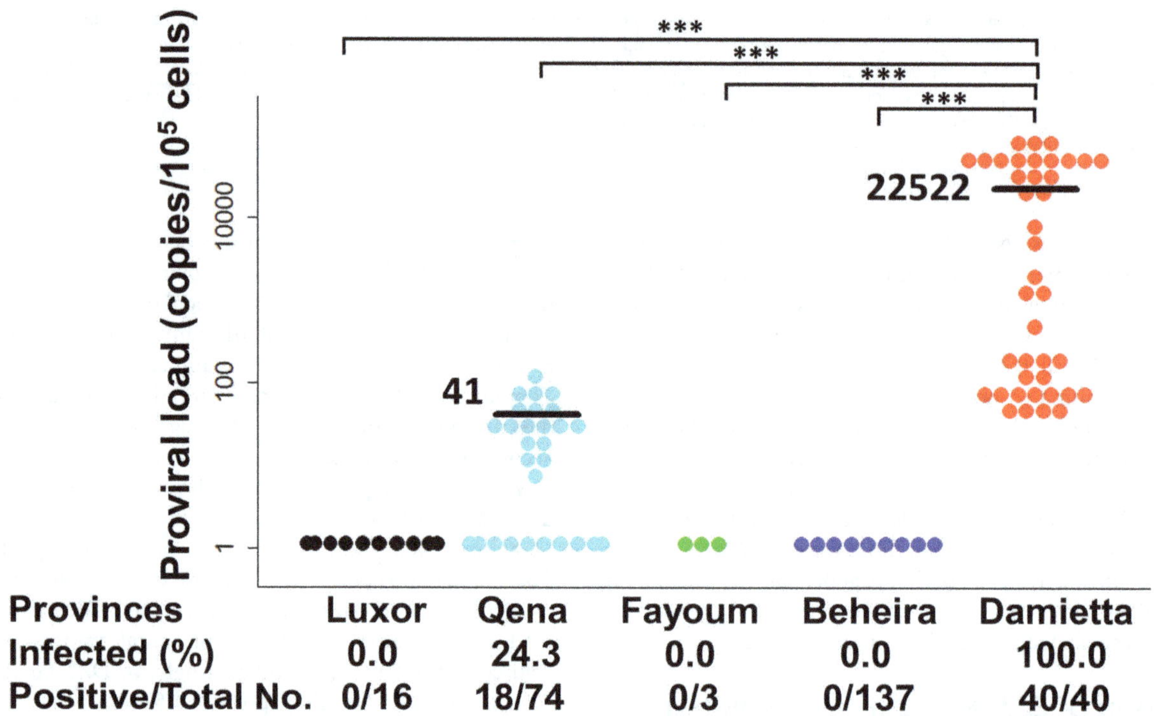

FIGURE 5 | Estimation of BLV proviral load (PVL) among Egyptian cattle. BLV PVL calculated using CoCoMo-qPCR-2 among cattle samples were tested in five different provinces in Egypt. Black bars show the main BLV PVL values. The actual number (No.) of cattle reported positive via BLV-CoCoMo-qPCR-2 per total No. of tested cattle and BLV-infected rate (%) are indicted at the bottom of each block. Significant differences between different geographic regions were calculated using Tukey's test. $P<0.05$ was considered significant. ***$P < 0.00$.

suppliers in Egypt (23). Indeed, phylogenetic analysis of the total 50 partial *env*-gp51 sequences detected here clearly showed that Egyptian BLV isolates were clustered into genotype-1 and-4, which have been detected worldwide. Genotype-1 is the most dominant genotype of BLV, distributed across almost all continents, including Europe, America, Asia, and Australia. Genotype-4 is the second most widely distributed genotype, primarily detected in Europe and some American countries (3). Noticeably, genotype-1 and-4 cover large geographic areas from Europe to America, suggesting the possibility of extensive trading between countries (47). Therefore, it is recommended to determine the risk factors for BLV infection that might have been introduced to Egypt from the imported cattle breeds or be specific for the management system employed for cattle in the field.

The phylogenetic analysis of the 420-bp sequences of *env*-gp51 region in this study showed that Egyptian BLV isolates were assigned to genotype-1 and-4 and alignment of the 501-bp sequences of *env*-gp51 region resulted in the identification of 18 nucleotide substitutions, of which 14 were silent and four were amino acid substitutions. The substitutions varied according to genotype. For example, phylogenetic tree based on the 501-bp sequence of *env*-gp51 region demonstrated four different strains (G1-a, G1-b, G1-c, and G1-d) with genotype-1 and two different strains (G4-x and G4-y) with genotype-4. Similarly, Marawan et al. (37) performed phylogenetic analysis and demonstrated the existence of 20 different BLV subgenotypes in Miyazaki prefecture of Japan based on their nucleotide sequences. Interestingly, the substitutions in genotype-1 strains were highly conserved and only one unique non-synonymous substitution was analyzed in the G1-d strain sequence, which is located at the residue 99 and changed an amino acid in the neutralizing domain (ND1) and the CD4+ epitope region of gp51 protein from glycine to lysine. Moreover, in the genotype-4 strains, G4-x strain exhibited two amino acid substitutions in residues 121 and 233, which were located in G and B epitopes, respectively, and G4-y strain exhibited three substitutions, two of them were identical to the aforementioned substitutions in G4-x strain and the third was an unique amino acid substitution in residue 239, which is located in the region between B and D epitopes of gp51 protein.

In this study, we noticed that, in a single farm DZ1, all the 40 samples collected were BLV-positive, with 35 of these BLV isolates being identical and classified as the same BLV strain (G4-x) with genotype-4. Two isolates were classified as G4-y strain having a 99.8% similarity with G4-x strain, but the remaining three isolates were classified as G1-a strain with genotype-1. Interestingly, as calculated by CoCoMo-qPCR2, BLV PVL of these BLV-infected cattle ranged from 45 to 98,725 copies/10^5 cells with a mean value of 22,522 copies/10^5 cells. Regarding horizontal BLV transmission, we previously detected BLV provirus in the nasal secretions and saliva of cattle with PVL $>$14,000 and $>$18,000 copies/10^5 cells in blood, respectively, and suspected that BLV-infected cells were present in nasal secretions and saliva, respectively (11). Furthermore, the BLV provirus was detected in milk samples from dams when the PVL in blood samples were approximately >10,000 copies/10^5 cells (12). It might infect healthy cattle via licking, sneezing, rubbing of noses, or milking. In this study, the PVL in 15 among the 35 infected cattle harboring G4-x strain in farm DZ1 appeared to be >10,000 copies/10^5 cells, indicating that they may be high-risk transmitters. Therefore, we hypothesized that the infected cattle with high PVL act as virus spreader and transmit genetically identical provirus to other cattle during long-time physical contact. Thus, the G4-x strain is widely spread in cattle from DZ1 farm. This result harmonized with those of Murakami et al. (38), who showed that three genetically distinct BLV strains co-existed among the infected cattle in one farm and described that the major viral strains were the source of infection spread in that farm. In contrast, BLV-infected cattle with low PVL are not a source of infection for BLV-free cattle (14). Therefore, it is recommended to isolate and monitor the BLV-infected cattle with high PVL to prohibit virus spread horizontally and vertically.

Here we detected BLV infectivity in two provinces: Qena and Damietta. We examined cattle from six dairy farms in Qena province and found cattle from all of them to be BLV-infected. Five of these farms (QB1, QB2, QB3, QB4, and QB5) are small-sized, but farm QC6 is large. The infection rate was higher in the small-sized farms than that in the large farm (**Table 2**). These findings concurred with those of other studies demonstrating that average BLV seroprevalence in small farms (less than 20 cattle) was higher than that in medium or large farms in Miyazaki prefecture, Japan (48). Several studies have described the risk factors for BLV transmission within herd and considered that physical contact (49), loose housing system (50), use of common sleeves during rectal palpation (51), blood sucking insects, blood-contaminated devices, and needle reuse (4) are the most dominant factors for virus transmission. Therefore, it is possible that in the small-sized farms, loose cattle housing system, presence of hematophagous insects, and poor managemental procedures may increase the chance for virus transmission from infected to uninfected cattle.

In contrast, in DZ1 farm located in Damietta province, we demonstrated the highest BLV infection rate (100%). It is a large dairy farm (~500 cattle) and depends on natural breeding for reproduction. Interestingly, the milking system of this farm depends on using a limited number of common portable milking machines, thus lacking sufficient cleaning during milking between individual cows. Therefore, the likelihood of bovine milk pathogen transmission is higher in herds using mobile milking machines than that in herds using fixed milking machines, as previously demonstrated (52). In addition, BLV has a broad tropism to the mammary tissue (53) and the milk or milk cells of infected cattle could be a source of infection (12, 54, 55). However, the role of milk in virus transmission is considered to be little (56). Thus, we hypothesized that there is a possibility for BLV transfer from infected to healthy receptive cattle during the milking process.

To gain insight into the fundamental nature of existence of each genetically distinct virus strain, we checked the virus strain spreading the infection between animals in each particular farm. In the five small-sized BLV-infected farms (QB1, QB2, QB3, QB4, and QB5) harboring Native and Mixed breed cattle located in El-Brahma, Qena, the BLV infection rate was ranged from 25 to 60%. These farms were neighbors and located very close to each other. Shettigara et al. (57) have proposed that at least 200 m distance should be maintained between farms to prevent transmission among herds. It is interesting that the cattle from three of these farms (QB1, QB3, and QB5) harbored genetically identical strains (G1-b and G4-x), as shown in **Table 2**. This result might be a good example for horizontal BLV transmission from one farm to its adjoining farm in the field. On the contrary, we identified two genetically different strains G1-c and G1-d in farms QB2 and QB4, respectively. The sixth farm (QC6) located in the capital town of Qena province was a large-sized dairy farm (~300 cattle) harboring Holstein breed cattle. Although the BLV infection rate in this farm was 12.8% (5/39) as determined by CoCoMo-qPCR, we successfully identified a single BLV isolate classified as G1-b strain. This might be due to the difference in sensitivity between CoCoMo-qPCR assay used for virus detection and nested PCR technique used for gp51 amplification (29).

In conclusion, the phylogenetic analysis based on partial BLV *env*-gp51 sequence revealed that there are at least six genetically distinct BLV strains present in Egyptian cattle, which belong to genotype-1 and-4 among the 11 globally detected genotypes. This study provides a new molecular characterization of BLV in Egyptian dairy cattle and calculated the PVL among BLV-infected cattle in Egypt. This study also showed that the BLV infection prevalence was 21.5% (58 out of 270 head) in five provinces located in the northern, central, and southern parts of Egypt. Further research should focus on determining the impact of BLV genetic diversity on viral pathogenicity and disease progression in dairy cattle on a large scale.

AUTHOR CONTRIBUTIONS

YA conceived of and designed the study. SM, AA, AA-H, and AM collected the samples. RH, SM, MP, LB, SW, and YA acquired, analyzed, and interpreted the data. YA contributed reagents, materials, and analysis tools. RH and YA drafted and revised the manuscript. All authors agree to be accountable for the content of the work.

ACKNOWLEDGMENTS

We thank the veterinarians and our collaborators for kindly assisting with sampling from many farms in Egypt. We are grateful to members of the Viral Infectious Diseases Field, RIKEN, for their technical assistance, help, and suggestions, and Support Unit at the Bio-material Analysis, RIKEN BSI Research Resources Center, for help with sequence analysis. We would like to thank Editage (http://www.editage.com) for English language editing.

REFERENCES

1. Gillet N, Florins A, Boxus M, Burteau C, Nigro A, Vandermeers F, et al. Mechanisms of leukemogenesis induced by bovine leukemia virus: prospects for novel anti-retroviral therapies in human. *Retrovirology*. (2007) 4:18. doi: 10.1186/1742-4690-4-18
2. Aida Y, Murakami H, Takahashi M, Takeshima SN. Mechanisms of pathogenesis induced by bovine leukemia virus as a model for human T-cell leukemia virus. *Front Microbiol.* (2013) 4:328. doi: 10.3389/fmicb.2013.00328
3. Polat M, Takeshima SN, Aida Y. Epidemiology and genetic diversity of bovine leukemia virus. *Virol J.* (2017) 14:209. doi: 10.1186/s12985-017-0876-4
4. Hopkins SG, DiGiacomo RF. Natural transmission of bovine leukemia virus in dairy and beef cattle. *Vet Clin North Am Food Anim Pract.* (1997) 13:107–28. doi: 10.1016/s0749-0720(15)30367-4
5. Kettmann R, Meunier-Rotival M, Cortadas J, Cuny G, Ghysdael J, Mammerickx M, et al. Integration of bovine leukemia virus DNA in the bovine genome. *Proc Natl Acad Sci USA*. (1979) 76:4822–6. doi: 10.1073/pnas.76.10.4822
6. Tajima S, Ikawa Y, Aida Y. Complete bovine leukemia virus (BLV) provirus is conserved in BLV-infected cattle throughout the course of B-cell lymphosarcoma development. *J. Virol.* (1998) 72:7569–76.
7. Jimba M, Takeshima SN, Matoba K, Endoh D, Aida Y. BLV-CoCoMo-qPCR: quantitation of bovine leukemia virus proviral load using the CoCoMo algorithm. *Retrovirology*. (2010) 7:91. doi: 10.1186/1742-4690-7-91
8. Sato H, Watanuki S, Murakami H, Sato R, Ishizaki H, Aida Y. Development of a luminescence syncytium induction assay (LuSIA) for easily detecting and quantitatively measuring bovine leukemia virus infection. *Arch Virol.* (2018) 163:1519–30. doi: 10.1007/s00705-018-3744-7
9. Lo C-W, Borjigin L, Saito S, Fukunaga K, Saitou E, Okazaki K, et al. BoLA-DRB3 Polymorphism is associated with differential susceptibility to bovine leukemia virus-induced lymphoma and proviral load. *Viruses*. (2020) 12:352. doi: 10.3390/v12030352
10. Ohno A, Takeshima SN, Matsumoto Y, Aida Y. Risk factors associated with increased bovine leukemia virus proviral load in infected cattle in Japan from 2012 to 2014. *Virus Res.* (2015) 210:283–90. doi: 10.1016/j.virusres.2015.08.020
11. Yuan Y, Kitamura-Muramatsu Y, Saito S, Ishizaki H, Nakano M, Haga S, et al. Detection of the BLV provirus from nasal secretion and saliva samples using BLV-CoCoMo-qPCR-2: comparison with blood samples from the same cattle. *Virus Res.* (2015) 210:248–54. doi: 10.1016/j.virusres.2015.08.013
12. Watanuki S, Takeshima SN, Borjigin L, Sato H, Bai L, Murakami H, et al. Visualizing bovine leukemia virus (BLV)-infected cells and measuring BLV proviral loads in the milk of BLV seropositive dams. *Vet Res.* (2019) 50:102. doi: 10.1186/s13567-019-0724-1
13. Takeshima SN, Kitamura-Muramatsu Y, Yuan Y, Polat M, Saito S, Aida Y. BLV-CoCoMo-qPCR-2: improvements to the BLV-CoCoMo-qPCR assay for bovine leukemia virus by reducing primer degeneracy and constructing an optimal standard curve. *Arch Virol.* (2015) 160:1325–32. doi: 10.1007/s00705-015-2377-3
14. Juliarena MA, Barrios CN, Ceriani MC, Esteban EN. Hot topic: bovine leukemia virus (BLV)-infected cows with low proviral load are not a source of infection for BLV-free cattle. *J Dairy Sci.* (2016) 99:4586–9. doi: 10.3168/jds.2015-10480
15. Mamoun RZ, Morisson M, Rebeyrotte N, Busetta B, Couez D, Kettmann R, et al. Sequence variability of bovine leukemia virus env gene and its relevance to the structure and antigenicity of the glycoproteins. *J Virol.* (1990) 64:4180–8.
16. Portetelle D, Couez D, Bruck C, Kettmann R, Mammerickx M, Van der Maaten M, et al. Antigenic variants of bovine leukemia virus (BLV) are defined by amino acid substitutions in the NH2 part of the envelope glycoprotein gp51. *Virology*. (1989) 169:27–33. doi: 10.1016/0042-6822(89)90037-8
17. Zhao X, Buehring GC. Natural genetic variations in bovine leukemia virus envelope gene: possible effects of selection and escape. *Virology*. (2007) 366:150–65. doi: 10.1016/j.virol.2007.03.058
18. Yu C, Wang X, Zhou Y, Wang Y, Zhang X, Zheng Y. Genotyping bovine leukemia virus in dairy cattle of Heilongjiang, Northeastern China. *BMC Vet Res.* (2019) 15:179. doi: 10.1186/s12917-019-1863-3
19. Agency US, Development I. *Livestock Production Systems Spotlight Cattle and Buffaloes and Poultry Sectors in Egypt*. Available online at: http://www.fao.org/ag/againfo/programmes/en/ASL2050.html
20. Delgado J V, Landi V, Martinez A, Elbeltagy A, Sharaf A, Elsaid U, et al. Integrating Local Egyptian Cattle Breeds in a National Breeding Strategy. A CATTLECONIKTA Proposal. *Viii Congr Ibérico Sobre Recur Genéticos Animais.* (2012) 15.
21. Galal S. Farm animal genetic resources in Egypt: factsheet. *Egypt J Anim Prod.* (2007) 44:1–23.
22. Faid-Allah E, Ghoneim E, Elbetagy AR, El-Dabour M. Genetic diversity and structure of native Egyptian cattle populations and French-Egyptian Cross via DNA-microsatellite. *J Ilmu Ternak dan Vet.* (2018) 23:1. doi: 10.14334/jitv.v23i1.1647
23. *Products UGL and USDA Staff and Not Necessarily Statements of Official U. S. Government Egypt Livestock and Products Annual 2017 Strengthening Egyptian Pound to Ease Beef Prices, Consumption and Imports to Rise in 2018* Approved By: Abdi, Ali. (2017). p. 1–10. Available online at https://www.fas.usda.gov/data/egypt-livestock-and-products-annual-3
24. Zaghawa A, Beier D, Abd El-Rahim IH, Karim I, El-ballal S, Conraths FJ, et al. An outbreak of enzootic bovine leukosis in upper Egypt: clinical, laboratory and molecular-epidemiological studies. *J Vet Med B Infect Dis Vet Public Health.* (2002) 49:123–9. doi: 10.1046/j.1439-0450.2002.00517.x
25. Abd El-Rahim IHA, El-Ballal SS. Introduction of bovine leukaemia virus (BLV) into Egypt. *Assiut Vet Med J.* (1999) 42:113–23.
26. OIE. *World Animal Health Information Data Before 2005 Handistatus II Archives of World Animal Health. HANDISTATUS II Multiannual Animal Disease Status Egypt / Enzootic Bovine Leukosis.* Paris: World organisation for animal Health (2005). Available online at: http://web.oie.int/hs2/sit_pays_mald_pl.asp?c_pays=56&c_mald=38
27. Zaher K S, Ahmed W M. Bovine leukemia virus infection in dairy cows in Egypt. *Acad J Cancer Res.* (2014) 7:126–30. doi: 10.5829/idosi.ajcr.2014.7.2.83265
28. Selim A, Marawan MA, Ali AF, Manaa E, AbouelGhaut HA. Seroprevalence of bovine leukemia virus in cattle, buffalo, and camel in Egypt. *Trop Anim Health Prod.* (2019)3–6. doi: 10.1007/s11250-019-02105-8
29. Polat M, Ohno A, Takeshima SN, Kim J, Kikuya M, Matsumoto Y, et al. Detection and molecular characterization of bovine leukemia virus in Philippine cattle. *Arch Virol.* (2015) 160:285–96. doi: 10.1007/s00705-014-2 280-3
30. Asfaw Y, Tsuduku S, Konishi M, Murakami K, Tsuboi T, Wu D, et al. Distribution and superinfection of bovine leukemia virus genotypes in Japan. *Arch Virol.* (2005) 150:493–505. doi: 10.1007/s00705-004-0433-5
31. Moratorio G, Obal G, Dubra A, Correa A, Bianchi S, Buschiazzo A, et al. Phylogenetic analysis of bovine leukemia viruses isolated in South America reveals diversification in seven distinct genotypes. *Arch Virol.* (2010) 155:481–9. doi: 10.1007/s00705-010-0606-3
32. Rovnak J, Boyd AL, Casey JW, Gonda MA, Jensen WA, Cockerell GL. Pathogenicity of molecularly cloned bovine leukemia virus. *J Virol.* (1993) 67:7096–105.
33. Kumar S, Stecher G, Tamura K. MEGA7: molecular evolutionary genetics analysis version 7.0 for bigger datasets. *Mol Biol Evol.* (2016) 33:1870–4. doi: 10.1093/molbev/msw054
34. Polat M, Takeshima SN, Hosomichi K, Kim J, Miyasaka T, Yamada K, et al. A new genotype of bovine leukemia virus in South America identified by NGS-based whole genome sequencing and molecular evolutionary genetic analysis. *Retrovirology*. (2016) 13:4. doi: 10.1186/s12977-016-0239-z
35. Polat M, Moe HH, Shimogiri T, Moe KK, Takeshima SN, Aida Y. The molecular epidemiological study of bovine leukemia virus infection in Myanmar cattle. *Arch Virol.* (2017) 162:425–37. doi: 10.1007/s00705-016-3118-y
36. Moe KK, Polat M, Borjigin L, Matsuura R, Hein ST, Moe HH, et al. New evidence of bovine leukemia virus circulating in Myanmar cattle through epidemiological and molecular characterization. *PLoS ONE*. (2020) 15:e0229126. doi: 10.1371/journal.pone.0229126
37. Marawan MA, Mekata H, Hayashi T, Sekiguchi S, Kirino Y, Horii Y, et al. Phylogenetic analysis of env gene of bovine leukemia virus strains

spread in Miyazaki prefecture, Japan. *J Vet Med Sci.* (2017) 79:912–6. doi: 10.1292/jvms.17-0055

38. Murakami H, Todaka H, Uchiyama J, Sato R, Sogawa K, Sakaguchi M, et al. A point mutation to the long terminal repeat of bovine leukemia virus related to viral productivity and transmissibility. *Virology.* (2019) 537:45–52. doi: 10.1016/j.virol.2019.08.015
39. Burgu I, Alkan F, Karaoglu T, Bilge-Dagalp S, Can-Sahna K, Gungor B, et al. Control and eradication program of enzootic bovine leucosis (EBL) from selected dairy herds in Turkey. *Dtsch Tierarztl Wochenschr.* (2005) 112:271–4.
40. Ababneh MM, Al-Rukibat RK, Hananeh WM, Nasar AT, Al-Zghoul MB. Detection and molecular characterization of bovine leukemia viruses from Jordan. *Arch Virol.* (2012) 157:2343–48. doi: 10.1007/s00705-012-1447-z
41. Kurdi A, Blankenstein P, Marquardt O, Ebner D. Serologic and virologic investigations on the presence of BLV infection in a dairy herd in Syria. *Berl Munch Tierarztl Wochenschr.* (1999) 112:18–23.
42. Hafez SM, Sharif M, Al-Sukayran A, Dela-Cruz D. Preliminary studies on enzootic bovine leukosis in Saudi dairy farms. *Dtsch Tierarztl Wochenschr.* (1990) 97:61–3.
43. OIE. *World Animal Health Information Database-Version: 1.* Paris: World organisation for animal Health (2012). Available online: https://www.oie.int/wahis_2/public/wahid.php/Diseaseinformation/statusdetail
44. Khudhair YI, Hasso SA, Yaseen NY, Al-Shammari AM. Serological and molecular detection of bovine leukemia virus in cattle in Iraq. *Emerg Microbes Infect.* (2016) 5:e56–6. doi: 10.1038/emi.2016.60
45. Gautam S, Mishra N, Kalaiyarasu S, Jhade SK, Sood R. Molecular characterization of bovine leukaemia virus (BLV) strains reveals existence of genotype 6 in cattle in India with evidence of a new subgenotype. *Transbound Emerg Dis.* (2018) 65:1968–78. doi: 10.1111/tbed.12979
46. Murakami K, Kobayashi S, Konishi M, Kameyama K, Tsutsui T. Nationwide survey of bovine leukemia virus infection among dairy and beef breeding cattle in Japan from 2009-2011. *J Vet Med Sci.* (2013) 75:1123–6. doi: 10.1292/jvms.12-0374
47. Lee E, Kim EJ, Joung HK, Kim BH, Song JY, Cho IS, et al. Sequencing and phylogenetic analysis of the gp51 gene from Korean bovine leukemia virus isolates. *Virol J.* (2015) 12:64. doi: 10.1186/s12985-015-0286-4
48. Mekata H, Sekiguchi S, Konnai S, Kirino Y, Horii Y, Norimine J. Horizontal transmission and phylogenetic analysis of bovine leukemia virus in two districts of Miyazaki, Japan. *J Vet Med Sci.* (2015) 77: 1115–20. doi: 10.1292/jvms.14-0624
49. Lassauzet ML, Thurmond MC, Johnson WO, Stevens F, Picanso JP. Effect of brucellosis vaccination and dehorning on transmission of bovine leukemia virus in heifers on a California dairy. *Can J Vet Res.* (1990) 54:184–9.
50. Kobayashi S, Tsutsui T, Yamamoto T, Hayama Y, Kameyama K, Konishi M, et al. Risk factors associated with within-herd transmission of bovine leukemia virus on dairy farms in Japan. *BMC Vet Res.* (2010) 6:1. doi: 10.1186/1746-6148-6-1
51. Hopkins SG, DiGiacomo RF, Evermann JF, Christensen JD, Deitelhoff DP, Mickelsen WD. Rectal palpation and transmission of bovine leukemia virus in dairy cattle. *J Am Vet Med Assoc.* (1991) 199:1035–8.
52. Azevedo C, Pacheco D, Soares L, Moitoso M, Maldonado J, Guix R, et al. Prevalence of bovine milk pathogens in Azorean pastures: mobile versus fixed milking machines. *Vet Rec Open.* (2016) 3:1–6. doi: 10.1136/vetreco-2016-000181
53. Buehring GC, Kramme PM, Schultz RD. Evidence for bovine leukemia virus in mammary epithelial cells of infected cows. *Lab Invest.* (1994) 71:359–65.
54. Ferrer JF, Kenyon SJ, Gupta P. Milk of dairy cows frequently contains a leukemogenic virus. *Science.* (1981) 213:1014–6.
55. Kuckleburg CJ, Chase CC, Nelson EA, Marras SA, Dammen MA, Christopher-Hennings J. Detection of bovine leukemia virus in blood and milk by nested and real-time polymerase chain reactions. *J Vet Diagn Invest.* (2003) 15:72–6. doi: 10.1177/104063870301500117
56. Ferrer JF, Piper CE. An evaluation of the role of milk in the natural transmission of BLV. *Ann Rech Vet.* (1978) 9:803–7.
57. Shettigara PT, Samagh BS, Lobinowich EM. Control of bovine leukemia virus infection in dairy herds by agar gel immunodiffusion test and segregation of reactors. *Can J Vet Res.* (1989) 53:108–10.

2

Monitoring *Coxiella burnetii* Infection in Naturally Infected Dairy Sheep Flocks throughout Four Lambing Seasons and Investigation of Viable Bacteria

Raquel Álvarez-Alonso [1], Ion I. Zendoia [1], Jesús F. Barandika [1], Isabel Jado [2], Ana Hurtado [1], Ceferino M. López [3] and Ana L. García-Pérez [1]*

[1] Animal Health Department, NEIKER-Instituto Vasco de Investigación y Desarrollo Agrario, Derio, Spain, [2] Laboratory of Special Pathogens, Instituto de Salud Carlos III, Centro Nacional de Microbiología, Madrid, Spain, [3] Department of Animal Pathology, Veterinary Faculty, University of Santiago de Compostela, Lugo, Spain

***Correspondence:**
Ana L. García-Pérez
agarcia@neiker.eus*

Progression of *Coxiella burnetii* infection in four naturally infected sheep flocks, and in their farm environment, was monitored throughout four lambing seasons. Flocks with an active infection were selected based on the presence of *C. burnetii* DNA in bulk-tank milk (BTM) and a high seroprevalence in yearlings during the previous milking period (Spring 2015). During four consecutive lambing seasons (2015/16–2018/19), samples were collected within 1 week after each lambing period from animals (vaginal swabs, milk and feces from ewes, and yearlings) and the environment (dust indoor sheep premises). BTM samples and aerosols (outdoors and indoors) were monthly collected between lambing and the end of milking. Real-time PCR analyses showed different trends in *C. burnetii* shedding in the flocks, with a general progressive decrease in bacterial shedding throughout the years, interrupted in three flocks by peaks of reinfection associated with specific management practices. A significant relationship was found between *C. burnetii* fecal shedding and the bacterial burden detected in dust, whereas shedding by vaginal route affected the detection of *C. burnetii* in indoor aerosols. Three genotypes were identified: SNP8 (three flocks, 52.9% of the samples), SNP1 (two flocks, 44.8% samples), and SNP5 (one flock, two environmental samples). *Coxiella burnetii* viability in dust measured by culture in Vero cells was demonstrated in two of the flocks, even during the fourth lambing season. The results showed that infection can remain active for over 5 years if effective control and biosafety measures are not correctly implemented.

Keywords: *Coxiella burnetii*, Q fever, sheep, genotypes, viability, lambing, environment

INTRODUCTION

Q fever is a widespread zoonosis caused by the intracellular bacterium *Coxiella burnetii*. Goats and sheep are considered the main reservoir of *C. burnetii*, and both have a significant role as source of human infection (1, 2). Q fever causes abortions in small ruminants (3), and once *C. burnetii* enters into a flock, infection spreads rapidly. Infected animals shed *C. burnetii* through birth products, vaginal fluids, feces, milk, and urine for several weeks after abortion or normal parturition

(4–10), but the bacterial load shed by aborted animals is higher than that shed by those that deliver normally (9). Abortion rates due to *C. burnetii* are especially high in goats (up to 70–90%) (4, 11) but lower in sheep (usually below 6%) (12). These low rates can be considered normal by the farmer, and consequently, samples of aborted animals are not submitted for diagnostic testing. Therefore, Q fever is not diagnosed, control measures are not implemented, and the infection can be maintained in a sheep flock throughout consecutive lambings. In a recent study carried out in dairy sheep flocks, *C. burnetii* shedding through milk was still observed in several flocks 10 years after first detection (13). This suggests that flock management practices together with lack of control measures implemented can cause periodical reactivation of *C. burnetii* infection (14–17).

Coxiella burnetii shedding by infected animals, together with their movements in indoor animal premises, promotes the formation of contaminated aerosols. Bacterial load in aerosols is the highest at the peak of abortions (4) and also correlates with the number of shedders in the flock (18). The progression of natural infection by *C. burnetii* in sheep flocks during several breeding seasons has not been fully investigated; thus, the length of time that the infection remains active in the flock is unknown. It is known that in the breeding seasons that follow an outbreak of abortion by Q fever, abortions decrease in sheep, and *C. burnetii* shedding naturally declines (19). Vaccination with phase I vaccine helped to limit bacterial shedding in ewes and yearlings from infected flocks in the two first years, resulting in a complete clearance of the infection after 4 years of vaccine implementation (20). However, *C. burnetii* DNA was still detected in dust samples in the fourth season after vaccination (20). Presence of *Coxiella* DNA in dust collected in farm premises has been reported in several studies (4, 9, 20, 21), but the time *Coxiella* remains viable has been scarcely investigated (4, 21). Kersh et al. (21) still found viable *Coxiella* in a goat farm in the kidding season that followed an abortion outbreak. In fact, the small-cell variant (SCV) is a spore-like form of *C. burnetii*, which can survive during long periods of time in the environment (22). Results pointed out that loads of viable *C. burnetii* are at the highest level during lambing/abortion period and progressively decrease thereafter until no viable bacteria are detected 2 months after the last parturition (4).

The genotype of *C. burnetii* could affect the course of infection (23, 24). In Spain, there is not much information about genotypes of *C. burnetii* involved in Q fever cases, neither in humans nor in animals. Recent studies carried out in Northern Spain identified goats rather than sheep as the main source of Q fever for humans, with pneumonia as the main symptom (4, 25–27), but interestingly, sheep and goats share the same *C. burnetii* genotypes in this area (4, 13, 27). Therefore, further studies are needed to better understand the epidemiological features of *C. burnetii* infection in sheep. This work was aimed at studying the progress of *Coxiella* infection throughout four lambing seasons in four dairy sheep flocks in semiextensive management systems in which no vaccination program was implemented. Genotyping of the strains involved and the investigation of *C. burnetii* viability in consecutive breeding seasons would help to better understand Q fever infection in sheep.

MATERIALS AND METHODS

Flocks Selection and Sampling Approach

Latxa is the dairy breed of sheep in the Basque Country. Lambing takes place once per year, between November and January for ewes and between March and April for yearlings. Animals are housed indoors in winter and at night and in rainy weather during the milking season, which ends in June–July. After that period, flocks are moved to communal mountain pastures where sheep share grazing areas with other sheep flocks, cattle, and horses, and wildlife, mainly wild boar, roe deer, badger, and foxes.

Four sheep flocks that tested real-time PCR positive to *C. burnetii* on bulk-tank milk (BTM) samples collected in March–April 2015 were selected. These flocks also showed a high seroprevalence against *C. burnetii* measured by ELISA in yearlings (**Table 1**). Both results suggested that *C. burnetii* infection was active in these flocks. Farmers were interested in collaborating and studying the evolution of the infection throughout four lambing seasons: 2015/2016, 2016/2017, 2017/2018, and 2018/2019. Flocks had never been vaccinated against this pathogen. It should be noted that, at the beginning of this study, there was a stock rupture in the production of the phase I inactivated vaccine, so vaccination could not be considered. A questionnaire was conducted to collect data on census, farm characteristics, management system, abortion history, and hygiene and biosecurity measures implemented in each farm. According to farmers' perception, significant abortions were not reported in the years prior to the study. However, one of them reported that a family member had suffered from pneumonia in the 2014/2015 production season, but since hospitalization was not needed, the etiological agent was not identified. For the correct management of the placentas, farmers were offered a freezer and biohazardous waste disposal containers, which, once filled, would be removed for incineration of infectious material. The goal was to quickly remove potentially infective material from the farm environment, thereby reducing possible environmental contamination. Three of the farmers performed this procedure, while the fourth (flock 2) had a type of slatted floor that resulted in placentas falling directly into the slurry pit. **Table 1** summarizes information about the selected flocks. Two of the flocks (flocks 2 and 3) used to buy animals from other flocks. Flock 4 had old animal premises and moved to a new farm in the lambing season 2018/2019.

Flocks were visited at lambing during four consecutive lambing seasons. During the first three seasons, samples were collected from ewes and yearlings and purchased animals (if any). During the last lambing season, only yearlings were sampled. Vaginal exudates (collected with swabs without medium), milk, and feces were taken from a maximum of 40 ewes and/or 40 yearlings within 1 week after parturition to evaluate *C. burnetii* shedding (**Table 1**). During these visits, environmental samples consisting of duplicates of 8–10 dust samples were taken from different surfaces of the animal premises to detect the presence of *C. burnetii* DNA and for further viability studies (one duplicate kept at −80°C). In addition, monthly visits were made until the end of the milking period, and a BTM sample was collected to monitor *C. burnetii* shedding at the flock level, as well as aerosols

TABLE 1 | General information of the sheep flocks included in the study.

	Flock 1	Flock 2	Flock 3	Flock 4
CENSUS				
Ewes	416	250	543	411
Yearlings	80	50	87	83
Communal pastures	Ewes	Ewes and yearlings	Ewes	Ewes and yearlings
Cattle in the farm	Yes	No	No	No
Goats in the farm	Yes	No	No	No
Purchase of animals	No	Yes	Yes	No
Abortions >3%	No	No	No	No
CHARACTERISTICS OF THE SHEEP PREMISES				
Year of construction	1995	2009	2007	1975*
Ventilation	Regular	Bad	Regular	Bad
Slatted floor	Yes	Yes	No	No
Straw bedding	Yearlings	No	Yes	Yes
Water source	Well	Well	Tap water	Tap water
Frequency of manure removal	Daily	1/year	2/year	2/year
BIOSECURITY MEASURES				
Management of placentas	Cremation	Manure	Cremation	Cremation
Exclusive cloth	No	No	No	No
Access of visits	Yes	Yes	Yes	Yes
Other measures	No	No	No	No
Q FEVER STATUS (2014/15)				
Seroprevalence (%)				
Ewes	26.7	40.0	13.3	26.7
Yearlings	66.7	46.7	46.7	53.3
BTM ELISA	Positive	Positive	Positive	Positive
BTM PCR	Positive	Positive	Positive	Positive
RANGE OF ANIMALS ANALYZED PER LAMBING SEASON				
Ewes†	30–40 (110)	30–61§ (131)	30–68§ (138)	30–40 (110)
Yearlings	28–40 (132)	7–28 (62)	7–28 (71)	30–40 (140)

**New sheep premises for the period 2018/19.*
†Ewes were not sampled in the 2018–2019 lambing season.
§Purchased ewes included.

collected indoor and outdoor sheep premises. The air sampler "MD8" Sartorius (Goettingen, Germany) was used, performing an aspiration of 100 L/min air for 10 min. The air passed through a gelatin filter adapted to the equipment, which was analyzed in the laboratory by real-time PCR in order to detect the presence of *C. burnetii* DNA in the aerosols generated at the farm.

Molecular Analyses

DNA Extraction and Real-Time PCR

DNA was extracted using the QIAmp DNA Blood Mini Kit (Qiagen Hilden, Germany) with some modifications. Briefly, milk or feces were mixed with 180 μl of ATL buffer (Qiagen, Hilden, Germany) and digested with 20 μl of proteinase K (8 mg/ml) for 30 min at 70°C before DNA extraction. Vaginal or dust swabs were treated with 300 μl of TE buffer (10 mM Tris base, 1 mM EDTA, pH 8) before being mixed with ATL and proteinase K for 1 h at 56°C. The initial treatment of the gelatin filters from the air sampler was done as previously described (18). Negative extraction controls were included every 10 samples to rule out DNA contamination. The presence of *C. burnetii* DNA was investigated by a real-time PCR procedure targeting the transposon-like repetitive region *IS1111* of *C. burnetii* genome (28). A commercial internal amplification control (IAC) (TaqMan® Exogenous Internal Positive Control, Thermo Fisher Scientific) was included in the assay to monitor for PCR inhibitors.

Genotyping

A selection of animal and environmental samples positive by real-time PCR with Ct < 31 were genotyped using a previously described single-nucleotide polymorphism (SNP) genotyping assay that detects 10 discriminatory SNPs by real-time PCR (29). SNPs were identified and selected by Huijsmans et al. (29) on the basis of both the consensus sequence generated from 100,000 bp of the five known whole genome sequences of *C. burnetii* (RSA493, RSA331, CbuG_Q212, Cbuk_Q154, and 5J108 111 Dugway) and an *in silico* investigation of their discriminatory power using BLAST (29). SNPs 769, 2287, 4439, 4557, 4844,

5423, and 6025 (positions indicated in the reference sequence RSA493, GenBank accession no. AE016828.2) are located within single-copy genes. SNPs 7087, 7726, and 7974 are located within the multicopy insertion sequence *IS1111* (positions within the first *IS1111* encountered, as indicated in the strain RSA493 reference sequence, GenBank accession no. AE016828.2), which is distributed throughout the *C. burnetii* genome. Ten real-time PCR reactions were performed per sample, each including two primers and two MGB® TaqMan probes to detect point mutations. Each 20 μl PCR mixture contained 625 nM of each primer, 125 nM of each probe, 1× Taq Mix ABsolute (Thermo Fisher Scientific), and 5 μl of template DNA. PCR reactions were run on a BioRad platform (CFX96™ RTi-PCR Detection System) using the following program: 15 min at 95°C, and 45 cycles of 3 s at 95°C, and 30 s at 60°C.

A selection of samples were also genotyped by multispacer sequence typing (MST) of eight spacers (Cox2, Cox5, Cox18, Cox22, Cox37, Cox51, Cox56, and Cox61) as previously described (30), with small modifications. Briefly, two four-plex PCR reactions were carried out followed by individual amplifications for each spacer region. Each amplicon was then purified and sequenced, and genotypes were identified by comparison with the database at https://ifr48.timone.univ-mrs.fr/mst/coxiella_burnetii/.

Serological Analyses: Enzyme-Linked Immunosorbent Assay

In order to evaluate seroprevalence against *C. burnetii*, individual milk samples were centrifuged, and milk sera were tested for Q fever antibodies using an ELISA test (LSIVET Ruminant Serum/Milk Q Fever kit; Thermo Fisher Scientific). An index (S/P) of the tested milk serum optical density to optical density of the positive control ratio was calculated according to the manufacturer's instructions. Individual milk samples with S/P indices ≤0.4 were considered negative, while samples with S/P >0.4 were considered positive.

Viability Studies

Ethics

Experimental studies were carried out in BSL3 facilities and consisted of experimental inoculations in 6-week-old BALB/c male mice combined with cell culture. Permission was obtained from the Ethical & Animal Welfare Committee (Bizkaiko Foru Aldundia, document 3/2017 v02, Reg. 32243 25 June 2018).

Isolation

Environmental viability of *C. burnetii* was assessed on dust samples collected after yearlings lambing under the assumption that dust deposited at that time would had been originated from aerosols generated during both ewes and yearlings lambing. Viability studies of C. *burnetii* in environmental samples were carried out by passage through mice and culture in Vero cells [African green monkey epithelial cells VERO C1008 (Vero 76, clone E6, Vero E6 ATCC® CRL-1586™)]. Dust samples were homogenized and prepared as detailed elsewhere (4). The quantification of *C. burnetii* genome equivalents (GE) in each homogenate was carried out by quantitative real-time PCR (qPCR) using 5 μl of DNA (in triplicates) and specific primers and a probe targeting the *IS1111* gene as described elsewhere (28). In each qPCR run, a standard curve was generated using 10-fold serial dilutions of a known concentration of Nine Mile (RSA439) phase II strain of *C. burnetii* DNA. After quantification, aliquots of 200–500 μl were prepared from each dust homogenate, containing approximately 10^2-10^3 *C. burnetii* GE. These aliquots were inoculated intraperitoneally in four mice each; a dust homogenate with viable *C. burnetii* (4) collected from a goat farm in 2017 and stored at −80°C was used as a positive control. As determined in previous studies (4, 31), mice were euthanized on days +14 and +21 p.i., and spleens were removed. The level of splenomegaly was determined from the ratio of the spleen weight to body weight. Half of the spleen from each mouse was processed for DNA extraction and real-time PCR amplification as fully detailed elsewhere (4). Positive samples were subjected to qPCR to quantify the number of *C. burnetii* GE detected in spleen in order to compare it with the number of GE inoculated; when the number of *C. burnetii* GE recovered from the spleen was equal or higher than the GE inoculated, *C. burnetii* was considered to have multiplied *in vivo*.

For qPCR-positive samples, the second half of the spleen was homogenized with 700 μl Dulbecco's modified Eagle's medium (DMEM) medium and 2% fetal bovine serum (FBS) in a TissueLyser. A hundred microliters of each homogenate were placed on shell vials (SV) containing Vero cells, as fully detailed elsewhere (4). Briefly, after harvesting *C. burnetii* from SV on day 6 p.i., three passages of 1,000 μl of harvested cells were transferred at weekly intervals into T25 culture flasks containing a Vero layer. At day 6 p.i. and before each passage, 200 μl was collected for DNA extraction and qPCR, following procedures described above. Cultures that maintained *C. burnetii* growth during the second or third passage were considered to be positive. Uninfected control cells were kept close to infected cells to rule out possible cross-contaminations.

Statistical Analyses

The possible influence of the different factors studied, i.e., flock (categorical; flock 1, flock 2, flock 3, flock 4), period of lambing (categorical; ewes/yearlings), and lambing season (categorical; 2015–2016, 2016–2017, 2017–2018, 2018–2019) over positive or negative *C. burnetii* animals shedding through vaginal fluids, feces, or milk was analyzed using a logistic regression. The final model was selected as the one with the lowest Akaike's information criterion (AIC) value from all of the models performed. Odds ratio values were computed by raising "e" to the power of the logistic coefficient over the reference category.

Cohen kappa statistics were used for assessing agreement between shedding by different excretion routes and ELISA results. The symmetry of disagreement between them was evaluated with McNemar's chi square test.

The risk of environmental (dust, indoor/outdoor aerosol) contamination by *C. burnetii* was evaluated with a data mining classification tree using "rpart" package (32); dust, indoor aerosols, and outdoor aerosols were continuous dependent variables (expressed in Ct values in real-time PCR). Classification and regression tree (CRT) identifies variables that divide

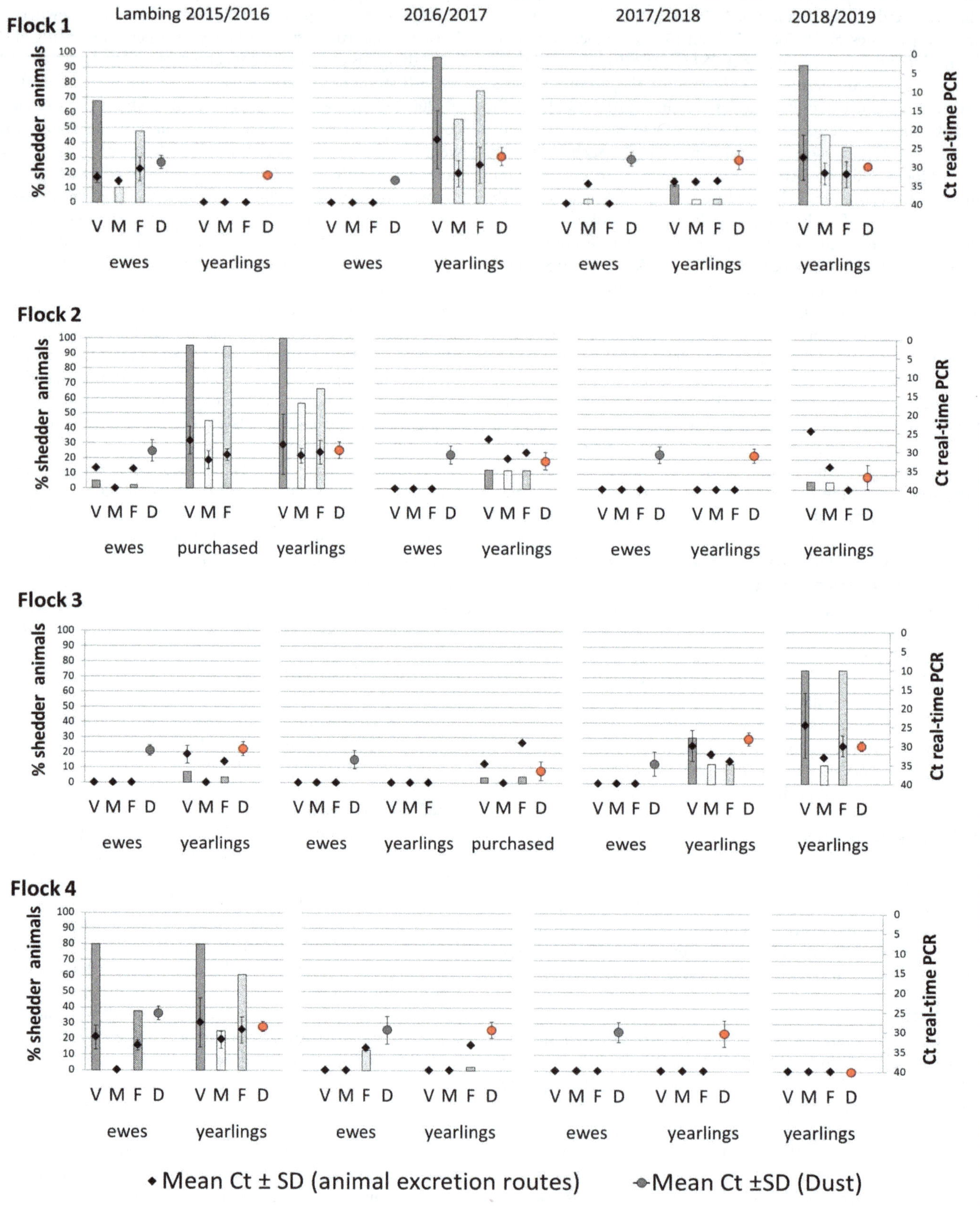

FIGURE 1 | Percentage of *Coxiella burnetii* shedders (ewes, yearlings, and, if applicable, purchased animals) throughout the four lambing seasons in the four studied flocks, through vaginal fluids (V), milk (M), and feces (F) with mean Ct values ± SD, represented with diamonds. The circles represent the mean of the Ct values ± SD obtained in real-time PCR from dust samples taken during ewes lambings (gray circles) and yearlings lambings (red circles). Ewes were not sampled in the fourth lambing season and are not represented.

environmental (dust/aerosols) results into homogeneous subgroups with distinct patterns of *C. burnetii* contamination. The CRT model provides a way to identify main factors. CRT evaluates all the values of the potential factor using, as a criterion, the significance of a statistical ANOVA test and split maximizing the between-groups sum of squares, selecting the best predictor variable to form the branch in a classification tree; successively splitting in data set makes increasingly homogeneous nodes in relation to the dependent variable. This process continues until the classification tree is fully grown. Figures for CRT were performed by "rpart.plot" package (33).

The degree of splenomegaly in experimental mice was evaluated with a Welch two sample *t* test to correct homoscedasticity. Linear regression was performed with the purpose of analyzing any relationship between *C. burnetii* GE load present in the inoculum injected to mice and the GE of *C. burnetii* recovered from the spleen of experimental animals. Log-transformed data were used in both analyses. All statistical analyses were performed using the statistical software R version 3.6.2 (34).

RESULTS

Coxiella burnetii Shedding and Serological Response in Ewes and Yearlings

Real-time PCR results showed different trends in *Coxiella* shedding throughout the 4-year study in the studied flocks (**Figure 1**). Overall, the percentage of *C. burnetii* shedders was significantly higher in the first lambing season (2015/2016) (**Table 2**). In the first lambing season, flock 1 showed a high-moderate percentage of ewes shedding *C. burnetii* by different routes (vaginal fluids > feces > milk), but no shedders were detected in the group of yearlings. The following lambing seasons (2016/2017 and 2017/2018) ewes barely shed *C. burnetii*, whereas yearlings showed a reactivation of the infection in the second and fourth lambing seasons. The situation in flock 2 was affected by the reported purchase of a group of 30 pregnant ewes in December 2015. These animals became infected when they entered into the contaminated animal premises and shed high *C. burnetii* loads at lambing. This caused the reactivation of infection in the flock, which mainly affected the yearlings while the proportion of ewe shedders of that season was low (**Figure 1**). Afterwards, in the following seasons, flock 2 showed a decrease in the percentage of animal shedders. Patterns of infection in flock 3 were the opposite, with a low proportion or absence of *C. burnetii* shedders during the first two lambing seasons and reactivation of infection in yearlings in the last two seasons. Flock 3 introduced a new group of pregnant ewes ($N = 62$) on the 20th March 2017, 1 week before the lambing of yearlings. Later on, purchased animals showed to be infected at lambing (7% animal shedders, 2/28, in samplings carried out between 27th March and 19th April). Flock 4 showed a high percentage of shedders during the first lambing season, in both ewes and yearlings, but a significant decrease occurred in the following lambings and no shedders were detected in the last two seasons (**Figure 1**). Overall, flock 4 had a significantly higher number of animal shedders than flocks 2 and 3, but lower than flock 1 (**Table 2**).

Shedders were more frequently found among yearlings than among ewes, but to a lesser extent than among newly introduced animals (purchased group) (**Table 2**). Regarding *C. burnetii* shedding loads expressed as Ct values in real-time PCR, the highest excretion levels (lowest Ct) were detected in yearlings, especially through vaginal fluids (**Figure 1**).

Comparison of seroprevalence in ewes throughout the lambing seasons showed marked differences between flocks (**Figure 2**). Thus, in flock 1, seroprevalence in ewes ranged between 58 and 80%; in flock 2, between 30 and 60%; in flock 3, 35–40%; and in flock 4, 13–63%. Thirty-two percent of the recently purchased ewes (9/28) in flock 3 had antibodies against *C. burnetii*, suggesting that ewes were already infected when introduced into the flock.

In yearlings, seroprevalence increased or decreased according to the trends of *C. burnetii* infection in each flock, showing in general lower seroprevalences than ewes. Flocks 2 and 4 showed a progressive decrease in seroprevalence during the study period (**Figure 2**). Independently of the shedding route (vaginal, feces, or milk), a high percentage of *C. burnetii* shedders was

TABLE 2 | Logistic regression model for the prevalence of shedders.

	Estimate	*Z* value	Pr (> |*t*|)	OR	95% CI
Intercept	0.4718	2.233	0.0255	1.60	1.06–2.43
Flock 4 (Ref.)					
Flock 1	0.6048	2.816	0.0050	1.83	1.20–2.80
Flock 2	−1.1090	−3.775	0.0001	0.33	0.18–0.58
Flock 3	−1.7177	−5.553	0.0001	0.18	0.10–0.32
Yearlings (Ref.)					
Ewes	−0.7806	−3.762	0.0001	0.46	0.30–0.68
Purchased	1.2847	4.353	0.0001	6.20	2.74–14.26
Lambing.season 2015–2016 (Ref.)					
Lambing.season 2016–2017	−1.7405	−7.708	0.0001	0.18	0.11–0.27
Lambing.season 2017–2018	−2.4730	−8.327	0.0001	0.08	0.05–0.15
Lambing.season 2018–2019	−0.6371	−2.166	0.0303	0.52	0.30–0.93

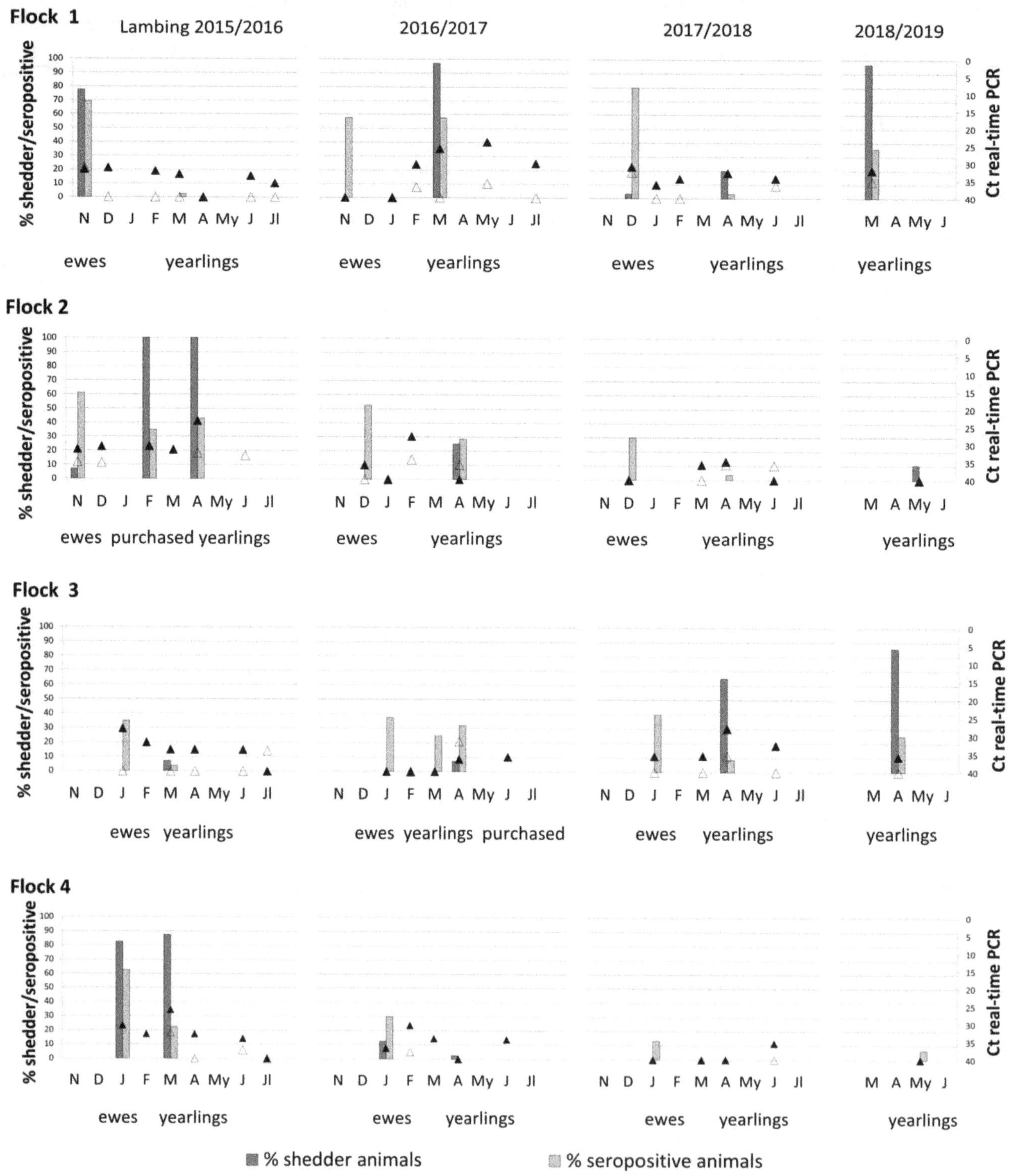

FIGURE 2 | Percentage of shedder animals by at least one excretion route (vaginal fluids, feces, or milk) and seroprevalence observed corresponding to ewes and yearlings of the four studied flocks during four lambing season (bars). *Coxiella burnetii* DNA present in aerosols taken outdoor (empty triangles) and indoor (black triangles) animal premises from lambing to the end of milking season are also represented. Ewes were not sampled in the fourth lambing season and are not represented.

not always positively correlated with seroprevalence (**Figure 2**). Cohen kappa (kappa = 0.142) and McNemar's test (McNemar's chi-squared = 10.75, $df = 1$, $P = 0.001$) statistics showed a poor relationship between *C. burnetii* shedding and ELISA results. Results of *C. burnetii* shedding as well as detection of antibodies in ewes and yearlings per flock and lambing season are compiled in **Table S1**.

The evolution of *C. burnetii* DNA presence in BTM samples during the four milking seasons is shown in **Figure 3**. In the first lambing season, bacterial shedding was very low in the four herds, always with Ct >30. In all milking seasons, bacterial load in BTM was higher after yearlings were included in milking (from February onwards). The highest bacterial load (Ct = 30) was found in flock 1 in the second lambing season. The reactivation of *C. burnetii* infection observed in yearlings from flocks 1 and 3 (see above) was also reflected in the bacterial load detected in BTM samples (**Figure 3** and **Table S1**).

Coxiella burnetii in Environmental Samples

Dust samples taken from different surfaces on animal premises during ewe and yearling lambings were *C. burnetii* DNA-positive throughout the 4 years of the study (ranges of Ct of 27–35), the only exception being flock 4, which became negative in the fourth lambing season. This flock had moved to new animal premises before lambing season 2018/2019 started, and *C. burnetii* DNA was not detected in dust thereafter. In the other three flocks, sporadic increases in dust bacterial load with respect to previous years were associated to increases in the number of shedders (**Figure 1**). The CRT algorithm stratified variables that played an important role in the amount of *C. burnetii* in dust (**Figure 4A**) and identified two determining factors for higher amounts of *C. burnetii* in dust (Ct = 29, 32% samplings), i.e., a percentage of fecal shedders higher than 1.2% (node 1), followed by the presence in the flock of more than 10% of shedders by vaginal route (node 3). When the presence of fecal shedders was low (node 2), the presence of *C. burnetii* in dust was determined by the lambing of ewes rather than yearlings (**Figure 4A**).

Results for the aerosols taken monthly indoor and outdoor of the farm from lambing until the end of the milking period are shown in **Figure 2**. Flocks 2 and 4 showed a progressive decrease in indoor environmental contamination during the course of the study, and in the fourth season, aerosols taken at yearling lambing were negative. On the contrary, flocks 1 and 3 showed sporadic increases in bacterial loads in aerosols due to reinfections in the flocks, and in the last lambing season, positive aerosols were still detected in the farm. The presence of *C. burnetii* in indoor aerosols was determined by the percentage of vaginal shedders (node 1) (**Figure 4B**), and when the percentage of shedders was below 10% (node 2), lambing season was identified as a determining factor (node 3); in the first lambing season, mean Ct value in indoor aerosols was lower than in the following seasons. From the second lambing period onwards, Ct values were determined by *C. burnetii* load shed through feces (node 5). Contamination of outdoor aerosols was less frequent, and when positive, the bacterial load was always lower (Ct > 32) than in aerosols taken indoors (**Figure 2**). Based on CRT algorithm results, rates of seroprevalence higher than 61% (node 1) determined the presence of positive aerosols outdoors (**Figure 4C**), and when seroprevalence in the flock was lower, a higher excretion of *C. burnetii* through feces (Ct < 40) (node 3) was the determining factor. Raw data of real-time PCR results obtained from dust and indoors/outdoors aerosols can be found in **Table S1**.

Genotypes of *C. burnetii*

A selection of samples (vaginal fluids, feces, milk, dust, and aerosols), with low Ct values in real-time PCR, was analyzed

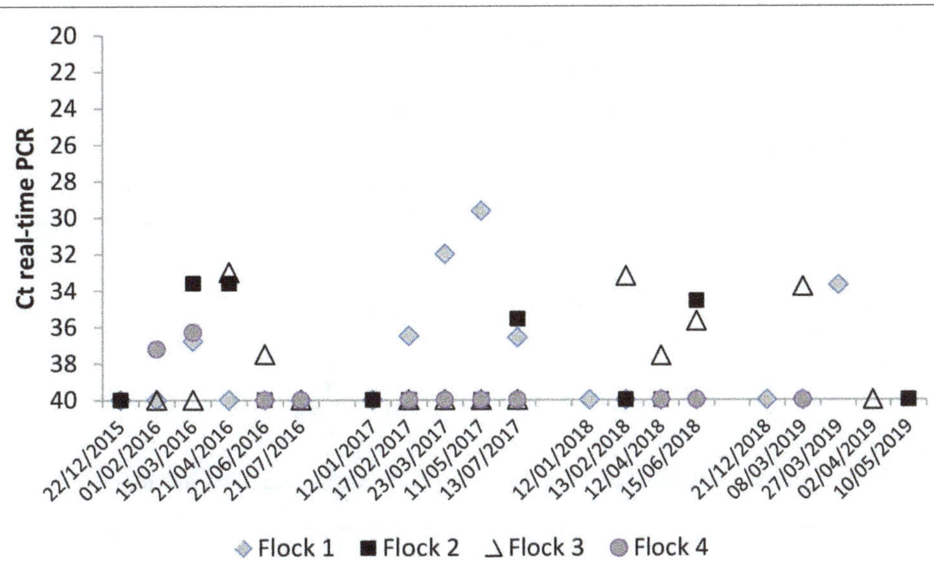

FIGURE 3 | Evolution of *C. burnetii* shedding through milk measured by bulk-tank milk (BTM) real-time PCR analyses throughout the four milking periods.

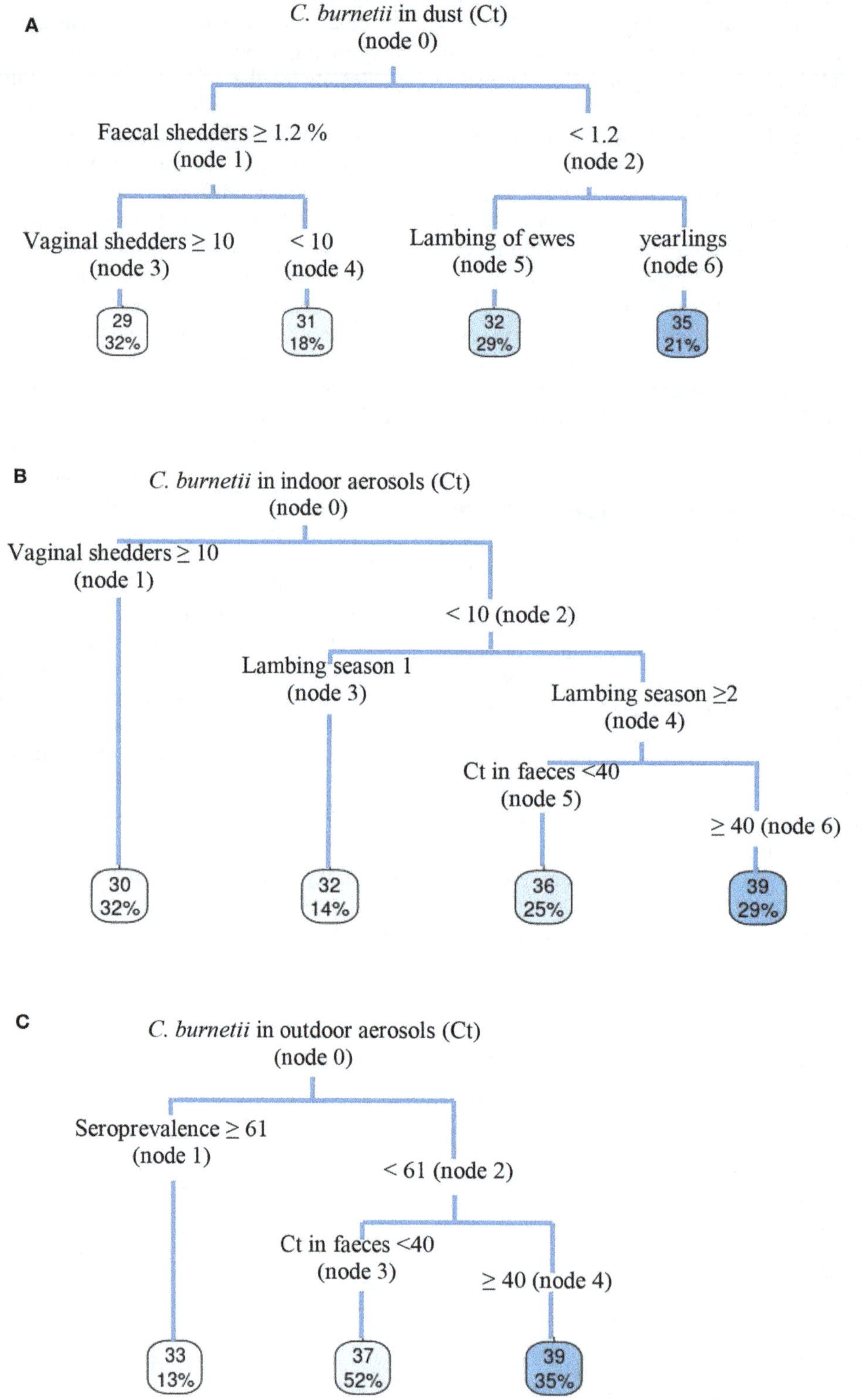

FIGURE 4 | Classification and regression tree (CRT) showing determining risk-factors for *C. burnetii* detection in **(A)** dust, **(B)** indoor aerosols, and **(C)** outdoor aerosols.

by SNP genotyping. The number of genotyped samples in each flock depended on the infection status shown in the course of the study. Thus, a total of 87 DNA samples could be genotyped (flock 1, 27 samples; flock 2, 25 samples; flock 3, 18 samples; flock 4, 17 samples), mainly from animals (61%) and dust (28%), and to a lesser extent, aerosols (11%) (**Table S2**). In flocks 1 and 4, only one genotype was identified (SNP8 in flock 1 and SNP1 in flock 4). In flock 2, three genotypes were identified (SNP1, SNP5, and SNP8), but SNP1 was the predominant genotype. In flock 3, two genotypes were identified (SNP1 and SNP8), but SNP8 was the predominant in both animal and environmental samples (**Table 3**). Overall, SNP8 was the most widespread genotype, found in three flocks and accounting for 52.9% of the samples; SNP1 was found in two flocks and 44.8% of the samples. For a selection of DNA samples ($N = 4$), the MST genotype was also determined. Two SNP1 samples from flocks 2 and 4 belonged to the MST13 genotype, while two SNP8 samples from flocks 1 and 2 corresponded with MST18. Unfortunately, no complete MST results were obtained from the only sample (dust) with SNP5 genotype.

Viability of *C. burnetii* in Dust

The duplicates of dust samples collected at each yearling lambing were pooled and processed to study *C. burnetii* viability using cell line culture. These accounted for 15 dust homogenates corresponding to the four lambings in flocks 1, 2, and 3, and three lambings in flock 4 (**Table 4**). Ct values of dust homogenates in real-time PCR ranged between 28.7 and 35.5 (**Table 4**). Prior to cell culture assays, each homogenate was inoculated into four 6-week-old male BALB/c mice. *C. burnetii* DNA was detected in the spleen of 20 of the 60 inoculated mice at +14 and +21 days p.i.; yet, in 3 of them, recovered GEs were below inoculated GEs. The presence of *C. burnetii* DNA was also confirmed in the four mice inoculated with the positive control (one mouse with lower GE than inoculated).

Comparisons among flocks suggested that viable *C. burnetii* were more widespread in flock 1, since 13 of the 16 mice spleens were positive after inoculation with dust collected in the four lambing seasons. In flock 2, only one mouse inoculated with a dust sample taken in the second lambing season was real-time PCR positive. In flock 3, six mice inoculated with dust collected in the first and fourth lambing seasons were positive in real-time PCR. Finally, mice inoculated with dust homogenates from flock 4 were all negative.

A significant correlation was observed between the *C. burnetii* GE inoculated and the *C. burnetii* GE recovered from spleen (adjusted $R^2 = 0.4398$, $P = 0.0042$). To assess splenomegaly, the ratio spleen of weight/live weight of mice was compared between positive mice (*C. burnetii* DNA detected in spleen by real-time PCR) and negative mice. Significant differences were observed ($t = -3.6449$; $df = 29.512$; $p = 0.0010$), and positive mice showed a ratio 1.53 times greater than negative mice.

Cultures in Vero cells of homogenates of spleens from the 20 real-time PCR-positive mice, as described above, resulted in *C. burnetii* growth in 7 mice (**Table 4**). Growth for at least two passages was only observed in those cases when shell vials were inoculated with at least 9.45×10^5 GE. *C. burnetii* isolates were successfully cultured from dust collected in flock 1 in the second and fourth lambing season, whereas in flock 3, viable *C. burnetii* was only recovered in dust collected in the fourth lambing seasons.

SNP genotypes were analyzed in positive spleens, and SNP8 was identified in mice inoculated with dust samples from flocks

TABLE 3 | Single-nucleotide polymorphism (SNP) genotyping results from selected DNA samples obtained in each flock from animals and the environment (dust and aerosols) during the four lambing seasons.

Lambing season	Origin of samples	Flock 1	Flock 2			Flock 3		Flock 4
		SNP8	SNP1	SNP5	SNP8	SNP1	SNP8	SNP1
2015–2016	Ewes/yearlings*	5	13	–	1	1	–	12
	Dust	–	3	–	–	–	3	3
	Aerosols	–	1	1	–	–	1	1
2016–2017	Ewes/yearlings	6	1	–	–	–	1	–
	Dust	2	1	1	–	–	1	1
	Aerosols	3	1	–	–	–	–	–
2017–2018	Ewes/yearlings	–	–	–	–	–	2	–
	Dust	2	–	–	1	–	2	–
	Aerosols	1	–	–	–	–	1	–
2018–2019	Ewes/yearlings	6	1	–	–	–	4	–
	Dust	2	–	–	–	–	2	–
	Aerosols	–	–	–	–	–	–	–

**Vaginal fluids/milk/feces.*

TABLE 4 | Investigation of viable *C. burnetii* in dust collected at yearling lambings in the studied flocks throughout the study using Balb/c mice and culture in Vero cell lines.

			BALB/c mice inoculation					Culture in cell lines (Vero E6) (GE/ml)					
Flock	**Lambing period**	**Ct real-time PCR (mean)**	**No. of GE[a] injected**	**No. of mice sacrificed at day +14 p.i.[b]**	**No. of mice sacrificed at day +21p.i.**	**No. of positive mice (day p.i.)**	**No. of GE in spleen**	**Inoculated**	**Day 6 p.i.**	**1st passage**	**2nd passage**	**3rd passage**	**Viable *C. burnetii***
1	2015–2016	32.9	3.8×10^2	2	2	2 (+14)	1.7×10^3	1.00×10^2	0.0	0.0	0.0	0.0	No
							1.0×10^3	1.00×10^2	0.0	0.0	0.0	0.0	No
						1 (+21)	1.3×10^4	1.00×10^2	0.0	0.0	0.0	0.0	No
	2016–2017	28.8	5.8×10^3	2	2	2 (+14)	3.4×10^4	1.54×10^2	3.44×10^2	0.0	0.0	0.0	No
							1.2×10^5	1.42×10^3	3.71×10^3	5.80×10^2	0.0	0.0	No
						2 (+21)	1.1×10^3	1.00×10^2	2.01×10^3	0.0	0.0	0.0	No
							9.8×10^6	9.50×10^5	8.16×10^5	1.43×10^6	2.88×10^5	2.26×10^5	Yes
	2017–2018	29.6	3.4×10^3	2	2	2 (+14)	2.5×10^2	1.00×10^2	0.0	0.0	0.0	0.0	No
							4.1×10^2	1.00×10^2	0.0	0.0	0.0	0.0	No
	2018–2019	28.7	6.2×10^3	2	2	2 (+14)	7.0×10^5	1.20×10^4	1.11×10^4	9.10×10^3	0.0	0.0	No
							4.5×10^7	9.45×10^5	4.23×10^5	1.94×10^5	2.22×10^5	0.0	Yes
						2 (+21)	2.7×10^6	3.82×10^6	2.18×10^6	4.70×10^5	5.24×10^5	1.00×10^5	Yes
							5.5×10^6	9.49×10^5	2.76×10^6	3.65×10^5	3.65×10^5	0.0	Yes
2	2015–2016	29.8	2.9×10^3	2	2	0	0						
	2016–2017	31.9	7.5×10^2	2	2	1 (+21)	8.8×10^3	2.52×10^3	2.10×10^3	0.0	0.0	0.0	No
	2017–2018	34.2	1.7×10^2	2	2	0	0						
	2018–2019	34.7	1.2×10^2	2	2	0	0						
3	2015–2016	30.5	2.0×10^3	2	2	1 (+14)	8.5×10^4	1.00×10^2	0.0	0.0	0.0	0.0	No
						2 (+21)	7.1×10^5	4.51×10^3	9.86×10^3	1.89×10^3	0.0	0.0	No
							1.2×10^4	5.19×10^3	1.42×10^4	1.85×10^4	0.0	0.0	No
	2016–2017	35.5	9.4×10^1	2	2	0	0						
	2017–2018	32.9	3.9×10^2	2	2	0	0						
	2018–2019	29.4	3.9×10^3	2	2	1 (+14)	7.1×10^7	4.45×10^6	1.11×10^6	4.63×10^5	4.46×10^5	1.00×10^5	Yes
						2 (+21)	1.5×10^7	3.79×10^6	1.25×10^6	1.99×10^6	3.30×10^6	1.32×10^6	Yes
							5.4×10^7	9.03×10^6	1.95×10^7	1.19×10^7	6.92×10^6	6.03×10^6	Yes
4	2015–2016	31.9	7.4×10^2	2	2	0	0						
	2016–2017	30.8	1.6×10^3	2	2	0	0						
	2017–2018	33.2	3.2×10^2	2	2	0	0						
Posit. Control (goats)	2017	20.9	10.7×10^5	2	2	2 (+14)	3.0×10^7	1.82×10^4	4.88×10^4	5.33×10^4	8.53×10^4	0.0	Yes
							9.1×10^6	2.88×10^6	6.90×10^5	8.37×10^5	2.76×10^5	6.91×10^5	Yes
						2 (+21)	4.8×10^6	2.30×10^4	2.05×10^4	2.86×10^4	0.0	0.0	No
							5.0×10^4	3.00×10^2	0.0	0.0	0.0	0.0	No

[a] *GE, genome equivalents of C. burnetii determined by quantitative real-time PCR targeting IS1111.*
[b] *p.i., postinoculation.*

1 and 3, whereas SNP1 was identified in the only mouse positive from flock 2. Interestingly, SNP5 detected in two environmental samples in flock 2 was not recovered from mice.

DISCUSSION

This study shows the patterns of *C. burnetii* infection in four naturally infected dairy sheep flocks throughout four lambing seasons. The presence of animal shedders in the previous milking season and high seroprevalence in yearlings suggested at the beginning of the study that infection was active in all flocks (1, 16). It is known that shedding of *C. burnetii* by vaginal fluids, feces, and milk can persist in the breeding season that follows infection onset in small ruminant farms, even when vaccination has been implemented (20). In this study, the low percentage or even the absence of shedders among ewes (flocks 2 and 3) and yearlings (flock 1) during the first lambing season supported the suspicion that *C. burnetii* infection had been present in these flocks before the 2014/2015 season. Besides, infection was still active in some flocks in the fourth lambing season (flocks 1 and 3), leading one to think that *C. burnetii* infection can remain in a flock for more than 5 years, probably due to periodical reinfections. In fact, a previous study hypothesized that infection could be maintained for 10 years (13). The outcome of infection showed the most desirable progression in flock 4, which started with the highest percentage of animal shedders and the highest bacterial shedding in ewes and yearlings during the first lambing season, followed by a significant decrease in the following years until the infection disappeared in the fourth lambing season. Movement of the flock to new uncontaminated farm premises before lambing season 2018/2019 undoubtedly helped to keep the flock free of infection.

The fact that the bacterial load shed throughout the 4 years of the study was lower in ewes than in yearlings also supports the idea that infection had established in the flocks some time before the study started. Had the infection onset occurred before, ewes would have had time to develop immunity, whereas yearlings would have been more susceptible to the infection (9).

This study also highlighted the risk of introducing naive animals into an infected flock, which, as shown in flock 2, can cause a reactivation of the infection. Purchasing infected animals also poses a risk when introduced into a negative flock (35, 36). This was probably the situation in flock 3, where purchased pregnant ewes could have been the source of a new infection. After lambings started, 1 week after purchase, the presence of shedders was detected and moderate seroprevalence was recorded, suggesting that those animals could have been infected previously and be the source of the infection observed in yearlings during the third and fourth lambing seasons.

The four flocks were managed under a semiextensive system where animals are housed during lambing and milking and, afterwards, graze on communal mountain pastures in contact with livestock and wildlife. In a region like the Basque Country, where Q fever is endemic and vaccination is not frequently implemented, this system poses a risk for infection and reinfection (14, 15, 17). Nevertheless, the infection peak observed in yearlings in flock 1 during the second and fourth lambing seasons is difficult to explain since yearlings did not share grazing pastures with other flocks. Roe deer frequented yearling grazing fields; however, their role as infection source was ruled out after testing *Coxiella* negative by PCR analysis of their feces (data not shown). However, 5.1% of the roe deer analyzed in the same region harbored *C. burnetii* DNA (37). Therefore, the role of roe deer and other wildlife species as source of *C. burnetii* infection as reported elsewhere (38) cannot be ignored. Besides, this was the only farm that also holds beef cattle and goats as potential source for yearling infection that unfortunately could not be tested. However, cattle and goats in the farm were managed under a year-round extensive system and did not share pastures with sheep, thus minimizing opportunities for sheep cross-infection. In any case, inappropriate implementation of biosafety measures is a risk factor for flock infections that cannot be ruled out (1, 16, 36).

The interpretation of the humoral immune response against *C. burnetii* is complex and has little value at individual level because a percentage of infected animals (25–50%) do not seroconvert (6, 39–41). In this study, a commercial ELISA kit was used to measure *C. burnetii* antibodies in milk samples, since a good correlation between the level of antibodies detected in individual milk with those present in blood serum has been reported (42, 43). The marked differences in seroprevalence observed in ewes and yearlings throughout the four lambing seasons among flocks were probably associated to the exposure of animals to different loads of viable bacteria. However, as seen in this study and others (16), seroprevalence is not correlated with bacterial shedding.

The abovementioned factors, such as animal purchase or grazing in communal pastures, can favor not only *C. burnetii* infection but also the probability of infection with more than one genotype. The presence of several *Coxiella* genotypes in a farm has been previously described (9, 44–46). Here, only one genotype was detected in flocks 1 and 4, whereas in flocks 2 and 3, three and two different genotypes were detected, respectively. Interestingly, flocks with more than one genotype were those that had purchased animals. Regardless of the flock, in all cases, the more frequently found genotypes were SNP1/MST13 and SNP8/MST18. Both genotypes had been found in the region in sheep flocks (13) or in Q fever outbreaks of caprine origin associated with pneumonia in humans (4, 27). In Europe, SNP1 and SNP8 genotypes have also been associated to Q fever outbreaks (29, 45), and SNP5, only detected here in two environmental samples (one dust, one aerosol) from flock 2, has been found in goats in Belgium and France (29, 45). Regarding any possible association between genotype and infection pattern, it is noteworthy that SNP1/MST13 was the predominant genotype in flocks where infection progressed toward a gradual decrease (flocks 2 and 4), whereas genotype SNP8/MST18 predominated in the two flocks where infection reactivated in yearlings (flocks 1 and 3). However, the effect of purchase of animals on that reactivation hampers any further conclusions. Similarly, since abortion rates were very low, no associations can be inferred between pathogenicity and genotype.

Inhalation of aerosols contaminated with *C. burnetii* is the main infection route in humans (23). Wind can easily spread *Coxiella* resistance forms when climatic conditions are favorable, and therefore, environmental contamination of the surroundings of infected farms is a hotspot of concern that has been addressed by many studies (4, 9, 21, 47, 48). In this study, *Coxiella* loads were higher in aerosols taken indoors than in those taken outdoors, and levels progressively decreased during the weeks that followed the lambing seasons. These results are in agreement with those found in similar studies (4, 18, 21, 47, 48). Interestingly, detection of *C. burnetii* in indoor aerosols was dependent on the proportion of animal shedders through vaginal fluids, as reported elsewhere (18). *C. burnetii* excretion by vaginal fluids is normally higher compared to feces or milk (9), especially when infection is recent in the flock. This study also pointed out that a high seroprevalence in the flock could be an indication of a recent infection by Q fever with a higher risk of detecting contaminated aerosols by *C. burnetii* outdoors.

Coxiella accumulates in the dust of infected farms, and its DNA remains in dust for long periods (20, 21). Here, levels of *C. burnetii* in dust seemed to depend mainly on the number of fecal shedders, and to a lesser extent of shedders by vaginal exudates. Nevertheless, the bacterial loads detected in dust samples were low in all four sheep flocks (ranges of Ct, 27–35) compared to the loads found in other goat and sheep flocks (4, 21, 49), but similar to the Ct values obtained in some farms from the Netherlands during the large Q fever outbreak (47, 48). The fact that, in the study herein, farmers rapidly discharged the placentas contributed to reduce environmental contamination at the sheep premises. Even though the inoculation procedure in mice was carried out at the same time and using the same conditions for all samples, inoculation of dust homogenates collected during the first lambing season of yearlings in flocks 2 and 4 did not produce positive results. Inoculated GE loads (2.9×10^3 in flock 2 and 7.43×10^2 in flock 4) were similar to those used with samples collected from the other two flocks that multiplied in mice tissues. Interestingly, the genotype identified in these samples was SNP1, which might suggests that multiplication of low concentrations of this particular genotype is not enough to grow in mice tissues.

Despite these low contamination loads in dust, isolation of *C. burnetii* was obtained from dust collected in the second and fourth lambing seasons in flock 1 and the fourth lambing season in flock 3. These results suggest that environmental contamination on the premises and surrounding areas of farms where *C. burnetii* infection has been present for several years and the number of shedders is low is markedly lower than at farms suffering a Q fever outbreak (4). However, despite the low loads of *C. burnetii* in dust, infection risk was still present since viable *C. burnetii* were detected during the fourth lambing season in two of the studied sheep flocks.

In conclusion, this study provided valuable epidemiological data on *C. burnetii* infection in sheep and opened new questions that require further investigation. The results obtained demonstrated that if *C. burnetii* infection is not controlled using a combination of vaccination and implementation of adequate biosafety and managing procedures, an active infection and continuous shedding of viable bacteria can persist in sheep flocks for over 5 years.

AUTHOR CONTRIBUTIONS

JB and AG-P: conceptualization. JB, IJ, and AG-P: methodology. CL: statistical analysis. RÁ-A, IJ, IZ, JB, and AG-P: investigation. AG-P and IJ: resources. RÁ-A and JB: data curation. RÁ-A: writing—original draft preparation. AH and AG-P: writing—review and editing. JB, AH, and AG-P: supervision. AG-P: project administration and funding acquisition. All authors contributed to manuscript revision and have read and approved the final manuscript.

ACKNOWLEDGMENTS

We thank the collaboration of the farmers.

SUPPLEMENTARY MATERIAL

Table S1 | Compilation of results of *Coxiella burnetii* shedding and detection of antibodies in ewes and yearlings per flock and lambing season; real-time PCR results obtained from BTM samples and from dust and indoors/outdoors aerosols.

Table S2 | Results of SNP genotyping obtained from animal and environmental samples.

REFERENCES

1. EFSA. Scientific Opinion on Q fever. *EFSA J.* (2010) 8:1595. doi: 10.2903/j.efsa.2010.1595
2. van den Brom R, van EE, Roest HI, van der Hoek W, Vellema P. *Coxiella burnetii* infections in sheep or goats: an opinionated review. *Vet Microbiol.* (2015) 181:119–29. doi: 10.1016/j.vetmic.2015.07.011
3. Agerholm JS. *Coxiella burnetii* associated reproductive disorders in domestic animals-a critical review. *Acta Vet Scand.* (2013) 55:13. doi: 10.1186/1751-0147-55-13
4. Alvarez-Alonso R, Basterretxea M, Barandika JF, Hurtado A, Idiazabal J, Jado I, et al. A Q fever outbreak with a high rate of abortions at a dairy goat farm: *Coxiella burnetii* shedding, environmental contamination, and viability. *Appl Environ Microbiol.* (2018) 84:e01650-18. doi: 10.1128/AEM.01650-18
5. Astobiza I, Barandika JF, Hurtado A, Juste RA, García-Pérez AL. Kinetics of *Coxiella burnetii* excretion in a commercial dairy sheep flock after treatment with oxytetracycline. *Vet J.* (2010) 184:172–5. doi: 10.1016/j.tvjl.2009.01.017
6. Berri M, Souriau A, Crosby M, Crochet D, Lechopier P, Rodolakis A. Relationships between the shedding of *Coxiella burnetii*, clinical signs and serological responses of 34 sheep. *Vet Rec.* (2001) 148:502–5. doi: 10.1136/vr.148.16.502
7. Berri M, Rousset E, Hechard C, Champion JL, Dufour P, Russo P, et al. Progression of Q fever and *Coxiella burnetii* shedding in milk after an outbreak of enzootic abortion in a goat herd. *Vet Rec.* (2005) 156:548–9. doi: 10.1136/vr.156.17.548

8. Berri M, Rousset E, Champion JL, Russo P, Rodolakis A. Goats may experience reproductive failures and shed *Coxiella burnetii* at two successive parturitions after a Q fever infection. *Res Vet Sci.* (2007) 83:47–52. doi: 10.1016/j.rvsc.2006.11.001
9. Joulié A, Laroucau K, Bailly X, Prigent M, Gasqui P, Lepetitcolin E, et al. Circulation of *Coxiella burnetii* in a naturally infected flock of dairy sheep: shedding dynamics, environmental contamination, and genotype diversity. *Appl Environ Microbiol.* (2015) 81:7253–60. doi: 10.1128/AEM.02180-15
10. Rodolakis A, Berri M, Hechard C, Caudron C, Souriau A, Bodier CC, et al. Comparison of *Coxiella burnetii* shedding in milk of dairy bovine, caprine, and ovine herds. *J Dairy Sci.* (2007) 90:5352–60. doi: 10.3168/jds.2006-815
11. Rousset E, Durand B, Champion JL, Prigent M, Dufour P, Forfait C, et al. Efficiency of a phase 1 vaccine for the reduction of vaginal *Coxiella burnetii* shedding in a clinically affected goat herd. *Clin Microbiol Infect.* (2009) 15(Suppl 2):188–9. doi: 10.1111/j.1469-0691.2008.02220.x
12. Dijkstra F, van der Hoek W, Wijers N, Schimmer B, Rietveld A, Wijkmans CJ, et al. The 2007-2010 Q fever epidemic in The Netherlands: characteristics of notified acute Q fever patients and the association with dairy goat farming. *FEMS Immunol Med Microbiol.* (2012) 64:3–12. doi: 10.1111/j.1574-695X.2011.00876.x
13. Alvarez-Alonso R, Barandika JF, Ruiz-Fons F, Ortega-Araiztegi I, Jado I, Hurtado A, et al. Stable levels of *Coxiella burnetii* prevalence in dairy sheep flocks but changes in genotype distribution after a 10-year period in northern Spain. *Acta Vet Scand.* (2018) 60:75. doi: 10.1186/s13028-018-0429-x
14. Barlozzari G, Sala M, Iacoponi F, Volpi C, Polinori N, Rombola P, et al. Cross-sectional serosurvey of *Coxiella burnetii* in healthy cattle and sheep from extensive grazing system in central Italy. *Epidemiol Infect.* (2020) 148:e9. doi: 10.1017/S0950268819002115
15. Muema J, Thumbi SM, Obonyo M, Wanyoike S, Nanyingi M, Osoro E, et al. Seroprevalence and factors associated with *Coxiella burnetii* infection in small ruminants in baringo County, Kenya. *Zoonoses Public Health.* (2017) 64:e31–43. doi: 10.1111/zph.12342
16. Plummer PJ, McClure JT, Menzies P, Morley PS, van den Brom R, Van Metre DC. Management of *Coxiella burnetii* infection in livestock populations and the associated zoonotic risk: a consensus statement. *J Vet Intern Med.* (2018) 32:1481–94. doi: 10.1111/jvim.15229
17. Rizzo F, Vitale N, Ballardini M, Borromeo V, Luzzago C, Chiavacci L, et al. Q fever seroprevalence and risk factors in sheep and goats in northwest Italy. *Prev Vet Med.* (2016) 130:10–7. doi: 10.1016/j.prevetmed.2016.05.014
18. Astobiza I, Barandika JF, Ruiz-Fons F, Hurtado A, Povedano I, Juste RA, et al. *Coxiella burnetii* shedding and environmental contamination at lambing in two highly naturally-infected dairy sheep flocks after vaccination. *Res Vet Sci.* (2011) 91:e58–63. doi: 10.1016/j.rvsc.2010.11.014
19. Berri M, Souriau A, Crosby M, Rodolakis A. Shedding of *Coxiella burnetii* in ewes in two pregnancies following an episode of *Coxiella* abortion in a sheep flock. *Vet Microbiol.* (2002) 85:55–60. doi: 10.1016/S0378-1135(01)00480-1
20. Astobiza I, Barandika JF, Ruiz-Fons F, Hurtado A, Povedano I, Juste RA, et al. Four-year evaluation of the effect of vaccination against *Coxiella burnetii* on reduction of animal infection and environmental contamination in a naturally infected dairy sheep flock. *Appl Environ Microbiol.* (2011) 77:7405–7. doi: 10.1128/AEM.05530-11
21. Kersh GJ, Fitzpatrick KA, Self JS, Priestley RA, Kelly AJ, Lash RR, et al. Presence and persistence of *Coxiella burnetii* in the environments of goat farms associated with a Q fever outbreak. *Appl Environ Microbiol.* (2013) 79:1697–703. doi: 10.1128/AEM.03472-12
22. Angelakis E, Raoult D. Q fever. *Vet Microbiol.* (2010) 140:297–309. doi: 10.1016/j.vetmic.2009.07.016
23. Eldin C, Melenotte C, Mediannikov O, Ghigo E, Million M, Edouard S, et al. From Q fever to *Coxiella burnetii* infection: a paradigm change. *Clin Microbiol Rev.* (2017) 30:115–90. doi: 10.1128/CMR.00045-16
24. Melenotte C, Caputo A, Bechah Y, Lepidi H, Terras J, Kowalczewska M, et al. The hypervirulent *Coxiella burnetii* Guiana strain compared in silico, *in vitro* and *in vivo* to the Nine Mile and the German strain. *Clin Microbiol Infect.* (2019) 25:1155. doi: 10.1016/j.cmi.2018.12.039
25. Alonso E, López-Etxaniz I, Hurtado A, Liendo P, Urbaneja F, Aspiritxaga I, et al. Q Fever outbreak among workers at a waste-sorting plant. *PLoS ONE.* (2015) 10:e0138817. doi: 10.1371/journal.pone.0138817
26. Alonso E, Eizaguirre D, López-Etxaniz I, Olaizola JI, Ocabo B, Barandika JF, et al. A Q fever outbreak associated to courier transport of pets. *PLoS ONE.* (2019) 14:e0225605. doi: 10.1371/journal.pone.0225605
27. Hurtado A, Alonso E, Aspiritxaga I, López E, I, Ocabo B, Barandika JF, et al. Environmental sampling coupled with real-time PCR and genotyping to investigate the source of a Q fever outbreak in a work setting. *Epidemiol Infect.* (2017) 145:1834–42. doi: 10.1017/S0950268817000796
28. Schets FM, de Heer L, de Roda Husman AM. *Coxiella burnetii* in sewage water at sewage water treatment plants in a Q fever epidemic area. *Int J Hyg Environ Health.* (2013) 216:698–702. doi: 10.1016/j.ijheh.2012.12.010
29. Huijsmans CJ, Schellekens JJ, Wever PC, Toman R, Savelkoul PH, Janse I, et al. Single-nucleotide-polymorphism genotyping of a *Coxiella burnetii* during a Q fever outbreak in The Netherlands. *Appl Environ Microbiol.* (2011) 77:2051–7. doi: 10.1128/AEM.02293-10
30. Glazunova O, Roux V, Freylikman O, Sekeyova Z, Fournous G, Tyczka J, et al. *Coxiella burnetii* genotyping. *Emerg Infect Dis.* (2005) 11:1211–7. doi: 10.3201/eid1108.041354
31. Barandika JF, Álvarez-Alonso R, Jado I, Hurtado A, García-Pérez AL. Viable *Coxiella burnetii* in hard cheeses made with unpasteurized milk. *Int J Food Microbiol.* (2019) 303:42–5. doi: 10.1016/j.ijfoodmicro.2019.05.010
32. Therneau T and Atkinson B. *rpart: Recursive Partitioning and Regression Trees.* R package version 4.1-15 (2019). https://CRAN.R-project.org/package=rpart (accessed March 24, 2020).
33. Milborrow S. *rpart.plot: Plot 'rpart' Models: An Enhanced Version of 'plot.rpart'.* R package version 3.0.8 (2019). https://CRAN.R-project.org/package=rpart.plot (accessed March 24, 2020).
34. R Core Team. *A Language and Environment for Statistical Computing.* (2019). https://www.R-project.org/ (accessed March 24, 2020).
35. Anderson AD, Szymanski TJ, Emery MP, Kohrs PH, Bjork AC, Marsden-Haug N, et al. Epizootiological investigation of a Q fever outbreak and implications for future control strategies. *J Am Vet Med Assoc.* (2015) 247:1379–86. doi: 10.2460/javma.247.12.1379
36. Pandit P, Hoch T, Ezanno P, Beaudeau F, Vergu E. Spread of *Coxiella burnetii* between dairy cattle herds in an enzootic region: modelling contributions of airborne transmission and trade. *Vet Res.* (2016) 47:48. doi: 10.1186/s13567-016-0330-4
37. Astobiza I, Barral M, Ruiz-Fons F, Barandika JF, Gerrikagoitia X, Hurtado A, et al. Molecular investigation of the occurrence of *Coxiella burnetii* in wildlife and ticks in an endemic area. *Vet Microbiol.* (2011) 147:190–4. doi: 10.1016/j.vetmic.2010.05.046
38. González-Barrio D, Ruiz-Fons F. *Coxiella burnetii* in wild mammals: a systematic review. *Transbound Emerg Dis.* (2019) 66:662-671. doi: 10.1111/tbed.13085
39. Berri M, Crochet D, Santiago S, Rodolakis A. Spread of *Coxiella burnetii* infection in a flock of sheep after an episode of Q fever. *Vet Rec.* (2005) 157:737–40. doi: 10.1136/vr.157.23.737
40. Reichel R, Mearns R, Brunton L, Jones R, Horigan M, Vipond R, et al. Description of a *Coxiella burnetii* abortion outbreak in a dairy goat herd, and associated serology, PCR and genotyping results. *Res Vet Sci.* (2012) 93:1217–24. doi: 10.1016/j.rvsc.2012.04.007
41. Rousset E, Berri M, Durand B, Dufour P, Prigent M, Delcroix T, et al. *Coxiella burnetii* shedding routes and antibody response after outbreaks of Q fever-induced abortion in dairy goat herds. *Appl Environ Microbiol.* (2009) 75:428–33. doi: 10.1128/AEM.00690-08
42. Joulié A, Rousset E, Gasqui P, Lepetitcolin E, Leblond A, Sidi-Boumedine K, et al. *Coxiella burnetii* circulation in a naturally infected flock of sheep: individual follow-up of antibodies in serum and milk. *Appl Environ Microbiol.* (2017) 83:e00222–17. doi: 10.1128/AEM.00222-17
43. Ruiz-Fons F, Astobiza I, Barandika JF, Juste RA, Hurtado A, García-Pérez AL. Measuring antibody levels in bulk-tank milk as an epidemiological tool to search for the status of *Coxiella burnetii* in dairy sheep. *Epidemiol Infect.* (2011) 139:1631–6. doi: 10.1017/S0950268810003134
44. Astobiza I, Tilburg JJ, Piñero A, Hurtado A, García-Pérez AL, Nabuurs-Franssen MH, et al. Genotyping of *Coxiella burnetii* from domestic ruminants in northern Spain. *BMC Vet Res.* (2012) 8:241. doi: 10.1186/1746-6148-8-241
45. Dal Pozzo F, Renaville B, Martinelle L, Renaville R, Thys C, Smeets F, et al. Single nucleotide polymorphism genotyping and distribution of *Coxiella burnetii* strains from field samples in Belgium. *Appl Environ Microbiol.* (2016) 82:81–6. doi: 10.1128/AEM.02799-15

46. Piñero A, Barandika JF, García-Pérez AL, Hurtado A. Genetic diversity and variation over time of *Coxiella burnetii* genotypes in dairy cattle and the farm environment. *Infect Genet Evol.* (2015) 31:231–5. doi: 10.1016/j.meegid.2015.02.006
47. de Bruin A, van der Plaats RQ, de Heer L, Paauwe R, Schimmer B, Vellema P, et al. Detection of *Coxiella burnetii* DNA on small-ruminant farms during a Q fever outbreak in the Netherlands. *Appl Environ Microbiol.* (2012) 78:1652–7. doi: 10.1128/AEM.07323-11
48. de Bruin A, Janse I, Koning M, de Heer L, van der Plaats RQ, van Leuken JP, et al. Detection of *Coxiella burnetii* DNA in the environment during and after a large Q fever epidemic in the Netherlands. *J Appl Microbiol.* (2013) 114:1395–404. doi: 10.1111/jam.12163
49. Carrié P, Barry S, Rousset E, de CR, Sala C, Calavas D, et al. Swab cloths as a tool for revealing environmental contamination by Q fever in ruminant farms. *Transbound Emerg Dis.* (2019) 66:1202–9. doi: 10.1111/tbed.13137

3

Isolation and Pathogenic Characterization of Pigeon Paramyxovirus Type 1 via Different Inoculation Routes in Pigeons

Han Chang[1,2†], *Shengyong Feng*[1,2†], *Yutian Wang*[3], *Fuhuang Li*[3], *Qianqian Su*[1,2], *Bo Wang*[1,2], *Juan Du*[1,2] *and Hongxuan He*[1*]

[1] *National Research Center for Wildlife-Borne Diseases, Institute of Zoology, Chinese Academy of Sciences, Beijing, China,* [2] *College of Life Sciences, University of Chinese Academy of Sciences, Beijing, China,* [3] *Department of Microbiology, Beijing General Station of Animal Husbandry, Beijing, China*

Correspondence:
Hongxuan He
hehx@ioz.ac.cn

† *These authors have contributed equally to this work*

Pigeon paramyxovirus type I (PPMV-1) causes regular outbreaks in pigeons and even poses a pandemic threat among chickens and other birds. The birds infected with PPMV-1 mainly show a pathological damage in the respiratory system, digestive system, and nervous system. However, there were few reports on the efficiency of the virus entering the host *via* routes of different systems. In the present study, a PPMV-1 strain was obtained from a dead wild pigeon in 2016 in Beijing, China. The mean death time (MDT) and the intracerebral pathogenicity (ICPI) of our isolate showed medium virulence. Phylogenetic analysis based on F gene sequence showed that the isolate belonged to subgenotype VIb, class II, which dominated in China in recent years. Then, we evaluated the infection efficiency of different routes. Pigeons were randomly divided into five groups of six as follows: intracephalic (IC), intranasal (IN), and intraoral (IO) infection routes, cohabitation infection (CO), and negative control (N negative). All pigeons were inoculated with 100 $\mu l \cdot 10^6$ EID_{50} PPMV-1 virus. After infection, pathological lesions, virus shedding, body weight change, survival rate, and tissue tropism were tested to compare the efficiency of the different infected routes. The mortality of groups IC, IN, IO, and CO were 100, 66.7, 50, and 33.3%, respectively. Weight loss in group IC was higher than the other groups, followed by groups IN and IO. The lesions observed in PPMV-1-infected pigeons were severe, especially in the lung and intestine in group IC. Viral shedding was observed from 2 dpi in groups IC and IN, but the shedding rate was higher in group IN than group IC. The longest period was in group CO. Tissue tropism experiment showed that our isolate has a wide range of tissue distribution, and the virus titer in the heart and intestine of group IC and in the brain of group IN was higher. Our data may help us to evaluate the risk of transmission of PPMV-1.

Keywords: pigeon, paramyxovirus, virus, Newcastle disease, pathogenicity, route

INTRODUCTION

Newcastle disease, caused by Newcastle disease virus (NDV), is classified as a notifiable disease by the World Organization for Animal Health (OIE), because of its high morbidity and mortality in avian species. At least 250 avian species, including chickens, ducks, and pigeons were reported to be susceptible to NDV (1–3). NDV is a single-stranded, negative-sense, and non-segment RNA virus, which belongs to the genus Orthoavulavirus, subfamily Avulavirinae, family Paramyxoviridae of the Mononegavirales order (4–7). NDV isolates have been classified into classes I and II. NDV of class I are mostly of low virulence and contain only one genotype (8), and class II virus consists of 18 genotypes (9–13) based on the phylogenetic analysis of nucleotide sequence of the F gene and genomic size (14, 15). Pigeon paramyxovirus type 1 (PPMV-1) found in birds of Columbidae family, mainly turtle dove (*Streptopelia turtur*) and Eurasian collared dove (*Stretopelia decaocto*) is a variant of Newcastle disease virus, and it is almost genotype VI, class II. PPMV-1 first reported in England during the late 1970s, affected racing pigeons with outbreaks in domestic chickens (16), which caused the third worldwide pandemics of NDV (17). In recent years, a high mortality (from 40 to 80%, even to 100% in some cases) caused by PPMV-1 has been observed in pigeons (18–22). Clinical signs of the infected birds involve nervous, respiratory, and digestive system symptoms (23), consisting of moderate to severe depression with neck twisting, ataxia, crouch, paralysis, eyelid edema, diarrhea, and green loose feces. NDV has been documented to remain infectious in feces and carcasses for at least a couple of weeks, several months in feathers, and up to 90 days in soil or water (24). Quite a few times, outbreaks in poultry have been ascribed to PPMV-1 (25–28). The virulence can be enhanced after serial passages in chickens (17, 21, 29, 30), which makes these pigeon-originated viruses a tremendous and continuous threat to the poultry industry (31–33). For these reasons, the potential transmission of the virus and the effective route where the virus will enter the host have been considered points of concern. In the present study, the pathogenicity of a PPMV-1, obtained from a dead wild pigeon in 2016 in Beijing, China, was investigated *via* different inoculation routes. Findings from our study showed intracephalic, intranasal, and intraoral infection routes were effective, but intracephalic was the most.

MATERIALS AND METHODS

Viral Isolation, Amplification, and Full-Length Genome Sequencing

A moribund pigeon with neck twisting, diarrhea, and leg paresis or paralysis was found in Beijing, 5 September 2016. We initially diagnosed that the pigeon was infected with PPMV or avian influenza virus based on clinical symptoms, then, the avian influenza virus was excluded and PPMV-1 infection was confirmed by RT-PCR. The identification of Newcastle disease and the separation of strains are as follows: viral RNA was extracted from the tissues of the pigeon (i.e., heart, liver, spleen, lung, kidney, stomach, brain, trachea, intestine, and pancreas) using Trizol reagent (ambition by Life Technologies, Beijing, China) according to the manufacturer's instructions. Reverse transcription was performed as described (34). The detection gene (a part of fusion gene, 486 bp) was amplified from the cDNA by PCR utilizing Taq DNA Polymerase (CWBIO 2× Taq MasterMix, Cat. CW0682M), and the primers were designed according to the conserved sequence (34) (Primer sequence: F:CAG CTGCGGCCCTAATACA; R:TGGATGCCCAAGAGTTGAG). The program was as follows: 95°C for 5 min; 35 cycles of denaturation at 95°C for 30 s, annealing at 55°C for 30 s, and extension at 72°C for 25 s; and a final extension at 72°C for 10 min. The PCR products were visualized by 1% agarose gel electrophoresis. Other pathogens (circovirus, avian influenza, and pathogenic bacteria) were negative. The viruses from different organs were plaque-purified three times on primary chicken embryo fibroblasts and inoculated into the allantoic cavity of 9-day-old specific-pathogen-free (SPF) eggs. The virus was isolated and RNA was extracted from the allantoic cavity, detected using PCR as abovementioned. The strain was designated as PPMV-1/pigeon/Beijing/China/01/2016 and abbreviated as PPMV-1/BJ-01/CH. Complete genome of our strain was amplified (primers are shown in **Supplementary Table 1**), sequenced, and submitted to GenBank (GenBank ID: MH807446).

Virulence-Test

There are three virulence evaluation indexes on Newcastle disease virus, and virulence is usually determined by no <2 indexes. The mean death time (MDT) was determined in 9-day-old SPF chicken embryo eggs, and the intracerebral pathogenicity index (ICPI) was determined in 1-day-old chick as previously described (35). The least-fatal dose and egg-infectious dose of the virus were tested in 9-day-old SPF chicken embryo eggs by multiple proportion dilution (from 10^{-3} to 10^{-9}) with five repeats per dilution and calculated using the Reed and Muench method.

Phylogenetic Analysis Based on Complete F Gene

To determine the genetic relationships of the PPMV-1/BJ-01/CH isolate to others, a phylogenetic tree was constructed using the MEGA 7.0 software with the maximum likelihood method *via* the Kimura two-parameter model based on the complete F gene from 21 different subgenotypes of the reference PPMV-1 isolates and 1 APMV-1 as outgroup (8, 12, 29). All complete sequences of the F gene were downloaded from GenBank and aligned utilizing ClustalW. Nucleotide sequences obtained in the present study were aligned with reference sequences available in the GenBank database to determine the subgenotypes.

Animal Experimental Infection

To further determine the pathogenicity of the virus, a total of 31-month-old pigeons, with approximately equal body weight of −5–5%, were used in our study. These pigeons were bought from a hatchery in Miyun District, Beijing, and certified by hemagglutination inhibition (HI) experiment to have no antibodies of NDV and AIV. These pigeons were randomly divided into five groups, and a marked group was placed in a separate cage in an animal room under biosafety conditions. Adequate food and drinking water were provided. Pigeons were inoculated with the virus by intranasal, intraoral, intracephalic, and cohabitation infections (signed as groups IN, IO, IC, and CO, placing groups CO and IC together), which represented through respiratory system, digestive system, nervous system, and natural infection, respectively. Additionally, the negative control group received phosphate-buffered saline (PBS) solution at pH 7.2. All infected groups were inoculated with a dose of 10^6 median embryo lethal dose (ELD50)/100 μl each, calculated using the Reed and Muench method. Subsequently, all pigeons were observed daily for clinical signs, and clinical symptoms, mortality, and morbidity were recorded. Oropharyngeal and cloacal swabs were taken every day, and body weight was determined every other day until day post-infection (dpi) 14 (0 day post-infection in group CO means the day the pigeons were infected), when there is only one group left to shed virus.

Virus Shedding

All of the oropharyngeal and cloacal swabs were collected, placed in tubes with phosphate-buffered saline solution and 2% fetal bovine serum and stored at −80°C until RNA extraction. RNA was extracted, and reverse transcription and RT-PCR were performed as above to test the virus shedding. In addition, cDNA of the isolate in this study and reagent-grade water were used as positive and negative control, respectively.

Gross Lesion

Lesion formation and lesion size are often used to quantify virulence (36). In our study, organs of all dead pigeons were collected on dpi 5 and 14. The collected tissues (including the heart, brain, lung, intestine, and liver) were pathologically lesion examined. Individuals that died ahead of time point were examined and recorded in advance. Positive rate was tallied by percentage.

Histopathology

Tissues from each group were collected and fixed with 10% neutral formalin. The sections were stained with hematoxylin and eosin (HE), and all HE stained sections were examined for the presence of microscopic lesions.

Tissue Distribution

To understand the distribution and virus load of PPMV-1 in organs from different groups at dpi 5 when clinical symptoms emerged, we randomly choose three from each group, and collected samples from the heart, brain, lung, intestine, and liver. The virus was isolated from tissues of the same weight, and $TCID_{50}$ in DF-1 cells (chicken fibroblast cell line) was used

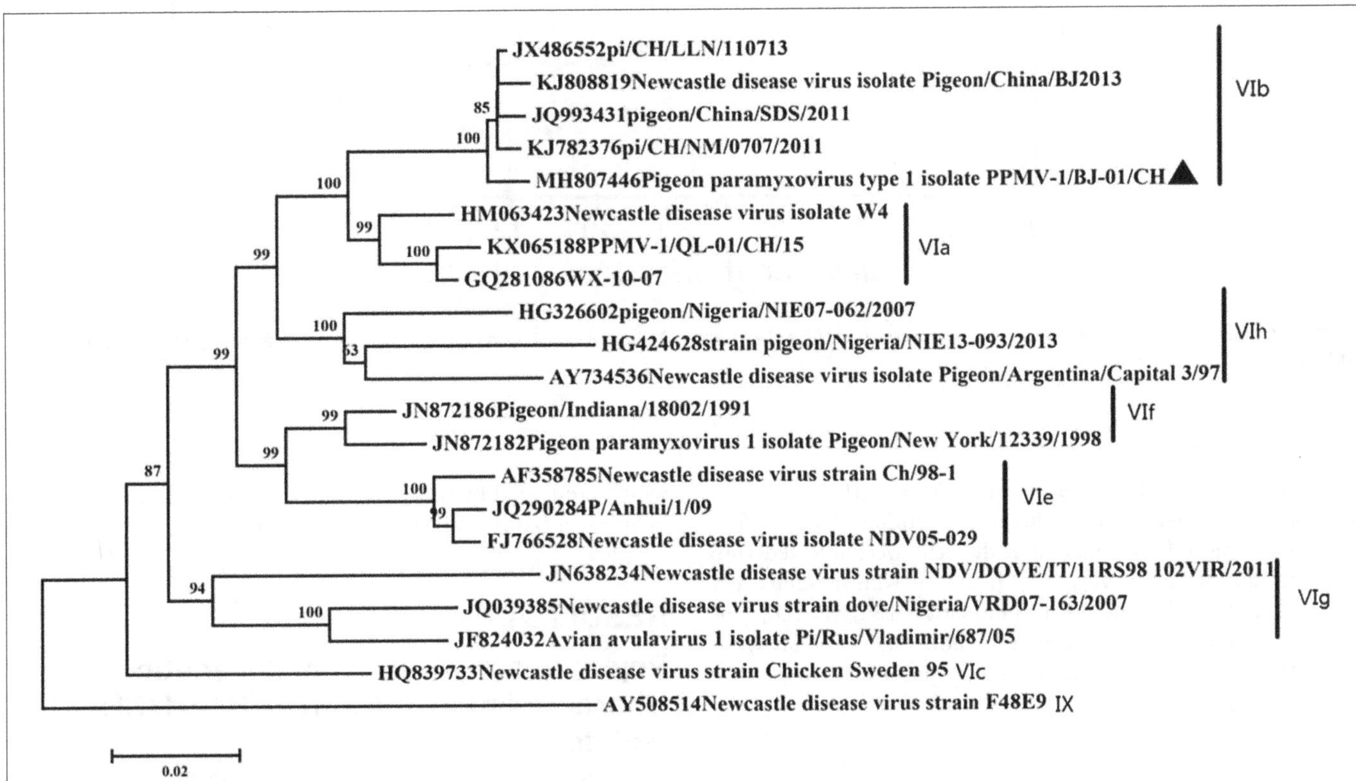

FIGURE 1 | Classification of the virus based on genotype criteria. A maximum likelihood tree of the complete F gene nucleotide sequence. The evolutionary analyses were conducted using the Kimura two-parameter method with 1,000 bootstrap replicates in MEGA7.0. Our isolate was marked with a black triangle.

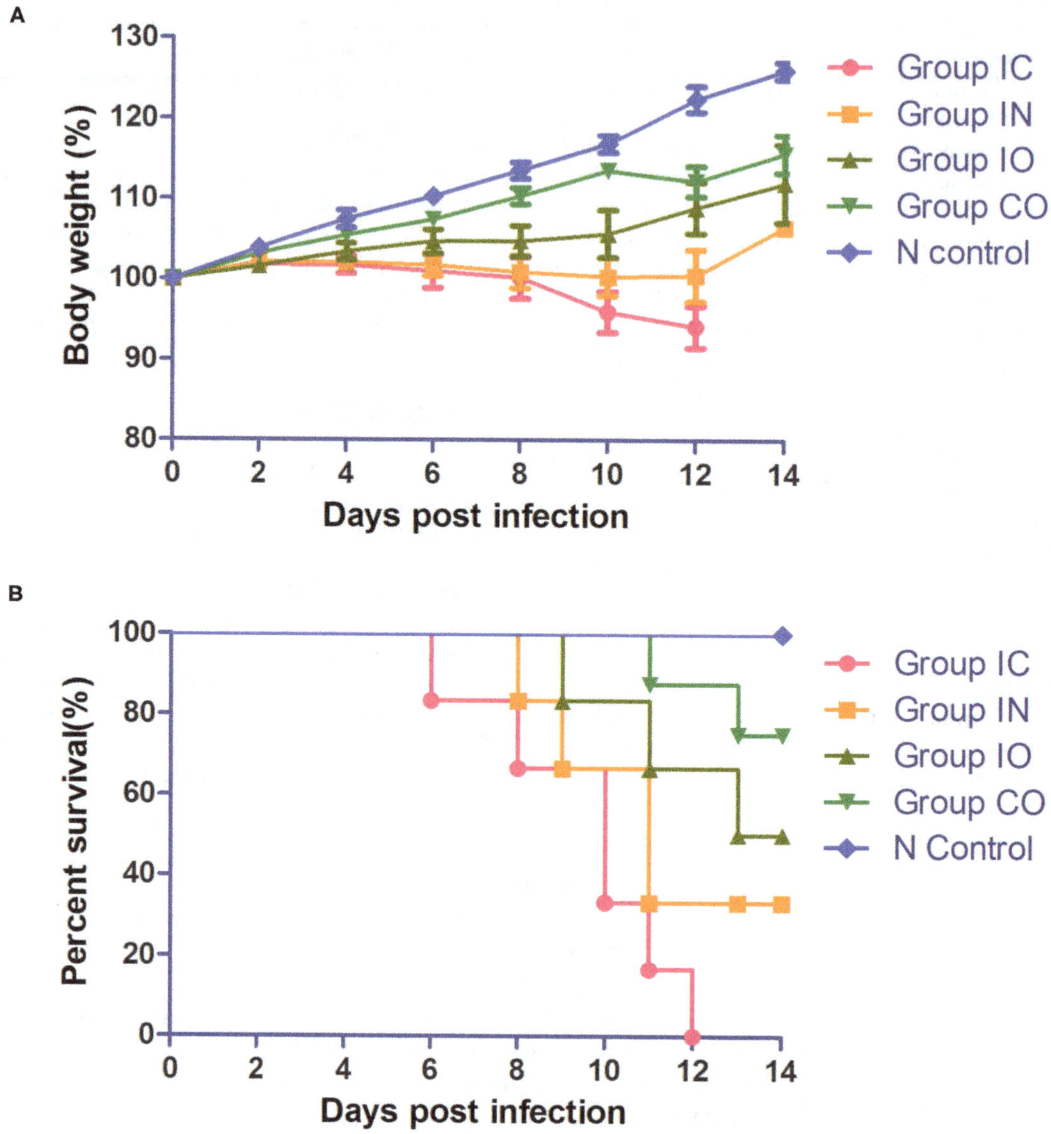

FIGURE 2 | Pathogenicity of the PPMV-1/BJ-01/CH in different routes of infection. **(A)** Body weight change of different groups post-infection. **(B)** Survival curve of different groups post-infection.

to estimate viral loads of the five groups; 3×10^4 DF-1 cells were seeded in 96-well plate with five repetitions 1 day before infection. Twenty-four hours later, the cells were infected with different dilutions of the virus for 1 h at 37°C with shaking every 12 h and confirmed by the hemagglutination assay. $TCID_{50}$ was calculated using the Reed-Muench method. Data were analyzed using Prism (v.5.01) software. Statistical significance was set at a P-value of <0.05.

Ethics Statement

These animal studies were performed in strict accordance with the Guidelines for the Care and Use of Animals in Research, which are issued by the Institute of Zoology, Chinese Academy of Sciences (Approval Number IOZ12017).

RESULTS

Phylogenetic Analysis and Genetic Characteristics of PPMV-1/BJ-01/CH Isolate

Phylogenetic analysis showed our isolate belonged to subgenotype VIb (**Figure 1**). Our isolate possessed an ^{11}2R-R-Q-K-RF^{117} segment at the cleavage site of F gene. This is characteristic of virulent NDVs. This motif is commonly found in NDV strains that are highly or moderately virulent in chickens, especially in genotypes VII and IX viruses and some pigeon paramyxovirus strains. Amino acid residues important for receptor recognition of HN is ^{174}R ^{175}I ^{198}D ^{236}K ^{258}E ^{299}Y ^{317}Y ^{401}E ^{416}R ^{498}R ^{516}R ^{526}Y ^{547}E (37), which is the same as most PPMV-1 strains.

Virulence of the PPMV-1/BJ-01/CH Isolate and Sequence Analysis

The MDT and ICPI were 72 h and 0.76, respectively. The results indicated that the PPMV-1 strain was medium according to the criteria (38). Moreover, the minimum lethal dose and 50% egg infection dose of the virus in chick embryo eggs were 10^{-3} and $10^{-5.37}$, respectively.

Pathogenicity of the PPMV-1/BJ-01/CH in Different Routes of the Infection

Clinical signs were observed in all pigeons from 5 dpi. The pigeons lost their weight sharply once clinical symptoms emerged, then soon died. The body weight change (**Figure 2A**) and survival curve (**Figure 2B**) showed the damage of the infected pigeons from group IC were much severer than other groups. A steady increase of body weight was found in negative control group. Post-mortem examination showed the congestion or hemorrhages on the meninx and in the brain. The tracheal

TABLE 1 | Percentage of PPMV-1 positive samples as determined by lesions examination.

Tissues	Groups									
	IC		IO		IN		CO		*N* control	
	D5	D14	D5	D14	D5	D14	D5	D14	D5	D14
Intestine	67	83	0	33	33	33	0	33	0	0
Lung	67	100	33	50	50	83	13	50	0	0
Brain	33	100	17	67	50	67	0	33	0	0
Liver	50	07	0	33	33	33	0	50	0	0
Heart	17	33	0	0	17	50	17	50	0	0

The lesions were shown in ***Supplementary Figure 1***.

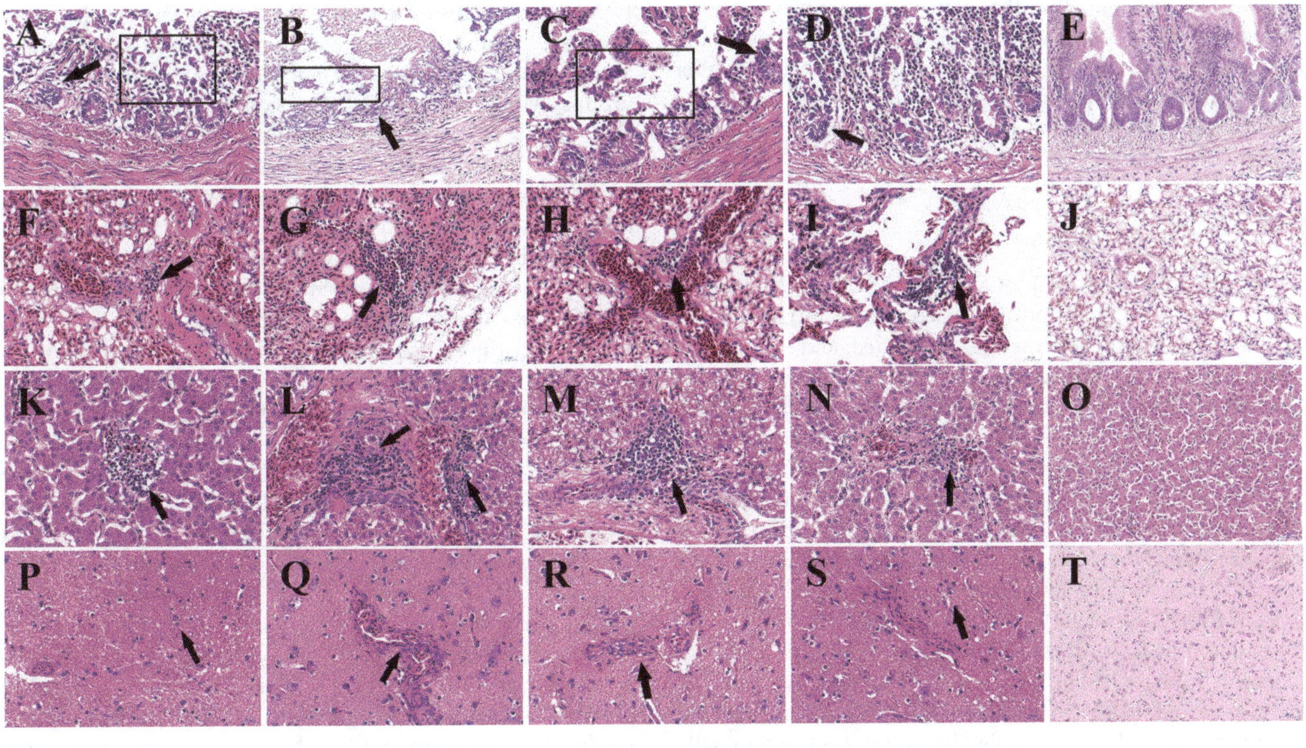

FIGURE 3 | Histopathologic lesions in pigeons of groups. The groups and tissues were marked in the figure. Black arrow indicated the severe histopathologic. **(A,F,K,P)** Histopathologic lesions in group IC. **(B,G,L,Q)** Histopathologic lesions in Group IN. **(C,H,M,R)** Histopathologic lesions in group IO. **(D,I,N,S)** Histopathologic lesions in group CO. **(E,J,O,T)** Histopathologic lesions in group N. **(A–E)** Small intestine. **(F–J)** Lung. **(K–O)** Liver. **(P–T)** Cerebrum. The pictures were magnified ×40.

mucosa was congested or hemorrhagic. Extensive hemorrhages were observed in the mucosa of the small intestine. The spleens were atrophic, friable, and hemorrhagic. Congestion and hemorrhage were found in the pancreas. Our data showed the most serious tissue lesion was discovered in group IC. Groups IO and CO caused less lesions on dpi 5 (**Table 1**).

Histopathological examination showed that the most severe lesions are found in group IC, including the desquamation of small intestine villi, lymphocyte infiltration, and severe epithelial cell loss in the intestine. The alveoli have been destroyed, and a small amount of lymphocyte infiltration and congestion were observed in the lungs. Hepatomegaly and the disappearance of hepatic cord structures were observed in the liver. A small amount of lymphocyte infiltration was also observed in the cerebrum. Milder lesions were observed in other groups (**Figure 3**).

Virus Shedding

The results and mortality of each group are compiled in **Table 2**. Pigeons shed virus from dpi 2 to dpi 14. The virus was detected from oropharyngeal swabs earlier than cloacal swabs in all groups. The earliest start time observed was in groups IC and IN in dpi 2, but the shedding rate was higher in group IN than group IC. The highest shedding rates were observed in group IN from the throat at 2 dpi and cloaca at 7 dpi. Viral shedding ceased at 14 dpi in all groups (**Table 2**).

Tissue Tropism of the PPMV-1/BJ-01/CH in Different Routes of Infection

In this study, we found that the virus can effectively replicate in different tissues, no matter which route of infection, and virus titer in the brain, lung, and intestine were higher than in other tissues. The highest titer of the virus was found in the intestine in group IC and brain in group in (**Figure 4**).

DISCUSSION

In the present study, a PPMV-1 was isolated from a dead pigeon. In order to better understand the genetic characteristics of the strain, the full-length genome was amplified and sequenced. Phylogenetic analysis showed that the isolate belonged to VIb, class II, which was consistent with most of the genotypes found in China (20, 21, 39–41). Amino acid sequence of F gene 112–117 is a typical virulent motif. But the MDT and ICPI showed medium virulence of our isolate. This contradiction often occurs on PPMV-1. Amino acid residues important for receptor recognition of HN are the same as most PPMV-1. All the characteristics of our strain consisted with current epidemic isolates in China (20, 42, 43).

The pathogenicity of the virus may relate to different inoculation routes. For example, the ducks infected intramuscularly with a virulent NDV strain showed the most severe clinical signs, while ducks infected intranasally and intraocularly sometimes also exhibited clinical signs but seldom died (44). To further understand the target system of the virus obtained in this study, several experiments were conducted to evaluate the pathogenicity *via* different system routes. Cohabitation infection was intended to mimic a natural-acquired infection. Intranasal infection was often used by labs as a substitute for aerosol infection of the virus. Oral infection mimic was used to simulate contaminated food and water. Inoculate intracranially was regularly used to evaluate NDV virulence, so it may be the most effective route of infection.

Viral shedding evaluates the effective replication and transmission of the virus in different groups. The results of our study showed infected pigeons of different groups except group CO which shed virus through the larynx from 2 dpi and through cloaca from 4 dpi. Pigeons shed virus through cloaca from 2 dpi after isolating NDV in previous studies (45, 46). The earliest start time observed was in groups IC and IN, and the shedding rate was higher in group IN than group IC; the highest shedding rates were observed in group IN from the throat at 2 dpi and cloaca at 7 dpi. The result indicated that the respiratory tract is the fastest way for PPMV-1 to spread. The shedding rate in group IC remained high, which may confirm that virus can efficiently enter into the hosts through the nervous system. All infection groups shed virus, and the longest persisted until 14 days. Continuous virus shedding may contribute to circulatory infection. Additionally, we used body weight and survival rate to test the pathogenicity. Death occurred in dpi 6, but previous study of a PPMV-1 was inoculated in pigeons through the intranasal route did not result in mortality up to 31 dpi. (47), it may be caused by the differences in virulence of the isolates used (48). The rate of body weight decline of group IC was higher than in the other groups, followed by groups IN and IO. According to the result of $TCID_{50}$ in DF-1 cells, PPMV-1 was able to cause systemic infection in a relatively short time, and virus titer in groups IC and IN was higher than in other groups, which was broadly consistent with gross lesions at dpi 5, resulting in an effective infection process. Groups IO and CO caused less lesions which might be due to lower viral load in the organs at these days. By comparison of the viral load in different tissues, the virus had a wide range of tissue distribution, especially in the lung, brain, and intestine. It can be inferred that the virus could replicate well in these three organs during early infection. At 14 dpi, the gross lesions were more severe in these groups, but the rate of virus shedding was reduced which may be due to higher mortality rates. The results indicated that the virus can effectively infect pigeon *via* different routes, and the most pathogenic was infection through the nervous system and respiratory system, but infection through the nervous showed stronger pathogenicity. Previous studies described neurological lesions in NDV-infected birds, and virulent virus was capable of replication in the brain, but not the avirulent virus (49–51), thus successful replication in the nervous system determines its pathogenicity.

Overall, pigeons play an important role in the epidemiology of PPMV-1. The routes of inoculation greatly influenced pathogenicity of the pathogenic strain isolated in the present study. Considering the growing number of PPMV-1 cases in recent years, it is necessary to develop effective vaccines or other prevention and control methods.

TABLE 2 | Virus shedding of groups.

Groups	**No. of positive samples/No. of pigeons tested Days post-infection**														
	0	**1**	**2**	**3**	**4**	**5**	**6**	**7**	**8**	**9**	**10**	**11**	**12**	**13**	**14**
Group IN	0/6[a]	0/6	6/6	6/6	6/6	6/6	6/6	4/6	3/5	2/4	2/4	1/2	1/2	0/2	0/2
	0/6[b]	0/6	0/6	0/6	0/6	0/6	0/6	3/6	2/5	2/4	2/4	0/2	0/2	0/2	0/2
Group IC	0/6	0/6	4/6	6/6	6/6	6/6	5/5	5/5	3/4	3/4	1/2	1/1			
	0/6	0/6	0/6	0/6	1/6	1/6	0/5	0/5	1/4	1/4	1/2	0/1			
Group IO	0/6	0/6	1/6	5/6	4/6	4/6	3/6	3/6	2/6	1/5	0/5	0/4	0/4	0/3	0/3
	0/6	0/6	0/6	0/6	1/6	1/6	2/6	2/6	3/6	3/5	3/5	3/4	3/4	0/3	0/3
Group CO	0/6	0/6	0/6	2/6	5/6	6/6	5/6	2/6	1/6	1/6	1/6	0/6	0/5	0/5	0/5
	0/6	0/6	0/6	0/6	0/6	2/6	2/6	5/6	5/6	4/6	4/6	4/6	3/5	3/5	0/5
N control	0/6	0/6	0/6	0/6	0/6	0/6	0/6	0/6	0/6	0/6	0/6	0/6	0/6	0/6	0/6
	0/6	0/6	0/6	0/6	0/6	0/6	0/6	0/6	0/6	0/6	0/6	0/6	0/6	0/6	0/6

[a] *Positive samples of oropharyngeal swabs.*
[b] *Positive samples of cloacal swabs.*

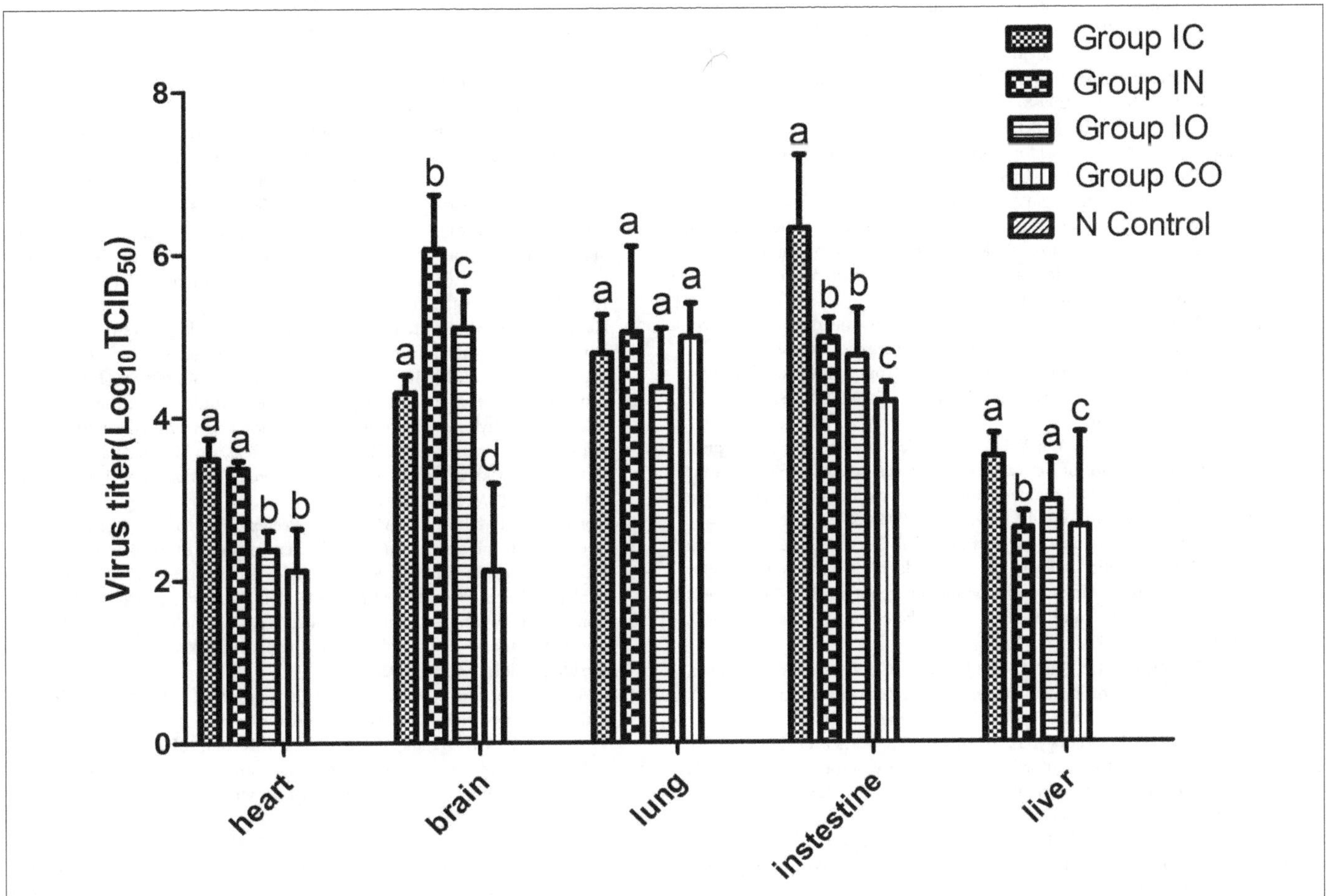

FIGURE 4 | Viral loads in different organs of pigeons post-infection. Virus titer of different tissues from dead pigeons [$\log_{10}$ median tissue culture infectious dose/ml (TCID50)] were quantified by serial end-point dilution in 96-well plates using DF-1 cells. The titer was calculated by one-way analysis of variance with standard error bars. Different lowercase letters over the bars denote statistically significant differences ($P < 0.05$) among different tissues after infection calculated by t-test. Non-significance ($P > 0.05$) was marked up by the same lowercase letters on different bars. Different lowercase letters marked up on the bars have no relationship among these five organs and represent one organ.

AUTHOR CONTRIBUTIONS

HH and HC designed the experiments. HC and SF conducted the experiments and analyzed the data. YW and FL provided the animals. BW performed the RNA extraction and PCR. HC wrote the manuscript. SF, QS, and JD revised the manuscript. All authors read and approved the final version of the manuscript.

REFERENCES

1. Alexander DJ. Newcastle disease and other avian paramyxoviruses. *Rev Sci Tech Oie.* (2000) 19:443–62. doi: 10.20506/rst.19.2.1231
2. Kaleta EF, Baldauf C. Newcastle disease in free-living and pet birds. *Dev Vet Virol.* (1988) 8:197–246. doi: 10.1007/978-1-4613-1759-3_12
3. Wan HQ, Chen LG, Wu LL, Liu XF. Newcastle disease in geese: natural occurrence and experimental infection. *Avian Pathol.* (2004) 33:216–21. doi: 10.1080/0307945042000195803
4. Amarasinghe GK, Ceballos, NG, Kuhn JH. Taxonomy of the order mononegavirales: update 2018. *Arch Virol.* (2018) 163:2283–94. doi: 10.1007/s00705-018-3814-x
5. Maes P, Gaya KA, Jens HK. Taxonomy of the order mononegavirales: second update 2018. *Arch Virol.* (2019) 164:1233–44. doi: 10.1007/s00705-018-04126-4
6. Dimitrov KM, Abolnik C, Afonso CL, Albina E. Updated unified phylogenetic classification system and revised nomenclature for Newcastle disease virus. *Infect Genet Evol.* (2019) 74:103917. doi: 10.1016/j.meegid.2019.103917
7. Kuhn JH, Wolf YI, Krupovic M, Zhang YZ, Maes P, Dolja VV, et al. Classify viruses—the gain is worth the pain. *Nature.* (2019) 566:318–20. doi: 10.1038/d41586-019-00599-8
8. Diel DG, Silva LH, Liu HL, Miller PJ, Afonso CL. Genetic diversity of avian paramyxovirus type 1: proposal for a unified nomenclature and classification system of Newcastle disease virus genotypes. *Infect Genet Evol.* (2012) 12:1770–9. doi: 10.1016/j.meegid.2012.07.012
9. Diel DG, Susta L, Stivalis CGA, Killian ML, Brown CC, Miller PJ, et al. Complete genome and clinicopathological characterization of a virulent Newcastle disease virus isolate from South America. *J Clin Microbiol.* (2012) 50:378–87. doi: 10.1128/JCM.06018-11
10. Kim LM, King DJ, Curry PE, Suarez DL, Swayne DE, Stallknecht DE, et al. Phylogenetic diversity among low-virulence Newcastle disease viruses from waterfowl and shorebirds and comparison of genotype distributions to those of poultry-origin isolates. *J Virol.* (2007) 81:12641–53. doi: 10.1128/JVI.00843-07
11. Liu XF, Wan HQ, Ni XX, Wu YT, Liu WB. Pathotypical and genotypical characterization of strains of Newcastle disease virus isolated from outbreaks in chicken and goose flocks in some regions of China during 1985–2001. *Arch Virol.* (2003) 148:1387–403. doi: 10.1007/s00705-003-0014-z
12. Snoeck CJ, Owoade AA, Couacy-Hymann E, Alkali BR, Okwen MP, Adeyanju AT, et al. High genetic diversity of Newcastle disease virus in Poultry in West and Central Africa: cocirculation of genotype XIV and newly defined genotypes XVII and XVIII. *J Clin Microbiol.* (2013) 51:2250–60. doi: 10.1128/JCM.00684-13
13. Dimitrov KM, Ramey MA, Qiu XT, Bahl J, Afonso, CL. Temporal, geographic, and host distribution of avian paramyxovirus 1 (Newcastle disease virus). *Infect Genet Evol.* (2016) 39:22–34. doi: 10.1016/j.meegid.2016.01.008
14. Czegledi A, Ujvari D, Somogyi E, Wehmann E, Werner O, Lomniczi B. Third genome size category of avian paramyxovirus serotype 1 (Newcastle disease virus) and evolutionary implications. *Virus Res.* (2006) 120:36–48. doi: 10.1016/j.virusres.2005.11.009
15. Dortmans JCFM, Rottier PJM, Koch G, Peeters BPH. The viral replication complex is associated with the virulence of Newcastle disease virus. *J Virol.* (2010) 84:10113–20. doi: 10.1128/JVI.00097-10
16. Meulemans G, Gonze M, Carlier MC, Petit P, Burny A, Long L. Antigenic and biological characterization of avian paramyxovirus type-1 isolates from pigeons. *Arch Virol.* (1986) 87:151–61. doi: 10.1007/BF01315295
17. Alexander DJ, Parsons G. Avian paramyxovirus type-1 infections of racing pigeons pathogenicity experiments in pigeons and chickens. *Vet Rec.* (1984) 114:466–9. doi: 10.1136/vr.114.19.466
18. Guo HB, Liu XL, Xu Y, Han ZX, Shao YH, Kong XG, et al. A comparative study of pigeons and chickens experimentally infected with PPMV-1 to determine antigenic relationships between PPMV-1 and NDV strains. *Vet Microbiol.* (2014) 168:88–97. doi: 10.1016/j.vetmic.2013.11.002
19. Perec-Matysiak A, Wesolowska M, Lesnianska K, Bunkowska-Gawlik K, Hildebrand J, Kicia M. Survey for zoonotic microsporidian pathogens in wild living urban rooks (*Corvus frugilegus*). *J Eukaryot Microbiol.* (2017) 64:721–4. doi: 10.1111/jeu.12402
20. Qiu XS, Meng CC, Zhan Y, Yu SQ, Li SC, Ren TT, et al. Phylogenetic, antigenic and biological characterization of pigeon paramyxovirus type 1 circulating in China. *Virol J.* (2017) 14:186. doi: 10.1186/s12985-017-0857-7
21. Wang JJ, Liu HL, Liu W, Zheng DX, Zhao YL, Li Y, et al. Genomic characterizations of six pigeon paramyxovirus type 1 viruses isolated from live bird markets in China during 2011 to 2013. *PLoS ONE.* (2015) 10:e0124261. doi: 10.1371/journal.pone.0124261
22. Zhao BH, Yuan-Hua FU, Fan JH, Bu XU, Zhu BU, Gao MY, et al. Development of bivalent inactivated oil-emulsion vaccine against Pigeon Paramyxovirus disease. *Jiangsu J Agric Sci.* (2010) 26:1293–7.
23. Vindevogel H, Marlier D. Viral infections in pigeons. *Vet J.* (2006) 172:40–51. doi: 10.1016/j.tvjl.2005.02.026
24. Leighton FA and Heckert RA. Newcastle disease and related avian paramyxoviruses. *Infect Dis Wild Birds.* (2008) 1–16. doi: 10.1002/9780470344668.ch1
25. Kim LM, King DJ, Guzman H, Tesh RB, Travassos da Rosa AP, Bueno R, Jr., et al. Biological and phylogenetic characterization of pigeon paramyxovirus serotype 1 circulating in wild North American pigeons and doves. *J Clin Microbiol.* (2008) 46:3303–10. doi: 10.1128/JCM.00644-08
26. Abolnik C, Gerdes GH, Kitching J, Swanepoel S, Romito M, Bisschop SP. Characterization of pigeon paramyxoviruses (Newcastle disease virus) isolated in South Africa from 2001 to 2006. *Onderstepoort J Vet Res.* (2008) 75:147–52. doi: 10.4102/ojvr.v75i2.13
27. Hassan W, Khair SAM, Mochotlhoane B, Abolnik C. Newcastle disease outbreaks in the Sudan from 2003 to 2006 were caused by viruses of genotype 5d. *Virus Genes.* (2010) 40:106–10. doi: 10.1007/s11262-009-0424-4
28. Pedersen JC, Senne DA, Woolcock PR, Kinde H, King DJ, Wise MG, et al. Phylogenetic relationships among virulent Newcastle disease virus isolates from the 2002–2003 outbreak in California and other recent outbreaks in North America. *J Clin Microbiol.* (2004) 42:2329–34. doi: 10.1128/JCM.42.5.2329-2334.2004
29. Dortmans JCFM, Rottier PJM, Koch G, Peeters BPH. Passaging of a Newcastle disease virus pigeon variant in chickens results in selection of viruses with mutations in the polymerase complex enhancing virus replication and virulence. *J Gen Virol.* (2011) 92:336–45. doi: 10.1099/vir.0.026344-0
30. Kommers GD, King DJ, Seal BS, Brown CC. Virulence of pigeon-origin 404 Newcastle disease virus isolates for domestic chickens. *Avian Dis.* (2001) 45:906–21. doi: 10.2307/1592870
31. Collins MS, Strong I, Alexander DJ. Evaluation of the molecular-basis of pathogenicity of the variant Newcastle-disease viruses termed "Pigeon Pmv-1 Viruses". *Arch Virol.* (1994) 134:403–11. doi: 10.1007/BF01310577
32. Collins MS, Strong I, Alexander DJ. Pathogenicity and phylogenetic evaluation of the variant Newcastle disease viruses termed "pigeon PMV-1 viruses" based on the nucleotide sequence of the fusion protein gene. *Arch Virol.* (1996) 141:635–47. doi: 10.1007/BF01718322
33. Irvine RM, Aldous EW, Marvell RJ, Cox WJ, Ceeraz V, Fuller CM, et al. Outbreak of Newcastle disease due to pigeon paramyxovirus type I in grey partridges (Perdix perdix) in Scotland in October 2006. *Vet Rec.* (2009) 165:531–5. doi: 10.1136/vr.165.18.531
34. Qiu XS, Sun Q, Wu SA, Dong L, Hu SL, Meng CC, et al. Entire genome sequence analysis of genotype IX Newcastle disease viruses reveals their early-genotype phylogenetic position and recent-genotype genome size. *Virol J.* (2011) 8:117. doi: 10.1186/1743-422X-8-117
35. OIE (World Organisation for Animal Health). *Manual of Diagnostic Tests and Vaccines for Terrestrial Animals.* 5th ed. Paris: OIE (2008). p. 957. Available online at: http://www.oie.int/eng/en_index.htm

36. Tscharke DC, Reading PC, Smith GL. Dermal infection with vaccinia virus reveals roles for virus proteins not seen using other inoculation routes. *J Gen Virol.* (2002) 83:1977–86. doi: 10.1099/0022-1317-83-8-1977
37. Munir M, Abbas M, Khan MT, Zohari S, Berg M. Genomic and biological characterization of a velogenic Newcastle disease virus isolated from a healthy backyard poultry flock in 2010. *Virol J.* (2012) 9:46. doi: 10.1186/1743-422X-9-46
38. Zhang S, Wang X, Zhao C, Liu D, Hu Y, Zhao J, et al. Phylogenetic and pathotypical analysis of two virulent Newcastle disease viruses isolated from domestic ducks in China. *PLoS ONE.* (2011) 6:e25000. doi: 10.1371/journal.pone.0025000
39. Hongbo G, Xiaoli L, Zongxi H, Yuhao S, Jinding C, Shasha Z, et al. Phylogenetic analysis and comparison of eight strains of pigeon paramyxovirus type 1 (PPMV-1) isolated in China between 2010 and 2012. *Arch Virol.* (2013) 158:1121–31. doi: 10.1007/s00705-012-1572-8
40. Chen L, Gorman JJ, McKimm-Breschkin J, Lawrence LJ, Tulloch PA, Smith BJ, et al. The structure of the fusion glycoprotein of Newcastle disease virus suggests a novel paradigm for the molecular mechanism of membrane fusion. *Structure.* (2001) 9:255–66. doi: 10.1016/S0969-2126(01)00581-0
41. Hualei L, Zhiliang W, Cuiping S, Yongkun W, Bin Y, Dongxia Z, et al. Characterization of pigeon-origin Newcastle disease virus isolated in China. *Avian Dis.* (2006) 50:636–40. doi: 10.1637/7618-042606R1.1
42. Wang X, Ren S, Wang X, Wang CY, Fan M, Jia Y, et al. Genomic characterization of a wild-bird-origin pigeon paramyxovirus type 1 (PPMV-1) first isolated in the northwest region of China. *Arch Virol.* (2017) 162:749–61. doi: 10.1007/s00705-016-3156-5
43. Ren S, Wang C, Zhang X, Zhao L, Wang X, Yao W, et al. Phylogenetic and pathogenic characterization of a pigeon paramyxovirus type 1 isolate reveals cross-species transmission and potential outbreak risks in the northwest region of China. *Arch Virol.* (2017) 162:2755–67. doi: 10.1007/s00705-017-3422-1
44. Dai YB, Cheng X, Liu M, Shen XY, Li JM, Yu SQ, et al. Experimental infection of duck origin virulent Newcastle disease virus strain in ducks. *BMC Vet Res.* (2014) 10:164. doi: 10.1186/1746-6148-10-164
45. King D. Susceptibility and protection of naive and vaccinated racing pigeons (*Columba liva*) against exotic Newcastle disease virus from the California 2002–2003 outbreak. *Avian Dis.* (2006) 50:336–41. doi: 10.1637/7479-112905R.1
46. Wakamatsu N, King DJ, Kapczynski DR, Seal BS, Brown CC. Experimental pathogenesis for chickens, turkeys, and pigeons of exotic Newcastle disease virus from an outbreak in California during 2002–2003. *Vet Pathol.* (2006) 43:925–33. doi: 10.1354/vp.43-6-925
47. Liu M, Cheng X, ShenXY, Zhou S, Wei YY, Liu JS, et al. Pathogenicity of duck origin virulent Newcastle disease virus strain in ducks. *Chin J Vet Sci.* (2014) 10:164.
48. Awu A, Shao MY, Liu MM, Hu YX, Qin ZM, Tian FL, et al. Characterization of two pigeon paramyxovirus type 1 isolates in China. *Avian Pathol.* (2015) 44:204–11. doi: 10.1080/03079457.2015.1025255
49. Ecco R, Susta L, Afonso CL, Miller PJ, Brown C. Neurological lesions in chickens experimentally infected with virulent Newcastle disease virus isolates. *Avian Pathol.* (2011) 40:145–52. doi: 10.1080/03079457.2010.544289
50. Wang W, Chang X, Yao W, Wei N, Huo N, Wang Y, et al. Host CARD11 inhibits Newcastle disease virus replication by suppressing viral polymerase activity in neurons. *J Virol.* (2019) 93:e01499-19. doi: 10.1128/JVI.01499-19
51. Sánchez-Felipe L, Villar E, Muñoz-Barroso I. α2-3- and α2-6- N-linked sialic acids allow efficient interaction of Newcastle disease virus with target cells. *Glycoconj J.* (2012) 29:539–49. doi: 10.1007/s10719-012-9431-0

4

Global Comprehensive Literature Review and Meta-Analysis of Brucella spp. in Swine Based on Publications from 2000 to 2020

Qing-Long Gong[1,2], *Yu-Han Sun*[1], *Yang Yang*[1], *Bo Zhao*[2], *Qi Wang*[2], *Jian-Ming Li*[1], *Gui-Yang Ge*[2], *Zi-Yang Chen*[2], *Kun Shi*[1], *Xue Leng*[1], *Ying Zong*[1*] and *Rui Du*[1,3,4*]

[1] College of Chinese Medicine Materials, Jilin Agricultural University, Changchun, China, [2] College of Animal Science and Technology, Jilin Agricultural University, Changchun, China, [3] Laboratory of Production and Product Application of Sika Deer of Jilin Province, Jilin Agricultural University, Changchun, China, [4] Key Lab of Animal Production, Product Quality and Security, Ministry of Education, Jilin Agricultural University, Changchun, China

***Correspondence:**
Ying Zong
zongying@jlau.edu.cn
Rui Du
durui197101@sina.com

Background: Brucellosis, a zoonotic disease, infects various hosts, including swine and humans. It has reemerged in recent years as a public health concern, and current studies on brucellosis infection in swine have been conducted worldwide. However, no meta-analyses of global brucellosis infection in swine have been published. The aim of this study was to provide an overview of *Brucella* species (spp.) in swine worldwide and the factors associated with its persistence.

Results: We searched seven databases for published epidemiological studies on brucellosis in pigs, including the Chinese National Knowledge Infrastructure, Wanfang Data, SpringerLink, ScienceDirect, Web of Science, the VIP Chinese Journal Database and PubMed. We selected 119 articles published from January 1, 2000 to January 3, 2020 for inclusion in the meta-analysis and analyzed the data using a random-effects model. Funnel plots and Egger's test showed significant publication bias in the included studies. The results of the sensitivity analysis showed that our study was relatively stable and reliable. The prevalence of brucellosis in swine was 2.1% (95% CI: 1.6–2.6), of which the highest infection rate, which was found in Europe, was 17.4% (95% CI: 11.1–24.9). The prevalence in feral pigs (15.0%, 95% CI: 8.4–23.2) was higher than that in domestic pigs (1.1%, 95% CI 0.2–2.5). The prevalence in high-income countries (15.7%, 95% CI 8.0–25.3) was significantly higher than that in middle- (0.8%, 95% CI 0.5–1.1), and low-income countries (0.1%, 95% CI 0.0–0.2). The prevalence was highest in finishing pigs at 4.9% (95% CI 0.9–11.0), and lowest among suckling pigs at 0% (95% CI 0.0–0.5).

Conclusion: The *Brucella* prevalence in pig herds currently is distributed widely throughout the world. In some countries, swine brucellosis may be a neglected zoonotic disease. We recommend long-term monitoring of the prevalence of brucellosis in domestic and wild pig herds. Attention should also be paid to animal welfare on intensive pig farms; controlling the breeding density may play an important role in reducing the spread of brucellosis among pigs.

Keywords: brucellosis, brucella suis, meta-analysis, prevalence, swine

INTRODUCTION

Brucellosis is a serious zoonotic disease caused by the *Brucella* species (spp), which occurs worldwide, especially in developing countries (1, 2). Although some developed countries have achieved freedom from animal brucellosis, it has reemerged in Japan, Australia and some European countries (Germany, Finland, Austria, Belgium and Italy) during the past 3 years (3–7). Brucellosis has been found in more than 170 countries in six major regions of the world (8). More than 500,000 new human infections are estimated to occur every year and more than 850 million pigs are infected with *Brucella* spp. (9, 10). At present, the prevalence of swine brucellosis varies widely worldwide, with the highest rates in America, North Africa and southern Europe (11, 12). In South America, the positive rate of swine brucellosis antibodies is 9%, and some countries in the European Union have no swine brucellosis while other countries have a positive antibody rate of 22.7%. In China, the positive rate of swine brucellosis antibodies in some areas is 10% (13–15). The prevalence of the disease varies among different regions, but the overall prevalence has been on the rise since the 1990s, which has had a considerable impact on the health of humans and animals and on the economy (16).

In addition to *Brucella suis*, there are 12 *Brucella* spp. currently (*Brucella* ovis, *Brucella* abortus, *Brucella* canis, et al.) and other strains without standing in nomenclature (17). Most of these species mainly infect specific hosts. Although it has been reported that pigs can be infected with different types of *Brucella* besides *Brucella suis* (18), *B. suis* is responsible for brucellosis in pigs. *Brucella suis* is composed of five biovars referred to as 1 through 5 (19, 20). Among them, *Brucella suis* biovars 1, 2 and 3 cause brucellosis in domestic swine, cattle, sheep and even human beings. Although *Brucella suis* is less harmful than *Brucella melitensis* and *Brucella abortus*, brucellosis in pigs caused by it often leads to chronic infection that is not easily detected (21). It may infect the surrounding livestock and other animals, increasing its epidemic scope and widening its range of infection (22). Most human infections derived from swine are caused by *Brucella suis* biovars 1 and 3 (23–27), which easily infect humans through direct exposure, particularly abattoir workers, farmers and veterinarians (28, 29). To date, there is no effective vaccine for *Brucella* (30). More importantly, the antimicrobial resistance of *Brucella* is emerging in brucellosis endemic regions of the world, such as China, Malaysia, Iran, Qatar and Egypt (31). Therefore, we should pay greater attention to its ongoing spread worldwide.

Pigs play a key role globally in providing animal protein in animal husbandry production. Pork is the most consumed land-animal meat, accounting for more than 36% of the world's meat intake, and has maintained a steady growth over the past few decades (32). Brucellosis was once considered to be one of the main diseases affecting the pig industry. In many countries, especially those in the developing world, pig production is usually housed in low biosecurity environments (32). However, as far as we know, systematic analyses of the overall prevalence of brucellosis in pigs worldwide, are scarce. Hence, we conducted a systematic review and meta-analysis of *Brucella* spp. infection worldwide to analyze the pooled prevalence of brucellosis in pigs and to assess potential risk factors associated with brucellosis prevalence.

Abbreviations: WHO, World Health Organization; LPS, Lipopolysaccharide; S-LPS, Smooth lipopolysaccharide; CNKI, Chinese National Knowledge Infrastructure; PRISMA, Preferred Reporting Items for Systematic Reviews and Meta-Analyses; OIE, Office International Des Epizooties.

MATERIALS AND METHODS

Search Strategy

Six databases were used to search the published research literature related to porcine brucellosis, including PubMed, ScienceDirect, SpringerLink, Web of Science, CNKI, Wanfang Data, and the VIP Chinese Journal Database. We retrieved all papers on worldwide *Brucella* spp. infection in swine that were published from January 1, 2000 to January 3, 2020 (the actual sampling dates in those publications were from 1980 to 2019).

In PubMed, the search terms and formulas used were "("*Brucella suis*" [MeSH] OR *Brucella melitensis biovar suis*) AND ("Swine"[MeSH] OR Suidae OR Pigs OR Warthogs OR Wart Hogs OR Hog, Wart OR Hogs, Wart OR Wart Hog OR Phacochoerus)." In ScienceDirect, we used the terms, "*Brucella suis*," "swine," "pig" and "prevalence." In SpringerLink, we used the terms "*Brucella suis*" and "pigs." In Web of Science, we used the keywords "*Brucella suis*," "Swine" and "prevalence" to search for the "TOPIC" (the article topic). We used the term "*Brucella*" (in Chinese) or "*Brucella* spp." (in Chinese) or "Brucellosis" (in Chinese) in the CNKI database. In Wanfang Data, we used the terms "*Brucella*" (in Chinese) and "pigs" (in Chinese), or "*Brucella* spp." (in Chinese) and "pigs" (in Chinese), or "Brucellosis" (in Chinese) and "pigs" (in Chinese). The types of articles found in Wanfang Data were limited to "papers in journals, degree theses and conferences." The search formulas used in the VIP Chinese Journal Database consisted of "Title" or "keywords" = "*Brucella*" (in Chinese) or "Brucellosis" (in Chinese) and "pigs" (in Chinese). The search strategies and search restrictions are reported in **Supplementary Material 1**. We used different keywords ("*Brucella suis*," "brucellosis," "swine," "pigs," "prevalence" and "epidemiological investigation") in each database for search verification; however, no additional qualified studies were found. Endnote (version X9.3.1) was used to catalog the articles retrieved.

Eligible studies were selected in accordance with the following criteria (inclusion criteria):

- The subjects of the research must be swine.
- The study's aim must be to investigate the prevalence of *Brucella suis* in swine.
- Data must include information on the number of examined pigs and the number of *Brucella suis*-positive pigs.
- The study must be published in Chinese or English.

Articles with the following characteristics were excluded:

- Articles that did not match the titles and abstracts (see inclusion criteria).
- Repetition of articles or data.
- The hosts were not swine.
- The article was not research study.
- Unable to access the article's full text.
- Published before 2000.
- The article had one or more internal data conflicts.
- The number of samples was <30.

TABLE 1 | Normal distribution test of the original rates and the different transformations of the original rates.

Conversion form	W	P
PRAW	0.448	< 2.2e−16
PLN	NaN	NA
PLOGIT	NaN	NA
PAS	0.653	2.238e−15
PFT	0.647	1.653e−15

PRAW, original rate; PLN, logarithmic conversion; PLOGIT, logit transformation; PAS, arcsine transformation; PFT, double-arcsine transformation; NaN, meaningless number; NA, missing data.

Data Extraction and Quality Assessments of the Publications

The four reviewers used standardized data collection forms to extract data that were consistent with the criteria to qualify for inclusion in the meta-analysis (33). Any differences between the reviewers or uncertainty about the quality of the research were resolved through the intervention of the lead author (QLG). The following information was reported: first author, the sampling year, the year of publication, income level, geographical region of the study, detection method, age, gender, collection season, feeding mode, pig classification, total number of pig samples and the number of samples that tested positive for *Brucella*.

The quality of the publications was graded using a scoring approach (34). We scored each study, and assigned a score of 5 when the information was described in greater detail (i.e., random sampling, detection method used, sampling method, sampling year and analyses of four or more factors). All the papers were assigned 0-5 points based on the standards. The quality of the papers with 3, 4 or 5 points was considered to be high, papers with a score of 2 points were considered to be average and those with 0 or 1 point were considered to be of low quality.

Statistical Analysis

Based on a large number of studies, all calculations, including the prevalence of *Brucella* spp. in swine were performed using R software (version 3.5.2). We chose the double-arcsine transformation (PFT) to perform the rate conversions (**Table 1**), based on these results and those of previous studies (35). The formula of PFT was as followed:

$$\begin{aligned} t &= \arcsin\{\mathrm{sqrt}[r/(n+1)]\} + \arcsin\{\mathrm{sqrt}[(r+1)/(n+1)]\} \\ se(t) &= \mathrm{sqrt}[1/(n+0.5)] \\ p &= [\sin(t/2)]^2 \end{aligned}$$

Note: t: transformed prevalence; r = positive number; n = sample size; se = standard error.

We used forest plots to visualize the results of the analyses and to evaluate the heterogeneity between the studies. Heterogeneity was calculated using Cochran's *Q*-test, the I^2 statistic and the χ^2 test ($P < 0.05$), and the cutoff value for the I^2 statistic was 50%. These two methods were used to examine the degree of statistical significance of the heterogeneity between the selected studies. We used a random effects model for the meta-analysis when heterogeneity was apparent in the selected articles (36). The funnel plot, trim and fill method and Egger's test were used to evaluate the studies for publication bias. Studies have shown that different subgroups may generate different funnel plots because of prevalence changes over time (37). Therefore, a funnel plot and forest plot were used for further evaluation of each subgroup. A sensitivity analysis was conducted to check whether any one study would have a significant impact on the estimates (38).

Heterogeneity between studies is an important indicator in meta-analyses; thus, an accurate assessment of heterogeneity is necessary to finding the key for preventing *Brucella* spp. infection in pigs worldwide. In order to examine the potential sources of heterogeneity, we analyzed the research data using subgroup analyses and univariate regression analysis to identify factors predictive of heterogeneity. The investigated factors consisted of geographical region (comparisons between Asia and other regions), the period of data collection (2006 to 2010 compared to 2000 or before, 2001 to 2005, 2011 to 2015 and 2016 or later), income (comparisons of high- with low- and middle-incomes), detection methods (comparison of the RBPT & TAT with other serological or molecular biology-based methods), season (comparisons of summer with spring, autumn and winter), gender (comparison of boars with sows), pigs' age classifications (comparisons of suckling pigs with finishing, growing and weaning pigs), feeding modes (comparison of extensive farms with intensive farms), pig classification (comparison of feral with domestic pigs) and quality of studies (comparisons of high-quality studies with average-quality studies). This meta-analysis was performed in accordance with the PRISMA guidelines (**Supplementary Material 2**) (39–41). A correlation analysis was performed for each subgroup by detection method and country in order to track the source of heterogeneity. The heterogeneity of the covariates is represented by R^2. Our meta-analysis does not include a review agreement and is not registered in the Cochrane database. The code in R for this meta-analysis was presented in **Supplementary Material 3**.

RESULTS

Search Results and Quality of the Eligible Studies

A total of 2,530 studies were retrieved from the seven databases. We conducted the meta-analysis with 119 studies based on our

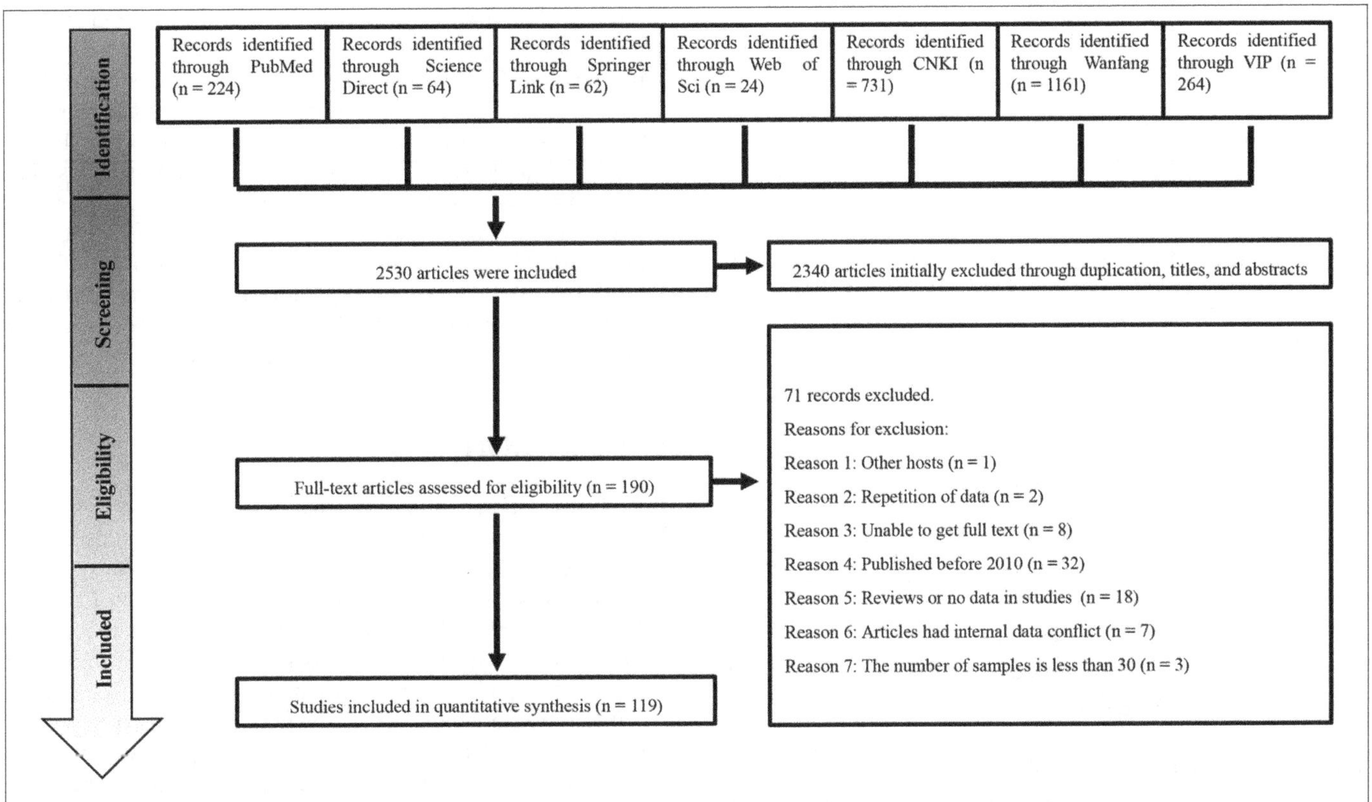

FIGURE 1 | Flow diagram of the search strategies and selection of studies.

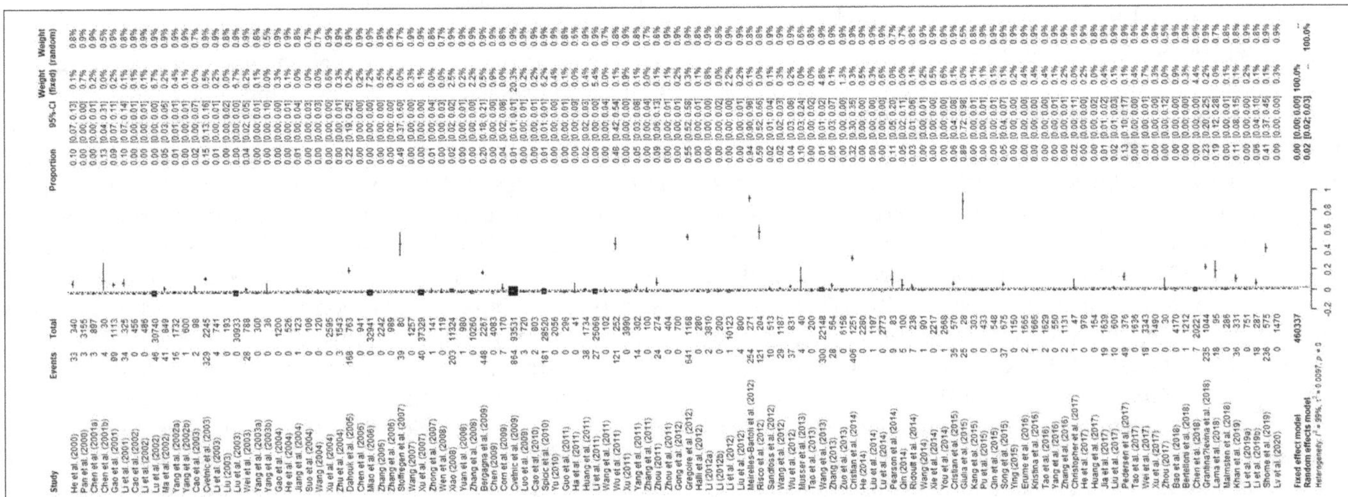

FIGURE 2 | Forest plot of the worldwide prevalence of *Brucella* spp. The length of the horizontal line represents the 95% confidence interval, and the diamonds represent the summarized effect.

inclusion and exclusion criteria (**Figure 1**). The included articles consisted of 41 high-quality publications (4 or 5 points), 78 average-quality publications (2 or 3 points) and no low-quality publications (0 or 1 point; **Supplementary Materials 4, 5**).

Results of Publication Bias

The results of the forest plot showed a high degree of heterogeneity between studies (I^2 = 99.3%, P = 0; **Figure 2**). The funnel plot showed that the graph was asymmetric, indicating the possibility of publication bias or small study effects (**Figure 3**). Egger's test showed significant publication bias in the included studies ($P < 0.05$; **Supplementary Materials 6, 7**). The results of the trim and fill method showed that some studies were filled, indicating publication bias or small study effects (**Supplementary Material 8**). In addition, we evaluated

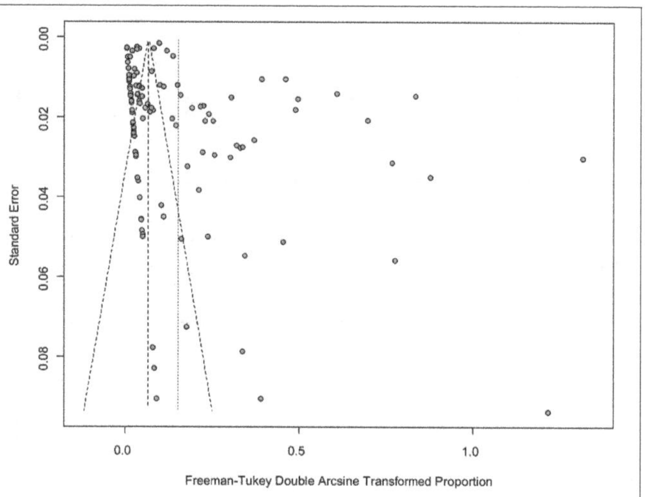

FIGURE 3 | Funnel plot with pseudo 95% confidence intervals for the publication bias test.

publication bias in all subgroups using funnel plots (**Supplementary Materials 9–18**).

Results of Sensitivity Analyses

The results of the sensitivity analysis showed that when a study was omitted, the analysis of the remaining studies yielded the same results as the previous analysis. Therefore, the results of our systematic review and meta-analysis were relatively stable and reliable (**Supplementary Material 19**).

Meta-Analysis of *Brucella* spp. in Swine worldwide

Our meta-analysis included five global geographic regions, namely Africa, America, Asia, Europe and Oceania. The pooled prevalence of *Brucella* spp. in swine worldwide was 2.1% (95% CI: 1.6–2.6; **Table 2**). Among the regional subgroups, the highest prevalence occurred in Europe, which was 17.4% (95% CI: 11.1–24.9; **Table 2**). Among the countries, Brazil had the highest rate of 93.73% (95% CI 90.5–96.3; **Table 2**), followed by Spain, with a rate of 59.3% (95% CI: 52.5–66.0; **Table 3**).

We conducted a subgroup analysis of sampling years, income level, detection method, season, gender, age, feeding mode, pig classification and quality of studies to explore their influence on the prevalence of *Brucella* spp. in swine. Among them, regions, sampling years, income level, detection method, age of pigs, pig classification and quality of the study were identified as risk factors for *Brucella* spp. infection in pigs ($P < 0.05$; **Table 2**). The combined prevalence of *Brucella* spp. in sampling years 2006 to 2010 was 2.7% (95% CI: 1.1–4.8; **Table 2**), which was higher than the other four periods. The estimate of prevalence in the high-income group was 15.7% (95% CI: 8.0–25.3; **Table 2**), which was higher than that of the low- and middle-income groups. In the detection methods subgroup, the CFT showed a prevalence of 26.5% (95% CI: 0.0–80.3; **Table 2**). The point estimate of the prevalence of *Brucella* spp. in pigs during the summer was the highest at 11.1% (95% CI: 0.0–63.0; **Table 2**). Compared with the other ages of the pigs, the prevalence of *Brucella* spp. among the finishing pigs (4.9%, 95% CI: 0.9–11.0; **Table 2**) was higher than that of the growing pigs, suckling pigs and weaning pigs. The prevalence of *Brucella* spp. in feral pigs (15.0%, 95% CI: 8.4–23.2) was significantly higher than that of domestic pigs. The subgroup analysis by quality of study showed the prevalence of *Brucella* spp. in swine was higher in the studies of high quality (5.0%, 95% CI: 3.5–6.7; **Table 2**). The heterogeneity of each subgroup was explained by detection method (the covariate), which ranged from 0–79.25% (R^2-method), and countries (the covariate), which was 60.97–97.04% (R^2-country).

DISCUSSION

Brucellosis is a zoonotic infectious disease caused by *Brucella*. It is the main cause of infertility, low litter size and miscarriage among sows (42) and an occupational hazard for farmers, slaughterhouse workers and veterinarians (43, 44). The OIE, WHO and Food and Agriculture Organization of the United Nations have classified brucellosis as one of the most important neglected occupational hazards in the world (45, 46). It has had a significant economic impact on the livestock industry and other industries (47). The prevalence of brucellosis plays an important role in the development of the world's pig herds (48). Therefore, we conducted the first meta-analysis to examine the prevalence of brucellosis in pig herds around the world and found that it was unevenly distributed among pigs.

Brucellosis in swine has been widely distributed worldwide for a long time, but in some high-income countries, including Canada, Australia, New Zealand and other countries, the eradication of brucellosis in animal husbandry has been successfully achieved (49, 50). Brucellosis has not been reported in domestic pigs in Belgium since 1969 (51). The United States has implemented reforms in pig management since 1950 to eliminate brucellosis in livestock, and efforts have been made to solve the problem of brucellosis infection in wild animals with almost complete eradication of it in livestock populations (52). However, in our study, the highest prevalence rates were found in America and Europe, and the prevalence rates in the high-income countries were higher than those in middle- and low-income countries. We attribute these results to several factors. First, most of the samples tested in these countries were feral or domestic pigs in contact with wild boars. This was confirmed in the subgroup analysis of pig classification, which showed the prevalence of feral pigs was significantly higher than that of domestic pigs. In recent decades, the population of wild boars has increased rapidly in the United States, which is caused mainly by natural population dynamics, and brucellosis has been reported in wild boars in 14 states (53). In Belgium, the increase in the wild boar population and the prevalence of brucellosis has led to an increased risk of infection in outdoor pig farms (54). Therefore, overabundance of wildlife is considered to be an important factor in the transmission of brucellosis between wildlife and livestock (55). After the first isolation of the *Brucella suis* biovar 2 strain from boars killed by hunters

TABLE 2 | Pooled worldwide prevalence of *Brucella* spp. by region.

	No. studies	No. tested	No. positive	% (95% CI*)	Heterogeneity			Univariate meta-regression		Joint analysis*	
					χ^2	*P*-value	I^2 (%)	*P*-value	Coefficient (95% CI)	R^2-method	R^2-country
Regions*											
Africa	3	3,661	39	1.7% (0.0–6.7)	111.64	< 0.01	98.2%				
America	9	2,570	382	16.5% (1.3–42.8)	1,580.03	0.00	99.5%				
Asia	90	320,164	1,429	0.5% (0.3–0.7)	4,029.49	0.00	97.8%	< 0.001	−0.295 (−0.3378 to −0.253)	0.00%	68.49%
Europe	15	133,621	3,575	17.4% (11.1–24.9)	7,805.04	0.00	99.8%				
Oceania	2	321	16	6.0% (0.5–16.0)	6.73	< 0.01	85.1%				
Sampling years											
2000 or before	41	81,246	922	0.7% (0.3–1.4)	2,252.12	0.00	98.2%				
2001 to 2005	42	140,647	1,182	0.7% (0.4–1.1)	2,182.60	< 0.01	98.1%				
2006 to 2010	35	55,798	1,095	2.7% (1.1–4.8)	4,111.44	0.00	99.2%	< 0.001	0.075 (0.039 to 0.112)	12.16%	67.09%
2011 to 2015	31	32,998	374	0.6% (0.1–1.3)	1,154.60	< 0.01	97.4%				
2016 or later	12	8,965	82	0.7% (0.0–2.0)	289.89	< 0.01	96.2%				
Income level*											
Low	2	3,330	3	0.1% (0.0–0.2)	0.27	–	–				
Middle	95	445,062	3,093	0.8% (0.5–1.1)	7,877.36	0.00	98.8%				
High	22	11,945	2,345	15.7% (8.0–25.3)	3,438.12	0.00	99.4%	< 0.001	0.297 (0.256 to 0.338)	19.42%	70.65%
Detection method*											
CFT	6	2,174	295	26.5% (0.0–80.3)	1,682.83	< 0.01	99.7%				
ELISA	11	35,170	1,216	9.4% (2.1–21.0)	3,647.44	0.00	99.7%				
PCR	3	623	101	16.3% (5.0–32.2)	41.30	< 0.01	95.2%				
RBPT	55	173,023	1,846	1.4% (0.8–2.1)	5,727.35	0.00	99.1%				
RBPT & TAT	23	105,223	162	0.2% (0.1–0.4)	479.88	< 0.01	95.4%	< 0.001	−0.152 (−0.206 to −0.103)	0.00%	36.46%
TAT	17	20,121	275	0.5% (0.0–1.4)	312.29	< 0.01	94.9%				
Others	26	112,102	3,169	11.0% (6.1–17.2)	6,830.99	0.00	99.6%				
Season*											
Spring	11	3,716	69	2.6% (0.0–3.8)	226.43	< 0.01	95.6%				
Summer	5	1,163	258	11.1% (0.0–63.0)	1,300.31	< 0.01	99.7%	0.077	0.195 (−0.021 to 0.411)	36.17%	37.04%
Autumn	6	1,452	12	0.7% (0.0–3.8)	46.65	< 0.01	89.3%				
Winter	6	3,444	21	1.2% (0.1–3.3)	63.17	< 0.01	92.1%				
Gender											
Boars	23	12,737	1282	7.9% (2.4–15.9)	3,594.80	0.00	99.4%	0.314	0.056 (−0.053 to 0.165)	75.00%	82.75%
Sows	29	51,698	1288	5.1% (2.8–8.1)	3,208.62	0.00	99.1%				
Age of pigs											
Finishing pigs	14	5,778	321	4.9% (0.9–11.0)	684.93	< 0.01	98.1%				
Growing pigs	18	31,454	411	2.1% (0.2–5.2)	1271.98	< 0.01	98.7%				

(Continued)

TABLE 2 | Continued

	No. studies	No. tested	No. positive	% (95% CI*)	Heterogeneity			Univariate meta-regression		Joint analysis*	
					χ^2	*P*-value	I^2 (%)	*P*-value	Coefficient (95% CI)	R^2-method	R^2-country
Suckling pigs	9	1,917	7	0.0% (0.0–0.5)	15.01	0.05	46.7%	0.045	−0.120 (−0.237 to −0.003)	79.25%	87.44%
Weaning pigs	5	1,015	28	1.0% (0.0–14.2)	98.67	< 0.01	95.9%				
Feeding mode											
Extensive	12	34,083	555	2.5% (0.4–5.9)	1,823.79	0.00	99.2%	0.065	0.076 (−0.005 to 0.156)	6.50%	68.57%
Intensive	35	55,196	468	0.5% (0.1–1.2)	1,790.10	0.00	98.9%				
Pig classification											
Domestic pigs	21	131,196	1,504	1.1% (0.2–2.5)	2,397.46	0.00	99.5%				
Feral pigs	21	9,186	2,085	15.0% (8.4–23.2)	1,838.57	0.00	99.0%	< 0.001	0.277 (0.197 to 0.357)	0.00%	74.40%
Quality level											
Middle	78	203,157	1,201	1.0% (0.6–1.3)	4,344.03	0.00	98.2%				
High	41	257,180	4,240	5.0% (3.5–6.7)	11,773.05	0.00	99.7%	< 0.001	0.117 (0.078 to 0.157)	9.21%	60.97%
Total	119	460,337	5,441	2.1% (1.6–2.6)	16,698.88	0.000	99.3%				

CI, Confidence interval; Joint analysis*, Joint analysis with prevalence of detection methods and provinces in China;* R^2*, Proportion of between-study variance explained.*
Region: Africa: India, Uganda; America: Brazil. USA; Asia: China. India; Europe: Belgium, Croatia, Finland, Germany, Italy, Latvia, Sweden; Oceania: Australia.*
Method: CFT: Complement fixation test; ELISA: Enzyme linked immunosorbent assay; PCR: Polymerase chain reaction; RBPT: Rose Bengal plate test; RBPT&TAT: Rose Bengal plate test and Tube agglutination test; TAT: Tube agglutination test.*
Season: Spring: Mar. to May.; Summer: Jun. to Aug.; Autumn: Sep. to Nov.; Winter: Dec. to Feb.*
Income level: High: Developed Country; Middle: Developing Country; Low: Least Developed Country.

TABLE 3 | Estimated pooled seroprevalence of *Brucella* spp. by country and region worldwide.

Countries	No. studies	Region	No. tested	No. positive	% Prevalence	% (95% CI)
Australia	2	Oceania	321	16	6.0%	0.5–16.0
Belgium	1	Europe	1,168	641	54.9%	52.0–57.7
Brazil	1	America	271	254	93.7%	90.5–96.3
China	89	Asia	319,589	1,193	0.3%	0.2–0.5
Croatia	3	Europe	124,296	1,374	3.5%	1.3–6.8
Egypt	1	Africa	331	36	10.9%	7.7–14.5
Finland	1	Europe	280	0	0.0%	0.0–0.6
Germany	1	Europe	763	168	22.0%	19.2–25.0
India	1	Asia	575	236	41.0%	37.1–45.1
Italy	5	Europe	5,328	915	22.6%	6.7–44.3
Spain	1	Europe	204	121	59.3%	52.5–66.0
Latvia	1	Europe	1,044	235	22.5%	20.0–25.1
Sweden	1	Europe	286	0	0.0%	0.0–0.6
Switzerland	1	Europe	252	121	48.0%	41.9–54.2
Uganda	2	Africa	3,330	3	0.1%	0.0–0.2
USA	8	America	2,299	128	8.7%	2.0–19.2
Total	119		460,337	5,441	2.1%	1.6–2.6

in 1994 (56), *Brucella suis* biovar 2 has been isolated from wild boars in many countries (57–61). Studies have reported that brucellosis among wild boars is widely distributed all over the world (51, 56, 57, 62–65). Second, different modes of feeding in different countries have led to different prevalence rate. Most developed countries mainly focus on intensive farming, while countries with lower incomes focus mainly focus on extensive farming. The prevalence of disease in countries with intensive farming is higher than that in countries with extensive farming, which has been confirmed in several studies (66–68). The increase in herd size results in higher stocking density and worse farm sanitation, thereby promoting the spread of *Brucella* among animals after abortion and parturition (69, 70). We recommend long-term monitoring of wildlife to implement preventive measures before an outbreak of brucellosis. Intensive farms need to control breeding density, pay attention to animal welfare, improve the prevention and control of epidemics and optimize the breeding environment to avoid the large-scale spread of disease. It is worth noting that among the studies we included, only a few on swine brucellosis were conducted in low-income countries. This may indicate that swine brucellosis has been overlooked in these countries and regions. Therefore, although our results show that the prevalence of brucellosis in low-income countries is lower than that of other countries, this finding may be due to these countries' neglect of surveillance and detection of brucellosis. Likewise, the farms in high-income countries are more capable of strengthening their detection of brucellosis, thus, showing a relatively high prevalence. We infer that the actual global infection rate of swine brucellosis may be higher. Although the disease has been controlled or eliminated in some developed countries (such as Canada, New Zealand, Australia and the majority of northern European countries) (71), brucellosis remains an intractable public health problem in poor and underdeveloped countries, especially in the Middle East (72). While strengthening the surveillance and prevention of swine brucellosis in high-incidence areas, we should also continue to strengthen the surveillance in lower incidence areas to prevent widespread infection of swine brucellosis.

The 2006-2010 prevalence of brucellosis was higher than that of the other sampling years. First, as reported in the included studies, an outbreak of swine brucellosis in Jaboticabal, Brazil in 2006 increased the prevalence to 93.7% (73). At the same time, brucellosis was found in Italy after collecting samples from pig farms with breeding problems for serological analysis. Furthermore, detection of suspected cases (non-random sampling) may overestimate the local prevalence of brucellosis (74, 75). Second, during this period, many countries began to analyze the situation of *Brucella* infection in feral pigs. Among the included articles, there were 21 studies on the prevalence of wild boars, and the prevalence of wild boars between 2006 and 2010 was 22.3% (881/3956). There were also studies on isolated *Brucella suis* biovar 2 from wild boars because of the substantial increase in the number of feral pigs (58–60, 76). Moreover, several *Brucella* outbreaks occurred in Germany due to infection of domestic pigs by feral pigs (77). After 2010, the prevalence of brucellosis gradually declined because the OIE proposed controls for *Brucella* farms, giving priority to the development of food safety standards for future animal production (78). Although the prevalence of brucellosis has shown a downward trend, its control should be continued.

The 119 selected studies that were analyzed included five main methods of brucellosis detection: CFT, ELISA, PCR, RBPT and TAT ($P < 0.001$; **Table 2**). We used detection method as a covariate to perform joint analysis with other risk factors, and the range of heterogeneity explained by the detection method was 0-100.00%, implying that different detection methods had a greater effect on some subgroups.

The analyses of the age and sex of pigs showed that the prevalence of finishing pigs was higher than that of the pigs in the other age groups, and the prevalence of sows was lower than that of the boars. This finding is mainly due to the adult males' contacts with these matrilineal groups during the mating season, while females live in matrilineal groups (60). The prevalence observed in the finishing pigs was higher than that in the other age groups, which was due to the higher involvement of the finishing pigs (79). Although the prevalence of boars was higher than that of sows, no significant differences were found between them, indicating that the relationship between the two animals warrants further examination. We recommend controlling the breeding density; planning a reasonable breeding process may play a positive role in the reduction of the spread of brucellosis in pigs.

The prevalence of brucellosis in the summer was higher than that in the other seasons, but the difference was not significant (**Table 2**). As far as we know, no research has shown a strong correlation between breeding season and prevalence of swine brucellosis. Studies have shown that the dryness of summer may lead to lack of food and water, increasing the trajectory coverage of animals (80). The correlation analysis showed that countries explained 97.04% of heterogeneity in the seasons subgroup. These results can be interpreted in the context of the world's vast territory with different countries having different characteristics during summer. Meta-analyses showed that the incidence rates of *Brucella* in cattle and deer were higher in hotter and more humid areas (81, 82). Therefore, we speculate that a similar phenomenon occurs in pigs with brucellosis. Thus, efforts to prevent epidemics should be increased in hot and humid areas to create a healthy environment for livestock and reduce the occurrence of disease.

Our study included 41 high-quality articles and 78 average-quality articles. We found that random sampling and detailed descriptions of sampling methods were not included in some of the articles by examining those of average quality. These findings may reflect sampling bias. We recommend that researchers provide detailed descriptions of their sampling and data collection methods to improve the reliability of the data.

This meta-analysis had the advantages of a long-time span, wide coverage and clear methods of analyses, yet it has some limitations. First, the language of the selected articles was limited to English or Chinese, and therefore, qualified articles in other languages might have been overlooked. Second, the articles were obtained from seven databases, which might have excluded qualified articles from other databases. Third, the inadequate information provided by the included studies (e.g., brucellosis classification and geographical factors) might have led to publication bias or other biases in the subgroups (**Supplementary Figures 3–12**). Fourth, some risk factors were examined in a small number of studies and samples, which might have resulted in small study effects leading to unstable results. We recommend that researchers conduct large-scale studies because the results of small-scale studies are often not representative of the population. Fifth, the research we have included covers only 14 countries, and some of those countries (e.g., Brazil) had few relevant reports. For these countries, we only presented data to reflect global trends, and the results presented are for reference only. The lack of articles from some countries might have led to inaccurate estimates of the prevalence of swine brucellosis in those countries. Prevalence surveys of *Brucella* spp. in more countries are recommended to clarify the true prevalence of swine brucellosis worldwide. Sixth, this study was not registered; however, it was carried out strictly in accordance with the PRISMA guidelines.

In conclusion, the *Brucella* infection rate in pig herds is distributed widely throughout the world. In addition, *Brucella* is common among wild boars in developed countries. Therefore, we suggest carrying out long-term detection of *Brucella* in wild animals and implementing reasonable isolation measures between livestock and wild animals to reduce the chance of contact between them. In addition, countries that do not pay much attention to swine brucellosis should disseminate information about *Brucella* infection, and epidemiological investigations should be conducted as soon as possible to establish better control of the disease. The high prevalence of swine brucellosis will cause serious economic losses to herdsmen, and increase the risk of infection. Therefore, attention to animal welfare on intensive pig farms is crucial, and control of the breeding density may play an important role in reducing the spread of brucellosis in pigs. This study can provide a theoretical basis for researchers to explore control schemes for brucellosis.

AUTHOR CONTRIBUTIONS

YZ and RD: idea contributions and funding. BZ, G-YG, Z-YC, and YY: data extraction. Y-HS: database establishment. QW and J-ML: data analysis. Q-LG: writing – original draft. Y-HS, KS, and XL: writing – review and editing. All authors contributed to the article and approved the submitted version.

ACKNOWLEDGMENTS

We thank the scientists and personnel of the College of Animal Science and Technology, Jilin Agricultural University and the College of Chinese Medicine Materials, Jilin Agricultural University, for their collaboration.

REFERENCES

1. Franco-Paredes C, Chastain D, Taylor P, Stocking S, Sellers B. Boar hunting and brucellosis caused by *Brucella suis*. *Travel Med Infect Dis.* (2017) 16:18–22. doi: 10.1016/j.tmaid.2017.03.006
2. Gusi AM, Bertu WJ, Jesús de Miguel M, Dieste-Pérez L, Smits HL, Ocholi RA, et al. Comparative performance of lateral flow immunochromatography, iELISA and Rose Bengal tests for the diagnosis of cattle, sheep, goat and swine brucellosis. *PLoS Negl Trop Dis.* (2019) 13:e0007509. doi: 10.1371/journal.pntd.0007509

3. Hammerl JA, Ulrich RG, Imholt C, Scholz HC, Jacob J, Kratzmann N, et al. Molecular survey on brucellosis in rodents and shrews - natural reservoirs of novel *Brucella* species in Germany? *Transbound Emerg Dis.* (2017) 64:663–71. doi: 10.1111/tbed.12425
4. Zhang N, Huang D, Wu W, Liu J, Liang F, Zhou B, et al. Animal brucellosis control or eradication programs worldwide: a systematic review of experiences and lessons learned. *Prev Vet Med.* (2018) 160:105–15. doi: 10.1016/j.prevetmed.2018.10.002
5. Buhmann G, Paul F, Herbst W, Melzer F, Wolf G, Hartmann K, et al. Canine brucellosis: Insights into the epidemiologic situation in Europe. *Front Vet Sci.* (2019) 6:151. doi: 10.3389/fvets.2019.00151
6. Kauffman LK, Petersen CA. Canine brucellosis: old foe and reemerging scourge. *Vet Clin North Am Small Anim Pract.* (2019) 49:763–79. doi: 10.1016/j.cvsm.2019.02.013
7. Kawakami N, Wakai Y, Saito K, Imaoka K. Chronic brucellosis in Japan. *Intern Med.* (2019) 58:3179–83. doi: 10.2169/internalmedicine.2961-19
8. Deng Y, Liu X, Duan K, Peng Q. Research progress on brucellosis. *Curr Med Chem.* (2018) 26:5598–608. doi: 10.2174/0929867325666180510125009
9. de Figueiredo P, Ficht TA, Rice-Ficht A, Rossetti CA, Adams LG. Pathogenesis and immunobiology of brucellosis: review of *Brucella*-host interactions. *Am J Pathol.* (2015) 185:1505–17. doi: 10.1016/j.ajpath.2015.03.003
10. Liu F. *Construction and evaluation of the immunogenicity of Brucella S2-BCSP31 deletion strain for vaccine* (In Chinese) (Doctoral Dissertation), Jilin Agricultural University, Changchun (2018).
11. Pappas G, Akritidis N, Bosilkovski M, Tsianos E. Brucellosis. *New Engl J Med.* (2005) 352:2325. doi: 10.1056/NEJMra050570
12. Buzgan T, Karahocagil MK, Irmak H, Baran AI, Karsen H, Evirgen O.Clinical manifestations and complications in 1028 cases of brucellosis: a retrospective evaluation and review of the literature. *Int J Infect Dis.* (2010) 14:e469–78. doi: 10.1016/j.ijid.2009.06.031
13. Sandfoss MR, DePerno CS, Betsill CW, Palamar MB, Erickson G, Kennedy-Stoskopf S. A serosurvey for *Brucella suis*, classical swine fever virus, porcine circovirus type 2, and pseudorabies virus in feral swine (Sus scrofa) of eastern North Carolina. *J Wildl Dis.* (2012) 48:462–6. doi: 10.7589/0090-3558-48.2.462
14. Grantina-Ievina L, Avsejenko J, Cvetkova S, Krastina D, Streikisa M, Steingolde Z, et al. Seroprevalence of *Brucella suis* in eastern Latvian wild boars (Sus scrofa). *Acta Vet Scand.* (2018) 60:19. doi: 10.1186/s13028-018-0373-9
15. Li L, Yan JH, Yan H, LI JP, MI JT, Di LXT. Research of prevention technology and prevalent in livestock brucellosis in Xinjiang (In Chinese). *Grass-Feeding Livestock.* (2012) 3:20–2. doi: 10.16863/j.cnki.1003-6377.2012.03.005
16. Avila-Granados LM, Garcia-Gonzalez DG, Zambrano-Varon JL, Arenas-Gamboa AM. Brucellosis in Colombia: Current status and challenges in the control of an endemic disease. *Front Vet Sci.* (2019) 6:321. doi: 10.3389/fvets.2019.00321
17. Acka PG, Zakowska D, Naylor K, Niemcewicz M, Bielawska-drozd A. Brucella -Virulence Factors, Pathogenesis and Treatment. *Pol J Microbiol.* (2018) 67:151–61. doi: 10.21307/pjm-2018-029
18. Stoffregen WC, Olsen SC, Wheeler CJ, Bricker BJ, Palmer MV, Allen E, et al. Diagnostic characterization of a feral swine herd enzootically infected with *Brucella*. *J Vet Diagn Invest.* (2007) 19:227–37. doi: 10.1177/104063870701900301
19. Sankarasubramanian J, Vishnu US, Gunasekaran P, Rajendhran J. A genome-wide SNP-based phylogenetic analysis distinguishes different biovars of *Brucella suis*. *Infect Genet Evol.* (2016) 41:213–7. doi: 10.1016/j.meegid.2016.04.012
20. More S, Bøtner A, Butterworth A, Calistri P, Depner K, Edwards S, et al. Assessment of listing and categorisation of animal diseases within the framework of the Animal Health Law (Regulation (EU) No 2016/429): paratuberculosis. *Efsa J.* (2017) 15:e04960. doi: 10.2903/j.efsa.2017.4960
21. Olsen SC, Tatum FM. Swine brucellosis: current perspectives. *Vet Med.* (2016) 8:1–12. doi: 10.2147/VMRR.S91360
22. Szulowski K, Iwaniak W, Weiner M, Złotnicka J. *Brucella suis* biovar 2 isolations from cattle in Poland. *Ann Agric Environ Med.* (2013) 20:672–5.
23. Menshawy AM, Perez-Sancho M, Garcia-Seco T, Hosein HI, García N, Martinez I, et al. Assessment of genetic diversity of zoonotic *Brucella* spp. *recovered from livestock in Egypt using multiple locus VNTR analysis Biomed Res Int.* (2014) 2014:353876. doi: 10.1155/2014/353876
24. Tian GZ, Cui BY, Piao DR, Zhao HY, Li LY, Liu X, et al. Multi-locus variable-number tandem repeat analysis of Chinese *Brucella* strains isolated from 1953 to 2013. *Infect Dis Poverty.* (2017) 6:89. doi: 10.1186/s40249-017-0296-0
25. De Massis F, Zilli K, Di Donato G, Nuvoloni R, Pelini S, Sacchini L, et al. Distribution of *Brucella* field strains isolated from livestock, wildlife populations, and humans in Italy from 2007 to 2015. *PLoS One.* (2019) 14:e0213689. doi: 10.1371/journal.pone.0213689
26. Liu ZG, Wang M, Zhao HY, Piao DR, Jiang H, Li ZJ. Investigation of the molecular characteristics of *Brucella* isolates from Guangxi province, China. *BMC Microbiol.* (2019) 19:292. doi: 10.1186/s12866-019-1665-6
27. Wang XM, Huang MH, Cui BY. Analysis on brucellosis epidemiological characteristics in Hainan province. *Chin J Epidemiol.* (2019) 40:350–3.
28. Galińska EM, Zagórski J. Brucellosis in humans–etiology, diagnostics, clinical forms. *Ann Agric Environ Med.* (2013) 20:233–8.
29. Zheng R, Xie S, Lu X, Sun L, Zhou Y, Zhang Y, et al. A systematic review and meta-analysis of epidemiology and clinical manifestations of human brucellosis in China. *Biomed Res Int.* (2018) 2018:5712920. doi: 10.1155/2018/5712920
30. Zriba S, Garcia-Gonzalez DG, Khalaf OH, Wheeler L, Chaki SP, Rice-Ficht A, et al. Vaccine safety studies of *Brucella* abortus S19 and S19ΔvjbR in pregnant swine. *Vaccine X.* (2019) 3:100041. doi: 10.1016/j.jvacx.2019.100041
31. Solís, J., and Solera, J. (2015). *Treatment of Human Brucellosis — Review of Evidence from Clinical* Trials.
32. Beltran-Alcrudo D, Falco JR, Raizman E, Dietze K. Transboundary spread of pig diseases: the role of international trade and travel. *BMC Vet Res.* (2019) 15:64. doi: 10.1186/s12917-019-1800-5
33. Wang W, Gong QL, Zeng A, Li MH, Zhao Q, Ni HB. Prevalence of *Cryptosporidium* in pigs in China: A systematic review and meta-analysis. *Transbound Emerg Dis.* (2020). doi: 10.1111/tbed.13806. [Epub ahead of print].
34. Ran X, Cheng J, Wang M, Chen X, Wang H, Ge Y, et al. Brucellosis seroprevalence in dairy cattle in China during 2008-2018: A systematic review and meta-analysis. *Acta Trop.* (2019) 189:117–23. doi: 10.1016/j.actatropica.2018.10.002
35. Barendregt JJ, Doi S, Lee YY, Pacella R, Vos T. Meta-analysis of prevalence. *J Epidemiol Commun H.* (2013) 67:974–8. doi: 10.1136/jech-2013-203104
36. Assefa A, Bihon A. Bovine cysticercosis in Ethiopia: A systematic review and meta-analysis of prevalence from abattoir-based surveys. *Prev Vet Med.* (2019) 169:104707. doi: 10.1016/j.prevetmed.2019.104707
37. Ni HB, Gong QL, Zhao Q, Li XY, Zhang XX. Prevalence of *Haemophilus parasuis* "*Glaesserella parasuis*" in pigs in China: A systematic review and meta-analysis. *Prev Vet Med.* (2020) 182:105083. doi: 10.1016/j.prevetmed.2020.105083
38. Gong QL, Li D, Diao NC, Liu Y, Li BY, Tian T, et al. Mink Aleutian disease seroprevalence in China during 1981-2017: A systematic review and meta-analysis. *Microb Pathog.* (2020) 139:103908. doi: 10.1016/j.micpath.2019.103908
39. Moher D, Liberati A, Tetzlaff J, Altman DG. Preferred reporting items for systematic reviews and meta-analyses: the PRISMA statement. *Int J Surg.* (2010) 8:336–41. doi: 10.1016/j.ijsu.2010.02.007
40. Moher D, Shamseer L, Clarke M, Ghersi D, Liberati A, Petticrew M, et al. Preferred reporting items for systematic review and meta-analysis protocols (PRISMA-P) 2015 statement. *Syst Rev.* (2015) 4:1. doi: 10.1186/2046-4053-4-1
41. Shamseer L, Moher D, Clarke M, Ghersi D, Liberati A, Petticrew M, et al. Preferred reporting items for systematic review and meta-analysis protocols (PRISMA-P) 2015: elaboration and explanation. *BMJ.* (2015) 350:g7647. doi: 10.1136/bmj.g7647
42. Megid J. Clinical manifestations of brucellosis in domestic animals and humans. *Open Vet Sci J.* (2010) 4:119–26. doi: 10.2174/18743188010040 10119
43. Radostits OM, Blood DC, Done SH. Veterinary medicine: a textbook of the diseases of cattle, sheep, pigs, goats and horses. *J Equine Vet Sci.* (1994) 20:625.
44. Swai ES, Schoonman L. A survey of zoonotic diseases in trade cattle slaughtered at Tanga city abattoir: a cause of public health concern. *Asian Pac J Trop Biomed.* (2012) 2:55–60. doi: 10.1016/S2221-1691(11) 60190-1
45. Musallam II, Abo-Shehada MN, Hegazy YM, Holt HR, Guitian FJ. Systematic review of brucellosis in the middle east: disease frequency in ruminants and humans and risk factors for human infection. *Epidemiol Infect.* (2016) 144:671–85. doi: 10.1017/S0950268815002575
46. Franc KA, Krecek RC, Häsler BN, Arenas-Gamboa AM. Brucellosis remains

a neglected disease in the developing world: a call for interdisciplinary action. *BMC Public Health.* (2018) 18:125. doi: 10.1186/s12889-017-5016-y
47. Singha BB, Dhandb NK, Gilla JPS. Economic losses occurring due to brucellosis in Indian livestock populations. *Prev Vet Med.* (2015) 119:211–5. doi: 10.1016/j.prevetmed.2015.03.013
48. Kreizinger Z, Foster JT, Rónai Z, Sulyok KM, Wehmann E, Jánosi S, et al. Genetic relatedness of *Brucella suis* biovar 2 isolates from hares, wild boars and domestic pigs. *Vet Microbiol.* (2014) 27:492–8. doi: 10.1016/j.vetmic.2014.05.031
49. Pappas G, Papadimitriou P, Akritidis N, Christou L, Tsianos EV. The new global map of human brucellosis. *Lancet Infect Dis.* (2006) 6:91–9. doi: 10.1016/S1473-3099(06)70382-6
50. McDermott J, Grace D, Zinsstag J. Economics of brucellosis impact and control in low-income countries. *Rev Sci Tech.* (2013) 32:249–61. doi: 10.20506/rst.32.1.2197
51. Godfroid J, Käsbohrer A. Brucellosis in the European Union and Norway at the turn of the twenty-first century. *Vet Microbiol.* (2002) 90:135–45. doi: 10.1016/S0378-1135(02)00217-1
52. Davis DS, Elzer PH. *Brucella* vaccines in wildlife. *Vet Microbiol.* (2002) 90:533–44. doi: 10.1016/S0378-1135(02)00233-X
53. Yagupsky P, Baron EJ. Laboratory exposures to brucellae and implications for bioterrorism. *Emerg Infect Dis.* (2005) 11:1180–5. doi: 10.3201/eid1108.041197
54. Grégoire F, Mousset B, Hanrez D, Michaux C, Walravens K, Linden A. A serological and bacteriological survey of brucellosis in wild boar (Sus scrofa) in Belgium. *BMC Vet Res.* (2012) 8:80. doi: 10.1186/1746-6148-8-80
55. Ferris RA, Schoenbaum MA, Crawford RP. Comparison of serologic tests and bacteriologic culture for detection of brucellosis in swine from naturally infected herds. *J Am Vet Med Assoc.* (1995) 207:1332–3.
56. Godfroid J, Michel P, Uytterhaegen L, Smedt CD, Rasseneur F, Saegerman C, et al. *Brucella* suis biotype 2 infection of wild boars (Sus scrofa) in Belgium. *Ann Med Vet.* (1994) 138:263–8.
57. Cvetnic Z, Mitak M, Ocepek M, Lojkic M, Terzić S, Jemersic L, et al. Wild boars (*Sus scrofa*) as reservoirs of *Brucella suis* biovar 2 in Croatia. *Acta vet Hung.* (2003) 51:465–73. doi: 10.1556/avet.51.2003.4.4
58. Leuenberger R, Boujon P, Thür B, Miserez R, Garin-Bastuji B, Rüfenacht J, et al. Prevalence of classical swine fever, Aujeszky's disease and brucellosis in a population of wild boar in Switzerland. *Vet Rec.* (2007) 160:362–8. doi: 10.1136/vr.160.11.362
59. Closa-Sebastià F, Casas-Díaz E, Cuenca R, Lavín S, Mentaberre G, Marco I. *Brucella* species antibodies and isolation in wild boar in north-east Spain. *Vet Rec.* (2010) 167:826–8. doi: 10.1136/vr.c5927
60. Muñoz PM, Boadella M, Arnal M, de Miguel MJ, Revilla M, Martínez D, et al. Spatial distribution and risk factors of brucellosis in Iberian wild ungulates. *BMC Infect Dis.* (2010) 10:46. doi: 10.1186/1471-2334-10-46
61. Wu N, Abril C, Hinić V, Brodard I, Thür B, Fattebert J, et al. Free-ranging wild boar: a disease threat to domestic pigs in Switzerland? *J Wildl Dis.* (2011) 47:868–79. doi: 10.7589/0090-3558-47.4.868
62. Garin-Bastuji B, Hars J, Calvez D, Thiébaud M, Artois M. Brucellose du porc domestique et du sanglier sauvage due ?? *Brucella suis* biovar 2 en France. *Epidémiol Santé Anim.* (2000) 38:1–5.
63. Hubálek Z, Treml F, Juricová Z, Hunady M, Halouzka J, Janík V, et al. Serological survey of the wild boar (*Sus scrofa*) for tularaemia and brucellosis in South Moravia, Czech Republic. *Vet Med.* (2002) 47:3–60. doi: 10.17221/5805-VETMED
64. Cvetnic Z, Toncic J, Spicic S, Lojkic M, Terzic S, Jemersic L, et al. Brucellosis in wild boar (*Sus scrofa*) in the republic of Croatia. *Vet Med.* (2004) 49:115–22. doi: 10.17221/5684-VETMED
65. Godfroid J, Cloeckaert A, Liautard JP, Kohler S, Fretin D, Walravens K, et al. From the discovery of the Malta fever's agent to the discovery of a marine mammal reservoir, brucellosis has continuously been a re-emerging zoonosis. *Vet Res.* (2005) 36:313–26. doi: 10.1051/vetres:2005003
66. Megersa B, Biffa D, Niguse F, Rufael T, Asmare K, Skjerve E. Cattle brucellosis in traditional livestock husbandry practice in Southern and Eastern Ethiopia, and its zoonotic implication. *Acta Vet Scand.* (2011) 53:24. doi: 10.1186/1751-0147-53-24
67. Terefe Y, Girma S, Mekonnen N, Asrade B. Brucellosis and associated risk factors in dairy cattle of eastern Ethiopia. *Trop Anim Health Prod.* (2017) 49:599–606. doi: 10.1007/s11250-017-1242-7
68. Bugeza J, Muwonge A, Munyeme M, Lasuba P, Godfroid J, Kankya C. Seroprevalence of bovine brucellosis and associated risk factors in Nakasongola district, Uganda. *Trop Anim Health Prod.* (2019) 51:2073–6. doi: 10.1007/s11250-018-1631-6
69. Omer MK, Asfaw T, Skjerue E, Tekleghiorgis T, Woldehiwot T. Risk factors for *Brucella spp.* infection in dairy cattle farms in Asmara, State of Eritrea. *Pre Vet Med.* (2000) 46:257–65. doi: 10.1016/s0167-5877(00)00152-5
70. Ibrahim N, Belihu K, Lobago F, Bekana M. Sero-prevalence of bovine brucellosis and its risk factors in Jimma zone of Oromia Region, South-western Ethiopia. *Trop Anim Health Prod.* (2010) 42:35–40. doi: 10.1007/s11250-009-9382-z
71. Abedi A, Hashempour-Baltork F, Alizadeh AM, Beikzadeh S, Hosseini H, Bashiry M, et al. The prevalence of *Brucella* spp. In dairy products in the middle east region: a systematic review and meta-analysis. *Acta Trop.* (2019) 202:105241. doi: 10.1016/j.actatropica.2019.105241
72. Goonaratna C. Brucellosis in humans and animals. *Ceylon Med J.* (2009) 52:66. doi: 10.4038/cmj.v52i2.1028
73. Meirelles-Bartoli RB, Mathias LA, Samartino LE. Brucellosis due to *Brucella suis* in a swine herd associated with a human clinical case in the State of São Paulo, Brazil. *Trop Anim Health Prod.* (2012) 44:1575–9. doi: 10.1007/s11250-012-0108-2
74. Barlozzari G, Franco A, Macrì G, Lorenzetti S, Maggiori F, Dottarelli S, et al. First report of *Brucella suis* biovar 2 in a semi free-range pig farm, Italy. *Vet Ital.* (2015) 51:151–4. doi: 10.12834/VetIt.50.3384.1
75. Pilo C, Tedde MT, Orrù G, Addis G, Liciardi M. *Brucella suis* infection in domestic pigs in Sardinia (Italy). *Epidemiol Infect.* (2015) 143:2170–7. doi: 10.1017/S0950268814003513
76. Ferreira AC, Tenreiro R, de Sá MIC, Dias R. Complete genome sequences of three iberian *Brucella* suis Biovar 2 strains isolated from wild boars. *Genome Announc.* (2014) 2:e00618–4. doi: 10.1128/genomeA.00618-14
77. Melzer F, Lohse R, Nieper H, Liebert M, Sachse K. A serological study on brucellosis in wild boars in Germany. *Eur J Wildlife Res.* (2006) 53:153–7. doi: 10.1007/s10344-006-0072-0
78. Knight-Jones TJ, Mylrea GE, Kahn S. Animal production food safety: priority pathogens for standard setting by the world organisation for animal health. *Rev Sci Tech.* (2010) 29:523–35. doi: 10.20506/rst.29.3.1994
79. Ruiz-Fons F, Vidal D, Höfle U, Vicente J, Gortázar C. Aujeszky's disease virus infection patterns in European wild boar. *Vet Microbiol.* (2007) 120:241–50. doi: 10.1016/j.vetmic.2006.11.003
80. Llario PF. *Ecología del Jabalí en Doñana: Parámetros Reproductivose Impacto Ambiental.* Cáceres: Univ of Extremadura (1996).
81. Tounkara K, Maiga S, Traoré A, Seck BM, Akakpo AJ. Epidemiology of bovine brucellosis in mali: serologic investigation and initial isolation of strains of *Brucella* abortus. *Rev Sci Tech.* (1994) 13:777–86. doi: 10.20506/rst.13.3.795
82. Jori F, Godfroid J, Michel AL, Potts AD, Jaumally MR, Sauzier J, et al. An assessment of zoonotic and production limiting pathogens in rusa deer (Cervus timorensis rusa) from Mauritius. *Transbound Emerg Dis.* (2014) 61(Suppl 1):31–42. doi: 10.1111/tbed.12206

5

One-Tube Nested Real-Time PCR Assay for Rapid Screening of Porcine Cytomegalovirus in Clinical Samples

Hye-young Wang [1], *Joong Ki Song* [2], *Seongho Shin* [2], *Ki Myung Choi* [1] *and Hyunil Kim* [1*]

[1] Optipharm, Inc., Cheongju, South Korea, [2] Optipharm Animal Disease Diagnostic Center, Cheongju, South Korea

***Correspondence:**
Hyunil Kim
hikim@optipharm.co.kr*

Porcine cytomegalovirus (PCMV) is a pathogen that must be removed from pigs for use as organ donors in xenotransplantation. Recently, it has been found that when donor pigs are infected with PCMV, a pig-to-non-human-primate xenotransplantation lower transplant survival by 2–3 times. Therefore, highly sensitive methods are needed to maintain designated pathogen free (DPF) pig and screen for xenografts. The purpose of this study was to evaluate the performance of commercially available method with one-tube nested real-time PCR assay to quickly detect PCMV infection in clinical samples and compare the results with those of sequence analysis. Molecular diagnostic methods were used to evaluate 127 samples, including tissues and blood samples from pigs suspected of PCMV infection. The detection rate for positive PCMV was 38.6% ($n = 49$), 23.6% ($n = 30$), and 12.6% ($n = 16$) in one-tube nested real-time PCR, nested PCR, and conventional PCR methods, respectively. All PCMV-positive samples in conventional PCR or nested PCR methods were also positive in the one-tube nested real-time PCR assay. All the PCR products in the three methods were checked for amplification of PCMV gene by PCR and subsequent direct sequencing. The results of one-tube nested real-time PCR were found to be consistent with those of sequence analysis for all the samples and showed good agreement ($\kappa = 1$). Our study found that the one-tube nested real-time PCR assay is more sensitive than the other two methods. This assay required approximately 1.5 h for completion. Therefore, we concluded that one-tube nested real-time PCR assay is a fast and reliable method for the characterizing pathogen responsible for PCMV infection.

Keywords: porcine cytomegalovirus, one-tube nested real-time PCR, xenotransplantation, designated pathogen free pig, diagnosis

INTRODUCTION

In order to alleviate the shortage of human donor organs available for allograft, xenotransplantation using pig cells, tissues, or organs have been proposed (1–3). This may be related to the transmission of porcine mediated disease, so the maintenance of designated pathogen free pigs is required for xenotransplantation (4–6).

Porcine cytomegalovirus (PCMV), also known as Suid herpesvirus 2 (SuHV2), is an enveloped virus with a double-stranded linear DNA genome. PCMV can cause fever, reduced general condition, loss of appetite, numbness, neurological signs, and respiratory symptoms (e.g., sneezing, coughing, and dyspnea), acute to subacute disease, and high mortality and morbidity in piglets (3, 7). In a previous studies, the virus have been reported to be immunosuppressive pathogen primarily affecting the immune function of the macrophages and T lymphocytes, which can cause preclinical infection in adult pigs and reproductive failure in pregnant sows (7, 8). PCMV infection is widespread worldwide and has a high prevalence in swine herds. For this reason, many researchers have continued to pay attention to the potential risk to public health in interspecies transmission of PCMV and human xenotransplantation (7). In addition, international xenotransplantation association has a guideline that resource pig for xenotransplantation should be free from PCMV (9). These data indicate that it is essential to quickly detect PCMV infection with high sensitivity and specificity in the early stages of the resource swine herds.

So far, some molecular diagnostic methods, including polymerase chain reaction (PCR) (10–12), enzyme-linked immunosorbent assay (ELISA) (13, 14), loop-mediated isothermal amplification assay (LAMP) (15), and western blot analysis (16) for the detection of PCMV infection has been reported. These assays have low sensitivity, need to agarose gel analysis for amplification products, or have a risk of contamination, which can lead to incorrect results. In addition, companies such as Novateinbio and MyBioSource have ELISA products that detect antibody or antigen of PCMV, there are no commercialized products using molecular diagnostic methods until now. Real-time fluorescent quantitative PCR technology has become a powerful alternative platform for detection and differentiation of pathogenic viruses (3, 17, 18).

In this study, we developed a highly sensitive one-tube nested real-time PCR assay (Opti PCMV-qPCR; Optipharm, Osong, Republic of Korea) that combines nested PCR and real-time PCR to detect PCMV targeting DNA polymerase gene and consists of two sequential reactions in a single tube. The performance of the one-tube nested real-time PCR assay was evaluated using clinical samples suspected of PCMV compared to conventional PCR and nested PCR, and the results were confirmed by sequence analysis.

METHODS

Preparation of DNA Samples

To evaluate the diagnostic performance of the PCR, nested PCR, and one-tube nested real-time PCR methods, a total of 127 field samples, including 37 lung tissues, 30 blood samples, 30 serums, and 30 feces samples, were provided by the Optipharm Animal Disease Diagnostic Center, which was commissioned from January to December 2019. In addition, 10 organs (lung, liver, pancreas, spleen, kidney, brain, heart, small intestine, nasal concha, and tonsil) of six pigs were analyzed to determine the infection rate of PCMV for each organ by one-tube nested real-time PCR assay. According to the manufacturer's recommendation, DNA was extracted from 200 μL of serum or 20 mg of organ tissue homogenate using a commercial automated system (Miracle-AutoXT Automated Nucleic Acid Extraction System, Intronbio, Seongnam, Republic of Korea). To avoid cross-contamination, all samples were individually processed and stored at −20°C. The content and purity of the extracted DNA was analyzed by measuring the absorbance at 260 and 280 nm by a spectrophotometer (Infinite 200 NanoQuant; Tecan, Switzerland).

Conventional PCR and Nested PCR

To evaluate the usefulness of one-tube nested real-time PCR assay, the results of conventional PCR and nested PCR were compared. PCR primers for the conventional PCR and nested PCR used in this study were selected from the nucleotide sequence of the PCMV DNA polymerase gene determined by Hamel (10) and Fryer (11), respectively. PCR was performed using 20 μL of reaction mixture (Genetbio, Daejeon, Korea) containing 2 × master mix, 1 × primer mixture, 3 μL of sample DNA, and ddH$_2$O added to achieve a final volume of 20 μL. The reaction conditions for conventional PCR and nested PCR using the outer primers (PCMVF1 and PCMVR1) were as follows: pre-denaturation at 94°C for 5 min; 40 cycles of 94°C for 30 s, 60°C for 30 s, 72°C for 30 s; and a final extension at 72°C for 10 min. For nested PCR using the inner primers (PCMVFB and PCMVR2), two microliters of the first-round PCR mixture was transferred to 20 μl of a premixed solution containing the PCR reagents at the same concentrations listed above. The amplification procedure was repeated for 40 cycles with the same time and temperature parameters as described above, except that annealing at 55°C for 30 s was used. The amplified target was visualized as a single band corresponding to a length of 413-bp for conventional PCR and 160-bp for nested PCR using the Chemi Doc system (Vilber Lourmat, Deutschland, Germany).

One-Tube Nested Real-Time PCR Assay

Oligonucleotide primers and probes corresponding to the two strands of the DNA polymerase gene of PCMV (**Figure 1**) were designed using Primer3Plus (http://www.bioinformatics.nl/cgi-bin/primer3plus/primer3plus.cgi). Primers were prepared as probes corresponding to the complementary strands and used exclusively thereafter. To verify the efficiency of the selected primers and probe, synthesized a positive control DNA sample (Bioneer, Daejeon, Republic of Korea) and amplified with custom PCR primers (forward, 5′-ATGACATTCTTAATCCATATAT-3′ and reverse, 5′-CACTGTCCCTAAAACTACTG-3′) resulting in amplicons of 3,010 bp. The resulting product was mutagenized after subcloning with pBHA vector. Detection of PCMV in clinical samples was performed with Opti PCMV real-time PCR (Optipharm), a quantitative one-tube nested real-time PCR-based assay, using a CFX-96 real-time PCR system (Bio-Rad, Hercules, CA, USA) for thermal cycling and fluorescence detection. Real-time PCR amplification was performed in a total reaction volume of 20 μL containing 10 μL of 2 × Thunderbird probe qPCR mix (Toyobo, Osaka, Japan), 2.5 μL of a mixture of 5 pmol each primers and 5 pmol TaqMan probe that were labeled with fluorophores (FAM-BHQ1), and 3 μL template DNA. The real-time PCR kit consisted of an internal control (IC) DNA and a primer set for IC DNA amplification included in the reaction mixture, which was used to indicate successful nucleic acid extraction, sample quality, and to confirm

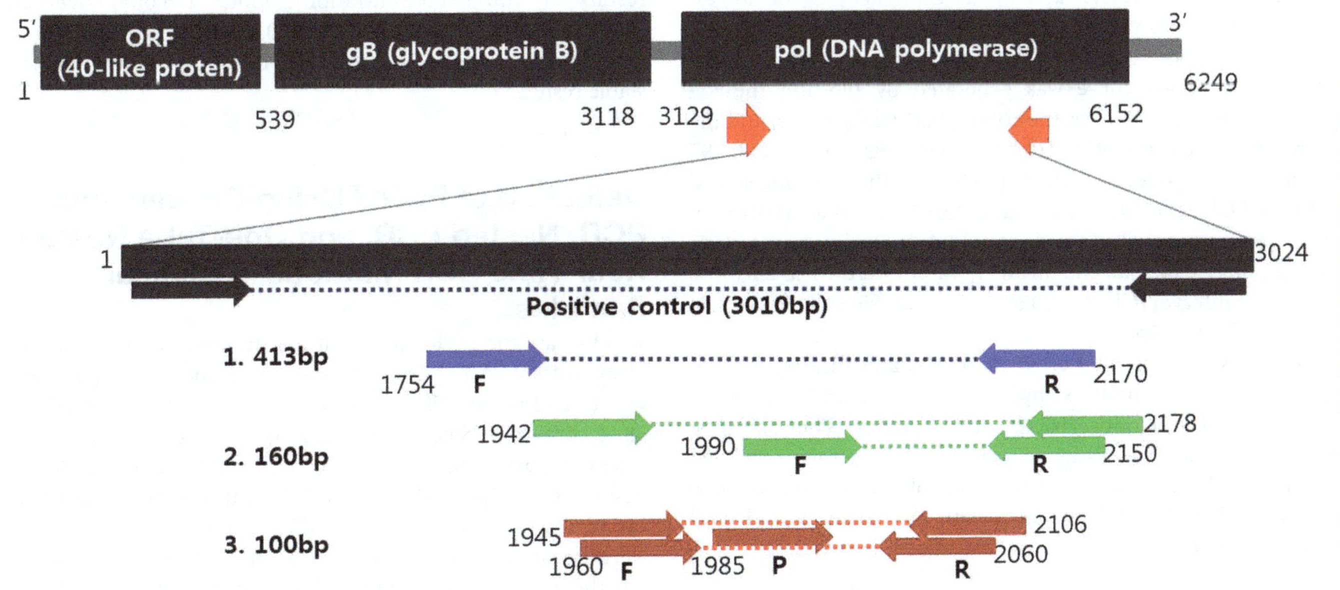

FIGURE 1 | Schematic diagram of the DNA polymerase gene to distinguish PCMV from positions of primers and probes. A positive control was synthesized to verify the efficiency of the developed primers and probes. Primer sequences for conventional PCR and nested PCR were selected from the PCMV DNA polymerase gene determined by Hamel (1) and Fryer (2), respectively. Primers and probe sequences for one-tube nested real-time PCR (3) used in this study were selected at differed locations from the human and mouse cytomegalovirus DNA polymerase gene.

the presence of PCR inhibitors in the reaction. Therefore, it does not compete directly with the amplification of species-specific targets in multiplex real-time PCR. Positive (plasmid PCMV DNA) and negative controls consisting of molecular grade (DNAse/RNAse-free) water (Ultra pure water; Welgene, Gyeongsan, Republic of Korea) without template DNA were included in each assay. The assay was carried out under the following conditions: 95°C for 3 min, then 10 cycles of 3 s at 95°C and 30 s at 60°C, and then by 40 cycles of 3 s at 95°C and 30 s at 55°C. Each sample was tested in duplicate by running the PCR cycle twice and a positive result was obtained when the C_T value was <35.

Interfering Reactions and Reproducibility Analysis

For interfering reactions, we used the following 7 substances by concentration: EDTA and sodium citrate (1, 10, 20, and 50 mM), and heparin (250, 300, 375, and 500 IU) for anticoagulants, phosphate buffered saline (PBS; 1, 5, 10, and 20X) for tissue emulsion, EtOH and xylene (1, 5, 10, 20, and 50%), and blood (1, 5, and 10%). The repeatability and reproducibility of this assay were performed with a total of 240 tests (10 days × 2 runs/day × 4 replicates × 3 lots). The coefficient of variation (CV) was calculated according to the form of the mean C_T values/standard deviation (SD).

Sequence Analysis

To confirm the results of the three molecular diagnostic methods, PCR amplicons of all clinical isolates were sequenced using an ABI 3730 automated DNA sequencer (Applied Biosystems, Foster City, CA, USA) and the ABI Prism BigDye Terminator (Applied Biosystems) system (CosmoGenetech, Republic of Korea). The primer sets used to amplify the target DNA polymerase gene were 5′-CCTGATCTTAAATGACGAGGACGTGAC-3′ (413F) and 5′-ACCGTCTGAGAGACTGAACTTCTCTGACAC-3′ (413R), 5′-AGGACCCTATGTTGGCAYTGATAC-3′ (1945F) and 5′-TCGTCTGCCTRAGCATGTCC-3′ (2106R), which resulted in a 413-bp and 162-bp PCR product, respectively. The obtained sequence was compared with that of the National Center for Biotechnology Information GenBank database. The primer sequences had been removed from alignment sequences before phylogenetic analysis. Multiple alignments of nucleotide sequences based on the PCR product of the PCMV DNA polymerase gene mentioned above were performed using MUSCLE within the Phylogeny.fr software (19). Then, Gblocks was used as a collection method to align the sequences, assess the phylogenetic relationships by the PhyML using the 49 strains isolated in this study, together with 12 PCMV strains deposited in the GenBank database, and finally visualized the phylogenetic tree by TreeDyn.

RESULTS

Analytical Sensitivity and Specificity of One-Tube Nested Real-Time PCR

The analytical sensitivity of the assay for PCMV detection was determined using a standard curve that 10-fold serially diluted (10^6 copies−1 copy) of plasmid DNA containing cloned PCMV gene (**Figure 2**). The sensitivity was estimated as the lowest PCMV gene copies yielding a positive result in all 20 replicates, and the corresponding C_T value were selected as the analysis cutoff. A standard curve was generated by plotting the log quantity of PCMV DNA vs. the corresponding C_T value, and the coefficient of determination (R^2) for linear regression was 0.997 with a slope of −4.082. The detection limit of the one-tube nested real-time PCR assay for PCMV was detected at a concentration of 1 copy per reaction. The C_T values of PCMV DNA concentration ranged from 1.2 to 28.5, and mean C_T values were 2.1 ± 2.2 (95% confidence interval [CI], 1.2–3) to 27.1 ± 1.7 (95% CI, 26.4–27.8) and the CV was <3%.

To assess the potential cross-reactivity, analytical specificity was performed with 40 samples with concentrations above 10^4 copies of individual bacterial/viral genes. The one-tube nested real-time PCR assay to detect PCMV-positive showed negative results in all strains except control PCMV. Hence, these primers and probes did not react with any bacterial and viral strains (**Table 1**).

Results of Interfering Reactions and Reproducibility Analysis by One-Tube Nested Real-Time PCR

We performed the interference reaction with 7 substances by concentration. As a result, there was no interference below 50 mM EDTA, 50 mM sodium, 375IU heparin, 10X PBS, 50% EtOH, 50% xylene, and 10% blood (data not shown). For repeatability and reproducibility, the measured number for the 3 concentrations of positive control was 240 (10 days × 2 runs/day × 4 replicates × 3 lots). As shown in **Table 2**, the CV for intra- and inter-assay variability ranged from 0.6 to 2.5% and 1.2 to 2.5%, respectively, which were all <3%. The intra-laboratory reproducibility results at cutoff concentration (about 1 copy) over time were 96.4% (κ = 0.96, 95% CI, 0.926–0.985). Based on the experimental results, we suggest that this assay may have stable results.

Detection of PCMV Using Conventional PCR, Nested PCR, and One-Tube Nested Real-Time PCR Methods in Clinical Samples

To evaluate the performance of one-tube nested real-time PCR assay, a total of 127 clinical samples, including lung tissues (n = 37, 29.1%), whole bloods (n = 30, 23.6%), serums (n = 30, 23.6%), and feces (n = 30, 23.6%), were used. The results were compared with those of conventional PCR (**Figure 3A**) and nested PCR (**Figure 3B**). Of the 127 clinical samples, 49 (38.6%) samples were positive for PCMV, while 78 (61.4%) samples were negative as detected by one-tube nested real-time PCR. On the other hand, 16 (12.6%) and 30 (23.6%) were detected by conventional PCR and nested PCR, respectively (**Table 3**). All clinical samples showed positive IC signals, and the C_T values of the 49 positive and 81 negative samples ranged from 17.6 to 22.5 (mean 20.6, SD ± 1) and 17.7 to 22.5 (mean 20.9, SD ± 0.8), respectively. In addition, the C_T values of PCMV-positive samples ranged from 14 to 28.8 (mean 22.8, SD ± 4.1). In a pilot study, we investigated detection for PCMV infection in 10 organs (lung, liver, pancreas, spleen, kidney, brain, heart, small intestine, nasal concha, and tonsil) of 6 pigs. As a result, the organs with the most prevalent PCMV detected were lung, spleen, and nasal concha (100%), followed by liver, small intestine, and tonsil (83.3%), kidney, heart, and pancreas (66.7%), and brain (50%), respectively (data not shown).

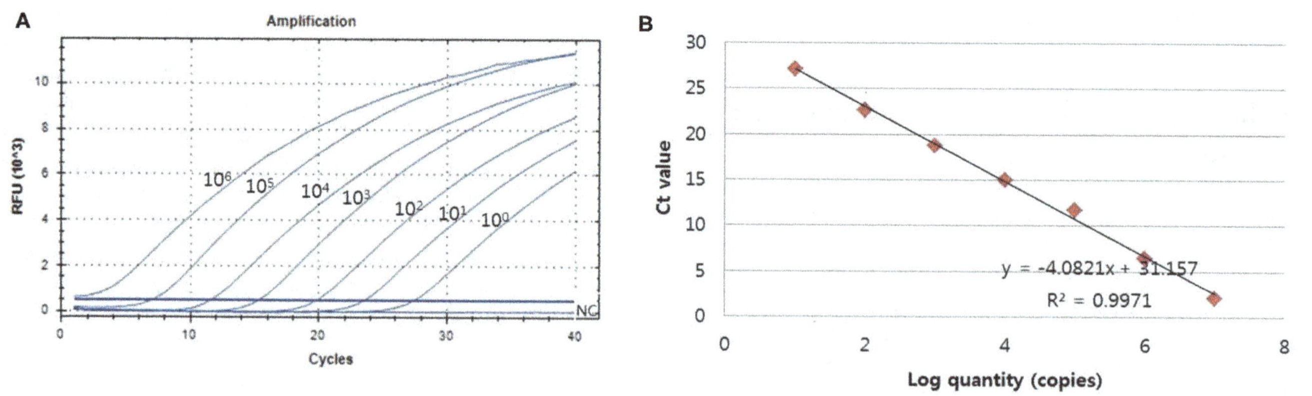

FIGURE 2 | The detection limit of the one-tube nested real-time PCR assay was evaluated using 10-fold serial diluted samples. Serially diluted PCMV control DNA ranging from 10^6 copies to 1 copy per reaction were used to determine the detection limit of the one-tube nested real-time PCR assay. In the one-tube nested real-time PCR assay, the amplification curve of the specific probe **(A)** for detecting PCMV is shown. The overall detection limit of this assay for the PCMV ranged from approximately 1 copy DNA per reaction. C_T was plotted against the input of the quantity of PCMV DNA (repeated 20 times). The linearity **(B)** was generated by plotting the log quantity of PCMV DNA vs. the corresponding C_T value, and the coefficients of determination of the linear regression were 0.997 with a slope of −4.082. The fluorescence intensity is displayed on the Y-axis (R^2 = reporter signal/passive reference signal). RFU, relative fluorescence unit; R^2, fluorescence units.

TABLE 1 | Analytical specificity of the one-tube nested real-time PCR assay to detect PCMV with 40 strains.

No.	Species	Isolate	Sample type	One-tube nested real-time PCR	
				PCMV (Ct)	IC (Ct)
1	*Porcine reproductive and respiratory syndrome virus*	Field isolate	Tissue	N/A	20.58
2	*Porcine reproductive and respiratory syndrome virus*	Field isolate	Tissue	N/A	21.46
3	*Porcine reproductive and respiratory syndrome virus*	Field isolate	Tissue	N/A	20.38
4	*Porcine reproductive and respiratory syndrome virus*	Field isolate	Tissue	N/A	20.54
5	*Swine Influenza virus*	Field isolate	Tissue	N/A	19.72
6	*Hemophilus parasuis*	Field isolate	Tissue	N/A	18.94
7	*Hemophilus parasuis*	Field isolate	Tissue	N/A	20.7
8	*Mycoplasma hyopneumoniae*	Field isolate	Tissue	N/A	22.2
9	*Mycoplasma hyopneumoniae*	Field isolate	Tissue	N/A	20
10	*Mycoplasma hyopneumoniae*	Field isolate	Tissue	N/A	22.28
11	*Porcine rotavirus*	Field isolate	Tissue	N/A	20.66
12	*Porcine rotavirus*	Field isolate	Stool	N/A	20.23
13	*Actinobacillus pleuropneumoniae*	Field isolate	Tissue	N/A	20.31
14	*Porcine epidemic diarrhea virus*	Field isolate	Stool	N/A	21.56
15	*Porcine epidemic diarrhea virus*	Field isolate	Sludge	N/A	20.46
16	*Porcine Parvovirus*	Field isolate	Collagen	N/A	22.21
17	*Porcine Parvovirus*	Field isolate	Collagen	N/A	21.13
18	*Porcine circovirus type 2*	Field isolate	Tissue	N/A	21.07
19	*Porcine circovirus type 2*	Field isolate	Tissue	N/A	21.1
20	*Porcine circovirus type 2*	Field isolate	Tissue	N/A	22.78
21	*Porcine circovirus type 2*	Field isolate	Tissue	N/A	21.19
22	*Porcine circovirus type 3*	Field isolate	Tissue	N/A	22.32
23	*Porcine circovirus type 3*	Field isolate	Tissue	N/A	21.41
24	*Porcine circovirus type 3*	Field isolate	Tissue	N/A	20.11
25	*Porcine circovirus type 3*	Field isolate	Tissue	N/A	20.84
26	*Porcine circovirus type 3*	Field isolate	Tissue	N/A	19.28
27	*Porcine circovirus type 3*	Field isolate	Tissue	N/A	22.45
28	*Escherichia coli*	ATCC 25922	Culture	N/A	21.33
29	*Escherichia coli*	ATCC 35150	Culture	N/A	21.1
30	*Salmonella enteritidis*	ATCC 13076	Culture	N/A	19.36
31	*Salmonella typhi*	ATCC 19430	Culture	N/A	21.13
32	*Salmonella paratyphi*	ATCC BAA-1250	Culture	N/A	20.66
33	*Salmonella Newport*	ATCC 6962	Culture	N/A	20.08
34	*Salmonella typhimurium*	ATCC 14028	Culture	N/A	18.58
35	*Staphylococcus aureus*	ATCC 25923	Culture	N/A	21.18
36	*Staphylococcus aureus*	ATCC 29213	Culture	N/A	21.55
37	*Staphylococcus aureus*	ATCC 6538	Culture	N/A	21.49
38	*Clostridium perfringens*	ATCC 13124	Culture	5.13	21.66
39	*Toxoplasma gondii*	ATCC 50853	Culture	10.74	21.9
40	*Bordetella bronchiseptica*	ATCC 4617	Culture	N/A	20.61
41	*Porcine cytomegalovirus*	PC	Culture0	10.38	20.24
42	*Porcine cytomegalovirus*	PC	Culture	10.74	20.61
43	NC	-	-	N/A	19.8

ATCC, American Type Culture Collection; PCMV, porcine cytomegalovirus.

TABLE 2 | Results of intra- and inter-assay for repeatability and reproducibility analysis.

Copies/$\mu\ell$	*N*	Total			Intra-assay			Inter-assay					
					Within-run			Between-run			Between-day		
		C_T avg	SD	CV(%)	C_T avg	SD	CV(%)	C_T avg	SD	CV(%)	C_T avg	SD	CV(%)
10^5	240	7.7	0.0	0.5	7.7	0.1	0.8	7.7	0.1	1.9	7.7	0.1	1.3
10^3	240	15.6	0.1	0.6	15.6	0.1	0.6	15.7	0.3	1.8	15.6	0.2	1.2
10^1	240	23.8	0.1	0.3	23.9	0.6	2.5	23.8	0.5	2.0	23.6	0.6	2.5

N, test number of inter- and intra- assay; avg, average; SD, standard deviation; CV, coefficients of variation.

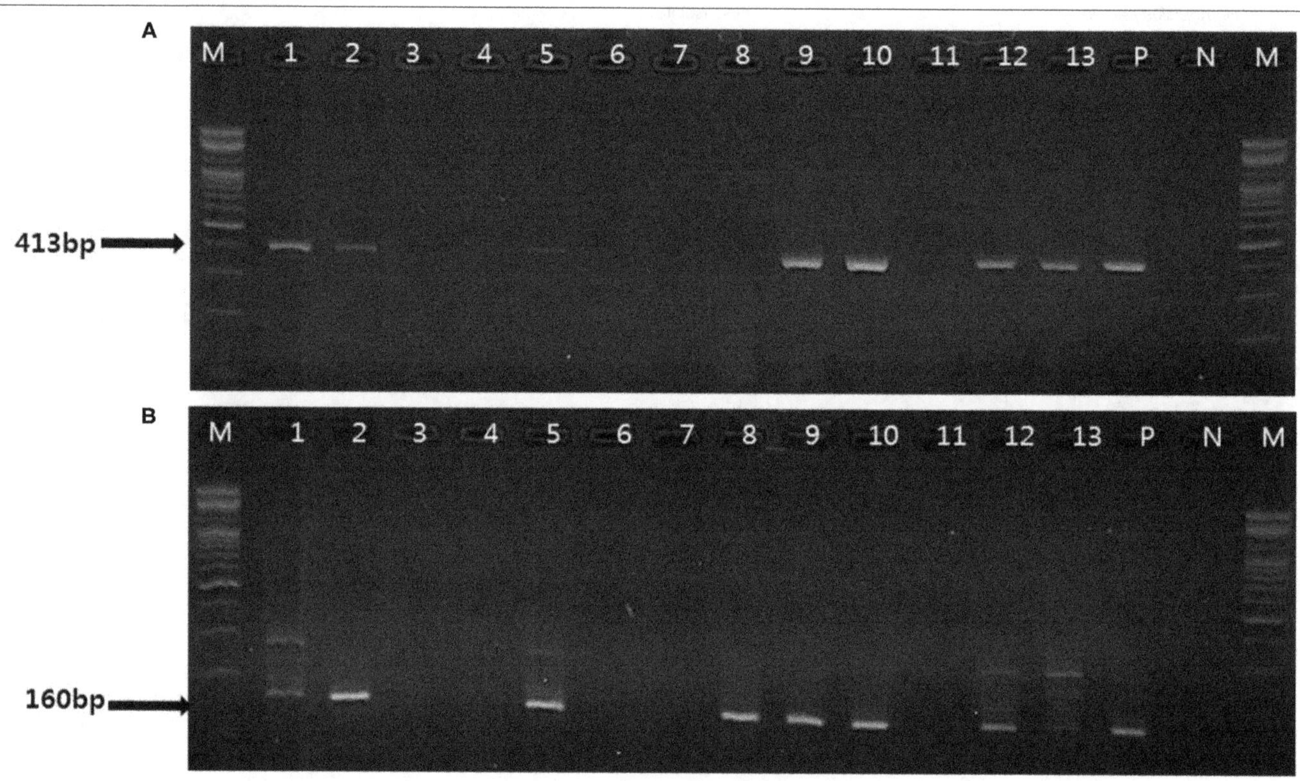

FIGURE 3 | Representative results of the conventional PCR and nested PCR with clinical samples. **(A)** Conventional PCR results. Lanes 1, 2, 5, 9, 10, 12–13: positive; M, 100 bp DNA ladder (Bioneer); P, positive control; N, negative control. **(B)** Nested PCR results. Lane 1, 2 5, 8–10, 12–13: positive; M, 100 bp DNA ladder (Bioneer); P, positive control; N, negative control.

Comparison of the Results Between the One-Tube Nested Real-Time PCR Assay and Sequence Analysis for the Detection of PCMV in Clinical Samples

To confirm the results obtained from the one-tube nested real-time PCR assay, sequence analysis was performed using the same clinical samples. All 49 samples detected as PCMV-positive by one-tube nested PCR assay were consistent with the sequencing results. Our study showed that nested PCR had a higher positive rate than conventional PCR (23.6% vs. 12.6%), but the one-tube nested real-time PCR assay (38.6%) was more sensitive than the other two methods. The agreement rate between one-tube nested real-time PCR assay and conventional PCR or nested PCR was 74% (95% CI 0.654–0.813, $p < 0.001$) and 85% (95% CI 0.776–0.907, $p < 0.001$), respectively (**Table 4**). In addition, the agreement rate of the one-tube nested real-time PCR assay and sequence analysis was 100% (95% CI 0.976–1.000, $p < 0.001$). Using sequence analysis, the sensitivity, specificity, and positive and negative predictive values of PCMV results by one-tube nested real-time PCR assay were 100% ($n = 49$, 95% CI 0.947–1.000, $p < 0.001$), 100% ($n = 78$, 95% CI 0.959–1.000, $p < 0.001$), 100% (95% CI 0.947–1.000, $p < 0.001$), 100% (95% CI 0.959–1.000, $p < 0.001$), respectively. All PCMV-positive samples in conventional PCR or nested PCR methods were also positive in the one-tube nested real-time PCR assay. The

TABLE 3 | Detection of PCMV DNA in 127 clinical samples suspected of PCMV infection using the conventional PCR, nested PCR, and one-tube nested real-time PCR assay.

Sample	Total no. (%) of samples	Detection of PCMV, no. (%) of isolates							
		Conventional PCR		Nested PCR		One-tube nested real-time PCR			
		Positive (%)	Negative (%)	Positive (%)	Negative (%)	Positive (%)	Negative (%)	IC ranged C_T value (mean ± SD)	PCMV ranged C_T value (mean ± SD)
Tissue	37 (29.1)	16 (43.2)	21 (56.8)	25 (67.6)	12 (32.4)	32 (86.5)	5 (13.5)	17.6–22.1 (20.5 ± 0.9)	14–27.3 (21.1 ± 3.9)
Blood	30 (23.6)	0 (0)	30 (100)	1 (3.3)	29 (96.7)	6 (20)	24 (80)	19.3–21.7 (21.1 ± 0.5)	23.1–28.1 (26.6 ± 1.8)
Serum	30 (23.6)	0 (0)	30 (100)	2 (6.7)	28 (93.3)	6 (20)	24 (80)	20.5–22.5 (21.6 ± 0.5)	20–28.5 (21.6 ± 0.5)
Feces	30 (23.6)	0 (0)	30 (100)	2 (6.7)	28 (93.3)	5 (16.7)	25 (83.3)	17.7–21.2 (20.1 ± 0.9)	25.4–28.8 (27.3 ± 1.4)
Total	127 (100)	16 (12.6)	111 (87.4)	30 (23.6)	97 (76.4)	49 (38.6)	78 (61.4)	17.6–22.5 (20.8 ± 0.9)	14–28.8 (22.8 ± 4.1)

PCMV, porcine cytomegalovirus; IC, internal control; SD, standard deviation.

TABLE 4 | Clinical sensitivity and specificity between the one-tube nested real-time PCR assay and conventional PCR, nested PCR, and sequence analysis methods stratified by PCMV suspected samples.

Molecular assays	One-tube nested real-time PCR		Sensitivity, % (*n*) (95% CI)	Specificity, % (*n*) (95% CI)	PPV, % (*n*) (95% CI)	NPV, % (*n*) (95% CI)	Agreement, % (*n*) (95% CI)	κ coefficient (95% CI)
	Positive	Negative						
Conventional PCR								
Positive	16	0	32.7 (16/49) (0.199–0.475)	100 (78/78) (0.959–1.000)	100 (16/16) (0.829–1.000)	70.3 (78/111) (0.608–0.785)	74 (94/127) (0.654–0.813)	0.373 (0.1893–0.5573)
Negative	33	78						
Nested PCR								
Positive	30	0	61.2 (30/49) (0.462–0.748)	100 (78/78) (0.959–1.000)	100 (30/30) (0.905–1.000)	80.4 (78/97) (0.711–0.877)	85 (108/127) (0.776–0.907)	0.659 (0.518–0.800)
Negative	19	78						
Sequence analysis								
Positive	49	0	100 (49/49) (0.947–1.000)	100 (78/78) (0.959–1.000)	100 (49/49) (0.947–1.000)	100 (78/78) (0.959–1.000)	100 (127/127) (0.976–1.000)	1 (0.963–1.000)
Negative	0	78						

PPV, positive predictive value; NPV, negative predictive value; 95% CI, 95% confidence interval.

phylogenetic tree was constructed using Phylogeny.fr software (19) after alignment of the 49 sequenced results. The 49 sequences obtained from direct sequence analysis of clinical samples were found that 69.4% ($n = 34$) in the FJ01 strain (Groups A; accession no. MG696113) groups and 30.6% ($n = 15$) in the B6 strain groups (Groups B; accession no. AF268039) were similar (**Figure 4**).

DISCUSSION

Pigs are frequently infected with PCMV, but infected adult animals do not always show symptoms of disease. Even though the virus remains latent, it can be transmitted the virus to anyone who receives a swine transplantation. Recently, pig-to-non-human-primate xenotransplantation have shown that transplant survival rates are 2–3 time lower when donor pigs were infected with PCMV (4). Therefore, highly sensitive methods are needed to select PCMV-free pigs and to screen for xenografts. The purpose of this study was to evaluate the analytical performance and clinical efficacy of newly developed high-sensitivity one-tube nested real-time PCR assay, taking advantage of conventional PCR and nested PCR for fast and accurate detection based on the DNA polymerase gene of PCMV. One-tube nested real-time PCR is a simple and sensitive method for the detection and identification of PCMV through sequential amplification of the DNA polymerase gene sequence of PCMV in a single tube (20). One-tube nested real-time PCR is about 100 times more sensitive than conventional PCR or nested PCR. Our results are consistent with previous reports indicated that nested PCR improved sensitivity significantly compared to conventional PCR, mostly due to two sequential amplification steps of the target gene (21–23). In addition, one-tube nested real-time

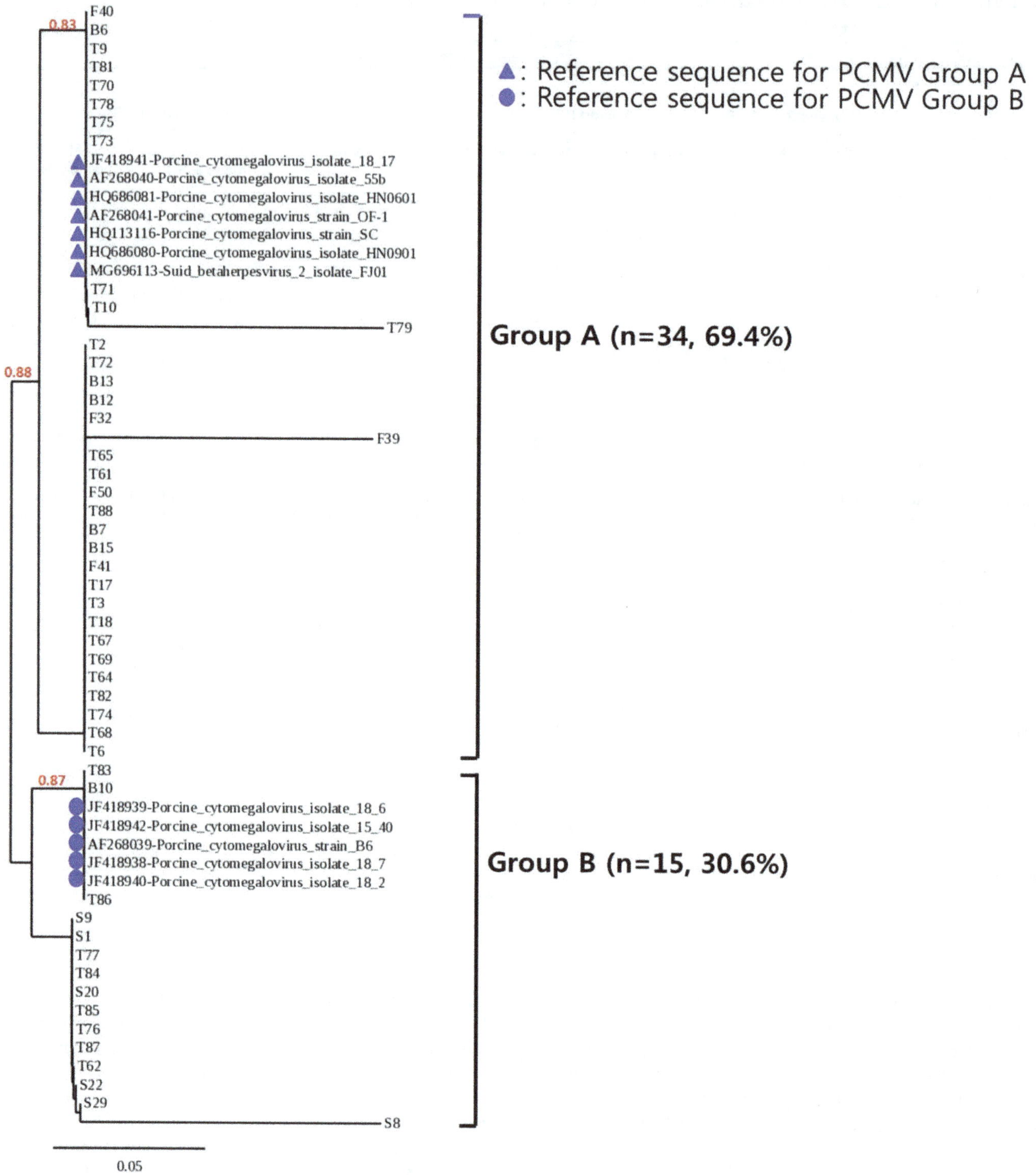

FIGURE 4 | Phylogenetic analysis of 49 PCMV isolates. The phylogenetic tree was constructed using Phylogeny.fr software after the alignment of the 49 sequenced results. The Phylogeny.fr software offers MUSCLE for multiple sequence alignments, Gblocks for alignment curation, PhyML for phylogenetic reconstruction, and TreeDyn for graphical representation of trees. Analysis of phylogenetic tree showed that the sequences obtained from the one-tube nested real-time PCR assay were similar to those of the reference strains FJ01 and B6, with two divided groups (Groups A and B) accounting for 69.4% (n = 34) and 30.6% (n = 15), respectively.

PCR has the same advantages as conventional real-time PCR, including ease, rapidity (turnaround time of 1.5 h), accuracy, low risk of cross-contamination due to sequential reactions in a single tube, reproducibility, and high-throughput capabilities allows quick screening of multiple samples (24, 25). Moreover, the development of fluorescence-based real-time monitoring allows PCR to be a quantitative method, and PCR amplification or quantification was performed in the same reaction tube to reduce possible errors. Owing to its high sensitivity, one-tube nested real-time PCR has been proposed as an excellent method for determining various diseases (24, 25). In Korea, performance evaluation data such as sensitivity, specificity, reproducibility, and repeatability are required for product approval. To evaluate the performance and accuracy of the one-tube nested real-time PCR assay, the synthesized PCMV plasmid DNA was used as a reference standard, and C_T values were repeatedly measured 20 times. The detection limit of the assay was determined to be 1 copy per reaction. The assay was tested using various strains, no cross-reactivity between strains was observed, and the presence of other samples in PCMV-infected strains was demonstrated to not affect the performance of the assay.

The DNA polymerase gene used in this study was proven to be a highly conserved sequence with no significant variation among several PCMV isolates (3), and showed a difference of 72.7 and 68.9% compared to that of human or mouse DNA polymerase genes, respectively. Nevertheless, the positive rate was high in samples from tissue other than sites. Thus, studies on areas with high PCMV infection in each organ should be conducted to gain further insights into xenotransplantation.

CONCLUSIONS

The one-tube nested real-time PCR assay generally showed high agreement and specificity with sequence analysis. This assay is a fast, accurate, and convenient tool for simultaneously detecting the presence of PCMV infection in many samples. Therefore, using the newly developed molecular diagnostic assay in PCMV screening can help detect the most important disease, while reducing false-positives or false-negatives. It is also likely to be used as a sensitive and specific tool for early detection and diagnosis of PCMV infection.

AUTHOR CONTRIBUTIONS

H-yW performed evaluation of the experiments, analyzed the data, and drafted the manuscript. JS and SS provided clinical samples and clinical information. KC and HK revised the manuscript. All authors have read and approved the final manuscript.

REFERENCES

1. Cooper DKC, Gaston R, Eckhoff D, Ladowski J, Yamamoto T, Wang L, et al. Xenotransplantation-the current status and prospects. *Br Med Bull.* (2018) 125:5–14. doi: 10.1093/bmb/ldx043
2. Kaufman CL, Bhutiani N, Ramirez A, Tien HY, Palazzo MD, Galvis E, et al. Current status of vascularized composite allotransplantation. *Am Surg.* (2019) 85:631–37. doi: 10.1177/000313481908500628
3. Chen R, Chen Q, Wu X, Che Y, Wang C, Wang L, et al. Development of a TaqMan based real-time fluorescent quantitative PCR assay for detection of porcine cytomegalovirus in semen. *Biomed Res Int.* (2020) 2020:5673145. doi: 10.1155/2020/5673145
4. Morozov VA, Plotzki E, Rotem A, Barkai U, Denner J. Extended microbiological characterization of *Göttingen minipigs*: porcine cytomegalovirus and other viruses. *Xenotransplantation.* (2016) 23:490–96. doi: 10.1111/xen.12265
5. Denner J. The porcine virome and xenotransplantation. *Virol J.* (2017) 14:171. doi: 10.1186/s12985-017-0836-z
6. McGregor CGA, Byrne GW. Porcine to human heart transplantation: is clinical application now appropriate? *J Immunol Res.* (2017) 2017:2534653. doi: 10.1155/2017/2534653
7. Gu W, Zeng N, Zhou L, Ge X, Guo X, Yang H. Genomic organization and molecular characterization of porcine cytomegalovirus. *Virology.* (2014) 460–1:165–72. doi: 10.1016/j.virol.2014.05.014
8. Liu X, Xu Z, Zhu L, Liao S, Guo W. Transcriptome analysis of porcine thymus following porcine cytomegalovirus infection. *PLoS ONE.* (2014) 9:e113921. doi: 10.1371/journal.pone.0113921
9. Rayat GR, Gazda LS, Hawthorne WJ, Hering BJ, Hosking P, Matsumoto S, et al. First update of the International Xenotransplantation Association consensus statement on conditions for undertaking clinical trials of porcine islet products in type 1 diabetes–Chapter 3: Porcine islet product manufacturing and release testing criteria. *Xenotransplantation.* (2016) 23:38–45. doi: 10.1111/xen.12225
10. Hamel AL, Lin L, Sachvie C, Grudeski E, Nayar GP. PCR assay for detecting porcine cytomegalovirus. *J Clin Microbiol.* (1999) 37:3767–8. doi: 10.1128/JCM.37.11.3767-3768.1999
11. Fryer JF, Griffiths PD, Fishman JA, Emery VC, Clark DA. Quantitation of porcine cytomegalovirus in pig tissues by PCR. *J Clin Microbiol.* (2001) 39:1155–6. doi: 10.1128/JCM.39.3.1155-1156.2001
12. Morozov VA, Morozov AV, Denner J. New PCR diagnostic systems for the detection and quantification of porcine cytomegalovirus (PCMV). *Arch Virol.* (2016) 161:1159–68. doi: 10.1007/s00705-016-2765-3
13. Tajima T, Hironao T, Kajikawa T, Suzuki Y, Kawamura H. Detection of the antibodies against porcine cytomegalovirus from whole blood collected on the blood sampling paper. *J Vet Med Sci.* (1994) 56:189–90. doi: 10.1292/jvms.56.189
14. Liu X, Zhu L, Shi X, Xu Z, Mei M, Xu W, et al. Indirect-blocking ELISA for detecting antibodies against glycoprotein B (gB) of porcine cytomegalovirus (PCMV). *J Virol Methods.* (2012) 186:30–5. doi: 10.1016/j.jviromet.2012.08.024
15. Yang JL, Zhang SH, Liu ZH, Yang R, Huang Y, Wen M. Development and evaluation of a loop-mediated isothermal amplification assay for the rapid detection of porcine cytomegalovirus under field conditions. *Virol J.* (2012) 9:321. doi: 10.1186/1743-422X-9-321
16. Plotzki E, Keller M, Ivanusic D, Denner J. A new Western blot assay for the detection of porcine cytomegalovirus (PCMV). *J Immunol Methods.* (2016) 437:37–42. doi: 10.1016/j.jim.2016.08.001
17. Morozov VA, Heinrichs G, Denner J. Effective detection of porcine cytomegalovirus using non-invasively taken samples from piglets. *Viruses.* (2017) 9:9. doi: 10.3390/v9010009
18. Sun SR, Ahmad K, Wu XB, Chen JS, Fu HY, Huang MT, et al. Development of quantitative real-time PCR assays for rapid and sensitive detection of two badnavirus species in sugarcane. *Biomed Res Int.* (2018) 2018:8678242. doi: 10.1155/2018/8678242
19. Dereeper A, Guignon V, Blanc G, Audic S, Buffet S, Chevenet F, et al.

Phylogeny.fr: robust phylogenetic analysis for the non-specialist. *Nucleic Acids Res.* (2008) 36:465–9. doi: 10.1093/nar/gkn180

20. Choi Y, Jeon BY, Shim TS, Jin H, Cho SN, Lee H. Development of a highly sensitive one-tube nested real-time PCR for detecting *Mycobacterium tuberculosis*. *Diagn Microbiol Infect Dis.* (2014) 80:299–303. doi: 10.1016/j.diagmicrobio.2014.08.009
21. Abrahão JS, Lima LS, Assis FL, Alves PA, Silva-Fernandes AT, Cota MM, et al. Nested-multiplex PCR detection of Orthopoxvirus and Parapoxvirus directly from exanthematic clinical samples. *Virol J.* (2009) 6:140. doi: 10.1186/1743-422X-6-140
22. Llop P, Bonaterra A, Penalver J, Lopez MM. Development of a highly sensitive nested-PCR procedure using a single closed tube for detection of *Erwinia amylovora* in asymptomatic plant material. *Appl Environ Microbiol.* (2000) 66:2071–8. doi: 10.1128/AEM.66.5.2071-2078.2000
23. Morris J, Clover GR, Harju VA, Hugo SA, Henry CM. Development of a highly sensitive nested RT-PCR method for Beet necrotic yellow vein virus detection. *J Virol Methods.* (2001) 95:163–9. doi: 10.1016/S0166-0934(01)00308-1
24. Shen XX, Qiu FZ, Zhao HL, Yang MJ, Hong L, Xu ST, et al. A novel and highly sensitive real-time nested RT-PCR assay in a single closed tube for detection of enterovirus. *Diagn Microbiol Infect Dis.* (2018) 90:181–5. doi: 10.1016/j.diagmicrobio.2017.11.015
25. Zhao L, Wang J, Li GX, Qiu FZ, Chen C, Zhao MC, et al. A highly sensitive 1-tube nested real-time RT-PCR assay using LNA-modified primers for detection of respiratory syncytial virus. *Diagn Microbiol Infect Dis.* (2019) 93:101–6. doi: 10.1016/j.diagmicrobio.2018.09.001

6

Evaluating the Risk Factors for *Porcine Epidemic Diarrhea Virus* Infection in an Endemic Area

Thi Ngan Mai [1,2], Thanh Phong Bui [3], Thi My Le Huynh [2], Yosuke Sasaki [4,5], Shuya Mitoma [1], Hala El Daous [1,6], Watcharapong Fahkrajang [7], Junzo Norimine [5,8] and Satoshi Sekiguchi [5,8]*

[1] Graduate School of Medicine and Veterinary Medicine, University of Miyazaki, Miyazaki, Japan, [2] Faculty of Veterinary Medicine, Vietnam National University of Agriculture, Hanoi, Vietnam, [3] Branch of Cargill Vietnam Co., Ltd, Dong Van II Industrial Zone, Ha Nam, Vietnam, [4] Department of Animal and Grassland Sciences, Faculty of Agriculture, University of Miyazaki, Miyazaki, Japan, [5] Center for Animal Disease Control, University of Miyazaki, Miyazaki, Japan, [6] Faculty of Veterinary Medicine, Benha University, Toukh, Egypt, [7] Department of Livestock Development, Ministry of Agriculture and Cooperatives, Bangkok, Thailand, [8] Department of Veterinary Science, Faculty of Agriculture, University of Miyazaki, Miyazaki, Japan

****Correspondence:***
Satoshi Sekiguchi
sekiguchi@cc.miyazaki-u.ac.jp

Porcine epidemic diarrhea virus (PEDV) causes enteritis, vomiting, watery diarrhea, and high mortality in suckling pigs, threatening the swine industry. Porcine epidemic diarrhea (PED) re-emerged globally in 2013 in many important swine-producing countries in Asia and the Americas. Several studies have identified the risk factors for the spread of PEDV in acute outbreaks. However, limited information is available on the risk factors for the transmission of PEDV in endemic regions. We hypothesized that poor biosecurity, location, and some social or cultural practices are the main risk factors for PEDV transmission in the Vietnamese pig population. The aim of this study was to evaluate the potential risk factors for the transmission of PEDV in an endemic area in Vietnam. In this case–control study, questionnaires containing 51 questions were completed for 92 PEDV-positive and 95 PEDV-negative farms. A logistic regression analysis was performed to assess the risk factors associated with PEDV infection. Province and the total number of pigs were included as random effects to determine their influence on the risk of PEDV infection. Twenty-nine variables of interest that have been associated with PEDV status were analyzed in a univariate analysis ($P < 0.20$), with backward stepwise selection. Only three of these 29 variables in four models remained significant PEDV risk factors in the final model: farrow-to-wean production type, distance from the farm to the slaughterhouse (< 1,000 m), and the presence of chickens on site ($P < 0.05$). This is the first study to identify the main risk factors for PEDV infection in an endemic area. Our findings suggest that hygiene measures should be strictly implemented on farms for the effective control and prevention of PEDV infection.

Keywords: *Porcine epidemic diarrhea virus*, case–control study, risk factor, endemic, Vietnam

INTRODUCTION

Porcine epidemic diarrhea virus (PEDV) causes enteritis, vomiting, watery diarrhea, and high mortality in < 10-day-old suckling pigs (almost 100%) and significant economic losses in the swine industry (1). PEDV re-emerged in 2013 and caused huge economic losses globally, in many important swine-producing countries in North America (USA, Canada, and Mexico) (2–4) and

Asia (South Korea, Japan, and Taiwan) (3, 5, 6). Direct contact between the pigs within farms is the primary transmission route of PEDV, via the fecal–oral route (7). Improvements in farm hygiene management and avoiding risky practices associated with contact with pig excrement are key factors in preventing the transmission of PEDV to farms (6). Several studies have comprehensively evaluated the risk factors for the spread of PEDV in the early phase of PEDV outbreaks (6, 8, 9). Indirect PEDV transmission through contaminated personal protection equipment occurs rapidly, within 24 h (10). In Japan, large-scale farms, proximity to an infected farm, number of feed trucks, short disinfectant contact time, and visiting veterinarians are factors strongly associated with the PEDV status of farms (11, 12). In the USA, transport is considered the main route of PEDV transmission (13, 14). In Italy, trucks have been shown to play an important role in the spread of PEDV (15). PEDV-contaminated feed was reported to be a significant risk factor for the transmission of PEDV between farms in the USA, Japan, and Canada (8, 9, 11, 16–18). Its transmission by transport vehicles was also reported to be a biological factor causing the rapid spread of PEDV in the USA and Japan (11, 13). Because PEDV is highly infectious and the infectious dose is low, it can be locally transmitted from PEDV-infected farms to neighboring PEDV-free farms through aerosol transmission or contaminated fomites (12, 19, 20). However, no study has analyzed the risk factors for PEDV spread in endemic areas or countries.

In Vietnam, PEDV was first observed in the southern provinces in 2009 (21). Published studies have demonstrated that PEDV is present in all major swine-producing regions in Vietnam (21–26). A descriptive survey recently provided evidence that northern Vietnam is an endemic area for PEDV, with a high proportion of PED-positive farms (30.89%) (Mai et al., unpublished). However, since its first detection, no specific PEDV control measures have been implemented by veterinary services to control the disease. Although vaccination or the feedback method has been applied on some pig farms, PEDV still occurs and frequently recurs. Our hypothesis is that the farm location and poor biosecurity measures for fomites, animals, and humans are the main risk factors for the nationwide transmission of PEDV in endemic areas. Some risk factors related to social and cultural practices in the Vietnamese swine industry could also play important roles in PEDV transmission among the pig population in Vietnam. Therefore, the objective of this study was to evaluate the potential risk factors for the widespread dissemination of PEDV in an endemic area with a case–control study. Theoutcome should extend our understanding of the dynamics of PEDV spread, in an effort to eliminate this economically important disease, which has emerged or re-emerged worldwide.

MATERIALS AND METHODS

Data Collection

In northern Vietnam, most piglets are produced and then transported to southernparts of the country. We have performed a survey between January 2018 and February 2019 to evaluate the proportion of PEDV-positive farms in a high-density pig population in northern Vietnam (**Figure 1**; the map was edited with PowerPoint from a screenshot of Google Maps [Map data©2020 Google]). The geographic location of Vietnam and the study area were mapped with the free, open-source Quantum Geographic Information System (QGIS) version 2.14.14 (https://www.qgis.org/en/site/). The required fecal sample size was estimated as 20 samples per farm. Therefore, on each farm, up to 20 fecal samples were collected from pigs in all ages. Then, 20 individual fecal samples from each farm were combined into two pooled samples (with a pooled size of 10 samples) for the test. Pooled samples were tested with reverse transcription (RT)–loop-mediated isothermal amplification (LAMP) (27). A "PEDV-positive farm" was defined as any swine herd with at least one positive result in two pooled samples from 20 samples collected from all-aged pigs. In total, 6,601 fecal samples were collected from 327 pig farms in northern Vietnam. The proportion of PEDV-positive farms was 30.9% (101 farms) and PEDV-positive farms were distributed throughout the study area. From the results of a PEDV survey of the pig population in northern Vietnam, there were 101 PEDV positive farms. All 101 PEDV-positive farms were selected as case farms, and 101 PEDV-negative farms, which were individually matched to a case farm based on the province in which they were located, were selected as the control farms for this study. The case and control farms were confirmed in 2018 with a PEDV survey to ensure that their management practices had not changed, even on the case farms, since 2018. We conducted a matched case–control study of the herd management practices for a period of 1 year (January—December, 2018). Questionnaires were sent to veterinarians or managers of these farms in July 2019, and the author (MTN) received the responses through the mail by the middle of August 2019.

Questionnaire

The questionnaire was developed based on known or published risk factors for PED and other infectious diseases of pigs (6, 9, 11, 13, 28). The designed questionnaire was checked by the authors (SS and YS) and then pre-tested with a selected number of veterinarians for the clarity and appropriateness of its content, questions, and responses in terms of the local situation, before the start of the study. Modifications were made if necessary.

Using a postal questionnaire survey, a case–control study was conducted on the PEDV-positive and -negative farms in northern Vietnam. The final version of the questionnaire contained 49 questions focusing on four main categories (**Table S1**).

Based on the actual data in Vietnam, PED frequently recurred in pig farms that had the presence of PEDV outbreaks in the past. To know whether there is a risk of the persistence of PEDV in these farms or not, only two questions applied specifically to the case farms. The first question concerned whether there had been an occurrence of PEDV in the preceding 2 years. If the answer was "yes," they were asked the second question, regarding how they dealt with PEDV on their farms.

Statistical Analysis

The outcome of interest for this study was the binary response variable "PEDV status," which took the value 1 if the farm was

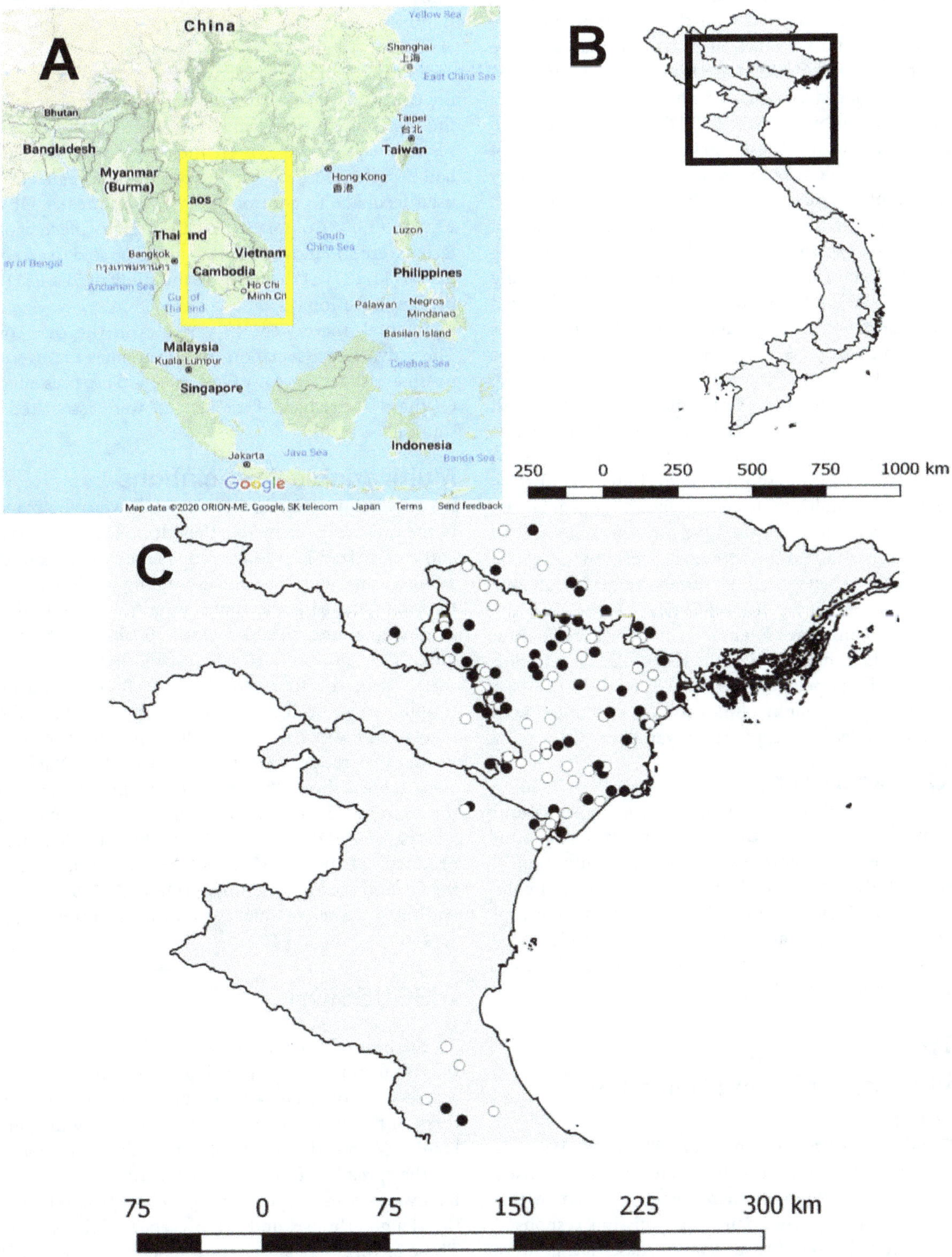

FIGURE 1 | Map of the study area. **(A)** Map is from Google Maps (Map data©2020 Google) and the yellow rectangle shows Vietnam. **(B)** Map of Vietnam; black square indicates the study area. **(C)** Locations of the 187 pig farms in northern Vietnam involved in this study. Black dots indicate PEDV case farms and white dots indicate PEDV control farms. Geographical locations of the farms were mapped with the Quantum Geographic Information System.

PEDV positive and 0 if the farm was PED negative according to RT–LAMP. The data captured with the questionnaire were entered into Microsoft Excel and all statistical analyses were performed with the statistical software R version 3.4.3 (CRAN, 2017). A univariate logistic regression analysis was performed to assess the association between PEDV status and each independent variable in the questionnaire. The significance of each explanatory variable was tested with the Wald test. Any variables significantly associated with PEDV status at the $P <$ 0.20 level were subsequently selected for multivariable modeling. Backwards stepwise explanatory variable selection, beginning with the least significant variable, was performed while observing the changes in Akaike's information criterion (AIC). The final model was obtained with P levels for the remaining variables of $<$ 0.05 and minimum AIC. After the main effects were identified, all possible two-way interactions were also examined. In this study, the total number of pigs did not correlate with PEDV status in the regression analysis. Therefore, to distinguish the influence of location (province) and the total number of pigs on the risk of PEDV, both variables were included as random effects in the multivariate model, by fitting generalized linear mixed-effects models. We used the lme4 package in R to analyze the fitted generalized linear mixed-effects models. The strengths of association between all the variables and the outcome were quantified by evaluating the odds ratios (ORs) and the corresponding 95% confidence intervals (CIs). The contribution of each variable in the final model of the risk of PEDV infection was quantified as the population attributable fraction (29). To avoid model convergence, multicollinearity was also tested with the variance inflation factor of explanatory variables (30).

Ethical Considerations

Informed consent was obtained in written form (by signature) or orally from all participants, who agreed to participate after they had received written information about the study. Ethical approval for the study was granted by the Hanoi School of Public Health Institutional Review Board, Hanoi, Vietnam (approval number 019-405/DD-YTCC) and the Animal Ethics Committee of the University of Miyazaki's Faculty of Agriculture, Miyazaki, Japan (approval number 2017–541).

RESULTS

Descriptive Statistics and Univariate Associations

In total, 187/202 (92.6%) respondents from 92/101 (91.1%) case farms and 95/101 (94.1%) control farms, located in a high-density pig-farming area in northern Vietnam, were included in this study (**Figure 1**). Some questionnaires had missing responses, which were excluded from the analysis. These farms were identified in a previous PEDV survey of the pig population in northern Vietnam. The data collected from these 187 farms were included in the analysis. In general, the number of pigs on the case farms was lower than the number on the control farms (mean numbers of pigs on the case and control farms were 1090 $\pm$ 1055.4 and 1533 $\pm$ 1661.4, respectively, $P > 0.05$). On average, the case farms had fewer vehicles visiting the farm per month than the control farms during the time of the study (mean numbers of vehicles per month on the case and control farms were 8.0 $\pm$ 4.3 and 8.4 $\pm$ 4.7, respectively, $P > 0.05$). However, the case farms contained more animal species other than pigs than the control farms (mean numbers of different animal species on the case and control farms were 3.6 $\pm$ 1.4 and 2.5 $\pm$ 1.5 species, respectively, $P < 0.05$). Of the 92 case farms, 52.17% (48/92) had experienced PEDV in the preceding 2 years and these farms used feedback to control the PEDV outbreaks. Of these farms, 27.08% (13/48) reported that the PEDV-infected pigs on their farms were still moved to other farms or sold to an abattoir. Only 5.88% (11/187) of the farms in the study used a PEDV vaccine to prevent infection.

In total, there were 49 variables in the case-control study. The univariate associations of 49 variables that were considered possible risk factors for PEDV infection are presented in **Table 1**. Of these 9 variables of interest, 29 were associated with PEDV status ($P < 0.20$).

Multivariable Associations

Because many variables (29 variables) were eligible for inclusion in the multivariable model, the selected variables were separated and categorized into four groups based on 4 main categories in **Table S1** and then four corresponding models were established. Backward stepwise selection was performed until the P-values of all the remaining variables were $<$ 0.1 in the four corresponding models. A new model was established using the remaining variables in the four models ($P < 0.1$) (6). Further stepwise simplification of the model has applied until the estimated regression coefficients for all the explanatory variables retained in the final model were significant on the Wald test at a $P <$ 0.05. **Table 2** shows the results of the final model. Only three of the 29 variables in these four models remained significant risk factors for PEDV infection in the final model: farrow-to-wean production (OR = 3.35, 95% CI: 1.51–7.43), close proximity of the farm to the slaughterhouse (OR = 7.15, 95% CI: 2.36–21.70), and the presence of chickens on the farm (OR = 3.36, 95% CI: 1.84–6.12) (AIC = 124.2).

DISCUSSION

To the best of our knowledge, this is the first study to quantify the risk factors for the spread of PEDV in an endemic area using a case–control strategy based on a questionnaire survey. Only three of the 49 variables tested remained significant risk factors for PEDV spread in the final model. The three main risk factors for the spread of PEDV in an endemic area in Vietnam are the farrow-to-wean production type, close proximity of the farm to the slaughterhouse, and the presence of chickens on the farm. These factors were significantly associated with the PEDV status of the farms.

In this study, there was a strong relationship between the distance from the farm to the slaughterhouse and the PEDV status of the farm. Close proximity to the slaughterhouse ($<$ 1,000 m) increased the risk of PEDV infection 7.15-fold relative to that on farms further from the slaughterhouse. Population attributed fraction is the proportion of disease in the population

TABLE 1 | Results of a univariate analysis of location variables in the risk of *Porcine epidemic diarrhea virus* infection in a case–control study of northern Vietnamese pig farms in 2018.

Groups	Variables	Category	No. of cases	Proportion of response (%)	No. of controls	Proportion of response (%)	OR (95% CI)	*P*-value
Farm location ($n = 8$)	Distance from farm to the closest farm	<200 m	24	26.1	17	17.9	1.96 (0.82–4.67)	0.127
		201–500 m	16	17.4	17	17.9	1.31 (0.52–3.26)	0.565
		501–1,000 m	34	37.0	36	37.9	1.31 (0.61–2.82)	0.487
		>1,000 m	18	19.6	25	26.3	Ref	
	Distance from farm to the main road	<200 m	24	26.1	14	14.7	3.31 (1.34–8.21)	0.009
		201–500 m	26	28.3	15	15.8	3.35 (1.38–8.16)	0.007
		501–1,000 m	27	29.3	37	38.9	1.41 (0.64–3.13)	0.396
		>1,000 m	15	16.3	29	30.5	Ref	
	Distance from farm to the residential area	<200 m	19	20.7	9	9.5	4.10 (1.53–10.98)	0.004
		201–500 m	24	26.1	25	26.3	1.86 (0.83–4.19)	0.13
		501–1,000 m	32	34.8	28	29.5	2.22 (1.02–4.81)	0.042
		>1,000 m	17	18.5	33	34.7	Ref	
	Distance from farm to the irrigation system	<200	54	58.7	40	42.1	2.16 (1.08–4.32)	0.028
		201–500 m	18	19.6	23	24.2	1.25 (0.54–2.88)	0.596
		>500 m	20	21.7	32	33.7	Ref	
	Distance from farm to the slaughterhouse	<=1,000 m	22	23.9	4	4.2	5.35 (1.68–17.07)	0.002
		Unknown	33	35.9	55	57.9	0.58 (0.31–1.10)	0.093
		>1,000 m	37	40.2	36	37.9	Ref	
	Distance from farm to local market	<500 m	12	13.0	2	2.1	9.27 (1.73–49.66)	0.004
		500–1,000 m	26	28.3	21	22.1	1.91 (0.74–4.96)	0.179
		1,001–5,000 m	43	46.7	55	57.9	1.21 (0.51–2.85)	0.665
		>5,000 m	11	12.0	17	17.9	Ref	
	Distance from barn to living room	<10 m	21	22.8	18	18.9	1.71 (0.69–4.25)	0.246
		10–20 m	21	22.8	23	24.2	1.34 (0.55–3.24)	0.517
		21–50 m	35	38.0	32	33.7	1.60 (0.71–3.62)	0.253
		>50 m	15	16.3	22	23.2	Ref	
	Distance from barn to the pig loading/unloading place	<=50 m	62	67.4	49	51.6	1.94 (1.07–3.51)	0.028
		>50 m	30	32.6	46	48.4	Ref	
Farm management ($n = 20$)	Farm status	Private	28	30.4	29	30.5	1.00 (0.53–1.86)	0.989
		Company	64	69.6	66	69.5	Ref	
	Production type	FF	20	21.7	26	27.4	0.99 (0.49–1.98)	0.97
		FW	26	28.3	10	10.5	3.33 (1.46–7.61)	0.003
		WF	46	50.0	59	62.1	Ref	
	Total pigs	<500	28	30.4	28	29.5	Ref	
		500–1,000	31	33.7	24	25.3	1.29 (0.61–2.73)	0.502
		1,000–1,500	18	19.6	15	15.8	1.20 (0.51–2.84)	0.679
		>1,500	15	16.3	28	29.5	0.54 (0.24–1.21)	0.133
	All-in/all-out policy in each barn	No	27	29.3	23	24.2	1.30 (0.68–2.49)	0.427
		Yes	65	70.7	72	75.8		
	Pig movement	Pig addition	10	37.0	4	17.4	Ref	
		Pig removal	9	33.3	11	47.8	0.33 (0.08–1.40)	0.127
		Both	8	29.6	4	17.4	0.8 (0.15–4.24)	0.793
	Separate place for pig movement	No	21	22.8	17	17.9	1.36 (0.66–2.78)	0.402
		Yes	71	77.2	78	82.1		
	Pig movement place is located on farm's property	No	17	18.5	15	15.8	1.21 (0.56–2.59)	0.625
		Yes	75	81.5	80	84.2		
	Truck through the same route at entrance and exit	Yes	89	96.7	87	91.6	2.73 (0.7–10.62)	0.134
		No	3	3.3	8	8.4		

(Continued)

TABLE 1 | Continued

Groups	Variables	Category	No. of cases	Proportion of response (%)	No. of controls	Proportion of response (%)	OR (95% CI)	*P*-value
	Source of trucks for the pig transport to the slaughterhouse	Slaughterhouse trucks	48	52.2	38	40.0		0.095
		Business operator trucks	44	47.8	57	60.0	1.64 (0.92–2.92)	
	Having a separate worker in isolation barn	No	64	69.6	57	60.0	1.52 (0.83–2.79)	0.171
		Yes	28	30.4	38	40.0		
	Opened barn type	Yes	18	19.6	14	14.7	1.41 (0.65–3.03)	0.381
		No	74	80.4	81	85.3		
	Water source	Direct	49	53.3	25	26.3	3.19 (1.73–5.89)	<0.001
		Indirect	43	46.7	70	73.7	Ref	
	Feeding swill to pigs	Yes	4	4.3	0	0.0	Inf	0.04
		No	88	95.7	95	100.0		
	Having workers in farm	Yes	76	82.6	71	74.7	1.61 (0.79–3.27)	0.189
		No	16	17.4	24	25.3		
	Changing workers	Monthly	6	6.5	2	2.1	1.98 (0.37–10.44)	0.414
		6 months	12	13.0	7	7.4	1.13 (0.40–3.19)	0.816
		Yearly	17	18.5	33	34.7	0.34 (0.16–0.71)	0.004
		No	47	51.1	31	32.6	Ref	
	Living place of workers after finishing work on the farm	Staying at farms	46	50.0	45	47.4	Ref	
		Go home	8	8.7	5	5.3	1.13 (0.40–3.19)	0.458
		Both	32	34.8	38	40.0	0.34 (0.16–0.71)	0.543
	Waste treatment applies in your farm	No	9	9.8	3	3.2	3.33 (0.87–12.70)	0.065
		Yes	83	90.2	92	96.8		
	Manure application	Feed for fish	7	7.6	3	3.2	7.58 (1.75–32.78)	0.003
		Applied on land inside farm	25	27.2	17	17.9	4.78 (2.08–10.99)	<0.001
		Mixed type	44	47.8	23	24.2	6.22 (2.93–13.21)	<0.001
		Sold	16	17.4	52	54.7	Ref	
	Share boars with other farms	Yes	10	10.9	11	11.6	0.93 (0.38–2.31)	0.878
		No	82	89.1	84	88.4		
	Addition ingredients in feed	Antibiotic	36	39.1	49	51.6	0.69 (0.29–1.60)	0.381
		Probiotic	4	4.3	4	4.2	0.93 (0.20–4.47)	0.931
		Both	37	40.2	28	29.5	1.23 (0.51–2.97)	0.64
		None	15	16.3	14	14.7	Ref	
Biosecurity practice and health management ($n = 11$)	Disinfection of environment on premises	Monthly	4	4.3	4	4.2	1.03 (0.25–4.26)	0.963
		Weekly	88	95.7	91	95.8		
	Biosecurity practices apply to people inside farm	High	67	72.8	69	72.6	Ref	
		Intermediate	23	25.0	21	22.1	1.13 (0.57–2.23)	0.729
		Low	2	2.2	5	5.3	0.41 (0.08–2.20)	0.285
	Biosecurity practices apply to visitors	High	55	59.8	63	66.3	Ref	
		Intermediate	21	22.8	17	17.9	1.41 (0.68–2.95)	0.353
		Low	16	17.4	15	15.8	1.22 (0.55–2.70)	0.62
	Biosecurity practices apply at pig loading/unloading place	High	54	58.7	50	52.6	Ref	
		Intermediate	26	28.3	22	23.2	1.09 (0.55–2.17)	0.797
		Low	12	13.0	23	24.2	0.48 (0.22–1.07)	0.071
	Time that vehicles must wait after disinfection to get into the farm	≤2 h	71	77.2	82	86.3	0.54 (0.25–1.15)	0.105
		>2 h	21	22.8	13	13.7	Ref	

(Continued)

TABLE 1 | Continued

Groups	Variables	Category	No. of cases	Proportion of response (%)	No. of controls	Proportion of response (%)	OR (95% CI)	*P*-value
	Time that vehicles must wait after disinfection to get into the farm	<30 min	15	16.3	20	21.1	Ref	
		30–60 min	55	59.8	46	48.4	1.59 (0.73–3.46)	0.237
		>60 min	22	23.9	29	30.5	1.01 (0.42–2.41)	0.979
	Diseases happen in farm	High	40	43.5	33	34.7	1.73 (0.59–5.05)	0.311
		Intermediate	45	48.9	52	54.7	1.24 (0.43–3.52)	0.69
		Low	7	7.6	10	10.5	Ref	
	Vaccination applying in farm	High	42	45.7	47	49.5	Ref	
		Intermediate	39	42.4	43	45.3	1.01 (0.56–1.85)	0.961
		Low	11	12.0	5	5.3	2.46 (0.79–7.67)	0.112
	Source of human food	Local market	78	84.8	72	75.8	1.69 (0.69–4.13)	0.25
		Supermarket	5	5.4	9	9.5	0.86 (0.22–3.43)	0.835
		Inside farm	9	9.8	14	14.7	Ref	
	Human food including pig products	Yes	21	22.8	16	16.8	1.46 (0.71–3.02)	0.304
		No	71	77.2	79	83.2		
	Cook human food before entering farm	No	81	88.0	80	84.2	1.38 (0.60–3.19)	0.449
		Yes	11	12.0	15	15.8		
People, animal and vehicle contact ($n = 10$)	Visiting of vet	Daily	6	6.5	5	5.3	1.37 (0.29–6.53)	0.691
		Weekly	29	31.5	28	29.5	1.18 (0.38–3.70)	0.772
		Monthly	50	54.3	54	56.8	1.06 (0.36–3.13)	0.919
		No	7	7.6	8	8.4	Ref	
	Other visitors	Yes	47	51.1	37	38.9	1.64 (0.92–2.93)	0.095
		No	45	48.9	58	61.1		
	Presence of wild birds inside farm	Yes	47	51.1	32	33.7	2.06 (1.14–3.71)	0.016
		No	45	48.9	63	66.3		
	Presence of rodents inside farm	Yes	86	93.5	59	62.1	8.75 (3.57–22.07)	<0.001
		No	6	6.5	36	37.9		
	Presence of chicken in farm	Yes	58	63.0	32	33.7	3.36 (1.84–6.12)	<0.001
		No	34	37.0	63	66.3		
	Presence of ducks in farm	Yes	31	33.7	23	24.2	1.59 (0.84–3.01)	0.152
		No	61	66.3	72	75.8		
	Presence of dog in farm	Yes	78	84.8	80	84.2	1.04 (0.47–2.31)	0.914
		No	14	15.2	15	15.8		
	Presence of cat in farm	Yes	31	33.7	14	14.7	2.94 (1.44–6.0)	0.002
		No	61	66.3	81	85.3		
	Vehicles visit another farm on the same day/trip	Yes	7	7.6	8	8.4	1.01 (0.34–2.97)	0.986
		Unknown	33	35.9	27	28.4	1.41 (0.75–2.65)	0.284
		No	52	56.5	60	63.2	Ref	
	Number of truck vehicles visit to farm/month	High	14	15.2	22	23.2	0.58 (0.27–1.28)	0.177
		Intermediate	29	31.5	28	29.5	0.95 (0.49–1.84)	0.882
		Low	49	53.3	45	47.4	Ref	

TABLE 2 | Results of the final multivariate model of risk factors associated with *Porcine epidemic diarrhea virus* in a case–control study on northern Vietnamese pig farms in 2018.

Variables	OR	95% CI	Coefficient	SE	Z-Statistic	*P*-value
Intercept			−0.9694	0.4587	−2.113	0.0346
Production type (FW)	3.35	1.51–7.43	1.6194	0.6473	2.502	0.0124
Near distance to the slaughterhouse (<1,000 m)	7.15	2.36–21.70	1.9391	0.7085	2.737	0.0062
Presence of chicken	3.36	1.84–6.12	1.1282	0.5646	1.998	0.0457

that is due to expose (29, 31). The population attributable fraction for this risk factor was 20.57% (95% CI 10.26–29.70), so eliminating or completely preventing its effects would reduce the incidence of PEDV by 20.57%. Cross-contamination of farm vehicles is reported to occur at slaughterhouses (11, 13). There are few central slaughterhouses in Vietnam, and pigs are commonly slaughtered at a slaughtering point near the house of a butcher or pig trader to supply meat to traditional markets. This partly explains why 47.06% (88/187) of the farms in this study reported "unknown distance" in response to the question on this variable. In this study, 27.08% (13/48) of the farms that had experienced PEDV in the preceding 2 years still moved or sold infected pigs to slaughterhouses or other farms. Moving the infected pigs to slaughterhouses could be a risk for environmental contamination of facility because of pigs shedding the virus in feces which can be tracked back to farms. Moving infected pigs has been shown to play a role in the spread of PEDV among farms (13, 14). The open transportation of pigs and pig products from the slaughterhouse to the local market on motorbikes, which is a popular transport method in Vietnam, could also explain why variables related to the farm location, such as the distance from the farm to the main road (< 500 m), the distance from the farm to the local market (< 500 m), and the distance from the farm to the residential area (< 200 m), were associated with the risk of PEDV infection in the univariate analysis. PEDV is known to persist on pig transportation vehicles especially if not disinfected post-use for transportation (13). All the reasons cited above could increase the risk of PEDV infection on farms close to slaughterhouses through the cross-contamination between animals, vehicles, fomites, and humans, and through the movement of animals or aerosol transmission. Increases in the risk of PEDV transmission have also been attributed to the movement of animals and aerosol transmission in previous studies (14, 32).

Another finding of the present study was the strong relationship between the presence of chickens on the farms and PEDV status (OR = 3.36, 95% CI: 1.84–6.12). Other animal species were also more frequently present on the case farms than on the control farms (average numbers of other animal species on the case and control farms were 3.6 ± 1.4 and 2.5 ± 1.5, respectively). Movements of animals between farms and other neighborhood features were indicated to be the most important factors associated with PEDV occurrence (33). Previous studies have also demonstrated that other animals on pig farms can transmit PEDV. PEDV was found in the tonsils in 4.2% of cats, suggesting that cats may play a role in the transmission of PEDV on swine farms (28). Experience in the USA suggests that the transmission of PEDV is related to bird traffic (32). Therefore, the transmission of PEDV on the case farms may be attributable to animal contact because animal species other than pigs were recorded on site. For example, 22.2% of the case farms had both cats and dogs, and another 22.2% of case farms had only cats (8). In our study, although the presence of other animal species (including wild birds, rodents, and cats) did not remain a risk factor in the final model, it was significantly associated with PEDV status in the univariate analysis. Furthermore, 31 of 92 (33.7%) case farms reported having ducks and 78/92 (84.78%) reported having dogs. Therefore, the presence of other animal species in general and especially the presence of chickens on the farms could play a role in the transmission of PEDV through animal contact and movement. Animal movement is an important mechanisms of pathogen transmission.

In this study, the farrow-to-wean production type was related to PEDV status, and had a 3.35-fold (95% CI: 1.51–7.43) higher risk of PEDV infection than other production systems. When PEDV infection occurs on a pig farm, it usually spreads among pigs of different ages. However, pigs display age-dependent resistance to pathogenic PEDV infection (34, 35). The virus accumulates and infects pregnant sows, and the subclinically infected sows transmit PEDV to the suckling piglets. The virus is then transferred to pigs of different ages (36). In another study, PEDV was considered to have been introduced in feeder pigs, fattening pigs, and adult pigs, and then spread to piglets (37). In the early phase of PEDV outbreaks, sow farms have had the highest incidence of PEDV (80.0%) (19, 32). However, after an acute outbreak, PEDV may remain in the farrowing unit because of poor biosecurity or persist in pigs in weaning or growing–finishing units, where the virus circulates (32). The number of sows on a farm is thought to play a role in the persistence of PEDV after the original outbreak (37). Of the case farms in the present study, 52.17% (48/92) had experienced PEDV in the preceding 2 years, and 68.75% (33/48) of these were sow farms (farrow-to-finish and farrow to wean production types). These outbreaks could have been caused by PEDV that was still circulating on these farms after the previous outbreak, which acted as the source of the recurrent epidemic outbreaks. This may explain why PED outbreaks occur periodically in endemic regions.

The application of manure as a biosecurity issue did not remain a risk factor for PEDV spread in the final model. However, there was a strong relationship between manure application and PEDV status in the univariate analysis. A previous study indicated that PEDV may persist in a herd long after its clinical impact (32). Previous studies have also provided evidence that PEDV can survive for up to 28 days in manure between −20 and 4 °C, and for up to 9 months in infected earthen manure stored at temperatures ranging from −30 to 23 °C (32, 38). In the present study, 68/187 farms sold manure from the farm, which could be a risk factor for the wide transmission of PEDV to other farms if the virus was present in the manure. Risk factors based on social or cultural practices, such as water sources (direct from drilled wells or irrigation systems), were not included in the final model, but were associated with PEDV status in the univariate analysis. In Vietnam, water for pig rearing can be taken from the irrigation system surrounding the farm, drilled wells, or fish ponds. Dead pigs are often thrown into the river. Therefore, there is a high risk of introducing PEDV into the irrigation system or groundwater, which could then be dispersed by the water flow. Therefore, to prevent further transmission of PEDV, it is necessary to raise public awareness about the risk entailed by social and cultural practices in pig raising in Vietnam.

Our study had several limitations. The accuracy of the information depended partly on the professional ability of each veterinarian or farm manager, whose knowledge of the epidemiology of PEDV could be limited. Second, bias may have been introduced by the time lag between the PEDV occurrence on farms and the questionnaire survey. Third, the respondents may have answered questions involving sensitive issues incorrectly. Typical examples are how sick pigs (selling) or dead pigs (throw away) are dealt with. In addition, the selection of PEDV-negative farm could affect the analysis for the identification of risk factors.

CONCLUSIONS

This is the first study to identify the three main risk factors for the spread of PEDV in an endemic area: the presence of chickens on the farm, close proximity to the slaughterhouse, and the farrow-to-wean production type. It is also the first study to show the distance to the slaughterhouse can play an important role in transmitting PEDV and to indicate this was the principal risk factor associated with the endemic area. In addition, the mechanical transmission by the presence of chicken in the farm that caused by the movement of chicken could be some way to explain the widespread of PEDV.

ETHICS STATEMENT

The studies involving human participants were reviewed and approved by Informed consent was obtained in written form (by signature) or orally from all participants, who agreed to participate after they had received written information about the study. Ethical approval for the study was granted by the Hanoi School of Public Health Institutional Review Board, Hanoi, Vietnam (Approval Number 019-405/DD-YTCC) and the Animal Ethics Committee of the University of Miyazaki's Faculty of Agriculture, Miyazaki, Japan (Approval Number 2017–541). The patients/participants provided their written informed consent to participate in this study.

AUTHOR CONTRIBUTIONS

TM designed the questionnaire, performed the study, analyzed the data, and drafted the manuscript. TB participated in the distribution and collection the questionnaires. YS participated in the design of the questionnaire, reviewed the drafts of the manuscript, and suggested revisions. TH, SM, HD, WF, and JN reviewed the drafts and suggested revisions. SS conceptualized and supervised the study, and analyzed and revised the manuscript. All authors read and approved the final manuscript.

ACKNOWLEDGMENTS

We are grateful to all the veterinarians and farm managers who participated in this study. We thank Janine Miller, Ph.D., from Edanz Group (www.edanzediting.com/ac) for editing a draft of this manuscript.

REFERENCES

1. Sun R, Cai RJ, Chen YQ, Liang PS, Chen DK, Song CX. Outbreak of porcine epidemic diarrhea in suckling piglets, China. *Emerg Infect Dis.* (2012) 18:161–3. doi: 10.3201/eid1801.111259
2. Kochhar HS. Canada: porcine epidemic diarrhea in Canada: an emerging disease case study. *Can Vet J.* (2014) 55:1048–9.
3. Lee C. *Porcine epidemic diarrhea virus*: an emerging and re-emerging epizootic swine virus. *Virol J.* (2015) 12:193. doi: 10.1186/s12985-015-0421-2
4. Niederwerder MC, Hesse RA. Swine enteric coronavirus disease: a review of 4 years with *Porcine epidemic diarrhoea virus* and porcine deltacoronavirus in the United States and Canada. *Transbound Emerg Dis.* (2018) 65:660–75. doi: 10.1111/tbed.12823
5. Lin CN, Chung WB, Chang SW, Wen CC, Liu H, Chien CH, et al. US-like strain of *Porcine epidemic diarrhea virus* outbreaks in Taiwan, 2013-2014. *J Vet Med Sci.* (2014) 76:1297–99. doi: 10.1292/jvms.14-0098
6. Toyomaki H, Sekiguchi S, Sasaki Y, Sueyoshi M, Makita K. Factors associated with farm-level infection of porcine epidemic diarrhea during the early phase of the epidemic in Japan in 2013 and 2014. *Prev Vet Med.* (2018) 150:77–85. doi: 10.1016/j.prevetmed.2017.12.008
7. Kim SH, Lee JM, Jung J, Kim IJ, Hyun BH, Kim HI, et al. Genetic characterization of *Porcine epidemic diarrhea virus* in Korea from 1998 to 2013. *Arch Virol.* (2015) 160:1055–64. doi: 10.1007/s00705-015-2353-y
8. Perri AM, Poljak Z, Dewey C, Harding JCS, O'Sullivan TL. An epidemiological investigation of the early phase of the porcine epidemic diarrhea (PED) outbreak in Canadian swine herds in 2014: a case-control study. *Prev Vet Med.* (2018) 150:101–9. doi: 10.1016/j.prevetmed.2017.12.009
9. Pasick J, Berhane Y, Ojkic D, Maxie G, Embury-Hyatt C, Swekla K, et al. Investigation into the role of potentially contaminated feed as a source of the first-detected outbreaks of porcine epidemic diarrhea in Canada. *Transbound Emerg Dis.* (2014) 61:397–410. doi: 10.1111/tbed.12269
10. Kim Y, Yang M, Goyal SM, Cheeran MCJ, Torremorell M. Evaluation of biosecurity measures to prevent indirect transmission of *Porcine epidemic diarrhea virus*. *BMC Vet Res.* (2017) 13:89. doi: 10.1186/s12917-017-1017-4
11. Sasaki Y, Alvarez J, Sekiguchi S, Sueyoshi M, Otake S, Perez A. Epidemiological factors associated to spread of porcine epidemic diarrhea in Japan. *Prev Vet Med.* (2016) 123:161–7. doi: 10.1016/j.prevetmed.2015.11.002
12. Sasaki Y, Toyomaki H, Sekiguchi S, Sueyoshi M, Makita K, Otake S, et al. Spatial dynamics of porcine epidemic diarrhea (PED) spread in the southern Kyushu, Japan. *Prev Vet Med.* (2017) 144:81–8. doi: 10.1016/j.prevetmed.2017.05.025
13. Lowe J, Gauger P, Harmon K, Zhang J, Connor J, Yeske P, et al. Role of transportation in spread of *Porcine epidemic diarrhea virus* infection, United States. *Emerg Infect Dis.* (2014) 20:872–4. doi: 10.3201/eid2005.131628
14. O'Dea EB, Snelson H, Bansal S. Using heterogeneity in the population structure of U.S. swine farms to compare transmission models for porcine epidemic diarrhoea. *Sci Rep.* (2016) 6:22248. doi: 10.1038/srep22248
15. Boniotti MB, Papetti A, Bertasio C, Giacomini E, Lazzaro M, Cerioli M, et al. *Porcine epidemic diarrhoea virus* in Italy: disease spread and the role of transportation. *Transbound Emerg Dis.* (2018) 65:1935–42. doi: 10.1111/tbed.12974
16. Dee S, Neill C, Singrey A, Clement T, Cochrane R, Jones C, et al. Modeling the transboundary risk of feed ingredients contaminated with *Porcine epidemic diarrhea virus*. *BMC Vet Res.* (2016) 12:51. doi: 10.1186/s12917-016-0674-z
17. Bowman AS, Krogwold RA, Price T, Davis M, Moeller SJ. Investigating the

introduction of *Porcine epidemic diarrhea virus* into an Ohio swine operation. *BMC Vet Res.* (2015) 11:38. doi: 10.1186/s12917-015-0348-2
18. Dee S, Clement T, Schelkopf A, Nerem J, Knudsen D, Christopher-Hennings J, et al. An evaluation of contaminated complete feed as a vehicle for *Porcine epidemic diarrhea virus* infection of naive pigs following consumption via natural feeding behavior: proof of concept. *BMC Vet Res.* (2014) 10:176. doi: 10.1186/s12917-014-0176-9
19. Alvarez J, Goede D, Morrison R, Perez A. Spatial and temporal epidemiology of porcine epidemic diarrhea (PED) in the Midwest and Southeast regions of the United States. *Prev Vet Med.* (2016) 123:155–60. doi: 10.1016/j.prevetmed.2015.11.003
20. Alvarez J, Sarradell J, Morrison R, Perez A. Impact of porcine epidemic diarrhea on performance of growing pigs. *PLoS ONE.* (2015) 10:e0120532. doi: 10.1371/journal.pone.0120532
21. Do TD, Nguyen TT, Suphasawatt P, Roongroje T. Genetic characterization of *Porcine epidemic diarrhea virus* (PEDV) isolates from Southern Vietnam during 2009–2010 outbreaks. *Thai J Vet Med.* (2011) 41:55–64. doi: 10.1002/vms3.256
22. Vui DT, Thanh TL, Tung N, Srijangwad A, Tripipat T, Chuanasa T, et al. Complete genome characterization of *Porcine epidemic diarrhea virus* in Vietnam. *Arch Virol.* (2015) 160:1931–8. doi: 10.1007/s00705-015-2463-6
23. Vui DT, Tung N, Inui K, Slater S, Nilubol D. Complete genome sequence of *Porcine epidemic diarrhea virus* in Vietnam. *Genome Announc.* (2014) 2:e00753-14. doi: 10.1128/genomeA.00753-14
24. Kim YK, Lim SI, Lim JA, Cho IS, Park EH, Le VP, et al. A novel strain of *Porcine epidemic diarrhea virus* in Vietnamese pigs. *Arch Virol.* (2015) 160:1573–7. doi: 10.1007/s00705-015-2411-5
25. Diep NV, Sueyoshi M, Izzati U, Fuke N, Teh APP, Lan NT, et al. Appearance of US-like *Porcine epidemic diarrhoea virus* (PEDV) strains before US outbreaks and genetic heterogeneity of PEDVs collected in Northern Vietnam during 2012–2015. *Transbound Emerg Dis.* (2018) 65:e83–93. doi: 10.1111/tbed.12681
26. Choe SE, Park KH, Lim SI, Le VP, Hien NB, Thach PN, et al. Complete genome sequence of a *Porcine epidemic diarrhea virus* strain from Vietnam, HUA-14PED96, with a large genomic deletion. *Genome Announc.* (2016) 4:e00002-16. doi: 10.1128/genomeA.00002-16
27. Mai T, Nguyen VD, Yamazaki W, Okabayashi T, Mitoma S, Notsu K, et al. Development of pooled testing system for porcine epidemic diarrhoea using real-time fluorescent reverse-transcription loop-mediated isothermal amplification assay. *BMC Vet Res.* (2018) 14:172. doi: 10.1186/s12917-018-1498-9
28. Truong QL, Seo TW, Yoon BI, Kim HC, Han JH, Hahn TW. Prevalence of swine viral and bacterial pathogens in rodents and stray cats captured around pig farms in Korea. *J Vet Med Sci.* (2013) 75:1647–50. doi: 10.1292/jvms.12-0568
29. Whittemore AS. Statistical methods for estimating attributable risk from retrospective data. *Stat Med.* (1982) 1:229–43. doi: 10.1002/sim.4780010305
30. O'brien RM. A Caution regarding rules of thumb for variance inflation factors. *Qual Quant.* (2007) 41:673–90. doi: 10.1007/s11135-006-9018-6
31. Brooks-Pollock E, Danon L. Defining the population attributable fraction for infectious diseases. *Int J Epidemiol.* (2017) 46:976–82. doi: 10.1093/ije/dyx055
32. Beam A, Goede D, Fox A, McCool MJ, Wall G, Haley C, et al. A *Porcine epidemic diarrhea virus* outbreak in one geographic region of the United States: descriptive epidemiology and investigation of the possibility of airborne virus spread. *PLoS ONE.* (2015) 10:e0144818. doi: 10.1371/journal.pone.0144818
33. Machado G, Vilalta C, Recamonde-Mendoza M, Corzo C, Torremorell M, Perez A, et al. Identifying outbreaks of *Porcine epidemic diarrhea virus* through animal movements and spatial neighborhoods. *Sci Rep.* (2019) 9:457. doi: 10.1038/s41598-018-36934-8
34. Shibata I, Tsuda T, Mori M, Ono M, Sueyoshi M, Uruno K. Isolation of *Porcine epidemic diarrhea virus* in porcine cell cultures and experimental infection of pigs of different ages. *Vet Microbiol.* (2000) 72:173–82. doi: 10.1016/S0378-1135(99)00199-6
35. Koike N, Mai TN, Shirai M, Kubo M, Hata K, Marumoto N, et al. Detection of neutralizing antibody against *Porcine epidemic diarrhea virus* in subclinically infected finishing pigs. *J Vet Med Sci.* (2018) 80:1782–6. doi: 10.1292/jvms.18-0132
36. Wang D, Fang L, Xiao S. Porcine epidemic diarrhea in China. *Virus Res.* (2016) 226:7–13. doi: 10.1016/j.virusres.2016.05.026
37. Pensaert MB, Martelli P. Porcine epidemic diarrhea: a retrospect from Europe and matters of debate. *Virus Res.* (2016) 226:1–6. doi: 10.1016/j.virusres.2016.05.030
38. Tun HM, Cai Z, Khafipour E. Monitoring survivability and infectivity of *Porcine epidemic diarrhea virus* (PEDv) in the infected on-farm earthen manure storages (EMS). *Front Microbiol.* (2016) 7:265. doi: 10.3389/fmicb.2016.00265

7

Concept of an Active Surveillance System for Q Fever in German Small Ruminants—Conflicts between Best Practices and Feasibility

Fenja Winter[1*], Clara Schoneberg[1], Annika Wolf[2], Benjamin U. Bauer[2], T. Louise Prüfer[3], Silke F. Fischer[4], Ursula Gerdes[5], Martin Runge[3], Martin Ganter[2] and Amely Campe[1]

[1] Department of Biometry, Epidemiology and Information Processing, WHO Collaborating Centre for Research and Training for Health at the Human-Animal-Environment Interface, University of Veterinary Medicine Hannover Foundation, Hanover, Germany, [2] Clinic for Swine, Small Ruminants and Forensic Medicine, University of Veterinary Medicine Hannover Foundation, Hanover, Germany, [3] Lower Saxony State Office for Consumer Protection and Food Safety – Food and Veterinary Institute Braunschweig/Hannover, Hanover, Germany, [4] National Consulting Laboratory for Coxiella burnetii, State Health Office Baden-Württemberg, Stuttgart, Germany, [5] Animal Disease Fund of Lower Saxony, Public Law Institution, Hanover, Germany

***Correspondence:**
Fenja Winter
fenja.winter@tiho-hannover.de

Q fever is a zoonotic disease caused by the bacterium *Coxiella burnetii*. Inhalation of contaminated dust particles or aerosols originating from animals (esp. small ruminants) is the main source of human infection. Hence, an active early warning system for Q fever in German small ruminant livestock was conceptualized to prevent human infections. First, we describe the best practice for establishing this system before evaluating its feasibility, as the combination of both evokes conflicts. Vaginal swabs from all husbandry systems with a focus on reproductive females should pooled and investigated by PCR to detect *C. burnetii*-shedding animals. Multistage risk-based sampling shall be carried out at the flock level and within-flock level. At the flock level, all flocks that are at risk to transmit the pathogen to the public must be sampled. At the within-flock level, all primi- and multiparous females after lambing must be tested in order to increase the probability of identifying a positive herd. Sampling should be performed during the main lambing period and before migration in residential areas. Furthermore, individual animals should be tested before migration or exhibition to ensure a negative status. If a flock tests positive in at least one individual sample, then flock-specific preventive measures should be implemented. This approach implies huge financial costs (sample testing, action/control measures). Hence, taking the step to develop more feasible and affordable preventive measures, e.g., vaccinating small ruminant flocks, should replace testing wherever justifiable.

Keywords: surveillance system, *Coxiella burnetii*, small ruminants, one health, early warning

INTRODUCTION

Infectious Agent

Coxiella burnetii is a small, obligate intracellular, pleomorphic Gram-negative bacterium. Because of its high tenacity, *C. burnetii* can be infectious in raw milk for 90–273 days at 4–6°C as well as in raw milk products like butter and soft cheese for 42 days at 20°C. In dust and wool, it can be infectious over 7–24 months depending on the surrounding temperature. *C. burnetii* evokes a zoonotic and mainly airborne disease called Q fever (1, 2).

Affected Species

Humans become infected by inhalation of dust particles or aerosols contaminated with only a few *C. burnetii* organisms (3, 4). Human infections through consumption of raw milk or raw milk products like butter or soft cheese is possible but rare. There is no transmission from man to man except some rare exceptions, e.g., by blood transfusion or during childbirth (5). Infections with *C. burnetii* remain subclinical in nearly 50% of patients. However, unspecific flu-like symptoms, hepatitis, or atypical pneumonia are possible consequences of acute Q fever, which may led to hospitalization (6, 7). In addition, approximately 20% of the patients are at risk of developing chronic fatigue after an infection (Q fever fatigue syndrome, QFS) (8). In <1% of the infected patients, chronic Q fever manifests in the form of endocarditis or hepatitis with a high mortality rate. Furthermore, Q fever is a risk for pregnancy (6, 7).

In animals, many species such as wild or domestic mammals and ticks can be infected by *C. burnetii* and spread this pathogen into the environment (6, 7, 9, 10). In Germany, infected (small) ruminants kept as livestock are the main source of pathogen transmission to humans (1, 11, 12). (Small) ruminants are infected by inhalation of *C. burnetii*, while other transmission routes (e.g., sexual, intrauterine, oral, infestation with ticks) are still being studied (7, 13–16). Therefore, pathogen transmission may take place through reservoir animals, which may be part of a flock or external (e.g., wild mammals but also dogs, cats other ruminant species, or ticks). These reservoir species may have some importance in maintaining *C. burnetii* in livestock as the most important factors here are contamination of the environment by their excretes as well as direct contact with livestock on the pasture. Pathogen transmission from wildlife to humans is rarely documented but is possible and should be considered when the source of infection cannot be identified (6, 7, 10, 11, 15). Concentrating on livestock, *C. burnetii*-infected sheep excrete the bacterium mainly in high concentrations in amniotic fluid, placenta and lochia during physiological birth or abortion. Moreover, excretion in milk, feces, urine, or semen is possible (1, 13, 17, 18). Goats and cattle also excrete the pathogen at the highest concentrations in birth products or with abortion, although the excretion period is longest in milk (17, 19–22). Q fever in sheep is mostly asymptomatic with an abortion rate of approximately 5–20% (23). In contrast, Q fever in goats is connected to abortion in most cases (17, 18, 22). However, abortion in small ruminants can have several causes and is not pathognomonic for an infection with *C. burnetii*. The impact of *C. burnetii* on reproductive disorders in cattle is still under discussion (17, 19, 20).

Pattern of Disease Occurrence

Q fever in humans and animals can be found worldwide except New Zealand and Antarctica. In Europe, an increasing trend was observed between 2012 and 2016, while from 2017 the number of confirmed Q fever cases decreased again. In 2018, 29 EU/EEA countries reported 794 confirmed Q fever cases. The three countries with the most confirmed cases in 2018 were Spain, France and Germany (24). In Germany, outbreaks of Q fever in the human population occur regularly, without nationwide spread, but often in connection with infected small ruminants. The distribution of Q fever was previously described (25–27).

In summary, the number of notified human Q fever cases in Germany has increased over the years and peaked during outbreaks since reporting obligations were regulated in 1962 (25–27). Between 2005 and 2018, the notified cases ranged between 416 and 93 each year as mentioned by the German Robert Koch Institute (RKI), without any detectable trend (24, 28). Due to the concept of passive monitoring, the number of notified cases depends on awareness by the relevant stakeholder groups and may exceed average numbers by far in the case of larger outbreaks as seen in 2003, 2005, 2008, 2010, or 2014, for example (11, 24, 25). In Germany, sporadic cases are reported nationwide, but outbreaks in the human population are reported more frequently in southern federal states and can often be linked to Q fever in small ruminants (11, 25, 26).

In comparison, the average number of notified cases in German (small) ruminant flocks fluctuated between 1970 and 2000 (26). Between 2000 and 2018, a total of 9,920 official individual cases were reported (8,359 cattle; 1,349 sheep; 212 goats) (25). Most of the notified animals were cattle, which can not only be explained by the total numbers of animals, but by the legal requirements for routine diagnostics and the different disease progression in cattle, resulting in more frequent testing of this species instead of small ruminants (26). Again, awareness of the disease is important, as illustrated by the increase of notified cases in cattle, sheep, and goats followed by outbreaks in the human population in Bad Sassendorf/Soest in 2003 and in Jena in 2005 (25, 26, 29).

Supplementary to the official reported cases, only a few surveys were conducted in the past (25). For example, the German within-flock seroprevalence was estimated at 19.3% in cattle, 8.7% in sheep, and 2.5% in goats (11). Moreover, Wolf and colleagues estimated the serological flock prevalence for small ruminants in Germany between 26 and 36.6% [$n = 71$; 14]. In comparison, in a non-representative German study, 7.8% of cattle ($n = 21{,}191$), 1.3% of sheep ($n = 1{,}346$), and 2.5% of goats ($n = 278$) tested positive for *C. burnetii* by PCR (30). Wolf et al. (14) detected that 13.9% of tested sheep and goat flocks ($n = 71$) were positive by PCR. Other studies mainly aimed at sheep farming within German federal states. Therefore, their study results vary widely due to their study design and locations (25). However, it can be concluded that detection of *C. burnetii* antibodies and the pathogen itself differs between animal species, geographic areas, and time of sampling (25).

Zoonotic Potential

Humans are at highest risk of inhaling *C. burnetii* through distant and close contact with animals, especially small ruminants (1, 11, 12, 31). **Distant contact** may occur through geographical proximity to small ruminant flocks as well as by visits to farmers markets where small ruminants are exhibited (11, 29, 31). As Q fever is an airborne disease, the pathogen can be spread over longer distances by wind and may pose a risk for human infection (11, 31). Therefore, the greatest risk of infection is within a radius of 2–4 km from the source of the pathogen. Moreover, in gale force winds, *C. burnetii* may reach distances up to 18 km

(31). Migration of small ruminants through residential areas was identified as a potential risk factor (32). Therefore, it may be a challenge to identify the infection source in human cases that did not have any obvious or known contact with sheep or goats. A higher risk of transmission from small ruminants to humans can be observed in spring/early summer due to the out-of-season lambing of some sheep breeds on pasture (11, 31, 33). Furthermore, **close contact** with contaminated products such as afterbirth or contaminated wool during sheep shearing may also be sources for human infections that can occur sporadically, e.g., animal owners, their family members, or employees (33, 34). Moreover, employees of slaughterhouses or laboratories can become infected at the workplace. Infections by consumption of contaminated raw milk (products) is possible but rare (5). Also possible, but even rarer, is infection through live cell therapy (35).

Rules and Regulations

On an international level, the World Organization for Animal Health (OIE) lists Q fever in the category of multiple species diseases (36). Moreover, OIE recommends protocols for diagnostic testing and vaccination of Q fever in small ruminants to prevent human infections (5). On the level of the European Union, data sampling of zoonoses in humans is regulated under Decision No 211/98/EC and coordinated by the European Centre for Disease Prevention and Control (ECDC). Moreover, Q fever is included in the Community Summary Reports on zoonoses since 2005. To harmonize information about Q fever within the European Union, a scheme for the monitoring and reporting of Q fever in animals was developed in 2010 under Directive 2003/99/EG. This report was prepared by the European Food Safety Authority (EFSA) in collaboration with the ECDC and EFSA's Zoonoses Collaborating Centre (32).

On the national level, Q fever in humans is a notifiable disease with inception of the German Protection against Infection Act (IfSG) in 2001 (25, 37). In accordance with the German National Animal Health Act (TierGesG) and the German Regulation of Notifiable Animal Diseases (TKrMeldpflV), only the direct detection (by culture or PCR) of *C. burnetii* in small ruminants and cattle has to be reported to the local veterinary health authority (25, 38, 39). All notifications are reported in the Animal Disease Reporting System (TSN) by the local veterinary health authorities and contain the date of detection, the species, the flock and its owner as well as the county/city concerned (25). Apart from official rules and regulations, the RKI published recommendations for Q fever after a huge sheep-associated outbreak in 2006 (9, 29). Moreover, an interdisciplinary research association in the German federal state Baden-Wuerttemberg published recommendations for the management of Q fever cases and outbreaks (40). Furthermore, the German Federal Institute for Risk Assessment (BfR) recommends pasteurization of raw milk before consumption and food processing if a *C. burnetii* infection is diagnosed within a ruminant flock (2). A recommendation published by the German Ministry of Food and Agriculture (BMEL) is available that involves hygiene measures in the case of Q fever cases in (small) ruminants (41). However, these recommendations are not mandatory and cannot be imposed by the local veterinary health authorities. In comparison, the local public health authorities may impose regulatory measures for animals based on the IfSG if humans are infected.

Rationale for Using a Monitoring and Surveillance Systems

The German legislation underlines the rationale for using a monitoring and surveillance system (MOSS) for Q fever as it defines this zoonosis as a notifiable disease in both (small) ruminants and humans (37–39). Hence, both MOSS's that are currently in place can be defined as passive monitoring systems, which focus on human health as the predominant rationale instead of health or production effects on animals (25, 42). However, the passive monitoring system of Q fever in small ruminants does not serve as reliable protection for humans against infection. This is especially because infection in small ruminants may proceed with unspecific symptoms or even asymptomatically (17, 18). As a passive reporting system does not detect these kinds of diseases very well, we assume that the occurrence of Q fever in small ruminants is heavily underestimated in Germany (43, 44). To prevent new infections in humans, it is important to gather reliable information about the current Q fever status of small ruminant flocks. With this knowledge, flock-specific action and control measures can be induced, while these measures effectively prevent new cases in the human population, as transmission risk will be reduced (5, 38, 39). It could be discussed that the low number of notified cases in the human population does not directly impose the need for action. However, underreporting of Q fever in humans has to be assumed, as symptoms are unspecific, and zoonotic infections are not high on the list of differential diagnoses (30, 45). Due to the obvious risk for human infection, there is a need to improve passive monitoring in small ruminants toward active surveillance, including measures for the control of Q fever (5, 42, 44). Therefore, the objective of this paper was to conceptualize such a MOSS as an early warning system for Q fever in small ruminant livestock in Germany and to evaluate the concept with regard to feasibility.

METHODS

To comply with international standards, previously developed checklists for the design of a MOSS in the animal health sector were used and modified (42, 43, 46–48). Referring to these international standards, we summarized the main characteristics and the chosen options of our concept in **Tables 1, 2**. First, we started by defining the **hypothesis and aim** of our MOSS. Afterwards, we discussed the **type of system** in detail. All further options in terms of the described characteristics of this concept are contingent on this aim with regard to international literature about *C. burnetii*, national legislation and regional differences in husbandry of small ruminants. Next, we focused on the characteristics of the **target population** for this MOSS, which is split into the topics ***animal species***, ***sex and age***, ***region***, and ***husbandry***. After this, we determined the **dependent variables** including the topics ***disease stage***, ***unit of interest***, and

TABLE 1 | Concept of an active surveillance system for Q fever in German small ruminants—conflicts between best practices and feasibility.

Characteristics (Topics)	Chosen options
Hypothesis	Small ruminants are the main source for Q fever infections/epidemics in the human population in Germany
Aim	Early warning system for Q fever in small ruminant flocks to prevent Q fever infections in the human population
Type of system	(Voluntary) active surveillance system in small ruminants with individually adapted action and control plan
Target population	All female reproductive small ruminants within the flocks regardless of the husbandry systems in Germany
Dependent variable	The flock status of *C. burnetii* shedding detected by PCR of pooled vaginal swabs in female small ruminants in Germany—with the flock-status defined as positive by at least one pool-sample testing positive
Independent variables	Factors influencing the flock status of *C. burnetii* shedding: - Preliminary information (suspicious symptoms, antibody activity, vaccination) - Target population (sex and age)
Sampling technique and sample size	Multistage risked-based sampling
At the flock level	Testing all flocks at risk to transmit the pathogen to public (reproduction, close contact, distant contact)
At the within-flock level	Testing all primi- and multiparous females after lambing in order to increase the probability of identifying a positive herd
Sampling time	During the main lambing period and before migrating in residential areas
Bias	- Selection bias - Information bias
Action and control plan	(Voluntary) individually adapted control plan in positive tested flocks
In the case of positive flock status	- Prevention of close contact between flocks and the public - Prevention of distant contact between flocks and the public - Hygienic measures on the farm - Flock-vaccination - Continuous testing - Examination of the people living and working on the farm
In the case of negative flock status	Continuous testing

diagnosis. Then, the **independent variables and confounder** were discussed. In the next step, we focused on the **sampling technique and sample size** at the ***flock level*** and ***within-flock level*** as well as ***sampling time*** and ***bias***. As Q fever bears a serious risk for the human population, we discussed an **action and control plan** ***in case of a positive*** or ***negative flock status***. As **implementation and evaluation** of a MOSS are important issues at the time of concept planning, we discussed the involvement of ***stakeholders*** as well as ***economic considerations*** in the context of this concept.

TABLE 2 | Implementation and evaluation of an active surveillance system for Q fever in German small ruminants—conflicts between best practices and feasibility.

Characteristics (Topics)	Chosen options
Stakeholders	Small ruminant sector - Animal owners, their employees, family members - Regional/national/breeding associations - Animal traders, abattoirs, dairies, and sheepshearers Veterinary health professionals - Veterinary health authority - Veterinary practitioners/animal health services - Laboratorians Human health professionals - Human health authority - Physicians - Laboratorians Policy makers Animal Disease Funds Public
Economic considerations	Financial costs - MOSS coordination - Sample collection - Sample testing - Costs from modifying usual flock management and housing practices - Vaccination costs - Loss of income Financial benefits - Saved costs for physicians, laboratories, medicine, hospitalization - Saved non-productive time of humans - Quality awareness - Saved cost for action measures Emotional costs - Stigmatism of people in the small ruminants sector - Existential fear of people in the small ruminant sector - Panic in the public Emotional benefits - Knowledge about flock status and necessary consequences - Responsibility of animal owners toward their fellow humans - Gain in confidence of the public in the animal owners - Zoonosis prevention/One Health

The referred literature was assessed in a non-systematic search strategy using the search database Web of Science (http://apps.webofknowledge.com) performed in English. Investigated search terms were defined and combined with the Boolean Operators AND and OR.

To report about our concept of an active surveillance system for Q fever in small ruminants, the STROBE Statement was used as a guideline (49).

CONCEPT OF THE MOSS

In this paper, we compile a concept of an early warning system for Q fever in small ruminants in Germany. First, we describe the best practice for this MOSS before taking the next step to address feasibility, as the combination of both evokes conflicts. The basic points of the MOSS are summarized in **Tables 1, 2**.

Hypothesis and Aim

To conceptualize a MOSS, the hypothesis and the aim are mandatory to define first (42, 43). These generate the basis for every subsequent decision regarding the design of the concept. Q fever has a non-specific aetiopathology as well as little effect on the health status of small ruminants. Nevertheless, there is no active MOSS for Q fever in small ruminants, which is mandatory in all federal states. Based on these facts, we assume that the health status of most small ruminants and thus the potential sources of human Q fever infections in Germany are unknown. As only a few *C. burnetii* organisms can initiate active infection in humans (3), it is imperative to detect a possible source of transmission as soon as possible. Therefore, "early detection in a defined animal population" is the predominant purpose of the MOSS presented here (5, 36, 46).

Type of System

MOSSs are used to gather health data of a defined population (47, 48). However, it should be discussed whether "passive" or "active" data collection is desired and if action should follow a positive finding, i.e., "monitoring" or "surveillance."

In the case of our MOSS, "monitoring" would result in the observation of the Q fever status in small ruminants without any control activities in the case of positive findings (42, 43, 47). However, as we are concerned with a zoonotic agent with considerable human health impact, monitoring without control activities would foil the principles of risk prevention and veterinary public health. Hence, "surveillance" system is preferred here. Those control activities can be either mandatory or voluntary. For mandatory implementation of control activities, rules, and regulations are necessary. In the case of human outbreaks caused by small ruminants or cattle, veterinarians and human local health offices have to work closely together using the IfSG. However, German law does not regulate consistent control activities in the case of Q fever in small ruminants without a link to human Q fever cases (37–39). A competent public health authority can take necessary measures to avert imminent danger only if facts are established, which might lead to the occurrence of Q fever in humans, or if it can be assumed that such facts exist (37). Hence, regulations need modifications. In the meantime, surveillance is contingent upon the voluntary implementation of control activities by animal owners. However, a surveillance system with voluntary control activities calls on the responsibility of animal owners for people in their environment. For the success of this MOSS concept, further considerations presume a 100% participation rate.

Furthermore, it is important to decide whether a "passive" or "active" data collection must take place for this MOSS (42, 43, 47). In the case of a "passive" MOSS, a reporting cascade is necessary to gather health data (43). Such a "passive" method would be an inexpensive way to get information about the Q fever status of small ruminants in Germany because the veterinary health authorities would not need to plan data acquisition, to take diagnostic tests or finance the work of sampling and laboratories. However, this "passive" system contains many sources of error as it is based on the idea that animal owners and practicing veterinarians recognize clinical signs of Q fever very easily and screen the population of interest. Therefore, passive monitoring would overlook small ruminants with positive Q fever status. Furthermore, different knowledge about Q fever and different motivations to report positive flock status negatively influence the quality of health data (42, 43, 50). Animal owners may be less motivated if they distrust the system, especially if consequences after reporting a positive Q fever status are unforeseeable [e.g., stigmatzation; (43)]. Therefore, the reporting cascade would not work reliably for this disease. In contrast, an "active" MOSS collects health data in a systematic way or by regular recording (42). For the active collection method, it is typical to define a specific aim of the MOSS, to use a formal sampling process in a specific population and a specific time of collection as well as standard tests to detect positive findings (42, 43). In general, the local veterinary health authorities are responsible for the coordination of this regular and periodic collection of health data (43). It is important to invest both money and time in structured data acquisition to get valid information about Q fever status in a favorable cost-benefit ratio (46–48). Hence, this leads to an "active" system of data collection in the case of our MOSS. An active MOSS is not restricted to clinical cases with typical symptoms, which is an important advantage in the case of Q fever in small ruminants. Another positive effect for the quality of the data is the control of sampling scheme and information collection by a competent veterinary health authority that guarantees statistically based objectivity as well as increasing comparability of results (42, 43). In conclusion, this MOSS should be implemented as an active surveillance system.

Target Population

The target population is defined as the population that is the focus of a study (42, 51). For example, this can include the whole population at risk that is susceptible to a specifical disease or just a subgroup with special qualities of this population at risk (42). If the target population is not clearly defined, individual interpretation of study results can lead to bias and differential perception of the results (51). To define the target population of this MOSS, we divided their characteristics into the topics ***animal species***, ***sex and age***, ***region***, and ***husbandry*** (46–48).

Animal Species

Although various domestic and wild mammals can be reservoirs for *C. burnetii*, the focus of this approach is on small ruminant livestock (6, 7, 9, 10). On an international level, (aborting) dairy goats have been the reason for the biggest Q fever outbreaks in humans. However, in Germany most small-scale epidemics have been caused by nondairy sheep (25). Because sheep and goats are often kept together (especially in southern Germany) and because the number of goats is increasing across the country (14, 25), this MOSS has to focus on both species. The German Federal Statistical Office reported 19,556 farms with 1,834,275 sheep and 9,808 farms with 138,810 goats in 2016. Unfortunately, no official number about these farms keeping sheep and goats together is available (52, 53).

Sex and Age

Possible differences regarding the transmission risk to humans between sex and age groups have to be considered when defining the target population. Both female and male small ruminants can be infected by *C. burnetii* and shed the pathogen via different pathways (13, 14, 18, 21, 22, 54). However, the highest pathogen concentrations are shed in amniotic fluid, placenta, and lochia during physiological birth or abortion and in the milk of small ruminants (18, 21, 22, 54). Hence, female small ruminants after lambing are the subgroup with the highest risk for humans to acquire infection and therefore are focused on in this MOSS. In Germany, approximately 64.42% (n = 1,181,560) of the sheep population and 63.72% (n = 88,451) of the goat population are reproductive females (52).

Region

As the pattern of disease occurrence of Q fever in humans and small ruminants in Germany was previously described (25–27), the reported cases and studies show that Q fever is endemic in Germany (11, 25–27). Therefore, the MOSS should be implemented nationwide. In Germany, rules and regulations for the implementation of a MOSS are split into national, federal, and district tasks. In the districts, the lowest administrative level, veterinary and public health authorities are responsible for general coordination and implementation of disease prevention in animals as well as in humans. These veterinary and public health authorities on the district level can rely on (communication) structures between different stakeholders, which are needed for the implementation of this MOSS (see chapter "Implementation and evaluation"). As the wind and the distance between settlements and small ruminants have an impact on Q fever transmission (11, 31), this MOSS mentions urbanization, density of livestock, and individual weather conditions in different regions of Germany and appeals to the cooperation between neighboring districts in the case of positive findings. In conclusion, this MOSS must be implemented nationwide with the administrative districts as the lowest subregional structure being responsible for implementation of action and control activities.

Husbandry

The current situation of sheep and goat husbandry in Germany was previously described by Bauer et al. (25). In short, the distribution of animals, farms and breeds differs between German federal states (25). Moreover, most German small ruminant farms practice a combination of management systems including grazing enclosure, milk production, and shepherded and migrating flocks, which makes husbandry very inhomogeneous (50). In addition, small ruminant husbandry is mostly associated with **reproduction** for lamb production as well as with landscape conservation and protection. Both are connected with **distant contact** between small ruminants and the public due to lambing and grazing on pasture and the proximity to residential areas. Migrating flocks, which change their location regularly or even cross administrative district borders, are particularly noteworthy here. Furthermore, **close contact** between small ruminants and the public takes place in petting zoos, family farm vacations, and animal-assisted education or therapy. These risk factors for public health will be discussed in the "sampling technique and sample size" section of this manuscript. Finally, this MOSS needs to focus on the whole range of small ruminant husbandry, as there is an overall risk of transmission to humans.

Dependent Variable

Conceptualized as an early warning system, the dependent variable for this MOSS is the status of Q fever in small ruminants.

Disease Stage

To describe a disease status in general, a MOSS can focus on different disease stages such as the infection, the occurrence of symptoms, the presence of antibodies, or the excretion of the pathogen itself. As we have to consider the zoonotic potential of Q fever, pathogen shedding by small ruminants must be identified as early as possible. Since clinical symptoms or the presence of antibodies cannot be connected to the occurrence of pathogen shedding (12, 18, 21, 32, 44), this MOSS has to focus on the detection of pathogen shedding itself. As mentioned in the topic **sex and age,** the perinatal period is the time of highest risk for human infections (18, 21, 22), and this MOSS focuses on the detection of current pathogen shedding early after lambing.

Unit of Interest

"The individual (animal), pen, herd, flock, or farm" or another defined structure may be chosen as an unit of interest (42). Choosing the individual animal as the smallest unit of interest is useful to detect sporadic diseases. Therefore, this strategy is valuable for a disease that is not very contagious. However, Q fever is a contagious disease and can be spread easily within flocks. This means that the occurrence of more than one *C. burnetii* shedding individual within a group of animals is very probable. Choosing the status of pathogen shedding at the flock level, the probability of a positive flock status may change over time with the composition of individuals within the flock (51). As farms may manage more than one flock, and flocks may be housed and handled differently, flocks should be the most appropriate unit of interest here (5, 51, 55). Due to the high concentration and prolonged time of *C. burnetii* shedding, a single *C. burnetii*-infected individual may be a sufficient risk for human infections (3, 29). Therefore, a single animal testing positive is sufficient to designate the flock as positive for *C. burnetii* shedding (14, 44, 55). Conclusively, the unit of interest is the flock status of pathogen shedding defined by at least one individual-sample testing positive.

Diagnosis

Different diagnostic tests are available for direct detection of *C. burnetii.* Only specialized labs perform bacterial cultivation. However, PCR is the most feasible diagnostic test for this MOSS because primer and probe sequences as well as ready-to-use kits are commercially available, and results may be provided with high speed and accuracy (i.e., high specificity and sensitivity) (1, 5, 25). PCR has been used to detect *C. burnetii*-genome fragments in feces, however further research is necessary to confirm feces as adequate test material to detect acute pathogen shedding in small ruminants (56, 57). As an officially approved diagnostic test, PCR is able to detect *C. burnetii*-genome fragments in milk samples, organs of fetuses, birth products, vaginal swabs, and ticks (25, 58). However, milk production is present on only 2.68% ($n = 524$) of all sheep farms and comprises only 0.98% ($n = 17{,}999$) of the sheep population in Germany in 2016, making this sample material unsuitable for this MOSS (52). In addition to sampling of fetuses and birth products, sampling of vaginal swabs means additional effort and cost, but vaginal swabs provide a high-quality sampling material (5, 25, 59). Furthermore, a vaginal swab can be assigned to an individual animal, so that subsequent measures can be implemented individually (e.g., follow-up testing). In addition, pooled samples of vaginal swabs are applicable to reduce temporal expenditure and financial costs (42). Conclusively, diagnosis must be carried out by conducting pooled vaginal swabs testing by PCR.

Independent Variables and Confounder

Factors influencing the probability of a flock testing positive for pathogen shedding were already discussed before and are only listed here for reasons of clarity:

- Preliminary information: Flocks already known to show **suspicious symptoms such as abortion** at the flock level [the abortion rate ranges between 5 and 90% of pregnant females, while 5–20% is common in sheep flocks, and high abortion rates occur only in some goat flocks (23)] may be an indicator of current and ongoing infection and shedding. Moreover, previously known **antibody titers** in animals may be an indicator of current or ongoing infection and shedding in a flock. This may increase the probability of a flock testing positive for current shedding but there is no guarantee (1, 59). Although previous **vaccination** heavily influences the antibody activity, it also reduces the amount of pathogens shed (5).
- Target population: Female animals with perinatal status are most likely to shed high amounts of the pathogen (see chapter "Sex and age") (18, 21).

Sampling Technique and Sample Size

First, it has to be decided which procedure is applicable for the aim of this MOSS: a census or a sample. The main disadvantage of a census is its great cost in terms of time and money; conversely, an advantage of sampling is its low cost, while leading to reliable estimation of the target population if the sample is selected correctly (42, 51). A solution is to conduct a risk-based sample. This enables lower costs and monitoring of the most relevant samples. Due to the well-known cluster effect of (n) animals in (m) farms, multistage sampling has to be considered, where first the number of flocks and then the number of animals per flock are determined (51).

At the Flock Level

Concerning risked-based sampling, flocks with the following characteristics should be investigated predominantly:

- **Reproduction** in general, but especially when lambing will happen on pasture: Information about the flock management (lambing location i.e., lambing in stable vs. on pasture) as well as the time of parturition (estrus synchronization/artificial insemination, lambing season) must be queried (33).
- **Close contact** in general, but especially when female and pregnant small ruminants are to be exhibited: Information about exhibitions (i.e., conformation shows, farm vacations, open house days). Furthermore, all reproducing female small ruminants kept for petting zoos, animal-assisted education and therapy must be identified and investigated in particular (29).
- **Distant contact** in general, but especially when migration is performed in residential areas: Information about the migration of flocks must be acquired, and the migrating flocks must be tested regularly (31, 33).

As it can be assumed that these characteristics concern most of the German small ruminant flocks, this risked-based sampling may almost be a census.

At the Within-Flock Level

Concerning risked-based sampling, all females after lambing should be investigated predominantly. Assuming that the flock has a positive status given that one individual is shedding *C. burnetii*, we calculated the required sample size (n) to identify freedom from disease considering the absolute number of primi-/multiparous females per flock (N) [see **Supplementary Material**; (5, 36, 51)]. Our calculation shows that the difference between census and sample (N-n) is minimal and therefore this risked-based sampling is almost a census (see **Supplementary Material**).

Sampling Time

Flock level testing should be done during the main lambing period and before migrating into residential areas at least once a year. In addition, an ultrasound examination should be carried out before individual animals are exhibited or transported/slaughtered. Animals in the last trimester of pregnancy should not be exhibited to prevent spontaneous abortions or births near humans and should not be transported/slaughtered to prevent infection of animal traders and abattoirs.

Bias

A sampling process always leads to an uncertainty about the gathered information because a conclusive statement in response to a research question is only available for the sampled individuals (42). To assess the quality of this MOSS, this section discusses possible sources for bias.

Selection bias describes the difference between an estimation and the truth (60). In case of this MOSS, the selection bias may originate from the sampling technique described above. First, it is important to mention that this MOSS currently depends on voluntary participation of the different stakeholders. Poor participation by these stakeholders could introduce selection bias such that only interested animal owners participate. This could bias the percentage of flocks testing positive toward an overestimation, if these persons already know about their flock having a problem with Q fever. However, it could also bias toward an underestimation, if these persons focus their flock management on a perfect hygiene strategy and therefore participate to prevent further *C. burnetii* infections. A percentage over- or underestimation would not impede the aim of this MOSS, which is to identify as many herds as possible in total that shed *C. burnetii*. Furthermore, if the system becomes obligatory, this bias will be settled. Next, veterinary health officers have to administer the risk-based principle of flock selection and individuals within the flocks. For example, sampling of non-mated female small ruminants, which do not lamb, or sampling of mated female small ruminants during pregnancy and late after lambing also may lead to underestimation. Although this selection process can be supported by the use of a questionnaire, it depends on subjective decisions and may be a source of possible bias. Beyond this, correct assignment of high-risk flocks depends on animal owners' provision of correct information.

Information bias describes the difference between the estimation and the truth that originates from over- or underestimation of results (60). In the case of this MOSS, the greatest information bias is because a few animal owners do not know the time of lambing, as fertile male small ruminants are constantly in the herd. Therefore, the information about time of lambing can only be communicated to the veterinary health officers when it has already taken place. Very good communication between animal owners and veterinarians is therefore a prerequisite for obtaining samples in a timely manner. Further information bias may originate from error classification of pools resulting in false classification of the flock status. This depends on the sensitivity and specificity of the chosen diagnostic test (60), which are very high in the case of PCR testing (1, 5, 25). As *C. burnetii* shedding occurs sporadically, test results can miss a positive individual and therefore the positive status of a flock. By planning to test herds completely and during a time when identification of positive animals is most likely, single false-positive or negative test results can only modify the estimated disease status on the flock level if shedding occurs in very few animals or if the flock is small. Therefore, as the test accuracy is comparably high and pools instead of individual animals are investigated, the test performance does not have to be considered as relevant bias for the determination of disease status.

Action and Control Plan

Recommendations for action and control measures regarding Q fever in small ruminants have been published elsewhere (1, 5, 12, 25, 33, 40, 41). However, German flock management and husbandry vary considerably between each small ruminant (production) system, resulting in a varying risk of pathogen transmission to the human population (5). Therefore, individually adapted action and control plans are preferable over general recommendations and should be developed with the cooperation of veterinary and human health professionals and the animal owners.

In the Case of Positive Flock Status (Pathogen Shedding in a Flock)

If *C. burnetii* shedding is detected, immediate and long-term actions must be defined in a flock-specific action and control plan (41).

Most importantly, prevention of <u>close contact</u> between the positive flock and the public means that animal **exhibitions** as well as **unauthorized persons in the flock** (i.e., farm visits, vacations, open house days) have to cease until the flock is proven negative again. **Authorized persons working in the flock** (animal owners, their employees, animal traders, abattoirs, dairies, sheepshearers) must protect themselves with **personal protection equipment;** wearing FFP3 respirators is most important, and protective work clothing should only be worn within the specific flock (12, 33, 40, 41).

Similarly important is the prevention of <u>distant contact</u> between the flock and the public. Therefore, the animal owners have to organize **lambing inside a stable** and to **store contagious materials** such as afterbirth or aborted material in safe containers until rendering. In addition, **cleaning and disinfection** of lambing areas and stables are necessary to prevent pathogen dissemination. Furthermore, **dung and litter** have to be covered for 9 months before spreading it on farmland (12, 33, 40, 41). Although the alimentary infection pathway is unlikely (2), selling and consumption of **raw milk and raw milk products** must be prohibited (12, 40, 41). Small ruminants must not be used as a source for **live cell therapy** (35). No **migrating** should be allowed, and the flock should be **kept as far as possible from human habitation** until the flock is proven negative again (31). **Shearing and storage of wool** have to take place in a closed room while wearing personal protection equipment. Contaminated wool must be destroyed in a rendering plant (31, 33, 40, 41).

Moreover, an action that concerns the individual animals itself is **vaccination.** However, phase I vaccine should be preferred over phase II vaccine as it is more effective (61). Although phase I vaccination cannot stop the shedding of *C. burnetii*, it can reduce pathogen shedding (1, 17, 33, 61). Oxytetracycline treatment is not recommended in the case of Q fever in small ruminants, as it does not stop pathogen shedding (25, 61).

As Q fever occurs sporadically and may reoccur after some time, a flock with a positive status should be **retested** for at least the next two lambing seasons (22). To prevent further unnoticed pathogen spread, the possible source of infection should be investigated [**tracing on** and **tracing back**, **wildlife as pathogen reservoir**; (10, 12, 33, 34, 45, 54, 61)].

In the Case of Negative Flock Status

If the status of a flock is negative, *C. burnetii* shedding was not detected by PCR of vaginal swabs and transmission to the public is currently unlikely. However, as Q fever occurs sporadically, **annually recurrent testing** is necessary. In cases of **increased risk for transmission** to the public, additional testing should be applied. Furthermore, **animals in their last trimester**

of pregnancy must not be transported, e.g., for exhibition or slaughter, in order to avoid pathogen contamination by spontaneous lambing or slaughter. Accordingly, an ultrasonography examination to determine the pregnancy status of an individual animal has to be carried out prior to transportation.

Implementation and Evaluation

To implement and evaluate this MOSS, it is important to discuss which ***stakeholders*** are potentially concerned and which ***economic considerations*** should be regarded.

Stakeholders

Stakeholders who are affected in some way by this MOSS are different subgroups working in the small ruminant sector as well as veterinary and human health professionals, policy makers, Animal Disease Funds and the public itself (5, 29, 45, 55, 62–64).

The small ruminant sector first includes **sheep and goat owners, their employees, and family members**. Small ruminant owners are organized within **regional and national (breeding) associations.** These associations represent the opinions of their members and are important counterparts to get in contact with small ruminant owners and amplify information regarding MOSS implementation. As long as participation is voluntary, animal owners have to actively agree to take part. Participation will be influenced by the good communication between different stakeholder groups and awareness of the importance of this MOSS for public health. Therefore, we discussed the idea of closely linking voluntary Q fever monitoring to another already well-established (and mandatory) monitoring program for brucellosis with a group of representatives from small ruminant owner associations. It became clear that awareness about the impact of this disease for public health currently is not high enough to trigger willingness to participate. The representatives emphasized that small ruminant owners are already overloaded with regulations and legal documentations and cannot justify further workload and restrictions, which are not predictable in the case of a positive flock status. Hence, it has to be concluded that prior to and in parallel with implementation of this MOSS, great effort must be put into raising awareness, dismantling barriers and fears and increasing knowledge of Q fever and exactly how the MOSS will work. Furthermore, possible economic benefits of a negative test result need to be discussed and emphasized to create an incentive for participation (see chapter "Economic considerations").

Further groups in the small ruminant sector that have to be considered are **animal traders, abattoirs, dairies, and sheepshearers.** These groups need to know the status of flocks in order to adapt their working habits when handling positive flocks with regard to personal protection equipment (i.e., wearing FFP-3 breathing masks) or when processing material derived from small ruminants [i.e., pasteurization of raw milk, separate slaughter, handling and selling of wool; (33, 40, 41)]. Some professionals might even have to postpone or cancel their work in small ruminant flocks that tests positive (e.g., sheepshearers) due to self-protection.

Veterinary health professionals includes the **veterinary health authority officers** who have to organize steps such as selection of most relevant flocks as well as the documentation and analysis of test results. Elaboration of flock-specific action and control plans is another of their tasks. However, these steps must take place in cooperation with the animal owners. At this point, **veterinary practitioners** function as a link between the veterinary health authority and animal owners, as they know the animal owners as their customers and therefore can advise which measures have to be implemented for the affected flock. In addition, veterinary practitioners must perform the vaginal swab sampling on behalf of the veterinary health authority. Since an animal health service exists in most German federal states, these tasks can be transferred to the practicing veterinarians of this organizational unit. **Laboratories** are necessary to do the diagnostic testing of these swabs. To implement necessary safety measures at the laboratory, samples have to be packed safely and accompanied by meaningful preliminary reports.

As Q fever is a zoonosis, human health professionals are additional stakeholders in this MOSS. Therefore, the **public health authority officers** and their colleagues at the veterinary health authority must cooperate. In the case of a positive flock status, an exchange of information must take place automatically, as this provides an early warning to draw attention to possible Q fever cases in the human population. Hence, the public health authority officers should forward information to **physicians** to raise awareness and alertness, without stigmatizing the animal owners and their families. Furthermore, **laboratories** in the human health sector are involved if human cases occur, and they must be informed to be alert about the zoonotic potential as well.

Next, policy makers are an important group of stakeholders in this MOSS. Due to recent German legislation, Q fever is only monitored via a passive MOSS. Hence, implementation of any new surveillance attempts depends on the voluntary participation of animal owners and veterinary health professionals. Therefore, legislation needs to be revised, and an active MOSS has to become mandatory in order to protect the public effectively.

Furthermore, the revision has to include subsidies for animal owners in cases of positive herd status. This leads to the Animal Disease Funds as further stakeholders. These public-law institutions are regulated nationwide by the TierGesG, but within the federal states the reimbursement of costs for monitoring and combating animal diseases varies (38). Therefore, federal legislation is necessary to regulate the subsidization of animal owners by these institutions in the case of positive flock status.

Finally, the public has to be mentioned as a stakeholder group. If there is a risk of a Q fever outbreak in the population, the population should be informed about possible risk factors and preventive behavior. Therefore, it is important that the public relations department of each district cooperates with the local press to inform the public without generating panic or causing stigmatization of small ruminant owners (62, 63).

Economic Considerations

Decisions about this concept are driven by economic considerations that affect all different stakeholder groups.

Financial costs evolve from MOSS coordination, sample collection and testing as well as action and control measures (see **Supplementary Material**). Therefore, the conflict between best practice and feasibility is notable.

For **MOSS coordination**, labor costs for veterinary health authority employees have to be assessed prior to implementation. Here, the effort to collect basic information about the risk-status of the flocks within each governmental district is considered the most time-consuming task. Calculating the financial costs of **sample collection, sample testing,** and vaccination, as an **action and control** measure, we considered the German veterinary fee regulation (GOT), the fee regulation for administration/consumer protection and veterinary health authority (GOVV) in Lower Saxony and the German permanent vaccination commission for veterinary medicine (STIKO Vet) [see **Supplementary Material**; (65–67)]. As **sample collection** has to be carried out by veterinary practitioners on behalf of the veterinary health authority, labor costs, driving costs, materials (vaginal swabs) and sample shipment must be taken into account. Additionally, costs for **sample testing** by the laboratories must be considered, whereby pooling of samples saves costs (see **Supplementary Material**). Concerning **action and control**, all implemented measures have to be supervised by the veterinary authorities, which causes additional personnel costs. For **vaccination**, we assumed four euros per 2 ml dose for a small ruminant individual (25). Further, we assumed that only the gimmers, replacement animals, and purchases of the flock (replacement rate of 20%) need an initial immunization. Here, two doses at intervals of 3 weeks were calculated. If possible, vaccination has to be completed 4 weeks before mating (61), while the other 80% of the flock gets only one booster vaccination per year. **Sample collection, testing, and vaccination** of all reproductive females (n = 1,270,011) in the German small ruminant population include 26,090,430 euros per year in this calculation [see **Supplementary Material**; (52, 53)]. Moreover, animal owners would face (additional) **costs from modifying their usual flock management and housing practices** in order to ensure that pathogen transmission will be prevented. Rendering of contaminated materials may cause additional costs. Furthermore, and most importantly, the **loss of income** for the affected animal owners has to be considered before implementing this MOSS, as well. Financial damage may be substantial depending on the purpose of use and the market value of the flock and its products [i.e., prohibition of trade with wool, raw milk (products), or live animals]. Moreover, **loss of income and threatened jobs** also must be considered. Although Q fever is listed by the OIE, it is not included within "Recommendations applicable to OIE Listed diseases and other diseases of importance to international trade" (5, 36). Since we recommend stopping animal trade from a positive herd, this could result in loss of income for the animal owners. This calculation and summary of financial costs shows that it is not feasible to implement this concept of a best practice MOSS.

Finally, the following steps are necessary to reduce costs in order to make this MOSS feasible. **Preventive measures** should replace testing wherever justifiable. Therefore, the focus on **nationwide vaccination** would be most useful, as this would guarantee lower pathogen shedding by infected small ruminants. Assuming the vaccination costs as stated above for all reproductive females (n = 1,270,011) in the German small ruminant population, a nationwide vaccination of these would include approximately 7,722,000 euros per year. If sample collection and testing are omitted completely, this would result in a cost reduction of 18,368,430 euros per year compared to the best practice concept [see **Supplementary Material**; (52, 53)]. Moreover, current studies are investigating if the **vaccination dose for sheep can be reduced by half** (1 ml per dose) compared to goats (25). Other studies are looking at whether **exclusive vaccination of gimmers** would be sufficient to prevent a positive flock status (68). These approaches would also further reduce costs. Unfortunately, it is not possible to avoid **sample collection and testing in cases of close contact** between small ruminants and the public because vaccination does not prevent pathogen shedding completely (5). On the other hand, vaccination can greatly reduce the risk of Q fever infection in the human population. For further cost reductions, it must also be considered that testing such a large number of animals means that **costs for sample testing and vaccination can be negotiated** between the national veterinary health authority and the industry, resulting in lower costs for each district as in our calculation above. In addition, costs could be saved if the **sample collection** was carried out by independent persons, such as employees of the responsible chamber of agriculture or Animal Disease Founds, who have lower labor costs as veterinarians. However, it must be ensured that employees have the necessary knowledge to guarantee the quality of the samples. Furthermore, it could also be considered whether the animal owners themselves could collect the samples. However, this raises several problems. First, it would have to be ensured that all animal owners have the necessary knowledge to carry out the sampling correctly. Second, the animal owners are directly affected by the results of the samples, which could make them prejudiced in taking the samples.

Regarding MOSS coordination, sample collection and testing as well as vaccination costs, it has to be decided which stakeholder group should participate in the financing. **Animal owners** could be a possible group as it is their responsibility not to compromise public health by animal husbandry (69). On the other hand, animal owners cannot be expected to solely take over these high costs and the responsibility. Therefore, the costs should be shared or assumed. While goat owners may be more willing to accept financial costs, as Q fever leads to losses for their animals (i.e., higher abortion rate), in contrast, sheep owners might be less willing to pay as Q fever usually does not show any health problems in sheep. Given the previous approaches in Germany, it is most likely that financial coverage would be taken over by the **Animal Disease Funds**. In addition, the public health authorities and veterinary health authorities should be considered in regard to joint (cost) management. This is because measures can only be ordered by the public health authorities. This is based on the IfSG. However, veterinary expertise is needed for disease control measures in small ruminant flocks, too. Therefore, it is desirable that an interdisciplinary team coordinates measures. In addition to the legal basis of the IfSG, both public and veterinary health authorities are responsible for the maintenance of public health as a common good. Although infection with *C. burnetii* poses a greater risk to human health than to animal health, joint financing by animal owners, Animal Disease Founds as well as the public health authorities and the veterinary health authorities is a logical conclusion.

Financial benefits arise from the prevention of human Q fever cases. Therefore, each case that can be prevented by this MOSS saves costs for **physicians, laboratories, medicine, hospitalization, and nonproductive time of humans.** "Expressed in disease adjusted life years (DALYs), Q fever ranked 12th of 32 infectious diseases in the Netherlands over the period 2007–2011, using the methodology developed under the Burden of Communicable Diseases in Europe (BCoDE) project. ... The healthcare-associated costs of the Q fever epidemic in the Netherlands was estimated at €18.4–26.5 million and the productivity loss at an additional €1.3–10.3 million" (70). Hence, though not precisely estimable, costs can be high, and outbreaks may affect the health system considerably. Therefore, every preventive measure is financially preferable to ongoing passive monitoring as it is currently in place. The financial benefit to small ruminant owners and the associated incentive to participate is difficult to recognize at the beginning of MOSS implementation. Animal owners are afraid of the financial damage that a positive test will bring. At this point, however, it is very important to emphasize that an active MOSS also leads to **quality awareness**, which in turn brings financial benefits. Once MOSS is implemented nationwide and an awareness of this zoonosis among small ruminant owners, public, veterinary, and human health professionals is available, small ruminant owners can use a negative flock status to prove the quality of their action measures against Q fever. As a financial benefit, animal owners of flocks with a negative test result could sell raw milk (products) for a better price (e.g., by self-marketing or selling to dairies) and escape restrictions such as migrating ban or culling of animals. This MOSS can therefore be the basis for creating a quality mark "Q fever free" for small ruminant livestock in the future. In addition, this active MOSS ensures that Q fever in small ruminant livestock is controlled nationwide and thus also reduces the **risk of pathogen introduction** into Q fever free flocks, e.g., by additional purchases. Therefore, a financial benefit is that Q fever in small ruminant livestock will be less widespread after MOSS implementation and thus fewer costs for **action measures** will be necessary in future.

Emotional costs include **stigmatism** of people in the small ruminant sector, **existential fear** of animal owners and **anxiety of the public about infection**. These costs cannot be enumerated pecuniary, but they have to be considered during the implementation process and when communicating with stakeholders. This MOSS can only act with high efficiency if emotions of animal owners and the public are taken seriously and are addressed properly.

Finally, emotional benefits evolve from protection of the public against Q fever while cooperating with animal owners. Knowing about positive flock status enables animal owners to take safety measures and thus demonstrate their **sense of responsibility** toward their fellow humans. Negative flock status can gain the **confidence** of the public in the animal owners and lead to economic strengthening of their business. Small ruminants are a considerable component of German livestock production especially for landscape conservation and are popular in the private sector. This MOSS does not want to impair the husbandry of small ruminants in Germany. Rather, it intends to support the small ruminant sector with regard to their responsibility in **zoonosis prevention.** Therefore, an emotional benefit is that stakeholders will work together in reaching this aim in a One **Health approach.**

CONCLUSION

In conclusion, this concept of active surveillance of Q fever in small ruminant livestock focuses on an early warning system in order to prevent Q fever infections in the human population. Considering a best practice approach, the aim is to identify flocks currently shedding the pathogen. Flocks should be considered positive if at least one pool of vaginal swabs is positive by PCR. The surveillance approach culminates in flock-specific action and control measures for the affected flocks. If this best practice concept were to be implemented, a huge conflict between economic costs and feasibility would emerge. Therefore, to maintain the aim of this MOSS (prevention of human cases by detecting small ruminant shedders), modifications of the concept are necessary. The system has been developed to serve as a basis for the introduction of a nationwide mandatory surveillance system in the future. Even without the context of subsequent obligation to participate or implement control measures, it is always a challenge to balance necessities and practicability when developing a MOSS.

Currently, successful implementation of this early warning system depends on **voluntary** participation of animal owners. For nationwide and mandatory implementation of this MOSS, a revision of the German law is necessary. Only if the active MOSS is ordered by law can Q fever be prevented safely among the public. In the meantime, and after legal obligation, the most important prerequisite for successful prevention of pathogen transmission is close cooperation between public health authorities and veterinary health authorities at the national and local levels as well as willingness to learn about the possibilities and challenges of the other parties. Furthermore, good and trusting communication with other stakeholders, especially with the animal owners, is mandatory. After successful implementation of this concept focusing on Q fever in small ruminant livestock, a further monitoring and surveillance system for Q fever in other domestic and wild mammals as a target group should be considered. This further development could provide insights into a possible pathogen reservoir in Germany and expand health protection for the population.

In conclusion, this surveillance system is built at the interface of animal and public health, thereby acting as a veterinary public health tool. The responsibility of veterinary and human medicine for public health is already well-recognized, and the One Health concept should be put into practice with the early warning system for Q fever presented here.

AUTHOR CONTRIBUTIONS

All authors contributed to the article and approved the submitted version.

REFERENCES

1. Rodolakis A. Q fever, state of art: epidemiology, diagnosis and prophylaxis. *Small Rumin Res.* (2006) 62:121–4. doi: 10.1016/j.smallrumres.2005.07.038
2. Bundesinstitut für Risikobewertung (BfR) Stellungnahmen 2010. *Q-Fieber: Übertragung von Coxiella burnetii Durch den Verzehr von Lebensmitteln Tierischer Herkunft Unwahrscheinlich, Stellungnahme Nr. 018/2010 des BfR vom 15.* Available online at: https://www.bfr.bund.de/de/bfr_stellungnahmen_2010.html (accessed April 02, 2020).
3. Jones RM, Nicas M, Hubbard AE, Reingold AL. The infectious dose of *Coxiella burnetii* (q fever). *Appl Biosaf.* (2006) 11:32–41. doi: 10.1177/153567600601100106
4. Todkill D, Fowler T, Hawker JI. Estimating the incubation period of acute q fever, a systematic review. *Epidemiol Infect.* (2018) 146:665–72. doi: 10.1017/S095026881700303X
5. World Organisation for Animal Health (OIE). *Manual of Diagnostic Tests and Vaccines for Terrestrial Animals 2019 Chapter 3.1.16 Q Fever (NB: Version adopted in May 2018)* Available online at: https://www.oie.int/standard-setting/terrestrial-manual/access-online/ (accessed March 11, 2020).
6. Tissot-Dupont H, Raoult D. Clinical aspects, diagnosis, and treatment of Q fever. In: Raoult D, Parola P, editors. *Rickettsial Diseases.* Boca Raton, FL: CRC Press (2007). p. 291–9. doi: 10.3109/9781420019971.021
7. Angelakis E, Raoult D. Q fever. *Vet Microbiol.* (2010) 140:297–309. doi: 10.1016/j.vetmic.2009.07.016
8. Morroy G, Keijmel SP, Delsing CE, Bleijenberg G, Langendam M, Timen A, et al. Fatigue following acute q-fever: a systematic literature review. *PLoS ONE.* (2016) 11:e155884. doi: 10.1371/journal.pone.0155884
9. Robert Koch-Institut (RKI). RKI-ratgeber infektionskrankheiten - merkblätter für ärzte, Q-fieber. *Epidemiol Bull.* (2002) 37:313–6.
10. González-Barrio D, Ruiz-Fons F. *Coxiella burnetii* in wild mammals: a systematic review. *Transbound Emerg Dis.* (2019). 66:662–71. doi: 10.1111/tbed.13085
11. Georgiev M, Afonso A, Neubauer H, Needham H, Thiéry R, Rodolakis A, et al. Q fever in humans and farm animals in four European countries, 1982 to 2010. *Euro Surveill.* (2013) 18:13–25.
12. Plummer PJ, McClure JT, Menzies P, Morley PS, Van den Brom R, Van Metre DC. Management of *Coxiella burnetii* infection in livestock populations and the associated zoonotic risk: a consensus statement. *J Vet Intern Med.* (2018) 32:1481–94. doi: 10.1111/jvim.15229
13. Ruiz-Fons F, González-Barrio D, Aguilar-Ríos F, Soler AJ, Garde JJ, Gortázar C, et al. Infectious pathogens potentially transmitted by semen of the black variety of the manchega sheep breed: health constraints for conservation purposes. *Anim Reprod Sci.* (2014) 149:152–7. doi: 10.1016/j.anireprosci.2014.07.006
14. Wolf A, Prüfer TL, Schoneberg C, Campe A, Runge M, Ganter M, et al. Prevalence of *Coxiella burnetii* in German sheep flocks and evaluation of a novel approach to detect an infection via preputial swabs at herd-level. *Epidemiol Infect.* (2020) 148:e88. doi: 10.1017/S0950268820000801
15. Körner S, Makert GR, Mertens-Scholz K, Henning K, Pfeffer M, Starke A, et al. Uptake and fecal excretion of *Coxiella burnetii* by *Ixodes ricinus* and *Dermacentor marginatus* ticks. *Paras Vectors.* (2020) 13:1–11. doi: 10.1186/s13071-020-3956-z
16. Nusinovici S, Hoch T, Brahim ML, Joly A, Beaudeau F. The effect of wind on *Coxiella burnetii* transmission between cattle herds: a mechanistic approach. *Transbound Emerg Dis.* (2017) 64:585–92. doi: 10.1111/tbed.12423
17. Rodolakis A. Q fever in dairy animals. *Ann NY Acad Sci.* (2009) 1166:90–3. doi: 10.1111/j.1749-6632.2009.04511.x
18. Berri M, Souriau A, Crosby M, Crochet D, Lechopier P, Rodolakis A. Relationships between the shedding of *Coxiella burnetii*, clinical signs and serological responses of 34 sheep. *Vet Rec.* (2001) 148:502–5. doi: 10.1136/vr.148.16.502
19. Guatteo R, Joly A, Beaudeau F. Shedding and serological patterns of dairy cows following abortions associated with *Coxiella burnetii* DNA detection. *Vet Microbiol.* (2012) 155:430–3. doi: 10.1016/j.vetmic.2011.09.026
20. Agerholm JS. *Coxiella burnetii* associated reproductive disorders in domestic animals-a critical review. *Acta Vet Scand.* (2013) 55:13. doi: 10.1186/1751-0147-55-13
21. Bouvery N, Souriau A, Lechopier P, Rodolakis A. Experimental *Coxiella burnetii* infection in pregnant goats: excretion routes. *Vet Res BioMed Centr.* (2003) 34:423–33. doi: 10.1051/vetres:2003017
22. Berri M, Rousset E, Champion JL, Russo P, Rodolakis A. Goats may experience reproductive failures and shed *Coxiella burnetii* at two successive parturitions after a q fever infection. *Res Vet Sci.* (2007) 83:47–52. doi: 10.1016/j.rvsc.2006.11.001
23. Palmer NC, Kierstead M, Key DW, Williams JC, Peaceock MG, Vellend H. Placentitis and abortion in goats and sheep in ontario by *Coxiella burnetii*. *Can Vet J.* (1983) 24:60–1.
24. European Centre for Disease Prevention and Control. Q fever. In: *ECDC. Annual Epidemiological Report for 2018.* Stockholm: ECDC (2019).
25. Bauer BU, Runge M, Campe A, Henning K, Mertens-Scholz K, Boden K, et al. *Coxiella burnetii: A Review Focusing on Infections in German Sheep and Goat Flocks. Berl Münch Tierärztl Wochenschr 2020.* Available online at: https://vetline.de/icoxiella-burnetiii-ein-uebersichtsartikel-mit-fokus-auf-das-infektionsgeschehen-in-deutschen-schaf-und-ziegenherden/150/3216/111683 (accessed April 15, 2020).
26. Hellenbrand W, Schöneberg I, Pfaff G, Kramer M, Steng G, Reintjes R, et al. The relevance of *Coxiella burnetii* infections in animals for q fever in humans - measures for prevention and control. *Tierärztl Prax.* (2005) 33:5–11. doi: 10.1055/s-0038-1624108
27. Hellenbrand W, Breuer T, Petersen L. Changing epidemiology of q fever in Germany, 1947-1999. *Emerg Infect Dis.* (2001) 7:789–96. doi: 10.3201/eid0705.010504
28. Robert Koch-Institut (RKI). *Infektions Epidemiologisches Jahrbuch Meldepflichtiger Krankheiten für Das Jahr 2018.* Berlin: Robert Koch-Institut (2019).
29. Porten K, Rissland J, Tigges A, Broll S, Hopp W, Lunemann M, et al. A super-spreading ewe infects hundreds with q fever at a farmers' market in Germany. *BMC Infect Dis.* (2006) 6:147. doi: 10.1186/1471-2334-6-147
30. Federal Institute for Consumer Health Protection and Veterinary Medicine (BgVV). Bericht über die epidemiologische Situation der Zoonosen in Deutschland für 1998, Übersicht über die Meldungen der Bundesländer. In: Hartung M, editor. *BgVV-Hefte XX/1999.* Berlin: Federal Institute for Consumer Health Protection and Veterinary Medicine (BgVV) (1999). p. 172.
31. Clark NJ, Magalhaes RJS. Airborne geographical dispersal of q fever from livestock holdings to human communities: a systematic review and critical appraisal of evidence. *BMC Infect Dis.* (2018) 18:218. doi: 10.1186/s12879-018-3135-4
32. Sidi-Boumedine K, Rousset E, Henning K, Ziller M, Niemczuck K, Roest HIJ, et al. Development of harmonised schemes for the monitoring and reporting of q-fever in animals in the European Union. *EFSA Support Publ.* (2010) 7:1–48. doi: 10.2903/sp.efsa.2010.EN-48
33. Ganter M. Zoonotic risks from small ruminants. *Vet Microbiol.* (2015) 181:53–65. doi: 10.1016/j.vetmic.2015.07.015
34. Bond KA, Vincent G, Wilks CR, Franklin L, Sutton B, Stenos J, et al. One health approach to controlling a q fever outbreak on an Australian goat farm. *Epidemiol Infect.* (2016) 144:1129–41. doi: 10.1017/S0950268815002368
35. George M, Reich A, Cussler K, Jehl H, Burckhardt F. Live cell therapy as potential risk factor for q fever. *Emerg Infect Dis.* (2017) 23:1210–2. doi: 10.3201/eid2307.161693

36. World Organisation for Animal Health (OIE). *Animal Terrestrial Health Code.* (2019). Available online at: https://www.oie.int/index.php?id=169&L=0&htmfile=sommaire.htm (accessed March 11, 2020).
37. Infektionsschutzgesetz vom 20. *Juli 2000 (BGBl. I S. 1045), Das Zuletzt Durch Artikel 3 des Gesetzes Vom 27. März 2020 (BGBl. I S. 587) Geändert Worden IST.* Available online at: https://www.gesetze-im-internet.de/ifsg/BJNR104510000.html (accessed March 15, 2020).
38. Tiergesundheitsgesetz in der Fassung der Bekanntmachung vom 21. *November 2018 (BGBl. I S. 1938), Das Zuletzt Durch Artikel 100 des Gesetzes vom 20. November 2019 (BGBl. I S. 1626) Geändert Worden IST.* Available online at: https://www.gesetze-im-internet.de/tiergesg/BJNR132400013.html (accessed March 15, 2020).
39. Verordnung über meldepflichtige Tierkrankheiten in der Fassung der Bekanntmachung vom 11. *Februar 2011 (BGBl. I S. 252), Die Zuletzt Durch Artikel 381 der Verordnung vom 31. August 2015 (BGBl. I S. 1474) Geändert Worden IST.* Available online at: https://www.gesetze-im-internet.de/tkrmeldpflv_1983/BJNR010950983.html (accessed March 15, 2020).
40. Chemisches und Veterinäruntersuchungsamt (CVUA) Stuttgart. *Leitfaden zum Q-Fieber Baden-Württemberg: Empfehlungen zur Bekämpfung des Q-Fiebers bei kleinen Wiederkäuern in Baden-Württemberg.* Stuttgart (2017).
41. Federal Ministry of Food and Agriculture (BMEL). *Bekanntmachung von Empfehlungen für Hygienische Anforderungen an das Halten von Wiederkäuern vom 7 Juli 2014 (BAnz. AT 01.08.2014 BI) Geändert Durch Erste Bekanntmachung der Änderung der Bekanntmachung von Empfehlungen für Hygienische Anforderungen an das Halten von Wiederkäuern vom 19. August 2014 (BAnz AT 28.08.2014 B1).* Available online at: https://www.bmel.de/DE/Tier/Tiergesundheit/_texte/EmpfehlungenHygiene.html (accessed March 15, 2020).
42. Salman MD. *Animal Disease Surveillance and Survey Systems: Methods and Applications.* Iowa, IA: Iowa State Press (2003). p. 1–222. doi: 10.1002/9780470344866
43. Doherr MG, Audige L. Monitoring and surveillance for rare health-related events: a review from the veterinary perspective. *Philos Trans R Soc Lond B.* (2001) 356:1097–106. doi: 10.1098/rstb.2001.0898
44. Hilbert A, Schmoock G, Lenzko H, Moog U, Diller R, Fröhlich A, et al. Prevalence of *Coxiella burnetii* in clinically healthy German sheep flocks. *BMC Res Notes.* (2012) 5:152. doi: 10.1186/1756-0500-5-152
45. Roest HIJ, Tilburg JJHC, Van der Hoek W, Vellema P, Van Zijderveld FG, Klaassen CHW, et al. Review article, the q fever epidemic in The Netherlands: history, onset, response and reflection. *Epidemiol Infect.* (2011) 139:1–12. doi: 10.1017/S0950268810002268
46. Hoinville LJ. Animal health surveillance terminology, final report from Pre-ICAHS Workshop, July 2013 (version 1.2). In: *International Conference on Animal Health Surveillance (ICAHS).* La Havana: CUB (2013).
47. Hoinville LJ, Alban L, Drewe JA, Gibbens JC, Gustafson L, Häsler B, et al. Proposed terms and concepts for describing and evaluating animal-health surveillance systems. *Prev Vet Med.* (2013) 112:1–12. doi: 10.1016/j.prevetmed.2013.06.006
48. Comin A, Haesler B, Hoinville LJ, Peyre M, Dórea F, Schauer B, et al. RISKSUR tools: taking animal health surveillance into the future through interdisciplinary integration of scientific evidence. In: *Annual Meeting of the Society for Veterinary Epidemiology and Preventive Medicine.* Elsinore: DNK (2016).
49. Sargeant JM, O'Connor AM. Issues of reporting in observational studies in veterinary medicine. *Prev Vet Med.* (2014). 113:323–30. doi: 10.1016/j.prevetmed.2013.09.004
50. Runge M, Binder A, Schotte U, Ganter M. Investigations concerning the prevalenceof *Coxiella burnetii* and *Clamydia abortus* in sheep in correlation with management systems and abortion rate in Lower saxony in 2004. *Berl Munch Tierarztl Wochenschr.* (2012) 125:10–5. doi: 10.2376/0005-9366-125-138
51. Dohoo IR, Martin W, Stryhn H. *Veterinary Epidemiologic Research.* Charlottetown, PE: VER Inc. (2010). p. 1–865.
52. Federal Statistical Office of Germany (Destatis). *Ergebnis - 41141-0019 Landwirtschaftliche Betriebe mit Viehhaltung, Viehbestand: Bundesländer, Stichtag, Tierarten (01.03.2016).* Available online at: https://www-genesis.destatis.de/genesis/online/data;sid$=$BD01EDE95F2DAE53798F8BBFCB748D7D.GO_2_1?operation$=$abruftabelleBearbeiten&levelindex$=$1&levelid$=$1568200076966&auswahloperation$=$abruftabelleAuspraegungAuswaehlen&auswahlverzeichnis$=$ordnungsstruktur&auswahlziel$=$werteabruf&selectionname$=$41141-0019&auswahltext$=$&werteabruf$=$Werteabruf (accessed September 11, 2019).
53. Federal Statistical Office of Germany (Destatis), Federal Ministry of Food and Agriculture (BMEL). *Statistik und Berichte des BMEL, Landwirtschaft, Tierhaltung, Schafe, MBT-0117490-0000 Betriebe mit Schafhaltung nach Bestandsgrößenklassen.* Available online at: https://www.bmel-statistik.de/landwirtschaft/tierhaltung/schafhaltung/ (accessed March 24, 2020).
54. Debeljak Z, Medic S, Baralic M, Andric A, Tomic A, Vidanovic D, et al. Clinical, epidemiological and epizootic features of a Q fever outbreak in the border region between Serbia and Montenegro. *J Infect Dev Ctries.* (2018) 12:290–6. doi: 10.3855/jidc.9918
55. Anderson AD, Szymanski TJ, Emery MP, Kohrs PH, Bjork AC, Marsden-Haug N, et al. Epizootiological investigation of a q fever outbreak and implications for future control strategies. *JAVMA.* (2015) 247:1379–86. doi: 10.2460/javma.247.12.1379
56. Bauer B, Prüfer L, Walter M, Ganter I, Frangoulidis D, Runge M, et al. Comparison of *Coxiella burnetii* excretion between sheep and goats naturally infected with one cattle-associated genotype. *Pathogens.* (2020) 9:15. doi: 10.3390/pathogens9080652
57. Roest HJ, van Gelderen B, Dinkla A, Frangoulidis D, van Zijderveld F, Rebel J, et al. Q Fever in pregnant goats: pathogenesis and excretion of *Coxiella burnetii. PLoS ONE.* (2012). 7:e48949. doi: 10.1371/journal.pone.0048949
58. Friedrich-Loeffler-Institut (FLI). *Amtliche Methodensammlung Q-Fieber.* Greifswald-Insel Riems (2018).
59. Rousset E, Berri M, Durand B, Dufour P, Prigent M, Delcroix T, et al. *Coxiella burnetii* shedding routes and antibody response after outbreaks of q fever-induced abortion in dairy goat herds. *Appl Environ Microbiol.* (2009) 75:428–33. doi: 10.1128/AEM.00690-08
60. Kreienbrock L, Pigeot I, Ahrens W. *Epidemiologische Methoden.* Berlin; Heidelberg: Springer (2012). p. 492. doi: 10.1007/978-3-8274-2334-4
61. Arricau-Bouvery N, Souriau A, Bodier C, Dufour P, Rousset E, Rodolakis A. Effect of vaccination with phase I and phase II *Coxiella burnetii* vaccines in pregnant goats. *Vaccine.* (2005) 23:4392–402. doi: 10.1016/j.vaccine.2005.04.010
62. Rahaman MR, Milazzo A, Marshall H, Bi P. Is a one health approach utilized for q fever control? A comprehensive literature review. *Int J Environ Res Public Health.* (2019) 16:730. doi: 10.3390/ijerph16050730
63. de Vries DH, Kinsman J, Takacs J, Tsolova S, Ciotti M. Methodology for assessment of public health emergency preparedness and response synergies between institutional authorities and communities. *BMC Health Serv Res.* (2020) 20:411. doi: 10.1186/s12913-020-05298-z
64. Greiner M, Baumann M, Campe A, Doherr MG, Gareis M, Greif G, et al. Zur rolle der veterinärmedizin im bereich public health. *Deutsch Tierärzteblatt.* (2017) 65:158–61.
65. Tierärztegebührenordnung vom 28. *Juli 1999 (BGBl. I S. 1691), die Zuletzt Durch Artikel 1 der Verordnung vom 10. Februar 2020 (BGBl. I S. 158) Geändert Worden IST.* Available online at: https://www.gesetze-im-internet.de/got/BJNR169100999.html (accessed March 15, 2020).
66. Gebührenordnung für die Verwaltung im Bereich des Verbraucherschutzes und des Veterinärwesens (GOVV) vom 29. *November 2014, Letzte Berücksichtigte Änderung: Anlage Geändert Durch Verordnung vom 16.01.2020 (Nds. GVBl. S. 4).* Available online at: http://www.nds-voris.de/jportal/portal/t/1bqx/page/bsvorisprod.psml?pid=Dokumentanzeige&showdoccase=1&js_peid=Trefferliste&documentnumber=1&numberofresults=1&fromdoctodoc=yes&doc.id=jlr-VetVwGOND2014V11Anlage&doc.part=X&doc.price=0.0#focuspoint (accessed March 15, 2020).
67. Ständige Impfkommission Veterinärmedizin (StIKo Vet) am Friedrich-Loeffler-Institut (FLI). *Leitlinie zur Impfung von Rindern und kleinen Wiederkäuern.* Greifswald-Insel Riems (2018).
68. Bauer BU, Janowetz B, Turowski V, Ambros C, Alex M, Domes U, et al. *Verlauf*

der Coxiellose in Einer Schafherde Nach Jährlicher Grundimmunisierung der Zutreter [Internet]. Tagung der DVG-Fachgruppe Krankheiten kleiner Wiederkäuer: Greifswald - Insel Riems (2019). p. 83–5. Available online at: https://elib.tiho-hannover.de/receive/tiho_mods_00003290

69. Coors W. *Das Tierseuchenentschädigungsrecht*. Hamburg: Jur. Fakultät Universität Hamburg (1966).
70. Discontool - Research gaps for improving infectious disease control in animals. *Diseases - Q-Fever*. Available online at: https://discontools.eu/database/57-q-fever.html (accessed February 27, 2020).

8

Pan-Genome Analysis of *Vibrio cholerae* and *Vibrio metschnikovii* Strains Isolated from Migratory Birds at Dali Nouer Lake in Chifeng

Lin Zheng[1,2†], *Ling-Wei Zhu*[2†], *Jie Jing*[2], *Jia-yao Guan*[2], *Ge-Jin Lu*[2], *Lin-Hong Xie*[3], *Xue Ji*[2], *Dong Chu*[3], *Yang Sun*[2], *Ping Chen*[1*] and *Xue-Jun Guo*[2*]

[1] School of Food and Engineering, Jilin Agricultural University, Changchun, China, [2] The Key Laboratory of Jilin Province for Zoonosis Prevention and Control, Changchun, China, [3] Wild Animal Sources and Diseases Inspection Station, National Forestry and Grassl and Bureau, Beijing, China

***Correspondence:**
Ping Chen
1243377523@qq.com
Xue-Jun Guo
xuejung@yahoo.com*

†These authors have contributed equally to this work

Migratory birds are recently recognized as *Vibrio* disease vectors, but may be widespread transporters of *Vibrio* strains. We isolated *Vibrio cholerae (V. cholerae)* and *Vibrio metschnikovii (V. metschnikovii)* strains from migratory bird epidemic samples from 2017 to 2018 and isolated *V. metschnikovii* from migratory bird feces in 2019 from bird samples taken from the Inner Mongolia autonomous region of China. To investigate the evolution of these two *Vibrio* species, we sequenced the genomes of 40 *V. cholerae* strains and 34 *V. metschnikovii* strains isolated from the bird samples and compared these genomes with reference strain genomes. The pan-genome of all *V. cholerae* and *V. metschnikovii* genomes was large, with strains exhibiting considerable individual differences. A total of 2,130 and 1,352 core genes were identified in the *V. cholerae* and *V. metschnikovii* genomes, respectively, while dispensable genes accounted for 16,180 and 9,178 of all genes for the two strains, respectively. All *V. cholerae* strains isolated from the migratory birds that encoded T6SS and *hlyA* were non-O1/O139 serotypes without the ability to produce CTX. These strains also lacked the ability to produce the TCP fimbriae nor the extracellular matrix protein RbmA and could not metabolize trimetlylamine oxide (TMAO). Thus, these characteristics render them unlikely to be pandemic-inducing strains. However, a *V. metschnikovii* isolate encoding the complete T6SS system was isolated for the first time. These data provide new molecular insights into the diversity of *V. cholerae* and *V. metschnikovii* isolates recovered from migratory birds.

Keywords: *Vibrio cholerae*, *Vibrio metschnikovii*, comparative genomics, migratory bird, pathogenic

INTRODUCTION

Vibrio is an abundant bacterial genus in oceans and comprises numerous species including pathogenic types such as *Vibrio cholerae*, *Vibrio parahaemolyticus*, and *Vibrio metschnikovii.* They are often observed in high abundance in marine products. *Vibrio* are halophilic and naturally found ubiquitously in marine settings, and thus raw seafood naturally harbors these microorganisms and is the main food source responsible for gastroenteritis caused by *Vibrio* spp. (1). Cholera is caused by *V. cholerae* that carry the cholera toxin and has resulted in seven pandemics throughout human history. The seventh *V. cholerae* pandemic continues to present day, and exhibits evolved characteristics compared to previous pandemics, rendering it difficult to treat cholera disease outbreaks (2, 3). One commonality between the sixth and seventh pandemics has been observed to be associated with the CTXΦ bacteriophage that may have introduced the CTX toxin to *V. cholerae*. Nevertheless, the strains underlying the seventh pandemic did not directly evolve from those underlying the sixth pandemic (2). In contrast to *V. cholerae*, few reports have described characterizations of *V. metschnikovii*, with only some studies focused on detection and no reports on their pathogenicity.

Migratory birds have been considered potential vectors of *V. cholerae*, wherein colonization of their intestines may occur by ingesting water and marine animals infected with *V. cholerae* (4). Migratory birds travel over long distances and could carry pathogenic microorganisms from one region to another, spreading pathogenic microorganisms by excretion (5, 6). Therefore, migratory birds have been considered as important reservoirs of *Vibrio*, forming a fecal-food-mouth transmission route (3). Within intestinal environments, *Vibrio* are induced to evolve into treatment-resistant bacteria or pandemic strains due to stresses they are exposed to. Consequently, increased risk of bacterial spread and difficulty of bacterial source tracking occur due to the long migration distances of vector birds.

Consequently, it is important to analyze the pathogenicity of *V. cholerae* strains and whether they exhibit the potential to evolve into pandemic strains. The concept of a pan-genome was first proposed in 2005 and is a term that encompasses the sum of all genes of a species, including their core-genome, dispensable genome, and unique genome components (7). Importantly, the population-level evolutionary trends of a species can be evaluated by analyzing their pan-genome.

Migratory birds exhibiting malnutrition, wasting, diarrhea, and high mortality were observed in the Inner Mongolia region of China between 2017 and 2018. Dead birds comprised individuals from several species including *Larus ridibundus*, *Pluvialis squatarola*, *Tadorna ferrgina*, *Anas poecilorhyncha*, and *Aix galericulata*, in addition to other migratory birds. Moreover, 40 *V. cholerae* strains and 34 *V. metschnikovii* strains were isolated from the migratory bird epidemic materials and water environments. The *V. cholerae* strains were non-O1/O139 strains without the *ctxA/B* toxin, based on serotyping and PCR identification. To further investigate this die-off, we conducted a bacteriological examination again on migratory bird feces in Inner Mongolia, China, in 2019. However, *V. cholerae* strains were again not present in the samples, while only *V. metschnikovii* was present. In this study, we analyzed the core-/pan- genomes of *V. cholerae*/*V. metschnikovii* and compared them with previously sequenced strains to evaluate whether migratory birds harbor *Vibrio* spp. that have the potential to evolve into pandemic or drug-resistant strains. These analyses thus provide important data to inform the prevention and treatment of *V. cholerae* and *V. metschnikovii* infections and/or outbreaks.

Abbreviations: PCR, Polymerase chain reaction; MLST, Multilocus sequence typing; ARDB, Antibiotic Resistance Genes Database; VFDB, virulence factor database; CARD, Comprehensive Antibiotic Research Database; COG, Cluster of Orthologous Groups of proteins; GO, Gene Ontology; KEGG, Kyoto Encyclopedia of Genes and Genomes; NR, Non-Redundant Protein Database. T6SS, Type VI secretory system; T3SS, Type III secretory system; CTX, cholera toxin.

MATERIALS AND METHODS

Sampling

Thirty-six samples (including 10 water samples, 2 aquatic plant samples, 19 epidemic material samples, and 24 feace samples) were taken from birds in 2018 and 2019. DNA was obtained from each fecal sample by stool DNA kit, and molecular method to determine the host source of feaces (8). The visceral organ and intestinal tract samples used for this study were collected aseptically from 19 freshly dead migratory birds (not corrupt). Samples were cultivated via spread plates in triplicate and directly cultivated onto selective thiosulfate citrate bile salts sucrose (TCBS) agar plates and incubated for 24 h at 37°C. Isolates were identified using PCR amplification of *ompW*, *infC*, *ctxA*, *hlyA*, and *chxA* genes (9–13). The primers and conditions used for PCR amplification are described in **Supplementary Table 1**. In addition, *V. cholerae* isolates were subjected to O1/O139 antigen serotyping using *V. cholerae* O antisera (Tianjin Biochip Corporation). Isolates were sub-cultured at 37°C in brain heart liquid (Qingdao Haibo, China) or on CHROM agar *Vibrio* plates (CHROM, Paris, France) unless otherwise specified. Green colonies were again confirmed using serology and PCR assays (see **Supplementary Table 1** for primer sequences and PCR conditions). Isolates identified as *Vibrio* were then stored in a −80°C freezer.

Extraction of Genomic DNA and Library Construction

Genomic DNA was extracted from isolates using the Bacterial Genomic DNA Extraction Kit (Omega). Harvested DNA was then quantified using a Qubit® 2.0 Fluorometer (Thermo Scientific). A total of 1 μg of DNA per sample was used as input material for DNA library preparations. Sequencing libraries were generated using the NEBNext® Ultra™ DNA Library Prep Kit for Illumina (NEB, USA) following manufacturer's recommendations. In addition, indexing oligonucleotides were added to sequences to identify each sample. Briefly, DNA samples were fragmented by sonication to a size of 350 bp, followed by DNA fragment end-polishing, addition of poly A-tails, and ligation with full-length adaptors for Illumina sequencing, followed by additional PCR amplification. Finally, PCR products were purified (AMPure XP system), and the size distribution of the libraries was analyzed using an Agilent 2100 Bioanalyzer and quantified using real-time PCR. The whole-genomes of strains were sequenced using an Illumina NovaSeq PE150 platform at the Beijing Novogene Bioinformatics Technology Co., Ltd.

Genome Assembly

Reads containing Illumina PCR adapters and low-quality reads were filtered from the dataset using readfq (vision 10). The remaining good quality paired reads were assembled into scaffolds using the SOAP denovo (https://sourceforge.net/projects/soapdenovo2/files/SOAPdenovo2/), SPAdes (http://cab.spbu.ru/software/spades/), and ABySS (http://www.bcgsc.ca/platform/bioinfo/software/abyss) assemblers (14–17). The filtered reads were then used to close gaps in the scaffolds using Readfq with the options: –rq1 input_1.fq, –rq2 input_2.fq,–oq1 out_1.fq,–oq2 out_2.fq,–adp1 adapter_1.lst,–adp2 adapter_2.lst,– Q QUAL, PERCENT,–C QUAL, PERCENT,–N PERCENT,–alen INT,–amis INT,–dup,–gz,–check1 read1.check,–check2 read2.check.

Genome Feature Predictions

Genome component prediction included prediction of coding genes, repetitive sequences, non-coding RNAs, genomic islands, transposons, prophages, and clustered regularly interspaced short palindromic repeat sequences (CRISPRs). The Gene Mark program was used to identify coding genes, while interspersed repetitive sequences were predicted using the Repeat Masker (http://www.repeatmasker.org/). Tandem repeats were identified using the tandem repeats finder (TRF) program. Transfer RNA (tRNA) genes were predicted using tRNA scan-SE (18–21), while ribosomal RNA (rRNA) genes were identified using rRNAmmer (22). Small nuclear RNAs (snRNA) were predicted by BLAST searches against the Rfam database (23, 24). The Island Path-DIOMB program was used to predict genomic islands and the transposon PSI program was used to identify transposons based on the homologous blast method (25). Lastly, PHAST was used to predict prophages (http://phast.wishartlab.com/), and CRISPR Finder was used to identify CRISPRs (26, 27).

Gene Function Prediction

Four databases were used to predict gene functions, including the Gene Ontology (GO), Kyoto Encyclopedia of Genes and Genomes (KEGG), Clusters of Orthologous Groups (COG) (28), and non-redundant (NR) protein databases (29–32). In addition, whole-genome BLAST searches were performed against the above-mentioned four databases using an *E*-value threshold of <1e-5 and a minimum alignment length percentage >40% as criteria (33). Secretory proteins were predicted using the Signal P database, and the prediction of Type I-VII proteins secreted by pathogenic bacteria was based on the EffectiveT3software program (34, 35). To evaluate pathogenic factors, pathogenicity, and drug resistance analyses were also conducted using the Virulence Factors of Pathogenic Bacteria (VFDB) and Antibiotic Resistance Genes Database (ARDB) databases (36, 37).

Comparative Genomic Analyses

Comparative genomic analyses were conducted including analysis of genomic synteny, the distribution of core- and strain-specific genes, and phylogenetic analysis of gene families. Genomic alignment between the sample and reference genomes was performed using the MUMmer and LASTZ tools while including 41 *V. cholerae* strains and 4 *V. metschnikovii* strains as reference genomes (see **Supplementary Table 2** for additional details) (38). The analysis of genomic synteny was based on alignment results. Core- and strain-specific genes were identified based on rapid clustering of similar proteins with the CD-HIT program while specifying a threshold of 50% pairwise identity and a 70% length difference cutoff. A Venn diagram was then used to show the relationships of core- and strain-specific genes among samples. The MUSCLE software program was used to align multiple single-copy core-encoded proteins identified by the core-/pan-genome analysis. The aligned sequences were then subjected to phylogenetic analysis using the TreeBeST program, a neighbor-joining tree reconstruction algorithm, and 1,000 bootstrap replicates.

Multilocus gene sequence typing was conducted based on sequence analysis of eight housekeeping genes (*adk, gyrB, mdh, metE, pgm, pntA, purM,* and *pyrC*) using previously described PubMLST protocols (https://pubmlst.org/databases.shtml). The nucleotide sequences for each locus were analyzed with the BioNumerics software program (version 7.6; Applied Maths, Belgium) and compared against published sequences on the PubMLST website. Sequence types (STs) were then determined on the basis of the eight locus allelic profiles.

Nucleotide Sequence

Accession Numbers

The 74 sequences of *V. cholerae* and *V. metschnikovii* were submitted to FigShare under the public doi: 10.6084/m9.figshare.14417870. And C16-2-29, M13F, M9D, M21D, M28D, and M29D uploaded Genbank database at the same time, accession number GCA_014281135.1, GCA_014305065.1, GCA_014267955.1, GCA_014267965.1, GCA_014305075.1 and GCA_014305185.1, respectively.

RESULTS

Genome Sequencing

A total of 40 *V. cholerae* and 34 *V. Metschnikovii* strains were identified in this study using PCR identification and comparison of gene sequences against the non-redundant (NR) protein database. All of the strains lacked the *ctxA, tcpA,* and *chxA* genes, and were also non-O1/O139 serotypes by PCR. All isolates were completely turbid after dripping *V. cholerae* O antisera and no agglutination occurred, the result was the consistent as the PCR, and it was identified as non-O1/O139 *V. cholerae* (**Table 1**).

Core- and Pan-Genomic Analysis

The *V. cholerae* pan-genomes were analyzed by dividing them into core and dispensable genomes. A total of 40 *V. cholerae* strains isolated from migratory birds were used in comparison against 41 reference *V. cholerae* genomes retrieved from GenBank. The number of core genes and the pan-genome sizes of the *V. cholerae* strains are shown in **Figure 1A** as a function of the number of genes within the genomes. The number of core genes plateaued when plotting the number of core genes against the reciprocal of the number of genomes included in the estimates. In contrast, the pan-genome size steadily increased with the addition of each additional genome, suggesting that *V. cholerae* exhibited a large pan-genome. Overall, a total of 18,310 pan-genes, 2,130 core-genes, and 16,180 dispensable genes were identified among all *V. cholerae* strain genomes (**Supplementary Table 3**). In this study, the dispensable genome

TABLE 1 | Characteristics of *Vibrio cholerae* and *Vibrio metschnikovii* isolates identified in migratory birds.

Isolate name	Sampling date	Species identification	Host	Sample location
C1F_2	2018.8.23	*V. cholerae*	*Larus ridibundus* (lung)	Chifeng, Inner Mongolia, China
C1C_1	2018.8.23	*V. cholerae*	*Larus ridibundus* (intestines)	Chifeng, Inner Mongolia, China
C1S_2	2018.8.23	*V. cholerae*	*Larus ridibundus* (kidney)	Chifeng, Inner Mongolia, China
C2XS_1	2018.8.23	*V. cholerae*	*Larus ridibundus* (kidney)	Chifeng, Inner Mongolia, China
C4C_1	2018.8.23	*V. cholerae*	*Himantopus* (intestines)	Chifeng, Inner Mongolia, China
C5G	2018.8.23	*V. cholerae*	*Pochard* (liver)	Chifeng, Inner Mongolia, China
C5G_R	2018.8.23	*V. cholerae*	*Pochard* (liver)	Chifeng, Inner Mongolia, China
C7F_1	2018.8.23	*V. cholerae*	*Larus argentatus* (lung)	Chifeng, Inner Mongolia, China
C8C_1	2018.8.23	*V. cholerae*	*Tadorna ferruginea* (intestines)	Chifeng, Inner Mongolia, China
C8C_2	2018.8.23	*V. cholerae*	*Tadorna ferruginea* (intestines)	Chifeng, Inner Mongolia, China
C11G_R	2018.8.23	*V. cholerae*	*Anas zonorhyncha* (liver)	Chifeng, Inner Mongolia, China
C11C_1	2018.8.23	*V. cholerae*	*Anas zonorhyncha* (intestines)	Chifeng, Inner Mongolia, China
C11S_2	2018.8.23	*V. cholerae*	*Anas zonorhyncha* (kidney)	Chifeng, Inner Mongolia, China
C18S_a	2018.8.30	*V. cholerae*	*Tadorna ferruginea* (kidney)	Chifeng, Inner Mongolia, China
C18p_2	2018.8.30	*V. cholerae*	*Tadorna ferruginea* (spleen)	Chifeng, Inner Mongolia, China
C18F_2	2018.8.30	*V. cholerae*	*Tadorna ferruginea* (lung)	Chifeng, Inner Mongolia, China
C18x_2	2018.8.30	*V. cholerae*	*Tadorna ferruginea* (heart)	Chifeng, Inner Mongolia, China
C18s_b	2018.8.30	*V. cholerae*	*Tadorna ferruginea* (kidney)	Chifeng, Inner Mongolia, China
C18s_2	2018.8.30	*V. cholerae*	*Tadorna ferruginea* (kidney)	Chifeng, Inner Mongolia, China
C18c_3	2018.8.30	*V. cholerae*	*Tadorna ferruginea* (intestines)	Chifeng, Inner Mongolia, China
C18G_a	2018.8.30	*V. cholerae*	*Tadorna ferruginea* (liver)	Chifeng, Inner Mongolia, China
C18F_b	2018.8.30	*V. cholerae*	*Tadorna ferruginea* (lung)	Chifeng, Inner Mongolia, China
C18G_b	2018.8.30	*V. cholerae*	*Tadorna ferruginea* (liver)	Chifeng, Inner Mongolia, China
C18c_a	2018.8.30	*V. cholerae*	*Tadorna ferruginea* (intestines)	Chifeng, Inner Mongolia, China
C18x_b	2018.8.30	*V. cholerae*	*Tadorna ferruginea* (heart)	Chifeng, Inner Mongolia, China
C19p_c	2018.8.30	*V. cholerae*	*Tadorna ferruginea* (spleen)	Chifeng, Inner Mongolia, China
C19F_3	2018.8.30	*V. cholerae*	*Tadorna ferruginea* (lung)	Chifeng, Inner Mongolia, China
C19c_a	2018.8.30	*V. cholerae*	*Tadorna ferruginea* (intestines)	Chifeng, Inner Mongolia, China
C19c_B	2018.8.30	*V. cholerae*	*Tadorna ferruginea* (intestines)	Chifeng, Inner Mongolia, China
C19G_b	2018.8.30	*V. cholerae*	*Tadorna ferruginea* (liver)	Chifeng, Inner Mongolia, China
C19F_1	2018.8.30	*V. cholerae*	*Tadorna ferruginea* (lung)	Chifeng, Inner Mongolia, China
C19S_b	2018.8.30	*V. cholerae*	*Tadorna ferruginea* (kidney)	Chifeng, Inner Mongolia, China
C19x_a	2018.8.30	*V. cholerae*	*Tadorna ferruginea* (heart)	Chifeng, Inner Mongolia, China
C19c_1	2018.8.30	*V. cholerae*	*Tadorna ferruginea* (intestines)	Chifeng, Inner Mongolia, China
C19x_b	2018.8.30	*V. cholerae*	*Tadorna ferruginea* (heart)	Chifeng, Inner Mongolia, China
C19G_a	2018.8.30	*V. cholerae*	*Tadorna ferruginea* (liver)	Chifeng, Inner Mongolia, China
C19p_b	2018.8.30	*V. cholerae*	*Tadorna ferruginea* (spleen)	Chifeng, Inner Mongolia, China
C2W	2018.8.30	*V. cholerae*	Water	Chifeng, Inner Mongolia, China
C7W	2018.8.30	*V. cholerae*	Water	Chifeng, Inner Mongolia, China
C16_2_290	2017.8.4	*V. cholerae*	*Phalacrocorax*	Wuliangsuhai, Inner Mongolia, China
M4G_2	2018.8.23	*V. metschnikovii*	*Himantopus mexicanus* (liver)	Chifeng, Inner Mongolia, China
M5C_1	2018.8.23	*V. metschnikovii*	*Pochard* (intestines)	Chifeng, Inner Mongolia, China
M5C_2	2018.8.23	*V. metschnikovii*	*Pochard* (intestines)	Chifeng, Inner Mongolia, China
M7S_1	2018.8.23	*V. metschnikovii*	*Larus argentatus* (kidney)	Chifeng, Inner Mongolia, China
M7C_1	2018.8.23	*V. metschnikovii*	*Larus argentatus* (intestines)	Chifeng, Inner Mongolia, China
M9G_2	2018.8.23	*V. metschnikovii*	*Tadorna ferruginea* (liver)	Chifeng, Inner Mongolia, China
M11F_1	2018.8.23	*V. metschnikovii*	*Anas poecilorhyncha* (lung)	Chifeng, Inner Mongolia, China
M12C	2018.8.30	*V. metschnikovii*	*Pochard* (intestines)	Chifeng, Inner Mongolia, China
M13F	2018.8.30	*V. metschnikovii*	*Aix galericulata* (lung)	Chifeng, Inner Mongolia, China
M14Y	2018.8.30	*V. metschnikovii*	*Tadorna ferruginea* (pancreas)	Chifeng, Inner Mongolia, China

(Continued)

TABLE 1 | Continued

Isolate name	Sampling date	Species identification	Host	Sample location
M14Y_1	2018.8.30	*V. metschnikovii*	*Tadorna ferruginea* (pancreas)	Chifeng, Inner Mongolia, China
M17C_1	2018.8.30	*V. metschnikovii*	Migratory birds (intestines)	Chifeng, Inner Mongolia, China
M19C_2	2018.8.30	*V. metschnikovii*	*Tadorna ferruginea* (intestines)	Chifeng, Inner Mongolia, China
M19C_6	2018.8.30	*V. metschnikovii*	*Tadorna ferruginea* (intestines)	Chifeng, Inner Mongolia, China
M1W	2018.8.30	*V. metschnikovii*	Water	Chifeng, Inner Mongolia, China
M3W	2018.8.30	*V. metschnikovii*	Water	Chifeng, Inner Mongolia, China
MH3GW	2018.8.30	*V. metschnikovii*	Water	Chifeng, Inner Mongolia, China
MNW	2018.8.30	*V. metschnikovii*	Water	Chifeng, Inner Mongolia, China
MNW_3	2018.8.30	*V. metschnikovii*	Water	Chifeng, Inner Mongolia, China
M3X	2019.7	*V. metschnikovii*	*Larus ridibundus*	Chifeng, Inner Mongolia, China
M7D	2019.7	*V. metschnikovii*	*Larus ridibundus*	Chifeng, Inner Mongolia, China
M8D	2019.7	*V. metschnikovii*	*Larus ridibundus*	Chifeng, Inner Mongolia, China
M9D	2019.7	*V. metschnikovii*	*Larus ridibundus*	Chifeng, Inner Mongolia, China
M14D	2019.7	*V. metschnikovii*	*Larus ridibundus*	Chifeng, Inner Mongolia, China
M15D	2019.7	*V. metschnikovii*	*Larus ridibundus*	Chifeng, Inner Mongolia, China
M16X	2019.7	*V. metschnikovii*	*Larus ridibundus*	Chifeng, Inner Mongolia, China
M19X	2019.7	*V. metschnikovii*	*Larus ridibundus*	Chifeng, Inner Mongolia, China
M21D	2019.7	*V. metschnikovii*	*Larus ridibundus*	Chifeng, Inner Mongolia, China
M26X	2019.7	*V. metschnikovii*	*Larus ridibundus*	Chifeng, Inner Mongolia, China
M27D	2019.7	*V. metschnikovii*	*Larus ridibundus*	Chifeng, Inner Mongolia, China
M28D	2019.7	*V. metschnikovii*	*Larus ridibundus*	Chifeng, Inner Mongolia, China
M29D	2019.7	*V. metschnikovii*	*Larus ridibundus*	Chifeng, Inner Mongolia, China
M19_1W	2019.7	*V. metschnikovii*	Water	Chifeng, Inner Mongolia, China
M19_6WC	2019.7	*V. metschnikovii*	Aquatic plants	Chifeng, Inner Mongolia, China

was considered to comprise strain-specific genes. A heatmap was constructed to identify the distribution of dispensable genes among different *V. cholerae* strains. With the exception of the strain TSY216 genome that contained 984 dispensable genes, most other strains in the group C clade contained few dispensable genes.

To analyze the *V. metschnikovii* pan-genome, 34 *V. metschnikovii* strain genomes recovered from migratory bird isolates and four reference genomes of *V. metschnikovii* strains were used for comparative analysis. The size of the pan-genome steadily increased with the addition of each additional genome in the analysis (**Figure 1B**), suggesting that *V. metschnikovii* also exhibited a large pan-genome. A total of 10,530 pan-genes, 1,352 core-genes, and 9,178 dispensable genes were identified among all *V. metschnikovii* strains. Like the genomes of the *V. cholerae* strains, most *V. metschnikovii* genomes did not contain many dispensable genes, with the exception of strain M13F, whose genome contained 1,048 dispensable genes.

Phylogenetic Analysis

Phylogenetic analysis indicated the presence of similar branching patterns, wherein the *V. cholerae* genomes consistently grouped into two major clades. The first clade contained *V. cholerae* strains from the GenBank reference database and one strain (C16-2-29) from our study. All of the other reference strains, with the exception of strain NCTC30, were present in this clade. In the first clade, strains harboring the cholera toxin (CTX) were divided into group C, while the others in the first clade were considered as group A. All of the strains identified in this study, with the exception of strain C16-2-29 (Wuliangsuhai, 2017), were present in the second clade, which was designated as Group B (**Figure 2**).

MLST analysis of the pandemic *V. cholerae* strains was conducted using eight different loci (*adk, gyrB, mdh, metE, pgm, pntA, purM,* and *pyrC*). However, only seven different loci (*adk, gyrB, mdh, metE, pntA, purM,* and *pyrC*) were used for the MLST of the environmental *V. cholerae* strains (**Supplementary Table 3**), since *pgm* was not detected in the environmental strain genomes. With the exception of the C16-2-29 genome, most of the housekeeping genes of *V. cholerae* strains from migratory birds did not exhibit homology to known genotypes in the pubMLST database. In addition, the *pgm* gene was detected in the strain C16-2-29 genome, as observed for the pandemic strain genomes. ST69 was the common sequence typing classification for the pandemic strains, while the sixth pandemic strain, O395, exhibited an ST73 sequence type. ST69 was not observed for the *V. cholerae* strains derived from environments or migratory birds.

Phylognetically, the *V. metschnikovii* and *V. cholerae* strains were genetically highly distant. The *V. metschnikovii* genomes consistently grouped into two major clades, with the first comprising *V. metschnikovii* strains from different samples and

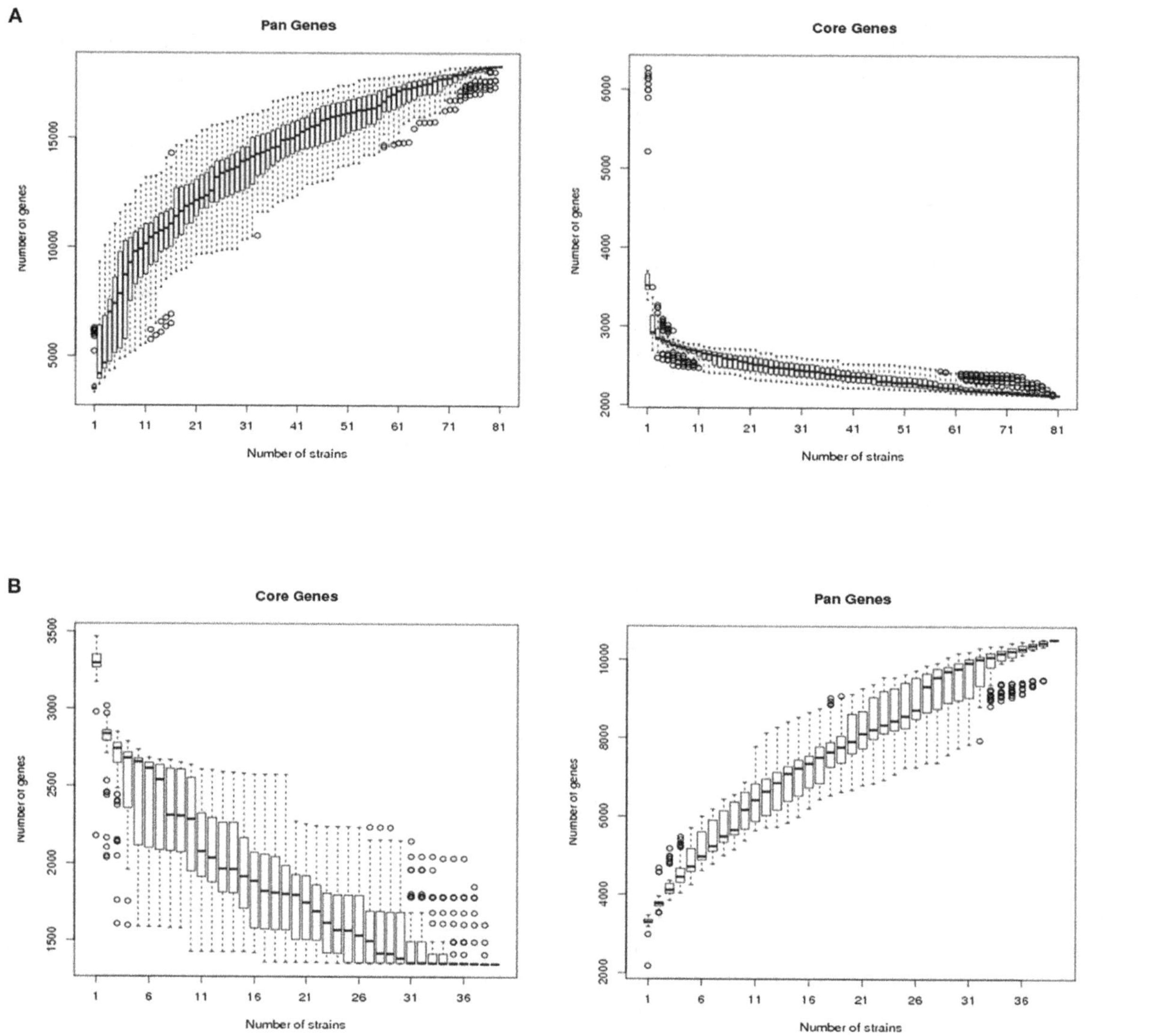

FIGURE 1 | *Vibrio cholerae* and *Vibrio metschnikovii* core-/pan-genome diversity curves. **(A)** The *V. cholerae* core- and pan-genomes are shown as a function of the number of genomes included in the counts. Boxes represent one standard deviation around the median number of genes within the subsets, while the whiskers indicate two standard deviations from the median. **(B)** The *V. metschnikovii* core- and pan-genomes are shown as a function of the number of genomes included in the counts. Boxes represent one standard deviation around the median number of genes within the subsets, while the whiskers indicate two standard deviations from the median.

the reference genomes. This first group was designated as Group D. The second clade comprised four strains (M21D, M28D, M9D, and M29D) designated as Group E (**Figure 3**). A *V. metschnikovii* MLST database has not been established yet, and thus the *V. metschnikovii* genomes were not subject to these analyses.

Comparison of Gene Functional Enrichment

Gene functions were predicted from the predicted genes and subjected to functional gene enrichment analysis. The *V. cholerae* core genes were enriched in numerous KEGG pathways including the "*E*," amino acid transport and metabolism, and "*T*," signal transduction mechanism pathways of the COG database. The numbers of genes within the "*T*," signal transduction mechanism pathway, were enriched in group C genomes relative to "*E*," amino acid transport and metabolism pathways. However, the other *V. cholerae* strain genomes exhibited opposite enrichment patterns (**Figure 4**).

To further investigate the functional differences encoded by the *Vibrio* genomes, we analyzed the "metabolism and environmental information processing" functional category encoded by different *V. cholerae* group genomes. Differences were observed in trimetlylamine oxide (TMAO) metabolism, in addition to two-component systems. Specifically, only group C genomes encoded complete TMAO systems. In addition, the genomes of the other groups lacked *TorA*, and these isolates are thus unable to metabolize TMAO. Differences

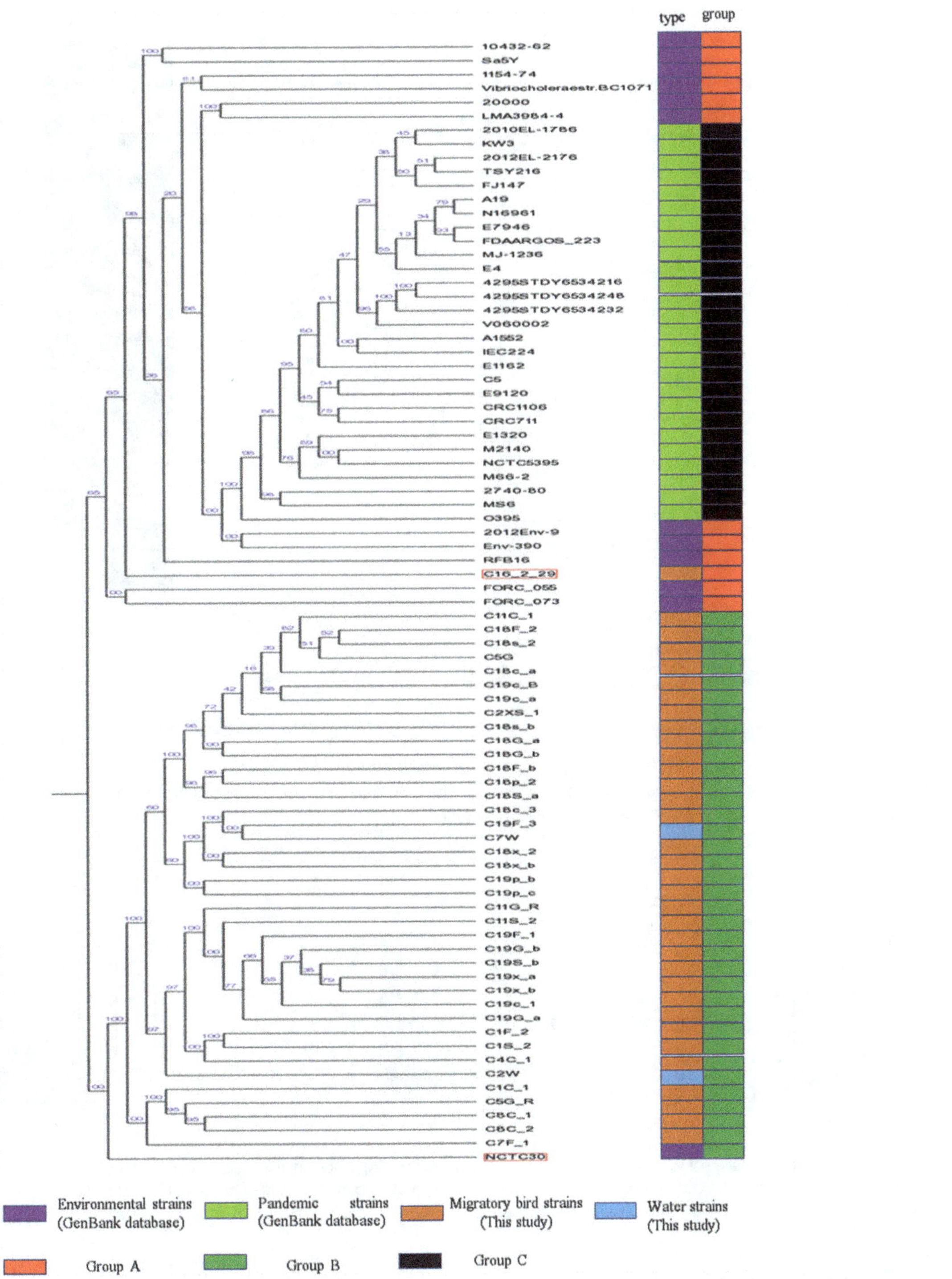

FIGURE 2 | Phylogenetic analysis of *V. cholera* strains. Different colored blocks are used to indicate types and groups of strains on the left of phylogenetic tree. The color legend is shown below the phylogenetic tree.

between the two groups of *V. metschnikovii* strain genomes were minimal, although all group genomes were particularly enriched in genes involved in the "*E*," amino acid transport and metabolism pathway.

Pathogenicity and Antibiotic-Resistance Potential

The *V. cholerae* genomes generated in this study only encoded partial RTX protein structures and not *rtxA*. In

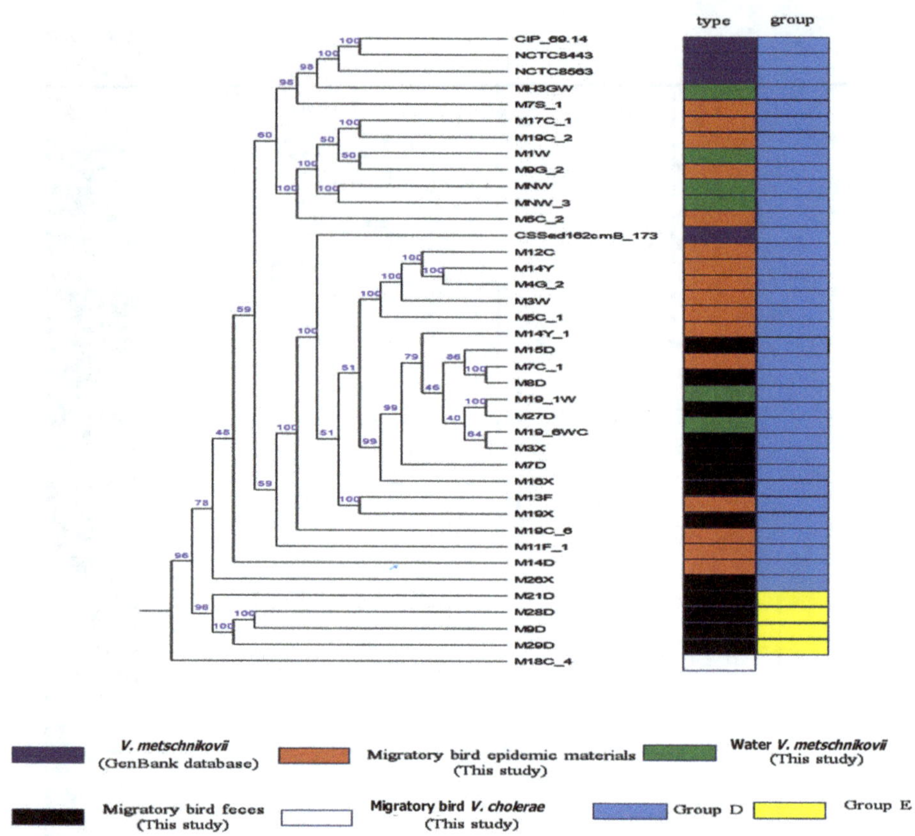

FIGURE 3 | Phylogenetic analysis of *V. metschnikovii* strain genomes. Different colored blocks are used to indicate types and groups of strains on the left of phylogenetic tree. The color legend is shown below the phylogenetic tree.

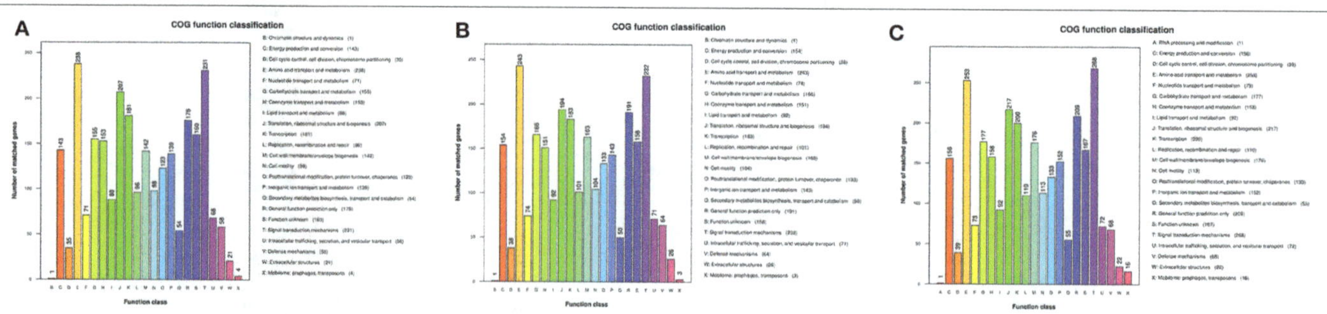

FIGURE 4 | Functional classification of *V. cholerae* core genome COG functions. **(A)** COG functional classification of the core genomes of reference environmental *V. cholerae* strains; **(B)** COG functional classification of the core genomes of migratory bird *V. cholerae* strains; **(C)** COG functional classification of the core genomes of *V. cholerae* pandemic strains retrieved from the GenBank database.

addition, all of the groups encoded complete type VI secretory systems (T6SS). The presence of drug resistance genes for *V. cholerae* in the genomes generated here exhibited low frequencies of resistance genes and the lack of plasmids (**Supplementary Table 4**). All *V. metschnikovii* strains lacked CTX, and RTX. However, the genomes of the four strains from migratory birds (M13F, M9D, M29D, and M28D) encoded a T6SS system. Among these, three strains (M9D, M29D, and M28D) lacked other genes involved in secreting proteins (e.g., *hcp* and *vgrG*), while only M13F encoded a complete T6SS system *V. metschnikovii.*

DISCUSSION

Vibrio cholerae acquired cholera toxin (CTX), which is the primary reason for their ability to cause global pandemics, and CTX acquisition occurred over a long evolutionary history (39).

CTX was likely introduced to *Vibrio* by the CTXϕ phage, while the toxin co-regulated pilus (TCP) is also a critical colonization factor of *V. cholerae* that serves as a receptor for CTXϕ (40). Other studies have indicated that AphA functions in a previously unknown step in the *ToxR* virulence cascade and helps activate the transcription of *tcpPH*. *TcpP/TcpH*, together with *ToxR/ToxS*, then activate *toxT* expression, ultimately resulting in the production of virulence factors like the cholera toxin and TCP (41–43). *Vibrio* strains isolated in this study exhibited unique combinations of virulence factor genes [e.g., *ctx*(-) *tcpA*(-) *hlyA*(+) *AphA*(+) *toxR*(+) *toxT*(-) *tcpP*(-) *tcpH*(-)], and thus they did not contain complete virulence factor regulatory networks based on the lack of *toxT*.

The group C genomes identified in this study also encoded the TMAO metabolic pathway, which differed from other *Vibrio* groups based on core-/pan-genome analysis. The TorR response regulator mediates TMAO induction of the *torCAD* operon expression and was intriguingly observed in all of the *V. cholerae* pandemic strains. With the exception of M66-2, all of the other strains in group C also encoded CTX. The original M66-2 strain did encode CTX, but CTX was knocked out of the strain in a previous study (44). The TMAO metabolic pathway exhibits a unique relationship with CTX production. Specifically, human intestines are anaerobic, and *V. cholerae*, as a facultative anaerobe, is able to grow by anaerobic respiration. CTX is a major virulence factor of *V. cholerae*, and its production is highly promoted during anaerobic growth using trimethylamine N-oxide (TMAO) as an alternative electron acceptor (45). The *V. cholerae* strains from environmental samples lacked the *torA* operon, which could lead to an inability to conduct TMAO respiration and thus produce CTX. However, the TMAO metabolic signaling pathway was not observed in the migratory bird *V. cholerae* strain genomes. Thus, it is likely that this metabolic pathway is not present in all *V. cholerae* strains. However, strain C16-2-29 shared very similar genomic attributes with the reference pandemic strains, unlike the other migratory bird *V. cholerae* strains. Specifically, the strain harbored the ability to encode a complete TMAO metabolic pathway, despite the apparent inability to produce CTX.

It should be noted that we were not able to exclude geographical factors that can influence bacterial evolution or differences in genomic contents. Strains that were isolated from the same host species but that exhibit differences in two-component systems will respond to external stresses differently. We speculated that conditionally pathogenic *V. cholerae* would unlike to evolve into a strain with CTX over a short period. Accordingly, the cholera pandemic strains have all been confirmed to be clonally related (2). The genomes of most strains belonging to group C contained fewer dispensable genes based on core-/pan-genomic analysis. A notable exception was the genome of TSY216, which contained more strain-specific genes. In addition to harboring two pairs of chromosomes, strain TSY216 also harbors a giant replicon that could explain its high strain-specificity relative to the others (46).

We additionally searched for other virulence genes in the genomes of *V. cholerae* from migratory birds by comparing them against the VFDB database. While the genomes contained some of the pathway components to produce the RTX toxin, they lacked the *rtxA* gene. *rtxA* deletion can cause a significant reduction in RTX toxin production (47). All strain genomes also encoded the T6SS system, while the *V. cholerae* genomes from migratory birds also harbored complete T6SS pathways based on KEGG analysis. T6SS was first discovered in *V. cholerae* in 2006 (48). Several of the *V. cholerae* groups encoded the T6SS system, and thus T6SS is probably a specific secretion system of *V. cholerae.* Only one of the three *V. metschnikovii* strain genomes contained the gene encoding the spike protein for T6SS. The *V. metschnikovii* strain encoding the spike protein of T6SS was isolated from migratory bird epidemic materials, while the *V. metschnikovii* strains that did not encode the spike protein of T6SS were isolated from healthy migratory bird feces in the second year. Importantly, T6SS without a spike protein does not confer pathogenic ability. Nevertheless, these results indicate that T6SS systems could have begun to evolve in *V. metschnikovii* strains. The M19X and M13F strains were closely related in the core genome phylogenetic analysis, although strain M13F did not encode a complete T6SS structure. Furthermore, strain M13F contained the HS I-I system that could activate T6SS, while M19X did not. Thus, different induction environments might activate the expression of HS I-I.

Phylogenetic analysis indicated that the *V. cholerae* strains from migratory birds (including strain NCTC30) were largely in group B, with the exception of C16-2-29. Strain NCTC30 was isolated from a World War One soldier with diarrhea (49). The strain harbored the T3SS-1 system, conferring it cytotoxicity (50). However, all of the migratory bird *V. cholerae* strains lacked the T3SS-1 system.

MLST analysis revealed a high degree of diversity among the strains that were evaluated. Indeed, these analyses indicated that the migratory bird strains harbored numerous new *V. cholerae* alleles and STs that have not been previously observed in databases. A total of seven different loci were used for MLST analysis of the environmental *V. cholerae* strains (excluding strain C16-2-29), while MLST analysis of the pandemic strains and C16-2-29 was performed using eight different loci (**Supplementary Table 2**). The combined phylogenetic analyses indicated that C16-2-29 was more closely related to the pandemic strains than to the strains isolated from the migratory birds.

In contrast to other migratory bird *V. cholerae* strains, C16-2-29 was classified within group A. The primary difference between the genome of this strain and other migratory bird *V. cholerae* strains was differences in the sequence of the Cbb3-type cytochrome oxidase. Accordingly, the genetic relationship between strain C16-2-29 and strains from group C was low. The COG group, "R," functional genes were specifically enriched in the C16-2-29 strain relative to the others. In addition, C16-2-29 harbored a complete biosynthesis pathway for siderophore group non-ribosomal peptides based on KEGG annotations, while the other strains did not. The C16-2-29 strain was isolated from the Wuliangsuhai area of the Inner Mongolia autonomous region of China in 2017, while the other migratory bird *V. cholerae* strains were isolated from the Chifeng area of the Inner Mongolia autonomous region of China in 2018. Consequently, it is unclear whether differences in geographic location influence the evolution of *V. cholerae* migratory bird strain genomes.

Transmissible elements similar to plasmids were not found integrated into the *V. cholerae* and *V. metschnikovii* genomes from migratory bird strains, indicating little chance of transmitting and spreading resistance genes. Rather, inherent resistance mechanisms were identified on the genomic chromosomes. For example, efflux pump-based inhibition is likely to be a viable strategy to overcome antibiotic resistance for V. *cholerae* and *V. metschnikovii* strains present in migratory birds. An important pathogenic characteristic to identify is whether *V. cholerae* can form biofilms based on complete formation pathways. All of the strains analyzed here exhibited this capacity, except for the environmental strains and those from migratory birds. Moreover, the biofilm formation capacity of the *V. metschnikovii* strains was the same as the environmental strains and *V. cholerae* strains from the migratory birds, wherein the basement protein-forming gene *RmbA* was absent. Thus, biofilms formed by these strains might be thinner than those of group C, or they may not develop a three-dimensional structure (51, 52). In addition, CTXϕ phage has been observed in biofilms (53), although it is yet unclear whether a relationship exists between biofilm thickness and the presence of CTXϕ phage.

Overall, our study demonstrates that *V. cholerae* strains isolated from migratory birds do not exhibit genomic features consistent with an ability to cause pandemics, or otherwise be pathogenic. Specifically, these strains were identified as non-O1/O139 serotypes and only conditional pathogens. In addition, we document the first isolation of *V. metschnikovii* strains with complete T6SS pathways. Both *V. cholerae* and *V. metschnikovii* strains may cause intestinal discomfort in migratory birds through the activities of T6SS and hemolysin. In contrast, all strains with an ability to form biofilms were identified in aquatic plant or animal intestine environments.

ETHICS STATEMENT

All migratory bird stool samples were collected under the supervision by the Wild Animal Sources and Diseases Inspection Station, National Forestry and Grassland Bureau of China, and did not cause any harm to the animals. All migratory bird epidemic material samples were provided by the local animal disease prevention and control center for bacteriological examination. The experimental protocol was established, according to the ethical guidelines of Helsinki Declaration and was approved by the Laboratory Animal Welfare and Ethics Committee of the Institute of Military Veterinary Science, the Academy of Military Medical Sciences (AMMS - 11 - 2020 - 11).

AUTHOR CONTRIBUTIONS

PC and X-JG conceived, directed, and carried out the study. L-WZ, DC, L-HX, JJ, YS, and G-JL prepared samples for sequence analysis. XJ, J-yG, and LZ acquired samples and analyzed the data. All authors have read and approved the final manuscript.

ACKNOWLEDGMENTS

We are grateful to members of Dali Nuoer Lake protected area, Chifeng city, Inner Mongolia autonomous region, China, which help for sampling.

REFERENCES

1. Rabbani GH, Greenough WB. Food as a vehicle of transmission of cholera. *J Diarrhoeal Dis Res.* (1999) 17:1–9.
2. Hu D, Liu B, Feng L, Ding P, Guo X, Wang M, et al. Origins of the current seventh cholera pandemic. *Proc Natl Acad Sci USA.* (2016) 113:E7730–9. doi: 10.1073/pnas.1608732113
3. Laviad-Shitrit S, Izhaki I, Arakawa E, Halpern M. Wild waterfowl as potential vectors of Vibrio cholerae and Aeromonas species. *Trop Med Int Health.* (2018) 23:758–64. doi: 10.1111/tmi.13069
4. Miyasaka J, Yahiro S, Arahira Y, Tokunaga H, Katsuki K, Kudo YH. Isolation of *Vibrio parahaemolyticus* and *Vibrio vulnificus* from wild aquatic birds in Japan. *Epidemiol Infect.* (2006) 134:780–5. doi: 10.1017/S0950268805005674
5. Dijk JG, Verhagen JH, Wille M, Waldenström J. Host and virus ecology as determinants of influenza A virus transmission in wild birds *Curr Opin Virol.* (2018) 28:26–36. doi: 10.1016/j.coviro.2017.10.006
6. Allarda SM, Callahan MT, Bui A, Ferelli AMC, Chopyk J, Sapkota AR, et al. Creek to table: tracking fecal indicator bacteria, bacterial pathogens, and total bacterial communities from irrigation water to kale and radish crops*Sci. Total Environ.* (2019) 666:461–71. doi: 10.1016/j.scitotenv.2019.02.179
7. Medini D, Donati C, Tettelin H, Masignani V, Rappuoli R. The microbial pan-genome. *Curr Opin Genet Dev.* (2005) 15:589–94. doi: 10.1016/j.gde.2005.09.006
8. Verma SK, Singh L. Novel universal primers establish identity of an enormous number of animal species for forensic application. *Molecular Ecology Notes.* (2003) 3:28–31. doi: 10.1046/j.1471-8286.2003.00340.x
9. Cao J, Xu J, Zheng Q, Yan P. Rapid detection of *Vibrio metschnikovii* in aquatic products by real-time PCR. *Folia Microbiol.* (2010) 55:607–13. doi: 10.1007/s12223-010-0098-2
10. Awasthi SP, Asakura M, Neogi SB, Hinenoya A, Ramamurthy T, Yamasaki S, et al. Development of a PCR-restriction fragment length polymorphism assay for detection and subtyping of cholix toxin variant genes of *Vibrio cholerae. J Med Microbiol.* (2014) 63(Pt 5):667–73. doi: 10.1099/jmm.0.070797-0
11. Li F, Du P, Li B, Ke C, Chen A, Chen J, et al. Distribution of virulence-associated genes and genetic relationships in non-O1/O139 *Vibrio cholerae* aquatic isolates from China. *Appl Environ Microbiol.* (2014) 80:4987–92. doi: 10.1128/AEM.01021-14
12. Nandi B, Nandy RK, Mukhopadhyay S, Nair GB, Shimada T, Ghose AC. Rapid method for species-specific identification of *Vibrio cholerae* using primers targeted to the gene of outer membrane protein OmpW. *J Clin Microbiol.* (2000) 38:4145–51. doi: 10.1128/JCM.38.11.4145-4151.2000
13. Alam M, Sultana M, Nair GB, Sack RB, Sack DA, Siddique AK, et al. Toxigenic *Vibrio cholerae* in the aquatic environment of Mathbaria, Bangladesh. *Appl Environ Microbiol.* (2006) 72:2849–55. doi: 10.1128/AEM.72.4.2849-2855.2006
14. Li R, Zhu H, Ruan J, Qian W, Fang X, Shi Z, et al. *De novo* assembly of human genomes with massively parallel short read sequencing. *Genome Res.* (2010) 20:265–72. doi: 10.1101/gr.097261.109

15. Li R, Li Y, Kristiansen K, Wang J. SOAP: short oligonucleotide alignment program. *Bioinformatics.* (2008) 24:713–4. doi: 10.1093/bioinformatics/btn025
16. Bankevich A, Nurk S, Antipov D, Gurevich AA, Dvorkin M, Kulikov AS, et al. SPAdes: a new genome assembly algorithm and its applications to single-cell sequencing. *J Computat Biol.* (2012) 19:455–77. doi: 10.1089/cmb.2012.0021
17. Simpson JT, Wong K, Jackman SD, Schein JE, Jones SJ, Birol I, et al. ABySS: a parallel assembler for short read sequence data. *Genome Res.* (2009) 19:1117. doi: 10.1101/gr.089532.108
18. Besemer J, Lomsadze A, Borodovsky M. GeneMarkS: a self-training method for prediction of gene starts in microbial genomes. *Implicat Finding Sequence Motifs Regulatory Regions Nucleic Acids Res.* (2001) 29:2607–18. doi: 10.1093/nar/29.12.2607
19. Saha S, Bridges S, Magbanua ZV, Peterson DG. Empirical comparison of ab initio repeat finding programs. *Nucleic Acids Res.* (2008) 36:2284–94. doi: 10.1093/nar/gkn064
20. Benson G. Tandem repeats finder: a program to analyze DNA sequences. *Nucleic acids research.* (1999) 27:573. doi: 10.1093/nar/27.2.573
21. Lowe TM, Eddy SR. tRNAscan-SE: a program for improved detection of transfer RNA genes in genomic sequence. *Nucleic Acids Res.* (1997) 25:955–64. doi: 10.1093/nar/25.5.955
22. Lagesen K, Hallin P, Rødland EA, Staerfeldt HH, Rognes T, Ussery DW. RNAmmer: consistent and rapid annotation of ribosomal RNA genes. *Nucleic Acids Res.* (2007) 35:3100–8. doi: 10.1093/nar/gkm160
23. Gardner PP, Daub J, Tate JG, Kolbe DL, Lindgreen S, Wilkinson AC, et al. Rfam: updates to the RNA families database. *Nucleic Acids Res.* (2009) 37:136–40. doi: 10.1093/nar/gkn766
24. Nawrocki EP, Kolbe DL, Eddy SR. Infernal 1.0: inference of RNA alignments. *Bioinformatics.* (2009) 25:1335–7. doi: 10.1093/bioinformatics/btp157
25. Hsiao W, Wan I, Jones SJ, Brinkman FS. IslandPath: aiding detection of genomic islands in prokaryotes. *Bioinformatics.* (2003) 19:418–20. doi: 10.1093/bioinformatics/btg004
26. Zhou Y, Liang Y, Lynch KH, Dennis JJ, Wishart DS. PHAST: a fast phage search tool. *Nucl Acids Res.* (2011) 39:347–52. doi: 10.1093/nar/gkr485
27. Grissa I, Vergnaud G, Pourcel C. CRISPRFinder: a web tool to identify clustered regularly interspaced short palindromic repeats. *Nucleic Acids Res.* (2007) 35:52–7. doi: 10.1093/nar/gkm360
28. Galperin MY, Makarova KS, Wolf YI, Koonin EV. Expanded microbial genome coverage and improved protein family annotation in the COG database. *Nucleic Acids Res.* (2015) 43:261–9. doi: 10.1093/nar/gku1223
29. Ashburner M, Ball CA, Blake JA, Botsein D, Butler H, Cherry JM, et al. Gene ontology: tool for the unification of biology. *Gene Ontol ConsortiumNature Genet.* (2000) 25:25–9. doi: 10.1038/75556
30. Kanehisa M, Goto S, Kawashima S, Okuno Y, Hattori M. The KEGG resource for deciphering the genome. *Nucleic Acids Res.* (2004) 32:277–80. doi: 10.1093/nar/gkh063
31. Kanehisa M, Goto S, Hattori M, Aoki-Kinoshita KF, Itoh M. From genomics to chemical genomics: new developments in KEGG. *Nucleic Acids Res.* (2006) 34:354–7. doi: 10.1093/nar/gkj102
32. Li W, Jaroszewski L, Godzik A. Tolerating some redundancy significantly speeds up clustering of large protein databases. *Bioinformatics.* (2002) 18:77–82. doi: 10.1093/bioinformatics/18.1.77
33. Cantarel BL, Coutinho PM, Rancurel C, Bernard T, Lombard V, Henrissat B. The carbohydrate-active EnZymes database (CAZy): an expert resource for glycogenomics. *Nucleic Acids Res.* (2009) 37:233–8. doi: 10.1093/nar/gkn663
34. Petersen TN, Brunak S, von Heijne GV, Nielsen H. SignalP 4.0: discriminating signal peptides from transmembrane regions. *Nature methods.* (2011) 8:785–6. doi: 10.1038/nmeth.1701
35. Eichinger V, Nussbaumer T, Platzer A, Jehl MA, Arnold R, Rattei T. Effective DB-updates and novel features for a better annotation of bacterial secreted proteins and Type III, IV, VI secretion systems. *Nucleic Acids Res.* (2016) 44:669–74. doi: 10.1093/nar/gkv1269
36. Chen L, Xiong Z, Sun L, Yang J, Jin Q. VFDB 2012 update: toward the genetic diversity and molecular evolution of bacterial virulence factors. *Nucleic Acids Res.* (2012) 40:641–5. doi: 10.1093/nar/gkr989
37. Liu B, Pop M. ARDB-antibiotic resistance genes database. *Nucleic Acids Res.* (2009) 37:443–7. doi: 10.1093/nar/gkn656
38. Kurtz S, Phillippy A, Delcher AL, Smoot M, Shumway M, Antonescu C, et al. Versatile and open software for comparing large genomes. *Genome Biol.* (2004) 5:R12. doi: 10.1186/gb-2004-5-2-r12
39. Clemens JD, Nair GB, Ahmed T, Qadri F, Holmgren J. Cholera. *Lancet.* (2017) 390:1539–49. doi: 10.1016/S0140-6736(17)30559-7
40. Kumar P, Thulaseedharan A, Chowdhury G, Ramamurthy T, Thomas S. Characterization of novel alleles of toxin co-regulated pilus A gene (*tcpA*) from environmental isolates of *Vibrio cholerae. Curr Microbiol.* (2011) 62:758–63. doi: 10.1007/s00284-010-9774-3
41. Skorupski K, Taylor RK. A new level in the *Vibrio cholerae ToxR* virulence cascade: AphA is required for transcriptional activation of the *tcpPH* operon. *Mol Microbiol.* (1999) 31:763–71. doi: 10.1046/j.1365-2958.1999.01215.x
42. Yu RR, DiRita VJ. Regulation of gene expression in *Vibrio cholerae* by ToxT involves both antirepression and RNA polymerase stimulation. *Mol Microbiol.* (2002) 43:119–34. doi: 10.1046/j.1365-2958.2002.02721.x
43. Ghosh C, Nandy RK, Dasgupta SK, Nair GB, Hall RH, Ghose AC. A search for cholera toxin (CT), toxin coregulated pilus (TCP), the regulatory element *ToxR* and other virulence factors in non-01/non-0139 *Vibrio cholerae. Microb Pathog.* (1997) 22:199–208. doi: 10.1006/mpat.1996.0105
44. Feng L, Reeves PR, Lan R, Ren Y, Gao C, Zhou Z, et al. A recalibrated molecular clock and independent origins for the cholera pandemic clones. *PLoS ONE.* (2008) 3:e4053. doi: 10.1371/journal.pone.0004053
45. Oh YT, Park Y, Yoon MY, Bari W, Go J, Min KB, et al. Cholera toxin production during anaerobic trimethylaminen-oxide respiration is mediated by stringent response in *Vibrio cholerae. J Biol Chem.* (2014) 289:13232–42. doi: 10.1074/jbc.M113.540088
46. Okada K, Natakuathung W, Na-Ubol M, Roobthaisong A, Wongboot W, Maruyama F, et al. Characterization of 3 megabase-sized circular replicons from *Vibrio cholerae. Emerg Infect Dis.* (2015) 21:1262–63. doi: 10.3201/eid2107.141055
47. Dolores J, Satchell KJ. Analysis of *Vibrio cholerae* genome sequences reveals unique *rtxA* variants in environmental strains and an *rtxA*-null mutation in recent altered El Tor isolates. *mBio.* (2013) 4:e00624. doi: 10.1128/mBio.00624-12
48. Pukatzki S, Ma AT, Sturtevant D, Krastins B, Sarracino D, Nelson WC, et al. Identification of a conserved bacterial protein secretion system in Vibrio cholerae using the Dictyostelium host model system. *Proc Natl Acad Sci USA.* (2006) 103:1528–33. doi: 10.1073/pnas.0510322103
49. Dorman MJ, Kane L, Domman D, Turnbull JD, Cormie C, Fazal MA, et al. The history, genome and biology of NCTC 30: a non-pandemic *Vibrio cholerae* isolate from World War One. *Proc R Soc B.* (2019) 286:2018–25. doi: 10.1098/rspb.2018.2025
50. Li S, Zhang Z, Pace L, Lillehoj H, Zhang S. Functions exerted by the virulence-associated type-three secretion systems during Salmonella enterica serovar Enteritidis invasion into and survival within chicken oviduct epithelial cells and macrophages. *Avian Pathol.* (2009) 38:97–106. doi: 10.1080/03079450902737771
51. Mattei MR, Frunzo L, D'Acunto B, Pechaud Y, Pirozzi F, Esposito G. Continuum and discrete approach in modeling biofilm development and structure: a review. *J Math Biol.* (2018) 76:945–1003. doi: 10.1007/s00285-017-1165-y
52. Tolker-Nielsen T. Biofilm development. *Microbiol Spectr.* (2015) 3:MB-001-2014. doi: 10.1128/microbiolspec.MB-0001-2014
53. Gallego-Hernandez AL, DePas WH, Park JH, Teschler JK, Hartmann R, Jeckel H, et al. Upregulation of virulence genes promotes *Vibrio cholerae* biofilm hyperinfectivity. *Proc Natl Acad Sci USA.* (2020) 117:11010–17. doi: 10.1073/pnas.1916571117

9

Quantitative Understanding of the Decision-Making Process for Farm Biosecurity among Japanese Livestock Farmers using the KAP-Capacity Framework

Kohei Makita[1*], *Elly Steenbergen*[1,2], *Lisa Haruta*[1], *Saddam Hossain*[1,3], *Yuki Nakahara*[1], *Yuto Tamura*[1], *Takuto Watanabe*[1], *Hazumu Kadowaki*[1] *and Shingo Asakura*[1]

[1] Veterinary Epidemiology Unit, School of Veterinary Medicine, Rakuno Gakuen University, Ebetsu, Japan, [2] Quantitative Veterinary Epidemiology Group, Wageningen University & Research, Wageningen, Netherlands, [3] Department of Medicine and Surgery, Faculty of Veterinary Medicine, Chittagong Veterinary and Animal Sciences University, Chittagong, Bangladesh

Correspondence:
Kohei Makita
kmakita@rakuno.ac.jp

In a globalized world, the frequency of transboundary livestock infectious diseases is increasing, and strengthening of farm biosecurity is vital to stabilize food production. The aim of this study was to understand the decision-making process for farm biosecurity among Japanese livestock farmers. Postal surveys using structured questionnaires were conducted on beef, dairy, pig, and layer farms in Hokkaido and Saitama Prefectures, which represent the principal production area and peri-urban Tokyo, respectively, as well as randomly selected broiler farms across Japan. The question items included the attributes of farms and owners, disease experiences, related associations and sources of hygiene information, attitude toward hygiene management, and compliance with the Standards of Rearing Hygiene Management (SRHM). The compliance rates were compared between livestock sectors. Univariable analyses were conducted using combined data from both prefectures, with the compliance rate as the outcome variable and the questionnaire items as explanatory variables, in generalized linear models. Exploratory factor analyses were conducted using the variables with $p <$ 0.2 in the univariable analyses. The factors identified were classified into knowledge, attitude, capacity, practice, and structural equation modeling (SEM) was performed. The questionnaires were completed and returned by 97 and 66 beef cattle, 86 and 136 dairy, 67 and 45 pig, 20 and 39 layer farmers in Hokkaido and Saitama Prefectures, respectively, and 95 broiler farms. The compliance rate was significantly higher among broiler farms (88.9%) compared with the other sectors, followed by pig (77.1%), layer (67.2%), dairy (63.8%), and beef (59.1%) farms in Hokkaido Prefecture, and layer (64.9%), pig (60.0%), dairy (58.5%), and beef (57.6%) farms in Saitama Prefecture. Based on SEM, the decision-making process from greater knowledge to higher attitude, and from higher attitude to greater compliance with the SRHM were significant ($p < 0.01$) in all sectors. Higher capacity was significantly associated with higher knowledge in dairy, pig,break and layer farms ($p < 0.01$), and with higher compliance in beef, pig, and layer farms ($p < 0.05$). These results suggest that the provision of targeted hygiene knowledge to livestock farmers and the support to smallholder farms would improve biosecurity through elevated attitudes and self-efficacy.

Keywords: KAP analysis, capacity, biosecurity, decision-making, structural equation modeling

INTRODUCTION

Infectious diseases remain a significant threat to the livestock industry in a globalized world. For example, African swine fever rapidly expanded from its original territory in sub-Saharan Africa to Georgia in 2007 (1), with subsequent outbreaks in the Caucasus, eastern and central Europe, and the Baltic countries (2, 3), as well as wide regions of east and southeast Asian countries, since 2018 (4, 5). Moreover, increased travel and trade, which also increases the chance of illegal importation of infected livestock products, pose an elevated risk of long-distance international transmission of infectious agents (6). Infectious animal disease epidemics not only cause severe economic damage, but also affect the mental well-being of farmers, veterinarians, and civilians in affected areas, as seen worldwide in the foot-and-mouth disease (FMD) epidemic (7–9).

Farm biosecurity is an integral part of livestock production (10). It prevents the introduction of infectious agents into farms thereby reducing the economic burden caused by infectious disease outbreaks in animals. In 2004, the Ministry of Agriculture, Forestry and Fisheries (MAFF) of Japan established the Standards of Rearing Hygiene Management (SRHM), specified by the Act on Domestic Animal Infectious Diseases Control in Japanese law (11, 12). The SRHM incorporated 10 basic on-farm standards for cattle, pig, and poultry farms as minimum hygiene standards, including hygienic rearing, disinfection at farm entrances and vehicles, quarantine upon animal introduction, and the acquisition of knowledge regarding infectious disease prevention. However, in 2010, major outbreaks of FMD and highly pathogenic avian influenza (HPAI) occurred in Japan, during which a total of 1.8 million chickens, 230,000 pigs, and 70,000 cattle were culled, causing serious losses to the livestock sectors (13, 14). After these major outbreaks, in 2011, the MAFF revised the SRHM by setting species-specific standards for (1) cattle, buffaloes, deer, sheep, and goats, (2) pigs and domesticated wild boars, (3) poultry, and (4) horses, and by increasing the number of hygiene standards from 10 to 22–25 items (15). Hereby, more emphasis was placed on the establishment of hygienic zones, farm entrance restrictions, the securing of land for burying carcasses after emergency culling, and the early detection and reporting of infectious diseases (12). Although substantial efforts were made to implement the SRHM on livestock farms, in 2013, porcine epidemic diarrhea (PED), which was causing a global pandemic, occurred in Japan, resulting in the deaths of over 500,000 pigs in the country (16). Reflecting on the findings of epidemiological investigations on PED (16) and critical discussions by experts (12), the SRHM were revised to include the prevention of contact between animal carcasses and wildlife, the establishment of a minimum temperature to heat human food waste for animal feeding, and the avoidance of leakage during the transportation of carcasses and animal excrement (17). The SRHM provided clear guidance to Japanese livestock farmers regarding biosecurity; however, compliance remains a challenge (18). The recent incursion of classical swine fever into the wild boar population has been causing infections on Japanese pig farms since 2018 (19, 20), and thus, improvements in farm biosecurity are becoming increasingly important.

Several frameworks have been proposed to understand the decision-making process in health-related practices. For example, the Health Belief Model (HBM), which consists of four components—perceived susceptibility to a health threat, severity of the threat, benefits to prevent the threat, and barriers to the preventive behavior (21)—has been reported in a review of 24 studies to affect preventive actions in the order of barriers, susceptibility, benefits, and severity (22). The Protection Motivation Theory (PMT) proposes that two cognitive processes—threat appraisal and coping appraisal—determine the conduct or inhibition of protective actions (23). Threat appraisal process evaluates the factors that increase or decrease the probability of making the maladaptive responses such as smoking or not wearing a seat-belt. Intrinsic (e.g., bodily pleasure) and extrinsic rewards (e.g., social approval) increase the probability of the maladaptive response, while assessed severity of the threat and perceived vulnerability to the threat reduce the probability. Coping appraisal is increased by judgments about the efficacy of a preventive response and one's ability to adapt the response successfully, and is decreased by the response cost (23). PMT has been applied in animal health to determine the factors associated with biosecurity practices during an equine influenza outbreak in Australia (24) and with the perception of vulnerability to future outbreaks (25) using logistic regression analysis. The Theory of Reasoned Action (TRA) states that an individual's behavior may be predicted by the strength of the intention, which depends on a combination of attitudes and subjective norms (26, 27). The Theory of Planned Behavior (TPB) is an extension of the TRA. In the TPB, in addition to attitudes and subjective norms, "perceived behavioral control (PBC)," which accounts for the belief in self-efficacy and perceived difficulties, is assumed to influence behavioral intentions (28). PBC not only affects behavioral intentions, but is also directly related to actual behaviors (27, 28). The TRA and TPB are applied in qualitative studies on the decision-making process of farm disease control (27–29). Another framework to identify knowledge gaps, cultural beliefs, or behavioral patterns that may be obstacles to the control of infectious diseases is the Knowledge, Attitudes, and Practice (KAP) framework (30). Numerous qualitative studies on the KAP framework have been carried out in animal health worldwide, and some studies, for example, on rabies, have applied this framework using uni- and multivariable linear analyses (31). The limitation of this approach is that linear analysis measures direct and indirect associations between factors and key disease preventive practice(s), but cannot infer complex mechanisms in the decision process. Toma et al. (10) modeled flows from several attitude nodes to the biosecurity behaviors of British cattle and sheep farmers, and Kadowaki et al. presented the flow of sociological factors to the KAP framework as a sequence (better livelihood enhances knowledge, higher knowledge leads to better attitudes, and better attitudes initiate good practices) in voluntary rabies control measures in Vietnam (32) using structural equation modeling (SEM). SEM is not intended to discover causes (33), but rather, to assess the soundness of causal relationships formulated a priori (10). SEM is useful for understanding decision-making mechanisms because it can distinguish latent variables (e.g., KAP) from observed variables (34) and assess the relationships between latent variables using observed variables.

The initial purpose of this study was to gain a better understanding of the influence of socioeconomic factors in the practice of biosecurity measures on livestock farms in Japan in order to further improve the level of biosecurity. During focus group discussions (FGDs) and an analysis of results from a postal survey using linear models, in addition to the KAP framework, the importance of the capacity of farmers, such as the size of the operation and the age of owners in family-owned farms, was perceived. A preliminary analysis on pig farmers, using the same data with the present study, is published in Japanese (35). Therefore, this study assesses the decision-making mechanism of farm owners in regard to biosecurity based on the KAP plus capacity (KAP-Capacity) framework.

MATERIALS AND METHODS

Study Areas

Studies on beef and dairy cattle, pig, and layer farm owners were conducted in Hokkaido and Saitama Prefectures, Japan, to compare livestock production (Hokkaido) and peri-urban areas (Saitama) (**Figure 1**). In Japan, broiler producers are no longer considered farmers, but rather, companies, so a study on these companies was conducted at the national level.

Focus Group Discussions

Between October 2013 and January 2014, at least one FDG was held for each of the livestock sectors, except for the broiler sector, to collect information that could be used to develop questionnaires. For the beef and dairy cattle, pig, and layer hen sectors, FDGs were held with people from both Hokkaido and Saitama Prefectures. For the broiler sector, semi-structured interviews were carried out with hygiene management veterinarians employed in broiler companies in Miyazaki and Hokkaido Prefectures. Each FGD, other than that for the broiler sector, was performed with a small group of people (5–6 persons) and included female farmers (or the wives of farm owners) and employees of livestock associations to gain different perspectives on the topics discussed. The discussions lasted a total of 80 min (two 40-min discussions with 10-min break in between), during which time, topics such as hygiene management, the influence of changes in the SRHM, livestock-related associations, and requirements for a questionnaire that could be easily interpreted and completed by farmers were discussed. All the FGDs were facilitated by an epidemiologist who was trained in participatory epidemiology and had 5-years' experience of the application in research.

Postal Surveys

Based on the results of the FDGs and semi-structured interviews, livestock sector-specific questionnaires were constructed and then pretested on farmers and veterinarians. **Table 1** shows a list of the question items with respect to farmer attributes, farm information, experience with animal diseases, cooperating associations, source of hygiene information, attitude toward hygiene information and management, and compliance with the SRHM. The questionnaire for the broiler sector was slightly different from that used in the other livestock sectors, as these are considered business companies owning several farms.

In Hokkaido Prefecture, questionnaires were sent to all beef cattle farmers belonging to Japan Agricultural Cooperatives (JA) in the Engaru and Yubetsu areas, those who attended technical workshops held in JA in the Tokachi area and the Hokkaido Dairy and Livestock Association (questionnaires were filled out at the workshops), all dairy farmers belonging to JA in the Engaru and Yubetsu areas, all pig farmers belonging to the Hokkaido Pig Farm Producers Association, and all layer farmers in Chitose, Ebetsu, Eniwa, and Ishikari cities, with assistance from the respective organizations. In Hokkaido, there were no integrated beef and dairy producers associations which can directly send questionnaires to farmers, and several intensive production areas were purposively selected. For layer farming, there were a few large scale companies, and there was no integrated farmers' association. Therefore, reachable cities from Rakuno Gakuen University were visited to enroll study participants. In Saitama Prefecture, questionnaires were sent to all beef and dairy cattle, pig, and layer farmers belonging to the Saitama Livestock Association, with assistance from the organization. For the broiler sector, sets of five questionnaires were sent to 50 randomly selected broiler-producing companies from a list published by the Japan Chicken Association, which has 81 member producers (36). The sample size for broiler companies was determined based on the available resources.

SRHM Compliance Rates

The SRHM compliance rates were calculated as a proportion of SRHM items complied out of all the SRHM items for livestock species. **Table 2** shows the SRHM items in the categories prepared following careful discussions by the authors: (1) prevention of disease incursion from fomites and animals, (2) limitation of access to a farm, (3) prevention of infection from wildlife, (4) prevention of within-farm spread, and (5) maintenance of preparedness. Some items such as provision of drinkable water and rearing animals with suitable density were associated with

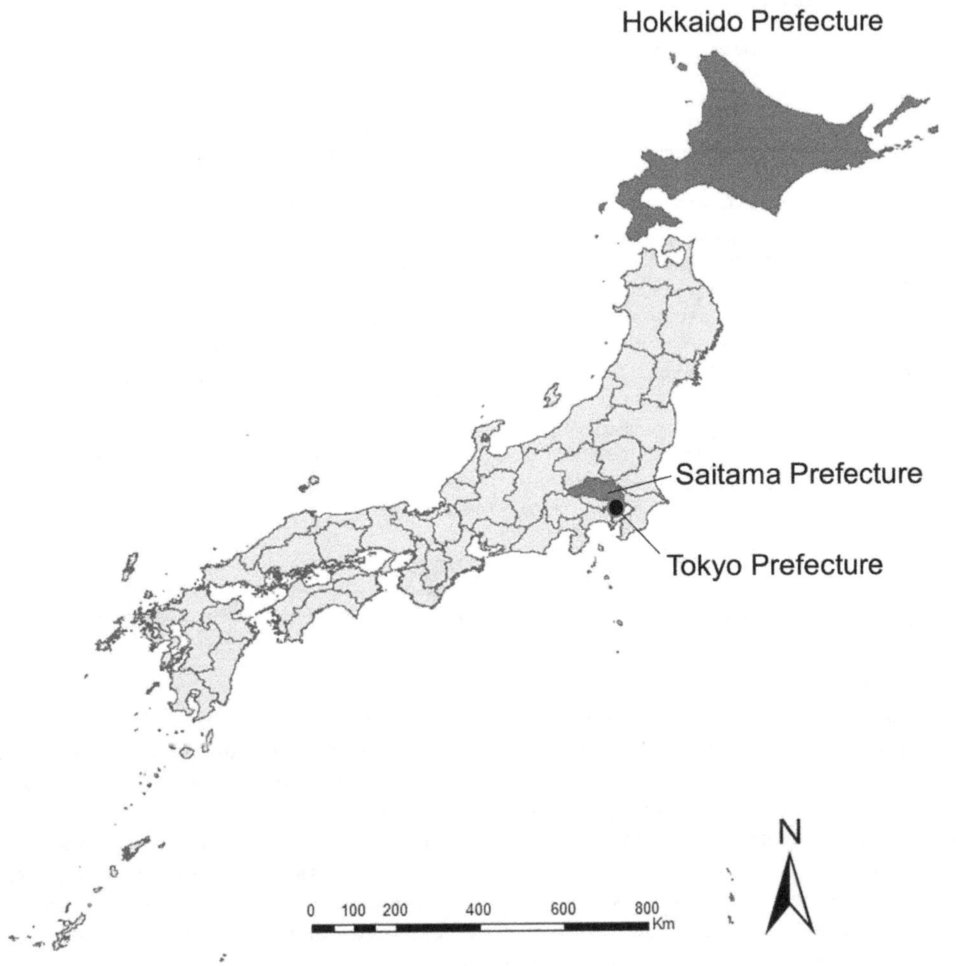

FIGURE 1 | A map of Japan indicating the locations of Hokkaido, Saitama, and Tokyo Prefectures.

TABLE 1 | Content of the questionnaire for farmers.

Category	Questionnaire item
Farmer's attributes	Age, gender, household size, schooling years, working time, and farming years of the farmer.
Farm information	Level of urbanization, year of farming since establishment, successor availability, number of livestock, housing facilities, management type, number of farm workers, whether the farm is adjacent to the main road, the density of neighboring farms, distance to the nearest farm, and the source of feed
Experience of diseases	Occurrence and impact of disease symptoms, a list of diseases experienced in last decade, and number of disease occurrences
Associations and information sources	Related associations, sources of hygiene information, and attendance of lectures and seminars about animal health
Attitudes toward hygiene information and management	Priority of information sources and activity, presence of change in attitude toward SRHM after its revision, and the reasons for this change, satisfaction level for hygiene management on the own farm and by the government, and the level of change in communication with other farmers after the revision of SRHM
Compliance with the Standards of Rearing Hygiene Management (SRHM)	Compliance with each standard described in the SRHM, categorized under five topics: the prevention of introduction with fomites, limitation of access to the farm, prevention of infection from wildlife, prevention of within-farm spread, and maintenance of preparedness

animal ethics and not necessarily with biosecurity; however they were classified into the most suitable categories. The SRHM included a few items specific to large-scale farms (adult cattle and buffalo: >300 heads; heifer, deer, sheep, and goats: >3,000 heads; poultry and quail: >100,000 birds; and ducks: >10,000 birds); however, for the purpose of analysis, in terms of compliance

TABLE 2 | Standards of rearing hygiene management.

Category	Hygiene standards
Prevention of disease incursion with fomites and animals	Disinfection of vehicles; Disinfection of hands and shoes of those who enter to the farm building; Provision of clothes and shoes only for hygiene control area (*only for pig and poultry farmers*); Cleaning or disinfection of materials directly used for animals when carry them in hygiene control area; Prohibition of carrying clothes and shoes used abroad into the farm; Quarantine of animals under segregation from other animals for certain period when introducing into the farm; Heat treatment of recycled feed (*only for pig farmers*)
Limitation of access to the farm	Segregation of hygiene control area from the other areas; Placement of a signboard indicating the hygiene control area; Limit of access for those who entered other farms or recently returned from abroad
Prevention of incursion from wildlife	Prevention of wildlife feces entering to feeding and water facilities; Provision of drinkable water; Placement of nets preventing entrance of wild birds (*only for poultry farmers*); Pest control, repair of damaged roof and walls (*only for poultry farmers*)
Prevention of within-farm spread	Change (disposal) or disinfection of materials to which body fluid of animals got attached, at each use; Cleaning and disinfection of a barn or cage after being emptied; Rearing animals with suitable density
Maintenance of preparedness	Collecting up-to-date information on prevention of animal infectious diseases; Immediate report of specific symptoms by law to the Livestock Hygiene Service Centre (LHSC) and restriction of animal movement; Immediate call of veterinarians when animals are sick without specific symptoms by law; Daily health check of animals; Removal of dirt and health check at selling out animals; Securing a land to bury culled animals; Record keeping for early identification of source of infection
Items for large scale farms (excluded from the analyses)	Designate one veterinarian or clinic, who tightly communicate with LHSM and regularly guide animal health management per farm, for all farms belonging to the company; Farm employees are aware that LHSC should be called without seeking permission of farm owner or manager immediately after the symptoms of specific diseases are detected

rate, these items for large-scale farms were excluded from the denominator to deal with all the respondents unweighted, regardless of farm size.

The compliance rates were compared among livestock species in Hokkaido and Saitama Prefectures separately using a generalized linear model (GLM) with quasi-binomial errors, as overdispersion was observed in the compliance rates. As broiler farms were sampled from the entire country, all broiler farm responses were included in the models for both prefectures. For dairy, beef, pig, and layer hen farmers, the compliance rates were compared between Hokkaido and Saitama Prefectures using GLMs.

Comparisons of Farm Capacity and Density Between Hokkaido and Saitama Prefectures

To understand the differences in farm capacity and farm density between Hokkaido and Saitama Prefectures, capacity-related factors—the age of the owners, number of animals raised, number of farm workers, including the owner, the availability of successors, and the shortest distance to a farm raising the same species were compared between the two prefectures for beef and dairy cattle, pig, and layer farms. Capacity related factors were identified during above mentioned FGDs; as the owner gets older physical ability would be weak; large-scale farms with large numbers of animals and workers have greater work force; and availability of successor would be a good motivation of investments. The age of the owners was compared using *t*-tests when the data were normally-distributed, and the Wilcoxon rank sum test otherwise. The total numbers of animals in dairy and layer farms were compared using GLMs with quasi-Poisson errors. Beef cattle and pig farms were categorized according to management types (farrow-to-finisher, fattening, growing, and reproduction for beef cattle farms; and farrow-to-finisher, fattening, and reproduction for pig farms), and the total numbers of animals within these types were compared using the Wilcoxon rank sum test. The numbers of farm workers were compared using GLMs with quasi-Poisson errors. The proportions of farms with a successor were compared using chi-squared tests. The shortest distance to a farm raising the same species was also compared using the Wilcoxon rank sum test.

Univariable Analysis of the Factors Affecting Compliance With the SRHM

We assumed that a decision making framework for implementing biosecurity measures would be common between Hokkaido and Saitama Prefectures, and as the sample sizes of the two prefectures were not so large, univariable analyses were conducted after combining both prefectures in terms of dairy and beef cattle, pigs, and layer farmers. For beef and dairy cattle, pigs, layer hen, and broiler producers, univariable analyses were conducted using GLMs with quasi-binomial errors, as overdispersion was commonly observed, selecting the compliance rate as the outcome variable and questionnaire items as the explanatory variables.

Exploratory Factor Analysis

For each livestock species, factors with $p < 0.2$ were used for the exploratory factor analysis. When variables with similar socioeconomic meanings were identified by the investigators, those with the most direct meaning were selected to keep the number of variables as small as possible. For the practice of the SRHM, category-specific compliance rates were used for the analysis. According to our hypothesis, higher knowledge (K) would foster a better attitude (A), and a better attitude would determine the decision to conduct biosecurity practices (P). In addition, we hypothesized that higher capacity (Capacity) would facilitate gaining animal health knowledge, and that capacity would be needed to implement practices. Using parallel analysis scree plots plotted with the fa.parallel() function in the package "psych" (37) in R, the validity of the number of factors—four for the KAP-Capacity framework—was checked. Exploratory factor analyses specifying four factors were performed using the fa() function in the "psych" (37) and "GPArotation" packages in R (38), and the factors were checked based on the variables grouped together in terms of whether they were representative of K, A, P, and Capacity.

Structural Equation Modeling

SEM was performed using the "lavaan" package in R (39). A path graph, which shows the structural part of the model, was designed selecting K, A, P, and Capacity as latent variables, and the remaining questionnaire variables from the exploratory factor analysis and category-specific SRHM compliance rates were used as the explanatory variables. To improve the model fit, in model tuning, non-significant variables in the exploratory factor analysis were either removed from the model or allocated to other factors based on the meanings of the variables. As the data sets included categorical and dichotomous variables and missing values, SEM was performed using mean-adjusted weighted least squares (WLSM) estimation, which is the robust version of weighted least squares (WLS) estimation (34). The fit indexes used were the significance of model chi-square (χ^2), Tucker–Lewis Index (TLI), root mean square error of approximation (RMSEA), and standardized root mean square residual (SRMR). For a satisfactory fit, a model should have a non-significant model-χ^2 ($p > 0.05$), TLI > 0.900, RMSEA < 0.08, and SRMR < 0.100 (40, 41). For all analyses, R statistical software version 3.6.1 (42) was used.

RESULTS

Questionnaire Responses

The response rates for beef cattle, dairy, pig, and layer farmers in Hokkaido and Saitama Prefectures were 33.3% (97/291) and 41.5% (66/159), 29.7% (86/290) and 44.2% (136/308), 34.5% (67/194) and 36.0% (45/125), and 33.3% (20/60) and 39.8% (39/98), respectively. The response rate for broiler farms belonging to commercial companies was 38.0% (95/250).

Compliance With the SRHM

Table 3 shows a comparison of SRHM compliance rates between livestock species in Hokkaido and Saitama Prefectures. In both prefectures, the mean compliance rates for beef cattle farms were the lowest among all livestock species (59.1 and 57.6% in Hokkaido and Saitama Prefectures, respectively). In Hokkaido Prefecture, the mean compliance rates of dairy (63.8%) and layer farms (67.2%) were not significantly different from that of beef cattle farms ($p > 0.05$), but the mean compliance rate of pig farms (77.1%) was significantly higher ($p < 0.001$). Conversely, in Saitama Prefecture, the mean compliance rate of layer farms (64.9%), but not those of dairy (58.5%) and pig farms (60.0%), was significantly higher than that of beef cattle farms (57.6%, $p = 0.001$). The compliance rate of broiler farms (88.9%) was significantly higher than any other species (the 95% confidence interval of the compliance rate did not overlap with any other species) in both prefectures.

When the SRHM compliance rates of the same livestock species were compared between the two prefectures, only pig farms showed a significant difference (Hokkaido > Saitama, difference in logit = 0.811, standard error [SE] = 0.214, $p < 0.001$); no significant differences were seen for beef, dairy, or layer farms ($p > 0.05$).

Figure 2 shows the category-specific SRHM compliance rates of the different livestock species in both prefectures and broiler. The beef cattle and dairy farms in both Hokkaido and Saitama Prefectures had particularly poor compliance with the SRHM items for the prevention of disease incursion from fomites compared with other categories. By contrast, the compliance rate associated with the SRHM category to maintain preparedness was high for both beef and dairy cattle farms in both prefectures. The SRHM categories to limit access and to prevent disease incursion with wildlife were particularly high for pig farms in Hokkaido Prefecture. A tendency toward poor prevention of within-farm

TABLE 3 | Comparison of the Standards of Rearing Hygiene Management compliance rates between livestock species in Hokkaido and Saitama Prefectures.

Livestock species	Compliance rate (%) (95% CI)	Estimate	Standard error	p-value
Hokkaido Prefecture				
Beef cattle farm	59.1 (54.6–63.5)	Reference	0.095	-
Dairy farm	63.8 (57.4–69.7)	0.196	0.136	0.150
Pig farm	77.1 (71.5–81.9)	0.846	0.151	<0.001
Layer farm	67.2 (57.5–75.7)	0.350	0.212	0.100
Broiler farm (entire Japan)	88.9 (85.4–91.7)*	1.714	0.160*	<0.001
Saitama Prefecture				
Beef cattle farm	57.6 (54.9–60.3)	Reference	0.056	-
Dairy farm	58.5 (55.2–61.7)	0.036	0.069	0.601
Pig farm	60.0 (55.8–64.0)	0.098	0.088	0.264
Layer farm	64.9 (60.7–68.8)	0.306	0.091	0.001
Broiler farm (entire Japan)	88.9 (87.1–90.5)*	1.776	0.088*	<0.001

Note that standard errors of the same dataset were estimated differently according to the models.

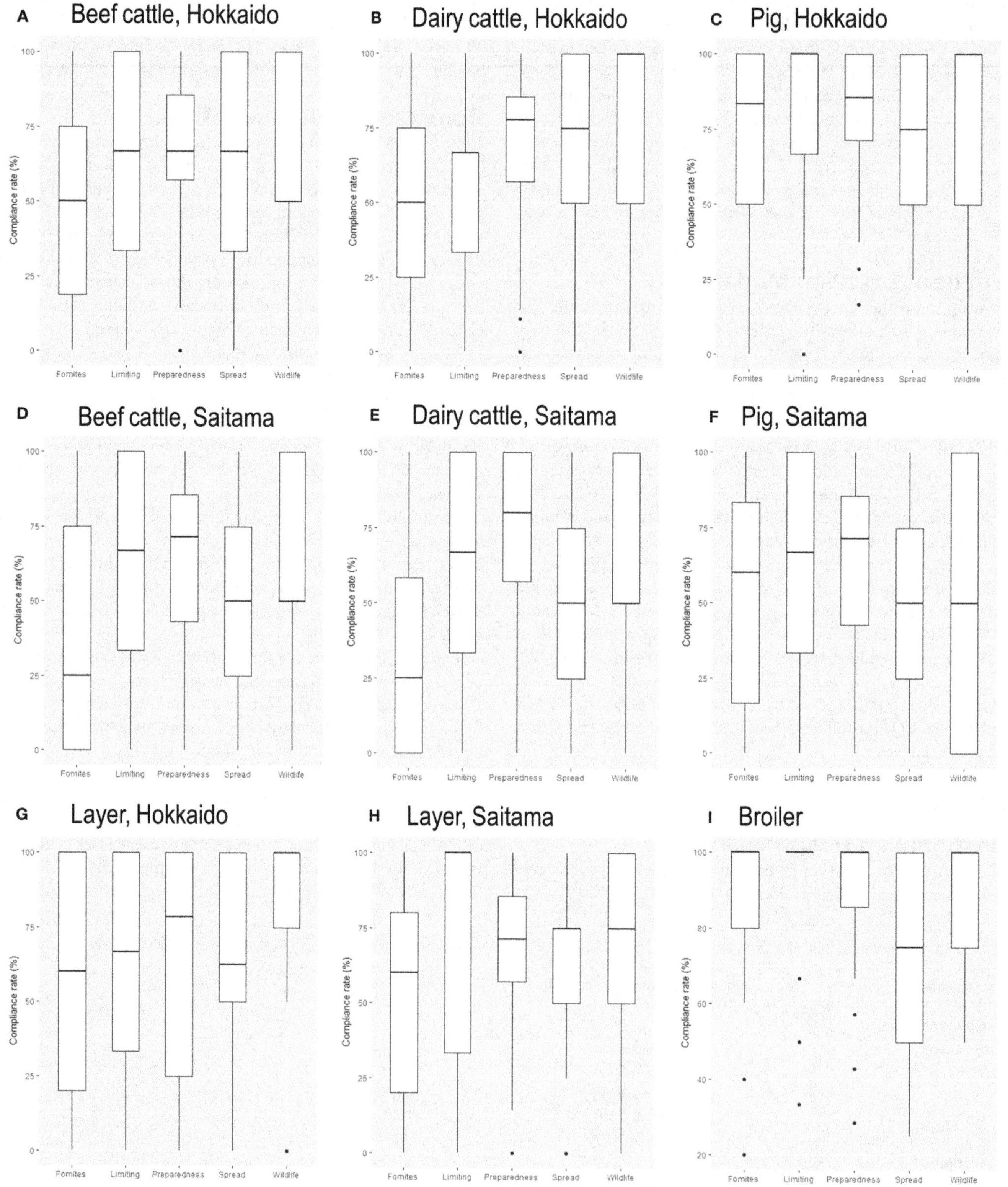

FIGURE 2 | Box plots of category-specific Standard Rearing Hygiene Management compliance rates for **(A,D)** beef cattle, dairy **(B,E)**, pig **(C,F)**, and layer farms **(G,H)** in Hokkaido and Saitama Prefectures, and broiler farms **(I)**. Categories include the prevention of disease incursion from fomites and animals, limitation of access to a farm, maintenance of preparedness, prevention of within-farm spread, and prevention of incursion from wildlife, from left to right.

TABLE 4 | Comparison of livestock farm capacity and density between Hokkaido and Saitama Prefectures.

Items	Hokkaido	Saitama	Statistics	p-value
Beef Cattle Farm				
Age of owner	48.5	63.6	$t = -7.4$, df = 139.2	<0.001
Number of animals (farrow-to-finisher)	161.4 ($n = 44$)	98.7 ($n = 10$)	W = 306	0.027
Number of animals (fattening)	64.0 ($n = 2$)	317.9 ($n = 28$)	-	-
Number of animals (growing)	44.3 ($n = 4$)	212.6 ($n = 7$)	W = 13	0.927
Number of animals (reproduction)	71.2 ($n = 44$)	20.6 ($n = 21$)	W = 813	<0.001
Total number of workers	3.5	2.9	Log = 0.18, se = 0.09	0.051
Availability of successor	61.8%	43.1%	$x^2 = 3.7$, df = 1	0.055
Nearest distance to other beef farm	1.6 km	2.3 km	W = 1893.5	0.026
Dairy Cattle Farm				
Age of owner	53.4	61.5	W = 2967.5	<0.001
Number of animals	113.6	44.7	Log = 0.93, se = 0.02	<0.001
Total number of workers	3.3	2.6	Log = 0.22, se = 0.08	0.005
Availability of successor	37.0%	31.9%	$x^2 = 0.4$, df = 1	0.528
Nearest distance to other dairy farm	1.4 km	2.1 km	W = 3747	0.026
Pig Farm				
Age of owner	55.8	60.0	W = 1055.5	0.028
Number of animals (farrow-to-finisher)	4,109.0 ($n = 59$)	1,024.5 ($n = 41$)	W = 1711.5	<0.001
Number of animals (fattening)	432.9 ($n = 7$)	774.3 ($n = 3$)	W = 17	0.628
Number of animals (reproduction)	62 ($n = 1$)	-	-	-
Total number of workers	6.4	3.0	Log = 0.77, se = 0.24	0.002
Availability of successor	46.2%	41.9%	$x^2 = 0.1$, df = 1	0.809
Nearest distance to other pig farm	7.0 km	2.5 km	W = 1883.5	0.013
Layer Farm				
Age of owner	56.5	62.3	$t = -1.24$, df = 14.3	0.235
Number of animals	242,146.0	40,375.6	Log = 1.79, se = 0.59	0.004
Total number of workers	10.1	8.4	Log = 0.18, se = 0.41	0.674
Availability of successor	23.1%	45.7%	$x^2 = 1.2$, df = 1	0.274
Nearest distance to other layer farm	8.4	4.1	W = 140	0.389

disease spread was observed for pig farms in Saitama Prefecture. While the compliance rate associated with preventing disease incursion with wildlife was high in layer farms in Hokkaido, the other category specific compliance rates varied greatly in layer farms in both prefectures. For broiler farms, the compliance rate associated with the prevention of within-farm spread was lower than any other category. The item-specific compliance rates for beef cattle, dairy, pig, layer, and broiler farms are described in **Supplementary Tables 1–5.**

Comparison of Farm Capacity and Density Between Hokkaido and Saitama Prefectures

Table 4 shows the results of comparisons of farm capacity and density between Hokkaido and Saitama Prefectures. For all livestock species, the farms in Hokkaido Prefecture were significantly larger than those in Saitama Prefecture in terms of the numbers of animals/birds. The numbers of workers were significantly larger in Hokkaido than in Saitama Prefecture for all livestock sectors except for in layer farms ($p = 0.674$). Farm owners were significantly younger in Hokkaido than in Saitama Prefecture for all livestock sectors except for layer farms ($p = 0.235$). The availability of a successor tended to be higher in beef cattle farms in Hokkaido than in Saitama Prefecture, but no difference was seen in the other sectors. Beef cattle and dairy farms were geographically closer to each other in Hokkaido than in Saitama Prefecture, but pig farms were more distant from each other in Hokkaido Prefecture.

Structural Equation Modeling (SEM)

Parallel analysis scree plots generally supported the number of factors (four factors) needed to consider the decision-making process structure, and the default SEM structure included the KAP-Capacity framework. **Figures 3–7** show the SEM path graphs on the structures of the decision-making process to practice the SRHM items for beef, dairy, pig, layer, and broiler farms, respectively, and **Supplementary Tables 6–10** show the detailed statistics. After excluding data with missing responses, 95, 192, 97, 36, and 84 responses from beef, dairy, pig, layer, and broiler farms were used in the SEM. The ellipses and rectangles in the figures indicate latent and measured variables, respectively. The measured variables connected to each latent variable were selected using exploratory factor analysis beforehand. The round arrows connecting to each of the latent and measured variables are disturbances, or in other words, variances. The values on the arrows in the figures show the SEM coefficients in tables, which are standardized factor loadings.

Regarding beef farms, flows in which better knowledge enhanced higher attitudes, and higher attitudes and greater capacity improved biosecurity practices, were significant ($p < 0.05$, **Figure 3** and **Supplementary Table 6**, respectively). Knowledge was explained by learning behavior (source of information and attendance to seminars), disease experience, and increased understanding of law and vigilance after the revision of the SRHM. Attitude was explained by the availability of a successor and the prioritization of hygiene. Capacity was explained by a younger owner, longer working hours, higher education levels, and in-house production of concentrate feed. Compliance with all SRHM categories was significantly associated with practice ($p < 0.05$, **Supplementary Table 6**).

Regarding dairy farms, flows were significant in which knowledge was enhanced by greater capacity, better knowledge enhanced higher attitudes, and higher attitudes induced biosecurity practices ($p < 0.001$, **Figure 4** and **Supplementary Table 7**). Capacity was explained by larger farm size (numbers of workers and buildings) and registration as a corporation, as compared with family-owned farms. Knowledge was explained by learning behavior (source of information and attendance to seminars) and disease experience. Attitude was explained by the availability of a successor, diligence (longer working hours), and increased understanding of the law after the revision of the SRHM. Practice was explained by compliance with all SRHM categories ($p < 0.001$, **Supplementary Table 7**).

Regarding pig farms, the decision-making process flow from knowledge and attitude to practice was similar to that for beef and dairy cattle farms, but capacity enhanced both knowledge and practice (**Figure 5** and **Supplementary Table 8**). Knowledge was explained by learning behavior (source of information and attendance to seminars) and relation with the Hokkaido Pig Producers' Association. Attitude was explained by lower satisfaction with own hygiene management, availability of a successor, and prioritization of hygiene among activities. Capacity was explained by registration as a corporation as compared with a family-owned farm, and located in a rural as compared with a peri-urban area. Practice was again explained by compliance with all SRHM categories ($p < 0.001$, **Supplementary Table 8**).

Regarding layer farms, the decision-making process showed exactly the same structure as that for pig farms (**Figure 6** and **Supplementary Table 9**). Knowledge was explained by learning behavior (source of information and attendance to seminars) and the number of related organizations regarding hygiene management. Attitude was explained by increased hygiene awareness and vigilance after the revision of the SRHM, as well as diligence (longer working hours and increased perceived workload). Capacity was explained by larger farm size (numbers of workers and buildings), registration as a corporation as compared with a family-owned farm, and located in rural area as compared with a peri-urban area. Practice was explained by compliance with all SRHM categories ($p < 0.001$, **Supplementary Table 9**).

Regarding broiler farms, the decision-making process flow from knowledge and attitude to practice was consistent with the other livestock sectors. However, capacity did not remain in the structure model (**Figure 7** and **Supplementary Table 10**). Knowledge was explained by the hygiene manager being a source of hygiene information and satisfaction with the animal health policy of the Japanese government. The categorical variable selection of a hygiene management planner was included because the model did not pass the fitness criteria when it was excluded. Attitude was explained by increased hygiene awareness, vigilance, and understanding of the law after the revision of the SRHM. Practice was explained by the prevention of incursion from fomites, introduced animals, and wildlife, the limitation of access to a farm, and the maintenance of preparedness ($p < 0.001$); however, the prevention of within-farm spread was not a significant factor (coefficient = 0.22, SE = 0.13, $p = 0.076$, **Supplementary Table 10**).

All the final models passed the criteria for the chi-square p-value, TLI, RMSEA, and SRMR (**Supplementary Tables 6–10**).

DISCUSSION

This study aimed to provide a better understanding of the decision-making process in biosecurity practices on Japanese livestock farms in order to develop an extension program to improve biosecurity engagement and compliance. Although the response rates were acceptable for a postal survey, both the rates and the actual number of respondents varied between species and areas. The response rates were higher in Saitama Prefecture than Hokkaido Prefecture for all the species (beef cattle, dairy, pig, and layer farms), and this might be due to the closer relationship with the Saitama Livestock Association, which covered all the sectors. The number of farmers responding was the smallest in layer farms in Hokkaido Prefecture, and this reflected the difficulty of access without farmers' association.

Comparisons between livestock sectors found that the already highly commercialized broiler sector had tighter biosecurity than any other sector. In comparisons between Hokkaido and Saitama Prefectures, the SRHM compliance rate was significantly different only for pig farms (higher in Hokkaido Prefecture), which may be explained by factors such as capacity, including a younger owner and larger numbers of workers and animals on a farm in Hokkaido, or potentially more active engagement by the Hokkaido Pig Farmers' Association (as shown in the SEM results). Hokkaido Prefecture is characterized by intensive food production; among Japan's 47 prefectures, it has the largest numbers of beef and dairy cattle, the fifth largest number of pigs, and ninth largest number of layer birds, compared with Saitama Prefecture, which had the 29th, 21st, 21st, and 16th largest numbers, respectively, according to the 2013 livestock census (43); however, the compliance rates did not differ between the two prefectures in other sectors. Although the age of the owner and farm size were significantly different, the causality

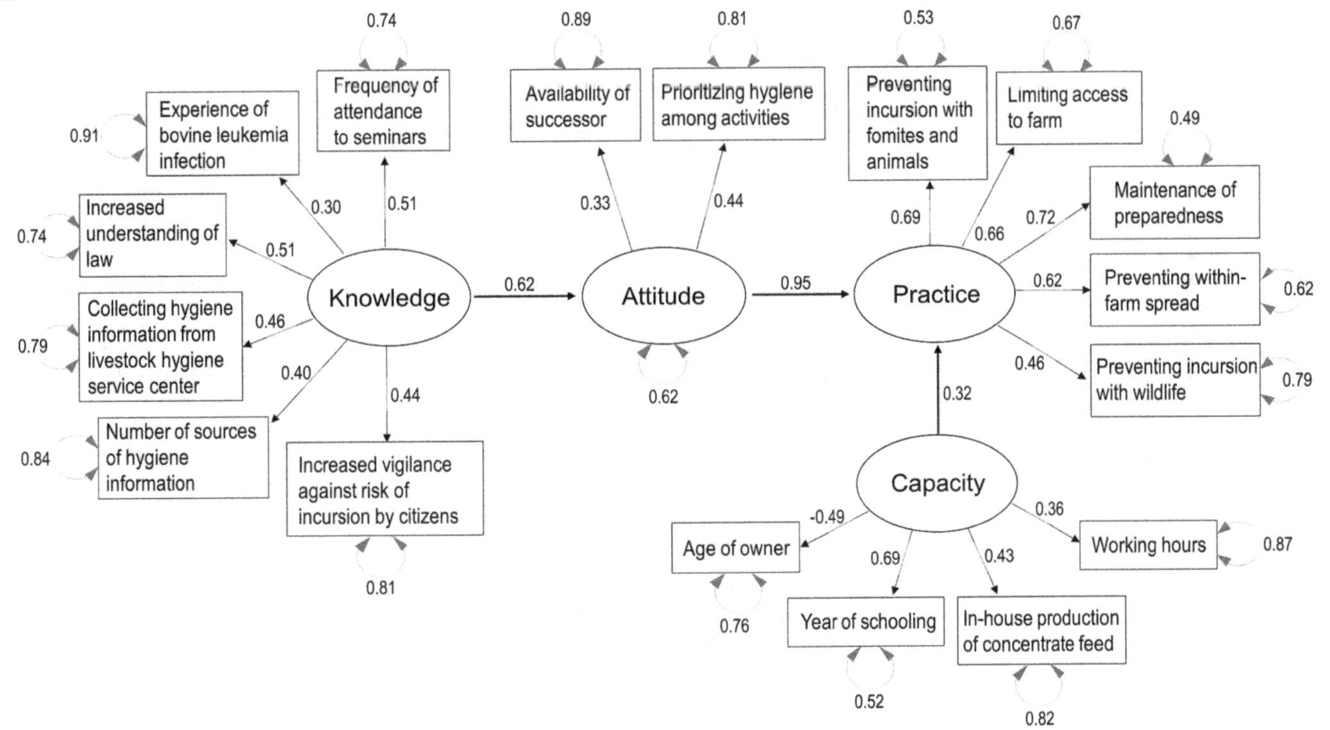

FIGURE 3 | Structural equation modeling path graph for beef cattle farms. The ellipses and rectangles indicate latent and measured variables, respectively, and the values on the arrows are standardized factor loadings. The round arrows connected to latent and measured variables indicate disturbances.

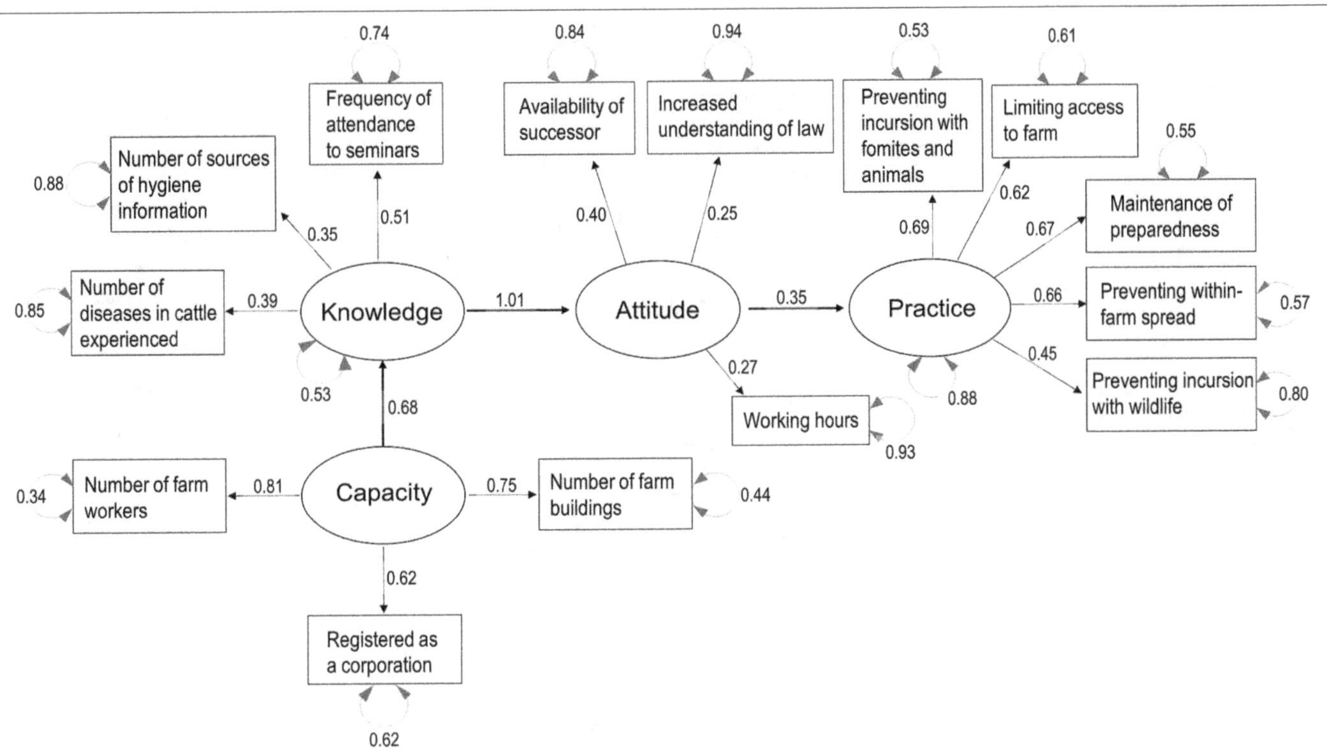

FIGURE 4 | Structural equation modeling path graph for dairy farms. The ellipses and rectangles indicate latent and measured variables, respectively, and the values on the arrows are standardized factor loadings. The round arrows connected to latent and measured variables indicate disturbances.

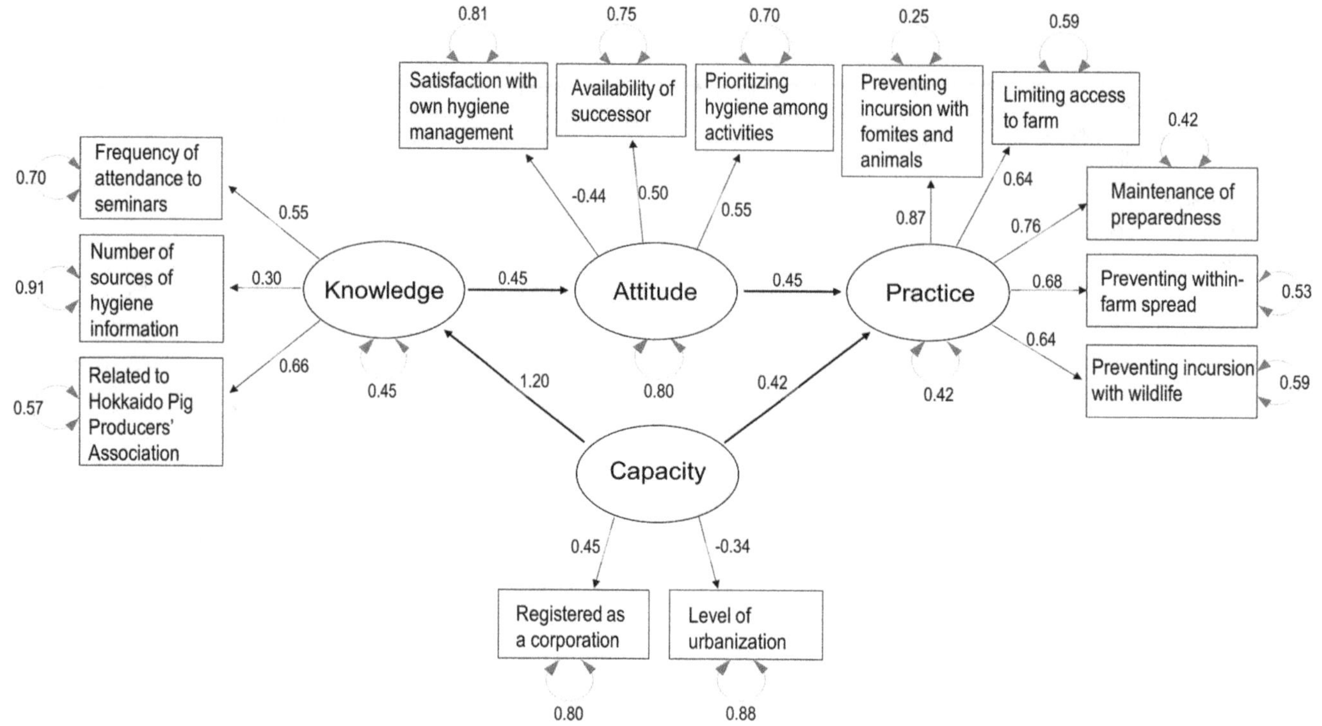

FIGURE 5 | Structural equation modeling path graph for pig farms. The ellipses and rectangles indicate latent and measured variables, respectively, and the values on the arrows are standardized factor loadings. The round arrows connected to latent and measured variables indicate disturbances.

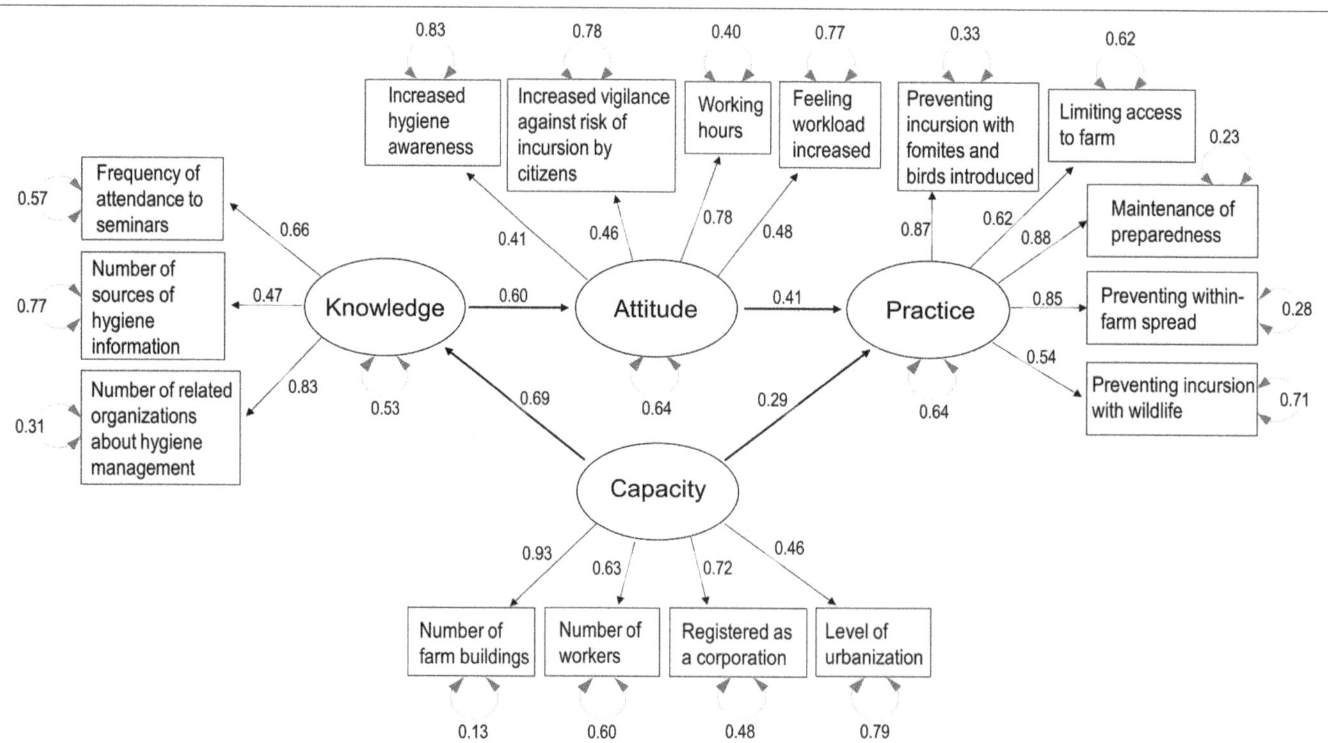

FIGURE 6 | Structural equation modeling path graph for layer farms. The ellipses and rectangles indicate latent and measured variables, respectively, and the values on the arrows are standardized factor loadings. The round arrows connected to latent and measured variables indicate disturbances.

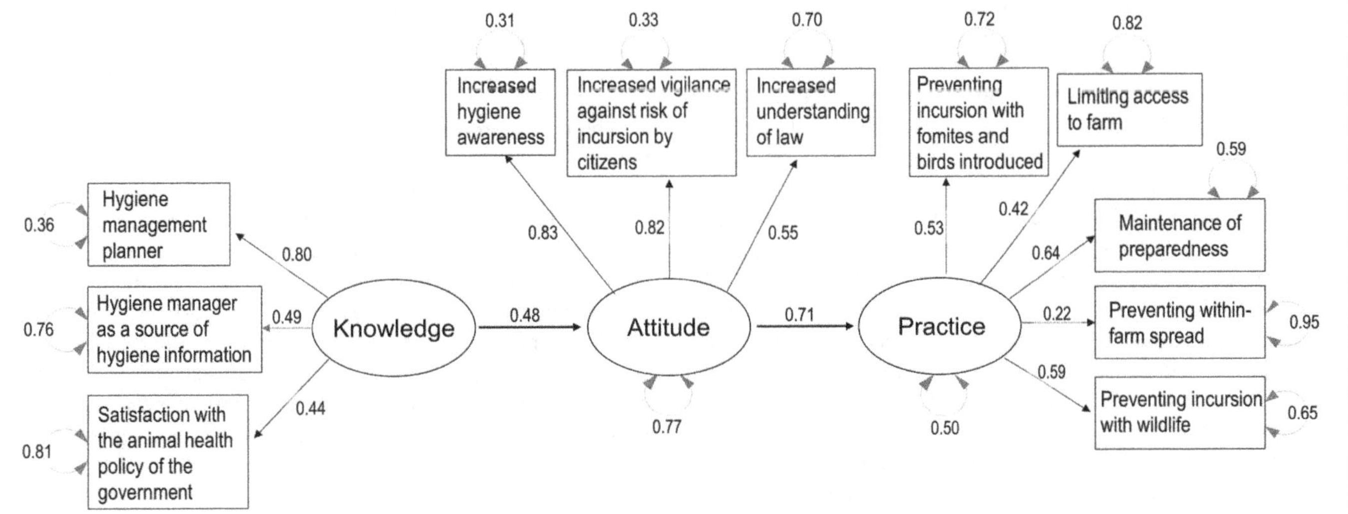

FIGURE 7 | Structural equation modeling path graph for broiler farms. The ellipses and rectangles indicate latent and measured variables, respectively, and the values on the arrows are standardized factor loadings. The round arrows connected to latent and measured variables indicate disturbances.

of the effect of socioeconomic factors on the difference in SRHM compliance rates between the two prefectures cannot be discussed further based on only these comparisons.

Comparisons between SRHM categories in each livestock sector suggested differences in biosecurity strategies between sectors. In beef cattle and dairy farms, while the preparedness for a disease outbreak was well-maintained, practices to prevent disease incursion from fomites and introduced animals, such as through the disinfection of vehicles, hands, and shoes of visitors, and the quarantining of introduced animals, were the most poorly conducted. Beef and dairy farmers complained about a lack of land and facilities to segregate animals for the quarantine period during FGDs. However, beef and dairy farmers should be aware that disease introduction can result in a greater economic burden than preparing an adequate quarantine facility. Intensive swine farms in Hokkaido made substantial efforts to prevent disease incursion from fomites and animals through biosecurity practices such as limiting access to a farm. This may be because farmers are aware of the apparent economic losses that can be incurred due to viral infectious diseases such as PED and porcine reproductive respiratory syndrome (44). Conversely, compliance with the SRHM category of preventing within-farm spread was weak, even for the intensive pig farms in Hokkaido Prefecture, which elucidated the challenges remaining in securing adequate space to reduce animal density and conduct all-in–all-out practices in intensive production systems. Layer farms in both prefectures did not have particularly high or low SRHM compliance categories, except preventing disease incursion from wildlife in Hokkaido, and this might have been due to their smaller sample size compared with other sectors. In Japan, the avian influenza vaccine is not used for layer hens, and thus, outbreaks of HPAI have been occurring in layer farms (14). As shown in **Figure 2**, the high compliance rate for the category of preventing incursion with wildlife in intensified layer farms in Hokkaido Prefecture was comparable to that of broiler farms. For broiler farms, systematic biosecurity strategies to prevent disease incursion from outside the farm are well-observed, but similar to pig farms, challenges remain in preventing within-farm spread, probably because of the intensity of the farming system.

The results of the SEM in all sectors studied suggest that greater knowledge of farm hygiene enhances positive attitudes toward hygiene, which determines the conduct of hygiene practice. In reality, attitude in itself may influence both knowledge uptake and behavior. However, our model assured the significant flow from knowledge *via* attitudes to practice. The KAP model has been applied in many countries for a wide variety of health and animal health problems (32, 45); however, during our FGDs, several farmers in different sectors described that even though they wanted to, they could not tighten biosecurity because farm labor and facilities are limited. We conceptualized that capacity, which is equivalent to self-efficacy in PMT (23) and PBC in the TPB (28), can be a prerequisite to high biosecurity performance. Although we hypothesized that knowledge, attitude, and capacity would be required to conduct biosecurity practices, these four components were not purposively selected in our statistical analyses. Parallel analysis scree plots indicated that four factors could generally explain the variance and covariance for livestock farming, and exploratory factor analyses identified the measured variables in the questionnaires to explain these factors; therefore, the KAP-Capacity decision-making structure was plausible, even statistically. Observation of the latent variable, capacity was useful in understanding the characteristics of the industries. The SEM results for the pig and layer farms suggested that in the default biosecurity decision-making structure, capacity is a driving force to increase the knowledge and feasibility needed to conduct the practices. A structure containing the flow from attitude to capacity, meaning that high motivation can increase capacity, was also tested (not indicated in the results), but the model fit was unacceptable, indicating that the SEM model cannot explain such a long-term effect of motivation on capacity development. For broiler farms, capacity did not remain in the model, probably because all the broiler producing companies studied had sufficient capacity to maintain high biosecurity. For dairy farms, even with sufficient capacity, the conduct of biosecurity measures may depend on better attitudes toward hygiene, as there was no significant linkage between capacity and practice. However, capacity enhanced knowledge, which would lead to better attitudes toward hygiene, and strengthening capacity would contribute to the higher SRHM compliance. Conversely for beef farms, limited capacity may be a physical obstacle to conduct these practices. Interestingly, the exchangeability of measured variables explaining different latent variables was observed between livestock sectors. For example, increased understanding of the law and vigilance after the revision of the SRHM explained knowledge in beef cattle farms, and attitude in other sectors, which suggests that knowledge, attitude, and even capacity are related and an experience or a response may constitute a personality that determines the strength of the KAP-Capacity process flow.

When planning policies to upgrade farm biosecurity, the provision of knowledge through networking with prefectural livestock hygiene centers, and of hygiene training by these centers, was identified as the most important step. The cost (46) and effectiveness (47) of biosecurity measures influence the motivation of farmers, and the provision of such evidence-based information should increase attitudes toward the SRHM. Policies to strengthen capacity, such as intensification through a shift to a corporate farm and support for smallholder farms, can also be effective. The standardized factor loads in the SEM models are useful for planning detailed intervention strategies and developing monitoring schemes for knowledge, attitude, and capacity; the variables with factor loads distant from zero have a strong relationship with the latent variables, and may be important factors for interventions and monitoring. However, the factor loads can be used as a guidance when developing monitoring schemes, but not as a direct manual or checklist, as each production system and biosecurity program must be addressed individually with practical knowledge. In addition, decision-making process frameworks for protective practices in health and animal health, such as the HBM, PMT, TRA, and TPB, have already described detailed qualitative factors, and thus, it is advisable that veterinary officers at both the national and local government levels understand these theories when carrying out detailed planning for hygiene guidance.

This study had three limitations: (1) the representativeness of farmers, (2) the use of self-administered questionnaires, and (3) the use of binary responses in the analyses. Regarding (1), due to budget constraints and the expected time required for coordination, postal surveys other than for broiler farms were conducted in only two prefectures. Among pig and beef cattle farms, there are reproduction farms, fattening farms, and farrow-to-finisher farms; however, due to the limited numbers of farmers who were reached to participate in this study, all farm types were analyzed together. In Japan, there are small numbers of sheep and goat farmers and those for indigenous breeds of chicken for eggs and meats, and these farmers were excluded from the present study. This study was initially designed to conduct statistics using GLMs, so a sample size calculation for the SEM was not conducted. However, the SEM models had adequate degrees of freedom and passed the model fit criteria, and thus, the results can be considered reliable. Regarding (2), our study used self-administered questionnaires and the results may be affected by information bias. Regarding (3), the default estimation method in SEM, maximum likelihood, assumes multivariate normality in between-variable relationships, and normal distributions of these variables (34). Therefore, in the SEM analyses, the WLSM was used. However, future studies should collect data using a Likert-type scale rather than binary responses. In addition, the postal surveys were conducted between 2013 and 2014, and the SRHM compliance rates in 2018, enumerated by the veterinarians at the prefectural livestock hygiene centers, were much higher (48).

CONCLUSIONS

The study results support the hypothesis that the decision-making process for conducting farm biosecurity starts from the acquisition of good hygiene knowledge, which enhances attitudes, and better attitudes are a trigger to conduct enhanced biosecurity practices. Capacity is an important factor to improve both hygiene knowledge and biosecurity practice. Intensification is a key factor for achieving tighter biosecurity, but well-designed facilities and management plans are needed to ensure the prevention of within-farm disease spread. SEM is a potentially powerful tool for collecting data to support the design of effective and well-targeted intervention programs to improve farm biosecurity.

AUTHOR CONTRIBUTIONS

KM planned, coordinated stakeholders, conducted fieldworks, analyses, supervised, and wrote the manuscript. ES and LH conducted analyses including SEM and wrote the manuscript. SH conducted univariable and multivariable analyses on poultry sectors. YN, YT, TW, and SA conducted fieldworks and analyses. HK conducted and supervised univariable and multivariable analyses. All authors contributed to the article and approved the submitted version.

ACKNOWLEDGMENTS

ES participated in this study in the Wageningen University and Research MSc Animal Sciences International Internship. Many thanks go to the Japan Agricultural Cooperatives (JA) and beef cattle farmers in the Engaru, Tokachi, and Yubetsu areas, the Hokkaido Dairy and Livestock Association, dairy farmers in the Engaru and Yubetsu areas, pig farmers belonging to the Hokkaido Pig Farm Producers Association, layer farmers in Chitose, Ebetsu, Eniwa, and Ishikari cities in Hokkaido

Prefecture, and beef and dairy cattle, pig, and layer farmers and the Saitama Livestock Association in Saitama Prefecture. We also thank the broiler farmers and Japan Chicken Association for the great facilitation and participation. We cordially thank Dr. Satoko Kubota and Professor Manabu Sawada at Obihiro University of Agriculture and Veterinary Medicine for the critical advice regarding the SEM.

REFERENCES

1. European Food Safety Authority. Scientific opinion on African swine fever. *EFSA J.* (2010) 8:1556. doi: 10.2903/j.efsa.2010.1556
2. Guinat C, Gogin A, Blome S, Keil G, Pollin R, Pfeiffer DU, et al. Transmission routes of African swine fever virus to domestic pigs: current knowledge and future research directions. *Vet Rec.* (2016) 178:262–7. doi: 10.1136/vr.103593
3. Pikalo J, Schoder ME, Sehl J, Breithaupt A, Tignon M, Cay AB, et al. The African swine fever virus isolate Belgium 2018/1 shows high virulence in European wild boar. *Transbound Emerg Dis.* (2020) 67:1654–9. doi: 10.1111/tbed.13503
4. Zhou X, Li N, Luo Y, Liu YE, Miao F, Chen T, et al. Emergence of African swine fever in China. *Transbound Emerg Dis.* (2018) 65:1482–4. doi: 10.1111/tbed.12989
5. Food and Agriculture Organization. *ASF Situation in Asia Update.* (2020). Available online at: http://www.fao.org/ag/againfo/programmes/en/empres/ASF/situation_update.html (accessed April 2, 2020).
6. Ito S, Jurado C, Sánchez-Vizcaíno, JM, Isoda N. Quantitative risk assessment of African swine fever virus introduction to Japan via pork products brought in air passengers' luggage. *Transbound Emerg Dis.* (2020) 67:894–905. doi: 10.1111/tbed.13414
7. Peck DF. Foot and mouth outbreak: lessons for mental health services. *Adv Psychiatr Treat.* (2005) 11:270–6. doi: 10.1192/apt.11.4.270
8. Hibi J, Kurosawa A, Watanabe T, Kadowaki H, Watari M. Post-traumatic stress disorder in participants of foot-and-mouth disease epidemic control in Miyazaki, Japan, in 2010. *J Vet Med Sci.* (2015) 77:953–9. doi: 10.1292/jvms.14-0512
9. Kadowaki H, Kayano T, Tobinaga T, Tsutsumi A, Watari M, Makita K. Analysis of factors associated with hesitation to restart farming after depopulation of animals due to 2010 foot-and-mouth disease epidemic in Japan. *J Vet Med Sci.* (2016) 78:1251–9. doi: 10.1292/jvms.15-0559
10. Toma L, Stott A, Heffernan C, Ringrose S, Gunn GJ. Determinants of biosecurity behaviour of British cattle and sheep farmers—a behavioural economics analysis. *Prev Vet Med.* (2013) 108:321–33. doi: 10.1016/j.prevetmed.2012.11.009
11. Ministry of Agriculture, Forestry, Fisheries of Japan. *Act on Domestic Animal Infectious Diseases Control.* (2012). Available online at: http://www.maff.go.jp/e/policies/ap_health/animal/attach/pdf/index-19.pdf (accessed March 10, 2020).
12. Ministry of Agriculture, Forestry, Fisheries of Japan. *Revisions of the Standards of Rearing Hygiene Management.* (2016). Available online at: https://www.maff.go.jp/j/council/seisaku/eisei/goudou_02/attach/pdf/index-14.pdf (accessed March 10, 2020).
13. Ministry of Agriculture, Forestry, Fisheries of Japan. *FY2010 Annual Report on Food, Agriculture and Rural Areas in Japan.* (2011). Available online at: https://www.maff.go.jp/e/annual_report/2010/pdf/e_all.pdf (accessed March 5, 2020).
14. Kishita Y. Outbreaks and control measures of notifiable avian influenza in Japan. *J Vet Epidemiol.* (2016) 20:S11–3. doi: 10.2743/jve.20.S11
15. Ministry of Agriculture, Forestry, Fisheries of Japan. *Standard Rearing Hygiene Management.* (2011). Available online at: https://www.maff.go.jp/j/syouan/douei/katiku_yobo/k_shiyou/attach/pdf/kako-12.pdf (accessed March 10, 2020).
16. Toyomaki H, Sekiguchi S, Sasaki Y, Sueyoshi M, Makita K. Factors associated with farm-level infection of porcine epidemic diarrhea during the early phase of the epidemic in Japan in 2013 and 2014. *Prev Vet Med.* (2018) 150:77–85. doi: 10.1016/j.prevetmed.2017.12.008
17. Ministry of Agriculture, Forestry, Fisheries of Japan. *Standard Rearing Hygiene Management.* (2017). Available online at: https://www.maff.go.jp/j/syouan/douei/katiku_yobo/k_shiyou/attach/pdf/index-2.pdf (accessed March 10, 2020).
18. Ministry of Agriculture, Forestry, Fisheries of Japan. *The Situation of Hygienic Management in Livestock Rearing in 2018.* (2018). Available online at: https://www.maff.go.jp/j/syouan/douei/katiku_yobo/k_shiyou/attach/pdf/index-49.pdf (accessed March 10, 2020).
19. Isoda N, Baba K, Ito S, Ito M, Sakoda Y, Makita K. Dynamics of classical swine fever spread in wild boar in 2018–2019, Japan. *Pathogens.* (2020) 9:119. doi: 10.3390/pathogens9020119
20. Hayama Y, Shimizu Y, Murato Y, Sawai K, Yamamoto T. Estimation of infection risk on pig farms in infected wild boar areas—epidemiological analysis for the reemergence of classical swine fever in Japan in 2018. *Prev Vet Med.* (2020) 175:104873. doi: 10.1016/j.prevetmed.2019.104873
21. Rosenstock IM. The health belief model and preventive health behavior. *Health Educ. Monogr.* (1974) 2:354–86. doi: 10.1177/109019817400200405
22. Janz NK, Becker MH. The Health Belief Model: a decade later. *Health Educ Q.* (1984) 11:1–47. doi: 10.1177/109019818401100101
23. Prentice-Dunn S, Rogers RW. Protection motivation theory and preventive health: beyond the health belief model. *Health Educ Res.* (1986) 1:153–61. doi: 10.1093/her/1.3.153
24. Schemann K, Taylor MR, Toribio JALML, Dhand NK. Horse owners' biosecurity practices following the first equine influenza outbreak in Australia. *Prev Vet Med.* (2011) 102:304–14. doi: 10.1016/j.prevetmed.2011.08.002
25. Schemann K, Firestone SM, Taylor MR, Toribio JALML, Ward MP, Dhand NK. Perceptions of vulnerability to a future outbreak: a study of horse managers affected by the first Australian equine influenza outbreak. *BMC Vet Res.* (2013) 9:152. doi: 10.1186/1746-6148-9-152
26. Fishbain M, Ajzen I. *Belief, Attitude, Intention, and Behaviour: An Introduction to Theory and Research.* Reading, MA: Addison-Wesley (1975).
27. Alarcon P, Wieland B, Mateus ALP, Dewberry C. Pig farmers' perceptions, attitudes, influences and management of information in the decision-making process for disease control. *Prev Vet Med.* (2014) 116:223–42. doi: 10.1016/j.prevetmed.2013.08.004
28. Ajzen I. The theory of planned behavior. *Organ Behav Hum Decis Process.* (1991) 50:179–211. doi: 10.1016/0749-5978(91)90020-T
29. Garforth CJ, Bailey AP, Tranter RB. Farmers' attitudes to disease risk management in England: a comparative analysis of sheep and pig farmers. *Prev Vet Med.* (2013) 110:456–66. doi: 10.1016/j.prevetmed.2013.02.018
30. Launiala A. How much can a KAP survey tell us about people's knowledge, attitudes and practices? Some observations from medical anthropology research on malaria in pregnancy in Malawi. *Anthropol Matters.* (2009) 11:1–13. doi: 10.22582/am.v11i1.31
31. Sambo M, Lembo T, Cleaveland S, Ferguson HM, Sikana L, Simon C, et al. Knowledge, attitudes and practices (KAP) about rabies prevention and control: a community survey in Tanzania. *PLoS Negl Trop Dis.* (2014) 8:e3310. doi: 10.1371/journal.pntd.0003310
32. Kadowaki H, Duc PP, Sato K, Phuong PTM, Hagiwara K, Makita K. Socio-economic factors associated with voluntary rabies control measures in Vietnam. *Prev Vet Med.* (2018) 157:105–14. doi: 10.1016/j.prevetmed.2018.06.006
33. Mueller R. *Basic Principles of Structural Equation Modeling.* New York, NY: Springer-Verlag (1996). doi: 10.1007/978-1-4612-3974-1
34. Kline RB. *Principles and Practice of Structural Equation Modeling.* 4th ed. New York, NY, London: The Guilford Press (2016).
35. Watanabe T, Nakahara Y, Asakura S, Makita K. Sociological factors influencing the practice and attitude towards pig farm hygiene in Hokkaido Prefecture, Japan. *J Vet Epidemiol.* (2015) 19:100–7. doi: 10.2743/jve.19.100
36. Japan Chicken Association. *A Member List of Japan Chicken Association in 2014.* Tokyo (2014).
37. Revelle W. *Procedures for Psychological, Psychometric, and Personality,*

Package "psych" Version 1.9.12.31. (2019). Available online at: https://cran.r-project.org/web/packages/psych/psych.pdf (accessed December 3, 2019).

38. Bernaads CA, Jennrich RI. Gradient projection algorythms and software for arbitrary rotation criteria in factor analysis. *Educ Psychol Meas.* (2005) 65:676–96. doi: 10.1177/0013164404272507
39. Rosseel Y. lavaan: an R package for structural equation modeling. *J Stat Softw.* (2012) 48:1–36. doi: 10.18637/jss.v048.i02
40. Hu LT, Bentler PM. Cutoff criteria for fit indexes in covariance structure analysis: conventional criteria versus new alternatives. *Struct Equ Modeling.* (1999) 6:1–55. doi: 10.1080/10705519909540118
41. Kline RB. *Global Fit Testing, Principles and Practice of Structural Equation Modeling.* 4th ed. New York, NY: Guilford Press (2005).
42. R Core Team. *R: A Language and Environment for Statistical Computing.* Vienna: R Foundation for Statistical Computing (2019). Available online at: https://www.R-project.org/ (accessed April 12, 2019).
43. Ministry of Agriculture, Forestry, Fisheries of Japan. *Raiser Households of Livestock or Chickens, Livestock or Chickens Raised, Production of Raw Milk and Hen Eggs by Prefecture.* Statistical Survey on Livestock (2013).
44. Iseki H, Morozumi T, Takagi M, Kawashima K, Shibahara T, Uenishi H, et al. Genomic sequence and virulence evaluation of MN184A-like porcine reproductive and respiratory syndrome virus in Japan. *Microbiol Immunol.* (2016) 60:824–34. doi: 10.1111/1348-0421.12455
45. Cloete A, Gerstenberg C, Mayet N, Tempia S. Brucellosis knowledge, attitudes and practices of a South African communal cattle keeper group. *Onderstepoort J Vet.* (2019) 86:1671. doi: 10.4102/ojvr.v86i1.1671
46. Fraser RW, Williams NT, Powell LF, Cook AJ. Reducing *Campylobacter* and *Salmonella* infection: two studies of the economic cost and attitude to adoption of on-farm biosecurity measures. *Zoonoses Public Health.* (2010) 57:109–15. doi: 10.1111/j.1863-2378.2009.01295.x
47. Gunn GJ, Heffernan C, Hall M, McLeod A, Hovi M. Measuring and comparing constraints to improved biosecurity amongst GB farmers, veterinarians and the auxiliary industries. *Prev Vet Med.* (2008) 84:310–23. doi: 10.1016/j.prevetmed.2007.12.003
48. Ministry of Agriculture, Forestry, Fisheries of Japan. *The Situation of Compliance to Standard Rearing Hygiene Management in Japan as of 2018 February 1st.* (2018). Available online at: https://www.maff.go.jp/j/syouan/douei/katiku_yobo/k_shiyou/attach/pdf/index-87.pdf (accessed March 10, 2020).

10

Establishment and Application of Multiplex PCR for Simultaneously Detecting *Escherichia coli*, *Salmonella*, *Klebsiella pneumoniae* and *Staphylococcus aureus* in Minks

Peng Li[1,2†], *Dingxiu Zhang*[1,2†], *Hongmei Li*[1,2†], *Jinying Pang*[1,2], *Huijun Guo*[1,2*] *and Jianhua Qiu*[1,2*]

[1] *College of Animal Science and Veterinary Medicine, Shandong Agricultural University, Tai'an, China,* [2] *Shandong Provincial Key Laboratory of Animal Biotechnology and Disease Control and Prevention, Shandong Provincial Engineering Technology Research Center of Animal Disease Control and Prevention, Shandong Agricultural University, Tai'an, China*

***Correspondence:**
Jianhua Qiu
qiujianhua@sdau.edu.cn
Huijun Guo
hjguo@sdau.edu.cn

† These authors have contributed equally to this work

To establish a multiplex PCR for simultaneous detection of *Escherichia coli* (*E. coli*), *Salmonella*, *Klebsiella pneumoniae* (*K. pneumoniae*), and *Staphylococcus aureus* (*S. aureus*), four pairs of specific primers were designed according to the conservative regions of *phoA* gene for *E. coli*, *invA* gene for *Salmonella*, *khe* gene for *K. pneumoniae*, *nuc* gene for *S. aureus*. The quadruple PCR system was established through optimization of multiplex PCR and detection of specificity, sensitivity, and stability. The results showed that target gene bands of *E. coli* (622 bp), *Salmonella* (801 bp), *K. pneumoniae* (303 bp), and *S. aureus* (464 bp) could be amplified by this method specifically and simultaneously from the same sample containing the four pathogens, with a detection sensitivity of 100 pg/μL. Meanwhile, no bands of common clinical bacteria, including *Clostridium perfringens*, *Pseudomonas aeruginosa*, *Pasteurella multocida*, *Streptococcus pneumoniae*, *Streptococcus pneumoniae*, *Proteus mirabilis*, *Staphylococcus sciuri*, *Staphylococcus pseudintermedius*, *Acinetobacter baumannii*, *Enterococcus faecalis,* and *Bacillus subtilis* were amplified. In addition, 380 tissue samples were detected by multiplex and single PCR established in current study, respectively. Among the 368 carcass samples, positive detection rates of *E. coli, K. pneumoniae, Salmonella,* and *S. aureus* were 33.7, 12.0, 10.6, and 13.9%. Among the 12 visceral tissue samples, positive detection rates of *E. coli, K. pneumoniae, Salmonella,* and *S. aureus* were 41.7, 25.0, 16.7, and 8.3%, respectively. Positive detection rates of multiplex PCR were consistent with that of single PCR. Compared with single PCR, the multiplex PCR method had the advantages of time-saving, high specificity and high sensitivity. The results showed that the minks in these farms had mixed infection of these four pathogens, and the method established in this study could be applied to the rapid and accurate detection and identification of these four bacteria. In conclusion, the multiplex PCR method has stable detection results, good repeatability, and short detection time. It is suitable for the rapid and accurate detection of four kinds of bacteria above the carcass of fur animals, which could be suitable in microbial epidemiology investigation. It can provide a reliable technical reference for rapid clinical diagnosis and detection.

Keywords: minks, *E. coli*, *Salmonella*, *K. pneumoniae*, *S. aureus*, multiplex PCR detection

INTRODUCTION

As a valuable economic fur animal, the domestic breeding of minks has been paid more and more attention. The scale of mink breeding in the world in 2014 is 100 million, while that in China is close to 80 million (1). And Shandong province is the largest province for mink breeding and skin production. The mink skins production in Shandong corresponded to 70% of all skins produced in China in 2016 (2). Although in recent years, due to the influence of foreign market demand, the breeding scale has declined, but mink breeding is still an important pillar industry in Shandong Province. However, a range of pathogenic microbes are causing a wide variety of infectious diseases in Shandong (3–8). Some of which may even have the risk of infecting people, and it would be a threat to mink breeding and public health. At the same time, bacterial disease is one of the main causes of mink death.

Escherichia coli (*E. coli*), *Salmonella*, *Klebsiella pneumoniae* (*K. pneumoniae*), and *Staphylococcus aureus* (*S. aureus*) are the most common pathogens or opportunistic pathogens in minks. They can infect not only minks, but also human, and other animals (9–12). In recent years bacterial diseases have been not only frequent, but also in the state of mixed infection or secondary infection in mink farms of Shandong (13, 14). Therefore, it is necessary to give timely and rapid diagnosis and treatment of multiple infection in mink culture.

The traditional method of bacterial pathogens identification mostly uses bacterial isolation and culture combined with biochemical characteristics detection and analysis. Although the traditional methods are reliable, there are still some shortcomings that affect their application, such as strong specialization and high requirements for operators, high risk, time-consuming, and expensive.

Modern molecular biology technology, such as polymerase chain reaction (PCR) combined with gel electrophoresis, is increasingly used in bacteria isolation and identification, which improves the detection efficiency. Compared with single PCR, multiplex PCR has higher detection efficiency, which can not only detect a variety of pathogens at the same time, but also reduce the cost and save the time. It can be seen that multiplex PCR detection is of great significance for the rapid diagnosis and detection of mixed infection (15–17). However, the research on the simultaneous detection of *E. coli*, *Salmonella*, *K. Pneumoniae*, and *S. aureus* in minks by quadruple PCR in Shandong has not been reported, and there is still a lack of relevant research data.

Therefore, the current study was conducted to design primers according to the published gene sequences of these four mink bacteria, and then to establish a multiplex PCR method for simultaneous detection of four bacteria. So as to provide a reference for the rapid identification of these four common or opportunistic pathogenic bacteria.

MATERIALS AND METHODS

Source of Bacterial Strains

Reference strains of *E. coli* (ATCC8739), *Salmonella* (ATCC13076), *K. pneumoniae* (CMCC46117), and *S. aureus* (ATCC6538) used in this study were all purchased from China microbial strain network. *Clostridium perfringens*, *Pseudomonas aeruginosa*, *Pasteurella multocida*, *Streptococcus pneumoniae*, *Streptococcus pneumoniae*, *Proteus mirabilis*, *Staphylococcus sciuri*, *Staphylococcus pseudintermedius*, *Acinetobacter baumannii*, *Enterococcus faecalis*, and *Bacillus subtilis* positive strains were all pathogenic bacteria isolated from minks, which were isolated, identified and preserved by the laboratory of College of Animal Science and Technology, Shandong Agricultural University.

Sampling and Isolation

During January 2017 to October 2018, 380 samples, including 368 carcass samples (from right hind leg) and 12 visceral tissue samples from diseased minks, were collected from 35 mink farms in the main mink-producing areas of Shandong Province, China, including Zhucheng, Wendeng, Liaocheng, Rizhao, Haiyang, and Dongping. Among the 12 diseased mink tissue samples, seven minks had obvious clinical symptoms of respiratory diseases, and the remaining five minks had clinical symptoms of digestive tract diseases. These samples were used for bacterial isolation by traditional clinical microbilologic methods, and then the established multiplex PCR method and the single PCR method were used to detect these bacterial isolation, and the multiplex PCR results were compared with the single PCR method to detect the specificity of multiplex PCR method.

Primers

The target genes chosen for their specificity were the *phoA* gene in *E. coli*, *invA* gene in *Salmonella*, *khe* gene in *K. pneumoniae* and *nuc* gene in *S. aureus* (6, 15–21). Four pairs of specific primers were designed by Premier 5.0 and Oligo 6.0 along with NCBI primer-BLAST comparison. All the primers used in current study were synthesized by Shanghai Sangon Biotech Co., Ltd. The primers and the respective amplification lengths are shown in **Table 1**.

DNA Extraction

The reference strains and the positive isolates identified by traditional clinical microbiologic methods were inoculated on 5 mL Tryptic soy broth (TSB), and then cultured by shaking at 37°C for 18~24 h. Bacterial genomic DNA was extracted from 1 mL bacterial solution with a TIANamp Bacterial DNA Kit (Tiangen, Beijing, China) according to the Kit instructions. The extracted bacterial DNA was detected

TABLE 1 | Primers used in multiplex PCR.

Bacteria	Primer sequences (5′-3′)	Target genes	Gene ID	PCR product size (bp)
K. pneumoniae	F-CGATGCTACTTATCCCGACA R-ACCACCAGCAGACGAACTT	*khe*	KX842080.1	303
S. aureus	F-AGGCATGGCTATCAGTAATGTTTC R-CATCAGCATAAATATACGCTAAGCCAC	*nuc*	DQ507382.1	464
E. coli	F-TACAGGTGACTGCGGGCTTATC R-CTTACCGGGCAATACACTCACTA	*phoA*	FJ546461.1	622
Salmonella	F-AAAAGAAGGGTCGTCGTTAG R-GGAAGGTACTGCCAGAGGTC	*invA*	MK017941.1	801

by nucleic acid analyzer and diluted to 10 ng/μL for subsequent test.

Genomic DNA of carcass samples and diseased mink visceral tissue samples were extracted using TIANamp Blood/Cell/Tissue DNA Kit (Tiangen, Beijing, China) according to the Kit instructions. The extracted DNA was stored at −20°C.

Control, Optimization, and Establishment of Multiplex PCR Conditions

Firstly, the genomic DNA of four standard positive strains was used as a template to screen the optimal annealing temperature by single PCR reaction. Ten annealing temperature gradients of 52, 52.9, 53.8, 54.9, 56, 57, 58.1, 59.2, 60.1, and 61°C were set to determine the optimal annealing temperature. Next, multiplex PCR was performed using the same volume mixture of genomic DNA of four standard strains as template. Thus, the concentration of primers and annealing temperature were optimized to determine the optimal multiplex PCR reaction conditions.

The results of the preliminary test showed the multiplex PCR reaction were carried out in 25 μL reaction mixtures containing 12.5 μL of 2×Es Taq MasterMix, 1 μL for each of the four bacterial DNA templates, 1 μL for each of the four pairs of primers with the best concentration ratio. Among which Taq MasterMix was composed of Es Taq DNA Polymerase (amplification efficiency: 2 kb/min), $MgCl_2$ (3 mM/L), dNTP(400 μM/L), PCR stabilizer, and enhancer. Finally, the volume of the reaction mixtures was filled up to 25 μL with sterilized double distilled water. The amplification conditions consisted of an initial denaturation at 94°C for 7 min, 30 cycles of denaturation at 94°C for 30 s, annealing at 52 61°C for 30 s, extension at 72°C for 30 s, and final extension for 5 min at 72°C. On the basis of four optimum concentration ratio primers, 10 annealing temperature gradients of 52, 52.9, 53.8, 54.9, 56, 57, 58.1, 59.2, 60.1, and 61°C were also set to select the annealing temperature and optimize the reaction conditions.

Sensitivity Test of Multiplex PCR

The DNA template was serially diluted to 10 ng/μL, 1 ng/μL, 100 pg/μL, 10 pg/μL, 1 pg/μL, 100 fg/μL by 10 fold gradient with sterile double distilled water, then amplified by the optimized single PCR reaction system. Subsequently, the DNA template was serially diluted to 100 ng/μL, 10 ng/μL, 1 ng/μL, 100 pg/μL, 10 pg/μL, 1 pg/μL by 10 fold gradient with sterile double distilled water, then amplified by the optimized multiplex PCR reaction system. Finally, the PCR products were electrophoresis to detect the sensitivity of each primer.

Specificity Test of Multiplex PCR

The mixed DNA or single DNA of four standard strains and the DNA of common bacteria samples in clinic, such as *Clostridium perfringens, Pasteurella multocida, Pseudomonas aeruginosa, Streptococcus pneumoniae, Streptococcus pneumoniae, Proteus mirabilis, Staphylococcus sciuri, Staphylococcus pseudintermedius, Acinetobacter baumannii, Enterococcus faecalis,* and *Bacillus subtilis* were used as templates in the optimized reaction system for multiplex PCR amplification to detect the specificity of primers.

Stability Test of the Multiplex PCR

In order to evaluate the stability of the multiplex PCR system, templates of the positive and negative samples, respectively, or mixed were added into reaction mixture, and then were amplified by the optimized multiplex PCR system. The positive control was four bacteria DNA (*E. coli, Salmonella, K. Pneumoniae,* and *S. aureus*), which were identified as positive by biochemical detection and 16S rRNA sequencing. The negative control was sterilized double distilled water. The stability test was repeated three times. In addition, the detection effect of multiplex PCR system was evaluated by comparing with single PCR.

RESULT

Establishment of Multiplex PCR Conditions

Single PCR test results of the each reference bacteria DNA showed that, the specific gene amplification products of the four bacteria DNA were obtained, which were 622 bp for *E. coli*, 801 bp for *Salmonella*, 303 bp for *K. Pneumoniae,* and 464 bp for *S. aureus,* respectively. The results of multiplex PCR combined with single PCR showed that when the annealing temperature was 56°C, the amplified bands of four target genes of *E. coli, Salmonella, K. Pneumoniae,* and *S. aureus* were uniform, concentrated and highly specific (**Figures 1, 2**). The subsequent tests were carried out at 56°C.

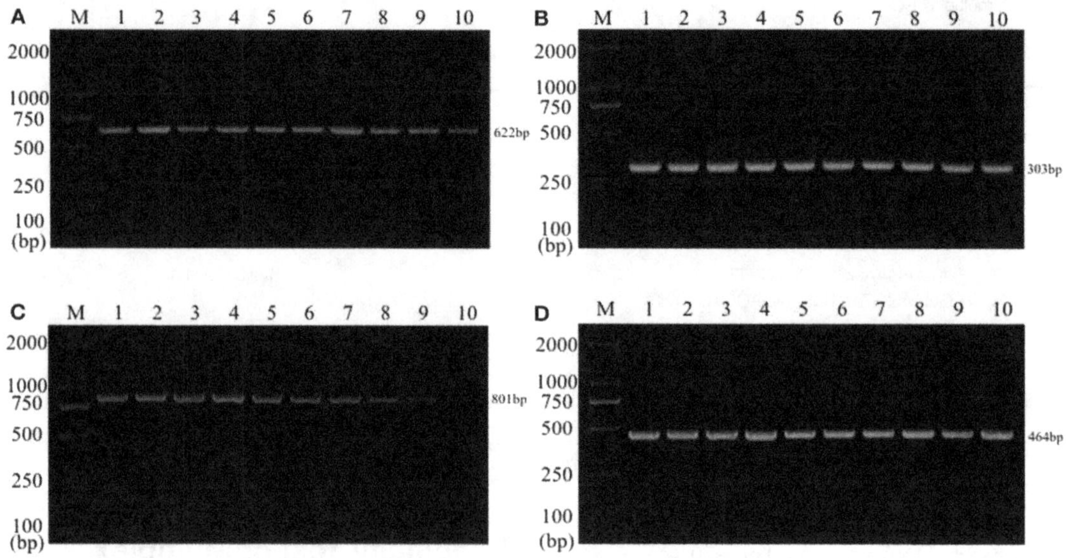

FIGURE 1 | Single PCR amplification at different annealing temperature. Lane M, D2000 DNA marker; Lane 1, 52.0°C; Lane 2, 52.9°C; Lane 3, 53.8°C; Lane 4, 54.9°C; Lane 5, 56.0°C; Lane 6, 57.0°C; Lane 7, 58.1°C; Lane 8, 59.2°C; Lane 9, 60.1°C; Lane 10, 61.0°C. **(A)** *E. coli*; **(B)** *K. pneumoniae*; **(C)** *Salmonella*; **(D)** *S. aureus*.

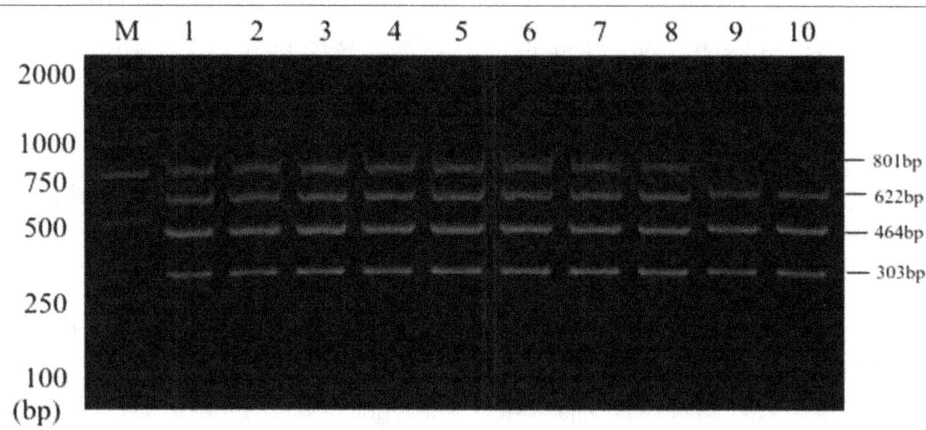

FIGURE 2 | Multiplex PCR amplification at different annealing temperature. Lane M, D2000 DNA marker; Lane 1, 52.0°C; Lane 2, 52.9°C; Lane 3, 53.8°C; Lane 4, 54.9°C; Lane 5, 56.0°C; Lane 6, 57.0°C; Lane 7, 58.1°C; Lane 8, 59.2°C; Lane 9, 60.1°C; Lane 10, 61.0°C.

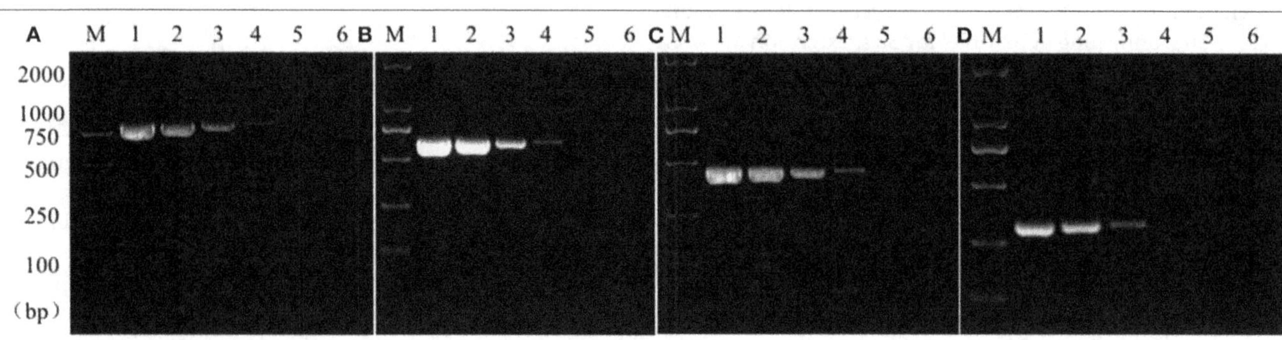

FIGURE 3 | Results of single PCR assay sensitivity experiment. Lane M, D2000 DNA marker; Lane 1~6: The concentration was 10 ng/μL, 1 ng/μL, 100 pg/μL, 10 pg/μL, 1 pg/μL, and 100 fg/μL, respectively; **(A)** *Salmonella*; **(B)** *E. coli*; **(C)** *S. aureus*; **(D)** *K. pneumoniae*.

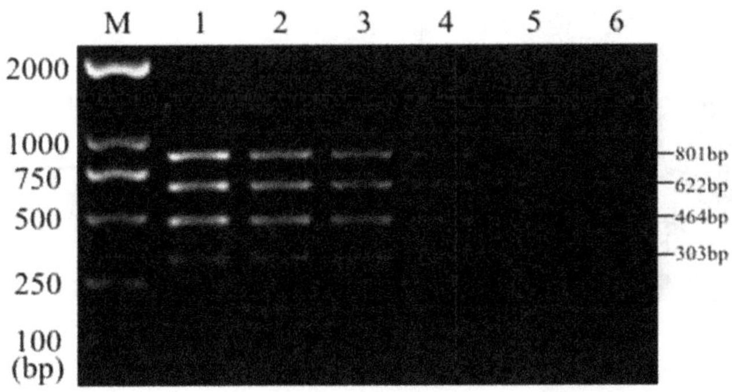

FIGURE 4 | Results of multiplex PCR assay sensitivity experiment. Lane M, D2000 DNA marker; Lane 1, 100 ng of DNA for each of *Salmonella, E. coli, S. aureus,* and *K. pneumoniae*; Lane 2, 10 ng; Lane 3, 1 ng; Lane 4, 100 pg; Lane 5, 10 pg; Lane 6, 1 pg.

Results of Multiplex PCR Sensitivity Experiment

Sensitivity test results of the reference bacteria DNA demonstrated that, the single PCR assay was capable of properly identifying the presence of bacteria at the following lowest concentration, 1.0 pg/μL for *S. aureus*, 10.0 pg/μL for *E. coli*, Salmonella, and *K. pneumoniae* (**Figure 3**). The multiplex PCR assay could properly identify the presence of bacteria at 100 pg/μL of DNA template for *S. aureus, E. coli, Salmonella,* and *K. pneumoniae* (**Figure 4**).

Results of Multiplex PCR Specificity Experiment

PCR specificity test results of bacteria DNA indicated that, the multiplex PCR assay could be capable to effectively identify the mixed DNA and the single DNA samples. Conversely, no bands of common clinical bacteria, including *Clostridium perfringens, P. aeruginosa, Pasteurella multocida, Streptococcus pneumoniae, Streptococcus pneumoniae, Proteus mirabilis, Staphylococcus sciuri, Staphylococcus pseudintermedius, Acinetobacter baumannii, Enterococcus faecalis,* and *Bacillus subtilis* were amplified by multiplex PCR (**Figure 5**). However, no amplification was achieved from control groups of other bacteria. The results suggested that the established multiplex PCR method showed good specificity.

Results of Multiplex PCR Stability Experiment

The stability test results displayed that the specific target bands were found in all the positive samples, while no amplification products were found in the negative samples (**Figure 6**). The above results were in line with our expectations and the experimental requirements. Together these results suggested that the established multiplex PCR method had good stability and repeatability.

Detection and Identification Results of Clinical Samples

Three hundred eighty samples were detected by multiplex and single PCR method established in current study. And the results were shown at **Tables 2, 3**. The results of the **Table 2** demonstrated that among the 368 carcass samples, positive detection rates of *E. coli, K. pneumoniae, Salmonella,* and *S. aureus* were 33.7% (124/368), 12.0% (44/368), 10.6% (39/368), and 13.9% (51/368), respectively. Among the 12 visceral tissue samples, positive detection rates of *E. coli, K. pneumoniae, Salmonella,* and *S. aureus* were 41.7% (5/12), 25.0% (3/12), 16.7% (2/12), and 8.3% (1/12), respectively. Positive detection rates of multiplex PCR were consistent with that of single PCR (**Table 2**). At the same time, the results also showed that there were four kinds of bacteria contamination in mink carcasses.

Co-contamination detection results of bacteria in 380 clinical tissue samples by multiplex PCR were shown at **Table 3**. From the results of **Table 3**, it could be seen that single and multiple contamination were present in these samples. Among the 368 carcass samples, positive detection rates of dual contamination for *E. coli, K. pneumoniae, E. coli,* and *Salmonella* were 6.0% (22/368) and 4.6% (17/368), respectively. Positive detection rates of dual contamination for *E. coli, S. aureus, Salmonella,* and *S. aureus* were 1.4% (5/368). Positive detection rate of triple contamination for *E. coli, K. pneumoniae,* and *Salmonella* was 1.4% (5/368). Positive detection rate of triple contamination for *E. coli, Salmonella,* and *S. aureus* was 0.8% (3/368). Positive detection rate of quadruple contamination was 0.8% (3/368). Among the 12 visceral tissue samples, positive detection rates of dual contamination for *E. coli, K. pneumoniae, E. coli,* and *Salmonella* were 8.3% (1/12). Together these results suggest that different degrees of double, triple, or quadruple bacterial infection were present in the minks used for tissue sampling. The multiplex PCR could detect four kinds of bacteria from contaminated mink carcasses.

DISCUSSION

Specific primers were designed for specific target genes of four kinds of bacteria in the current study. The *nuc* gene of *S. aureus* encodes an extracellular thermostable nuclease, which is often used to detect *S. aureus* rapidly and specifically (15, 17, 22, 23). The *invA* gene of *Salmonella* is responsible for encoding the surface protein of the infected epithelial cells, which is common within the genus and unique among the genera, and is closely related to the pathogenicity of *Salmonella* (24, 25). When using *invA* gene as the target gene to design primers for *Salmonella* detection, strong specificity and detection accuracy can be obtained (26). Housekeeper gene *phoA* is used as a specific target gene for detection of *E. coli* (16, 27, 28). *khe* gene encodes the unique hemolysin of *K. pneumoniae* and is widely used in its detection (29, 30). Four pairs of specific primers designed in this study were used for the multiplex PCR, and the size intervals of the expected amplification products were more than 100 bp, so that different target genes could be distinguished after agarose gel electrophoresis.

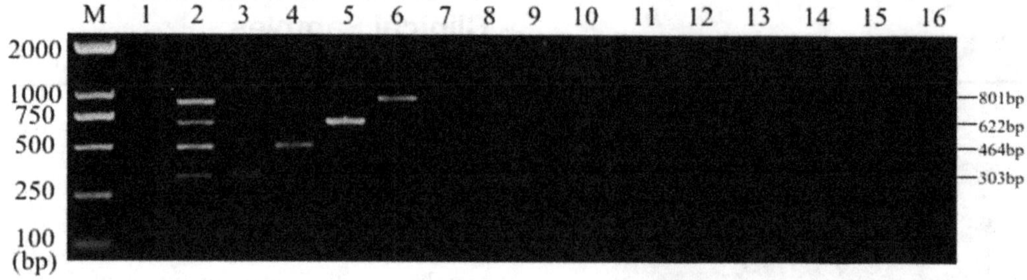

FIGURE 5 | Results of multiplex PCR specificity experiment. Lane M, D2000 DNA marker; Lane 1, Negative control; Lane 2, mixed DNA template of *Salmonella, E. coli, S. aureus* and *K. pneumoniae*; Lane 3, *K. pneumoniae*; Lane 4, *S. aureus*; Lane 5, *E. coli*; Lane 6, *Salmonella*; Lane 7, *Clostridium perfringens*; Lane 8, *Pasteurella multocida*; Lane 9, *P. aeruginosa*; Lane 10, *Streptococcus pneumoniae*; Lane 11, *Proteus mirabilis*; Lane 12, *Staphylococcus sciuri*; Lane 13, *Staphylococcus pseudintermedius*; Lane 14, *Acinetobacter baumannii*; Lane 15, *Enterococcus faecalis*; Lane 16, *Bacillus subtilis*.

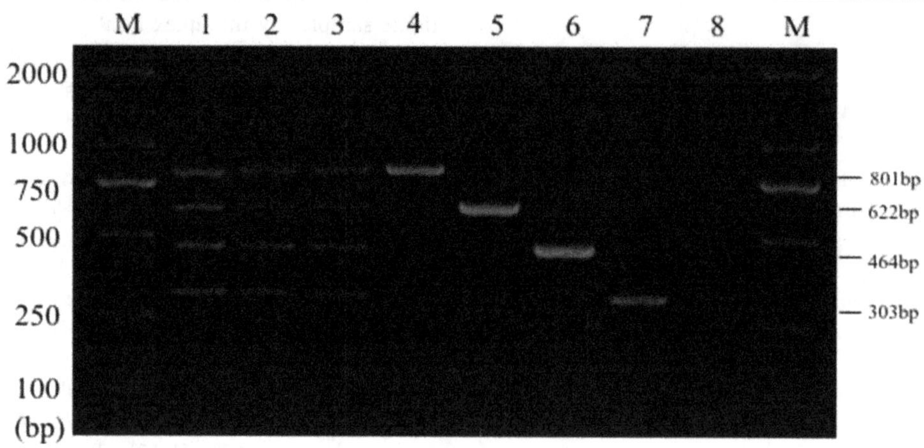

FIGURE 6 | Results of multiplex PCR stability experiment. Lane M, D2000 DNA marker; Lane 1~3: mixed DNA template; Lane 4, *Salmonella*; Lane 5, *E. coli*; Lane 6, *S. aureus*; Lane 7, *K. pneumoniae*; Lane 8, Negative control.

TABLE 2 | Multiplex and single PCR detection results of clinical samples from Shandong Province, China.

Samples	Pathogens	Proportion of positive samples (%)		Concordance rate (%)
		Multiplex PCR	Single PCR	
Carcass samples	*Salmonella*	39/368 (10.6)	39/368 (10.6)	100
	E.coli	124/368 (33.7)	124/368 (33.7)	100
	K. pneumoniae	44/368 (12.0)	44/368 (12.0)	100
	S. aureus	51/368 (13.9)	51/368 (13.9)	100
Visceral tissue	*Salmonella*	2/12 (16.7)	2/12 (16.7)	100
	E. coli	5/12 (41.7)	5/12 (41.7)	100
	K. pneumoniae	3/12 (25)	3/12 (25)	100
	S. aureus	1/12 (8.3)	1/12 (8.3)	100

The results of single PCR showed that the four pairs designed in this study could amplify the corresponding target genes specifically. Therefore, these primers can be used in multiplex PCR detection system. The optimization of reaction conditions is the key to the construction of multiplex PCR system, the most important of which is the optimization of annealing temperature. Generally, the annealing temperature is determined according to the chain breaking temperature of the upstream and downstream primers, but sometimes the results are not the same as expected (31). Although a single target gene fragment can be amplified specifically at 56–60°C, the annealing temperature of 4–6°C can be reduced in the multiplex PCR reaction, which is conducive to the amplification of all target gene fragments (32). The optimal annealing temperature is

TABLE 3 | Co-contamination detection results of pathogenic bacteria in 380 clinical samples by multiplex PCR.

Pathogens	Proportion of positive samples (%)	
	carcass samples (368)	visceral tissue (12)
E. coli + *K. pneumoniae*	22 (6.0%)	1(8.3%)
E. coli + *Salmonella*	17 (4.6%)	1(8.3%)
E. coli + *S. aureus*	5 (1.4%)	0 (0)
S. aureus + *Salmonella*	5 (1.4%)	0 (0)
E. coli + *K. pneumoniae* + *Salmonella*	5 (1.4%)	0 (0)
E. coli + *Salmonella* + *S. aureus*	3 (0.8%)	0 (0)
E. coli + *K. pneumoniae* + *Salmonella* + *S. aureus*	3 (0.8%)	0 (0)
Total	60 (16.4%)	2 (16.7%)

determined by designing the annealing temperature gradient, and the optimization of primer concentration, primer addition amount and addition proportion is also an important step of the optimization scheme (18). Our study showed that under the same cycle number, the amplification efficiency of specific primers for *E. coli* and *S. aureus* was higher than that for *Salmonella* and *K. pneumoniae*. The amplification efficiency of each pair of primers could be effectively balanced by reducing the concentration of primers with high amplification efficiency and increasing the concentration of primers with low amplification rate (33).

In this study, the sensitivity test results showed that the minimum detection amount of multiplex PCR for four pathogens reached 100 pg. The multiplex PCR sensitivity of *E. coli, Salmonella,* and *S. aureus* in this study is close to or higher than that reported by Xu et al. (34) and Wang et al. (16). The minimum detection concentration of single PCR for bacteria DNA could reach 10.0 pg/μL, even 1.0 pg/μL. The single PCR sensitivity of *E. coli* detection in the current study is the same as that of Xu et al. (34), and it is more convenient and time-saving than that of Guan et al. (35) and Liu et al. (36). In this study, 380 samples were detected by multiplex PCR and single PCR. The results showed that the positive detection rate, accuracy, and sensitivity of multiplex PCR were in agreement with that of single PCR. The multiplex PCR method established in this study can be used to identify and detect bacteria in mink tissue samples. This sensitivity can meet the needs of clinical detection. The specificity test results showed that the multiplex PCR system could not only amplify the mixed samples and single samples, but also could not amplify other kinds of common pathogens or opportunistic pathogens in minks which cause respiratory tract and digestive tract diseases. All of these show that the method is more specific and can be applied to the detection and identification of specific pathogenic bacteria. The research of Guan et al. (37) also showed good stability and repeatability of multiplex PCR, which was consistent with our results.

The detection results of clinical samples showed that the single and co-infection of bacteria in mink visceral tissue samples and carcass samples in Shandong are serious, which suggests that enough attention should be paid to these multiple and single infections. This is not consistent with the research results in pigs (35), which may be due to the different composition of sample pathogens caused by factors such as pre-mortem health status, feeding, and storage conditions.

CONCLUSIONS

In conclusion, the multiplex PCR method is designed to detect and analyze the pathogenic microorganisms in mink carcass and viscera, which provides a rapid, specific and sensitive detection method for the identification of pathogenic bacteria in minks. The establishment of the multiplex PCR is conducive to the harmless treatment, development and utilization of mink carcass resources, and provides technical support for the safe and accurate application of fur animal carcass resources.

AUTHOR CONTRIBUTIONS

HG conceived and designed the experiments. PL, DZ, and HL are mainly responsible for experimental implementation. JQ and JP are mainly responsible for sample collection and helped to do some experiments. PL and JQ wrote the manuscript. All authors have read and approved the final manuscript.

REFERENCES

1. Jiang CQ. *Epidemiological investigation of bacterial pneumonia from mink.* (Master's thesis). *Shandong Agricultural University, Tai'an city, China* (2016).
2. Yang ML, Wang FY, Jiang DH, Ma ZF. Investigation on the operation of special economic animal industry in Shandong Province, China Shangdong. *J Anim Sci Vet Med.* (2017) 8:47–9. doi: 10.3969/j.issn.1007-1733.2017.08.035
3. Diao FF, Zhao YF, Wang JL, Wei XH, Cui K, Liu CY, et al. Molecular characterization of feline panleukopenia virus isolated from mink and its pathogenesis in mink. *Vet Microbiol.* (2017) 205:92–8. doi: 10.1016/j.vetmic.2017.05.017
4. Li P, Chen C, Han KY, Zhang FX, Zhu YL, Ling ZS, et al. Molecular characterization of H9N2 influenza virus isolated from mink and its pathogenesis in mink. *Vet Microbiol.* (2015) 176:8–96. doi: 10.1016/j.vetmic.2015.01.009
5. Wang JL, Shang YY, Guo SY, Diao FF, Yu JY, Wei XH, et al. Serotype and virulence genes of *Klebsiella pneumoniae* isolated from mink and its pathogenesis in mice and mink. *Sci Rep.* (2017) 7:17291. doi: 10.1038/s41598-017-17681-8
6. Wang GS, Yin FF. Establishment of PCR detection for *Klebsiella pneumoniae*. *Shangdong J Anim Sci Vet Med.* (2017) 38:6–7. doi: 10.3969/j.issn.1007-1733.2017.04.003
7. Xue R, Tian Y, Hou T, Bao D, Chen H, Teng Q, et al. H9N2 influenza virus isolated from minks has enhanced virulence in mice. *Transbound Emerg Dis.* (2018) 65:904–10. doi: 10.1111/tbed.12805
8. Zhu Q, Peng H, Li H, Yang LZ, Zhang BS, Zhu J, et al. Serotypes and virulence genes of *Pseudomonas aeruginosa* isolated from

mink and its pathogenicity in mink. *Microbial Pathogenesis.* (2020) 139:103904. doi: 10.1016/j.micpath.2019.103904

9. Chiari M, Ferrari N, Giardiello D, Lanfranchi P, Zanoni M, Lavazza A, et al. Isolation and identification of *Salmonella* spp. from red foxes (Vulpes vulpes) and badgers (Meles meles) in northern Italy. *Acta Vet Scand.* (2014) 56:86. doi: 10.1186/s13028-014-0086-7
10. O'Gara JP. Into the storm: Chasing the opportunistic pathogen *Staphylococcus aureus* from skin colonization to life-threatening infections. *Environ Microbiol.* (2017) 19:3823–33. doi: 10.1111/1462-2920.13833
11. Sakaue T. Studies on the properties of *Escherichia coli* as an opportunistic pathogen. *Nihon Ika Daigaku Zasshi.* (1982) 49:759–66. doi: 10.1272/jnms1923.49.759
12. Wei S, Zhao H, Xian YY, Hussain MA, Wu XY. Multiplex PCR assays for the detection of Vibrio alginolyticus, Vibrio parahaemolyticus, Vibrio vulnificus, and Vibrio cholerae with an internal amplification control. *Diag Microbiol Infect Dis.* (2014) 79:115–8. doi: 10.1016/j.diagmicrobio.2014.03.012
13. Zhong SX, Chi SS, Wang Z, Jiang XD, Zhu FJ, Zhu RL. The etiology analysis of multiple infections in Shandong scale fur farms. *Chin J Vet Sci.* (2014) 34:1770–7. doi: 10.16303/j.cnki.1005-4545.2014.11.027
14. Yu J, Wang ZC, Zhang Y, Li WL, Ren HY. Identification of mink pathogens and detection of its sensitivity to antibiotics and Chinese Medicine. *Chinese Agricult Sci Bull.* (2015) 20:5–8. doi: 10.11924/j.issn.1000-6850.casb15010247
15. Gan C, Hu JF, Cao Q, Zhao RK, Li YC, Wang ZG, et al. Rapid identification of pathogens involved in pediatric osteoarticular infections by multiplex PCR. *Ann Transl Med.* (2020) 8:203. doi: 10.21037/atm.2020.01.34
16. Wang ZH, Zuo JK, Gong JS, Hu JG, Jiang W, Mi RS, et al. Development of a multiplex PCR assay for the simultaneous and rapid detection of six pathogenic bacteria in poultry. *AMB Express.* (2019) 9:185. doi: 10.1186/s13568-019-0908-0
17. Lee N, Kwon KY, Oh SK, Chang HJ, Chun HS, and Choi SW. A Multiplex PCR Assay for Simultaneous Detection of *Escherichia coli* O157:H7, *Bacillus cereus*, *Vibrio parahaemolyticus*, *Salmonella* spp., *Listeria monocytogenes*, and *Staphylococcus aureus* in Korean Ready-to-Eat Food. *Foodborne Pathog Dis.* (2014) 11:574–80. doi: 10.1089/fpd.2013.1638
18. Wei B, Cha SY, Kang M, Park IJ, Moon OK, Park CK, et al. Development and application of a multiplex pcr assay for rapid detection of 4 major bacterial pathogens in ducks. *Poult Sci.* (2013) 92:1164–70. doi: 10.3382/ps.2012-02823
19. Luo YQ. *The research of resistance phenotype chlormphenicols resistance gene in E. coli, Salmonella and S. aureus from livestock.* (Master's thesis). Southwest University, Chongqing city, China (2017).
20. Li J, Wang C. S. *Rapid detection of E coli, Salmonella and Pasteurella multocida in Langde goose by triple PCR. ShuiQin ShiJie.* (2016) 6:30–3. Available online at: http://d.wanfangdata.com.cn/periodical/sqsj201606018
21. Wei CJ, Zhong JL, Hu T, and Zhao XH. Simultaneous detection of Escherichia coli O157: H7, Staphylococcus aureus and Salmonella by multiplex PCR in milk. *3 Biotech.* (2018) 8:76. doi: 10.1007/s13205-018-1086-5
22. Coppens J, Heirstraeten LV, Ruzin A, Yu Li, Timbermont L, Lammens C, et al. Comparison of GeneXpert MRSA/SA ETA assay with semi-quantitative and quantitative cultures and nuc gene-based qPCR for detection of *Staphylococcus aureus* in endotracheal aspirate samples. *Antimicrob Resist Infect Control.* (2019) 8:4. doi: 10.1186/s13756-018-0460-8
23. Yang FL, Li XS, Liang XW, Zhang XF, Qin GS, Yang BZ. Detection of virulence-associated genes in Staphylococcus aureus isolated from bovine clinical mastitis milk samples in Guangxi. *Trop Anim Health Prod.* (2012) 44:1821–6. doi: 10.1007/s11250-012-0143-z
24. Siddique RA, Saxena M, Lakhchaura BD. PCR based rapid detection of Salmonella from poultry samples. *Indian J Public Health.* (2009) 53:226–8. Available online at: https://www.researchgate.net/profile/Mumtesh_Saxena/publication/44599180_PCR_based_rapid_detection_of_Salmonella_from_poultry_samples/links/5762283a08ae244d0372d3cd.pdf
25. D'souza DH, Critzer FJ, Golden DA. Real-time reverse-transcriptase polymerase chain reaction for the rapid detection of *Salmonella* using *invA* primers. *Foodborne Pathog Dis.* (2009) 6:1097–06. doi: 10.1089/fpd.2009.0322
26. Malorny B, Hoorfar J, Hugas M, Heuvelink A, Fach P, Ellerbroek L, et al. Interlaboratory diagnostic accuracy of a *Salmonella* specific PCR-based method. *Int J Food Microbiol.* (2003) 89:241–9. doi: 10.1016/S0168-1605(03)00154-5
27. Shome BR, Mitra SD, Bhuvana M, Krithiga N, Velu D, Shome R, et al. Multiplex PCR assay for species identification of bovine mastitis pathogens. *J Appl Microbiol.* (2011) 111:1349–56. doi: 10.1111/j.1365-2672.2011.05169.x
28. Kong RYC, So CL, Law WF, Wu RSS. A sensitive and versatile multiplex PCR system for the rapid detection of enterotoxigenic (ETEC), enterohaemorrhagic (EHEC) and enteropathogenic (EPEC) strains of Escherichia coli. *Mar Pollut Bull.* (1999) 38:1207–15. doi: 10.1016/S0025-326X(99)00164-2
29. Chen ZH, Liu MY, Cui YJ, Wang L, Zhang YQ, Qiu JF, et al. A novel PCR-based geno-typing scheme for clinical *Klebsiella pneumoniae. Future Microbiol.* (2014) 9:21–32. doi: 10.2217/fmb.13.137
30. Escobar Pérez JA, Olarte Escobar NM, Castro-cardozo B, Valderrama Marquez IA, Garzon Aguilar MIG, Barrera LM, et al. Outbreak of NDM-1-Producing *Klebsiella pneumoniae* in a Neonatal Unit in Colombia. *Antimicrob Agents Chemother.* (2013) 57:1957–60. doi: 10.1128/AAC.01447-12
31. Karlsen F, Kalantari M, Jenkins A, Pettersen E, Kristensen G, Holm R, et al. Use of multiple PCR primer sets for optimal detection of human papillomavirus. *J Clin Microbiol.* (1996) 34:2095–100. doi: 10.1128/JCM.34.9.2095-2100.1996
32. Henegariu O, Heerema NA, Dlouhy S. R., and Vance GH,Vogt, P. *H. Multiplex PCR: critical parameters and step-by-step protocol Biotechniques.* (1997) 23:504–11. doi: 10.2144/97233rr01
33. Stoeck T, Hayward B, Taylor GT, Varela R, Epstein SS. A multiple PCR-primer approach to access the microeukaryotic diversity in environmental samples. *Protist.* (2006) 157:31–43. doi: 10.1016/j.protis.2005.10.004
34. Xu XG, Yang LH, and Tong DW. Establishment and application of multiplex PCR detection method for Staphylococcus aureus, Streptococcus, Salmonella spp and Escherichia coli. *Chin J Vet Sci.* (2012) 32:534–8, 547. doi: 10.16303/j.cnki.1005-4545.2012.04.010
35. Guan ZP. *Simultaneous analysis of five pathogenic bacteria using multiplex PCR and predictive modelling of staphylococcus aureus growth on pork.* (Doctoral thesis). Nanjing Agricultural University. Nanjing city, China (2014).
36. Liu XD. *Development of multiplex PCR for diction of pathogenic bacteria.* (Master's thesis). Northeast Agricultural University, Harbin city, China (2013).
37. Guan N, Lu H, Fei DL, Wang SQ. Establishment and preliminary application of a multiplex PCR method for detection viruses induced reproductive failure of swine. *Chin J Vet Sci.* (2016) 36:5–1. doi: 10.16303/j.cnki.1005-4545.2016.01.02

11

Molecular Characteristics and Pathogenicity of *Porcine Epidemic Diarrhea Virus* Isolated in Some Areas of China in 2015–2018

Linyang Yu [1†]***, Yanling Liu*** [1†]***, Shuangyun Wang*** [1]***, Leyi Zhang*** [1]***, Pengshuai Liang*** [1]***, Lei Wang*** [1]***, Jianguo Dong*** [2*] ***and Changxu Song*** [1*]

[1] *College of Animal Science & National Engineering Center for Swine Breeding Industry, South China Agriculture University, Guangzhou, China,* [2] *School of Animal Husbandry and Medical Engineering, Xinyang Agriculture and Forestry University, Xinyang, China*

***Correspondence:**
Changxu Song
cxsong2004@163.com;
cxsong@scau.edu.cn
Jianguo Dong
dongjianguo213@163.com

[†] *These authors have contributed equally to this work*

Since 2010, *Porcine epidemic diarrhea virus* (PEDV) has caused severe diarrhea disease in piglets in China, resulting in large economic losses. To understand the genetic characteristics of the PEDV strains that circulated in some provinces of China between 2015 and 2018, 375 samples of feces and small intestine were collected from pigs and tested. One hundred seventy-seven samples tested positive and the PEDV-positive rate was 47.20%. A phylogenetic tree analysis based on the entire S gene showed that these strains clustered into four subgroups, GI-a, GI-b, GII-a, and GII-b, and that the GII-b strains have become dominant in recent years. Compared with previous strains, these strains have multiple variations in the SP and S1-NTD domains and in the neutralizing epitopes of the S protein. We also successfully isolated and identified a new virulent GII-b strain, GDgh16, which is well-adapted to Vero cells and caused a high mortality rate in piglets in challenge experiments. Our study clarifies the genetic characteristics of the prevalent PEDV strains in parts of China, and suggests that the development of effective novel vaccines is both necessary and urgent.

Keywords: PEDV, pig, phylogenetic analysis, S gene, pathogenicity

INTRODUCTION

Porcine epidemic diarrhea virus (PEDV) is the etiological agent of porcine epidemic diarrhea (PED), a severe diarrhea disease in piglets that is characterized by severe watery diarrhea, vomiting, dehydration, weight loss, and nearly 100% mortality (1). PED occurred sporadically around the world in 1990–2009, but in 2010, an acute and severe outbreak of PED in piglets occurred in China and spread to other Asian countries, causing large economic losses (2–8). In April 2013, PED suddenly erupted in the United States, causing many piglets to die, and the mortality rate in suckling piglets reached 100% (9, 10). The disease was shown to be caused by a highly pathogenic PEDV variant. The S genes of the classical CV777 strain and the new strain OH851 have the same insertions and deletions (S-INDEL strains), unlike those of the variant PEDV strains (11, 12).

The genome of PEDV is ∼28 kb in length and contains seven open reading frames (ORFs), which encode four structural proteins and three non-structural proteins (13). S is the largest structural protein, and contains neutralizing antibody epitopes and a specific receptor-binding site for viral entry (14). At present, four antigenic epitopes have been characterized in the S protein, including the CO equivalent (COE) domain (amino acids 499–638), the epitopes SS2 (amino acids 748–755) and SS6 (amino acids 764–771), and epitope 2C10 (1368-GPRLQPY-1374) (15, 16). Because the S protein plays a vital role and the S gene is extensively mutated, it is often used as the target gene in the analysis of viral genetic variation. Based on whether the S gene contains the INDEL sequence or not, PEDV strains can be classified into genogroup II (GII) or genogroup I (GI), respectively. GI is further divided into two subgroups (GI-a, GI-b) according to INDEL sequence differences. At present, most isolates recovered in China belong to GII (17). A new mutation in the S gene of PEDV has recently been reported (18). Different GI-b strains have also been reported in different areas of China (19, 20). Studies have shown that PEDV strains of different genotypes can coexist, in one province in particular. These findings indicate that PEDV has continued to spread widely to most areas of China and has caused serious economic losses in the pig industry, reflecting the complex evolution of the virus. Therefore, extensive research into the evolutionary pathogenic mechanism of these strains in China is essential.

To control the spread of PEDV, a classical-CV777-derived vaccine has been widely used in many areas of China. However, it does not provide adequate protection against PEDV invasion (6, 21). In contrast, the wide-scale use of vaccines has increased the environmental stress upon the virus, causing PEDV to mutate to escape its host's immune defenses. To further and fully understand the prevalence and evolution of PEDV in southern China, diarrhea samples were collected from piglets in this study, and the variation of the S genes of the PEDV-positive samples were analyzed with sequence alignment and a phylogenetic tree.

MATERIALS AND METHODS

Sample Collection

A total of 375 diarrheic samples from the small intestine tissues or feces were collected from suckling piglets on pig farms in eight provinces of China (Fujian, Guangdong, Guangxi, Guizhou, Jiangxi, Shandong, Hubei, Hu'nan, and Hainan) between June 2015 and October 2018. The piglets suffered severe watery diarrhea and dehydration. The diarrheic feces were resuspended in 1 mL of phosphate-buffered saline (PBS) in 1.5 mL Eppendorf tubes. After centrifugation at 10,000 × g for 5 min, 200 μL of each supernatant was transferred to a new tube for RNA extraction and virus isolation.

RNA Extraction and Sequencing

The total RNA from the collected supernatants was extracted with TRIzol Reagent (TaKaRa), according to the manufacturer's instructions. The extracted RNA was subjected to reverse transcription (RT–PCR) with three pairs of newly designed primers to amplify and detect the PEDV S gene (**Table 1**). The three overlapping PCR products were identified with 1.5% agarose gel electrophoresis. The positive PCR products were sequenced by Sangon Biological Engineering Co. Ltd, and the entire sequence of the S gene was determined with the DNAStar software. The complete S gene sequences were submitted to GenBank, under the accession numbers shown in **Table 2**.

TABLE 1 | Primers used for PEDV complete S gene amplification.

Primer name	Nucleotide sequence, 5′-3′	Size(bp)
PEDV S1-F	GGTAAGTTGCTAGTGCGTA	1,630
PEDV S1-R	CACAGAAAGAACTAAACCC	
PEDV S2-F	CTGCCATTCAGCGTATTCTTT	1,768
PEDV S2-R	CTGCGAGTTAACAACCTCTTGA	
PEDV S3-F	GTGCGCAGTATTACTCTGGT	1,559
PEDV S3-R	AAGAAGACGCTTTAAACAGTG	

S Gene Sequence Analysis

The complete genome sequences of reference strains available in GenBank were downloaded and used in a phylogenetic analysis (**Table 3**). A phylogenetic tree was constructed from all the S genes of the representative strains and isolates, using the neighbor joining method with 1,000 bootstrap replicates, with the Molecular Evolutionary Genetics Analysis (MEGA, version 6.0) software (22).

Virus Isolation

Vero cells grown in a 24-well cell culture plate were infected with the previously prepared supernatants and maintained in Dulbecco's modified Eagle's medium (Thermo Scientific) containing 7 μg/mL trypsin without EDTA (Thermo Scientific). The cells were monitored daily for a cytopathic effect (CPE). When the CPE appeared in 70% of the cells, the cells were fixed with anhydrous ethanol. An immunofluorescence assay (IFA) was then performed with an anti-N protein monoclonal antibody (mAb; cat. # PEDV12-F, Alpha Diagnostic International Inc., USA) diluted 1:1,000 and an Alexa-Fluor®-488-conjugated Affinipure goat anti-mouse IgG(H+L) secondary antibody (SA00013-1; Proteintech, USA) diluted 1:400.

Titer Determination for the Viral Proliferation Curve

Vero cells cultured in a 24-well cell culture plate were infected with PEDV at a multiplicity of infection (MOI) of 0.01. The cells and supernatants were collected at 12, 24, 36, 48, 60, 72, and 96 h post-infection (hpi). The cells were then frozen and thawed three times. After centrifugation at 10,000 × g for 5 min at 4°C, the supernatants were collected and the median tissue culture infective dose ($TCID_{50}$) was determined with a microtitration infection assay.

Piglet Challenge Experiment

To determine the virulence of the third-generation isolated strain GDgh16, six healthy 4-day-old colostrum-deprived suckling piglets were artificially fed bovine milk from birth. The colostrum-deprived piglets were randomly divided into two groups, with three piglets in each group. One group was challenged orally with 0.5 mL of PEDV at $10^{5.0}$ $TCID_{50}$/mL. The other group received cell-culture medium. Duplicate samples of small intestine were collected in from all piglets, which had been euthanized at 48 h postchallenge. One of the duplicate samples was crushed in a grinder with 2 mL of PBS. The crushed intestine

TABLE 2 | Information of S genes of 62 PEDV isolates.

No.	Designation	Area	Region	Year	S (bp)	Accession no
1	FJly15	Longyan	Fujian	2015	4161	MN368663
2	FJqz15	Quanzhou	Fujian	2015	4161	MN368664
3	FJzz15	Zhangzhou	Fujian	2015	4161	MN368665
4	GDgz15-1	Guangzhou	Guangdong	2015	4161	MN368666
5	GDgz15-2	Guangzhou	Guangdong	2015	4161	MN368667
6	GDhy15	Heyuan	Guangdong	2015	4161	MN368668
7	GDhz15	Huizhou	Guangdong	2015	4161	MN368669
8	GDjm15	Jiangmen	Guangdong	2015	4161	MN368670
9	GDmm15	Maoming	Guangdong	2015	4161	MN368671
10	GDsg15-1	Shaoguan	Guangdong	2015	4161	MN368672
11	GDsg15-2	Shaoguan	Guangdong	2015	4161	MN368673
12	GDsg15-3	Shaoguan	Guangdong	2015	4161	MN368674
13	GDzq15-1	Zhaoqing	Guangdong	2015	4161	MN368675
14	GDzq15-2	Zhaoqing	Guangdong	2015	4161	MN368676
15	GXnn15	Nanning	Guangxi	2015	4161	MN368678
16	GZgy15	Guiyang	Guizhou	2015	4161	MN368679
17	HBhg15	Huanggang	Hubei	2015	4161	MN368680
18	JXgz15	Ganzhou	Jiangxi	2015	4161	MN368681
19	JXyc15	Yichun	Jiangxi	2015	4161	MN368662
20	FJqz16	Quanzhou	Fujian	2016	4158	MN368683
21	GDfs16	Foshan	Guangdong	2016	4158	MN368684
22	GDhy16	Heyuan	Guangdong	2016	4161	MN368685
23	GDhz16	Huizhou	Guangdong	2016	4161	MN368686
24	GDjm16-1	Jiangmen	Guangdong	2016	4158	MN368687
25	GDjm16-2	Jiangmen	Guangdong	2016	4161	MN368688
26	GDjx16	Jiexi	Guangdong	2016	4158	MN368689
27	GDsg16-1	Shaoguan	Guangdong	2016	4158	MN368690
28	GDsg16-2	Shaoguan	Guangdong	2016	4158	MN368691
29	GDyj16	Ynagjiang	Guangdong	2016	4161	MN368692
30	GDgh16	Guanghui	Guangdong	2016	4158	MG983755
31	GDdg17	Dongguan	Guangdong	2016	4158	MN368693
32	FJfz17-1	Fuzhou	Fujian	2017	4161	MN368695
33	FJfz17-2	Fuzhou	Fujian	2017	4161	MN368696
34	FJqz17-1	Quanzhou	Fujian	2017	4161	MN368697
35	FJqz17-2	Quanzhou	Fujian	2017	4158	MN368698
36	GDhy17	Heyuan	Guangdong	2017	4158	MN368699
37	GDhz17	Huizhou	Guangdong	2017	4158	MN368700
38	GDjm17-1	Jiangmen	Guangdong	2017	4152	MN368701
39	GDjm17-2	Jiangmen	Guangdong	2017	4158	MN368702
40	GDjm17-3	Jiangmen	Guangdong	2017	4161	MN368703
41	GDmm17-1	Maoming	Guangdong	2017	4158	MN368704
42	GDmm17-2	Maoming	Guangdong	2017	4158	MN368705
43	GDsg17	Shaoguan	Guangdong	2017	4161	MN368706
44	HNcz17	Chenzhou	Hunan	2017	4161	MN368707
45	JXnc17	Nanchang	Jiangxi	2017	4158	MN368708
46	FJfz18-1	Fuzhou	Fujian	2018	4161	MN368710
47	FJfz18-2	Fuzhou	Fujian	2018	4158	MN368711
48	FJqz18	Quanzhou	Fujian	2018	4158	MN368712
49	GDhy18-1	Heyuan	Guangdong	2018	4158	MN368713
50	GDhy18-2	Heyuan	Guangdong	2018	4158	MN368714
51	GDhy18-3	Heyuan	Guangdong	2018	4158	MN368715

(Continued)

TABLE 2 | Continued

No.	Designation	Area	Region	Year	S (bp)	Accession no
52	GDhz18	Huizhou	Guangdong	2018	4158	MN368716
53	GDjm18-1	Jiangmen	Guangdong	2018	4158	MN368717
54	GDjm18-2	Jiangmen	Guangdong	2018	4149	MN368718
55	GDmm18-1	Maoming	Guangdong	2018	4158	MN368719
56	GDmm18-2	Maoming	Guangdong	2018	4158	MN368720
57	GDsg18-1	Shaoguan	Guangdong	2018	4158	MN368721
58	GDsg18-2	Shaoguan	Guangdong	2018	4158	MN368722
59	GDst18	Shantou	Guangdong	2018	4158	MN368723
60	GDzj18-1	Zhanjiang	Guangdong	2018	4155	MN368724
61	GDzj18-2	Zhanjiang	Guangdong	2018	4161	MN368725
62	SDbz18	Binzhou	Shandong	2018	4158	MN368709

was then centrifuged at 10,000 × g for 10 min at 4°C. The supernatant was collected and their RNA extracted. The PEDV N gene copies in the small intestine were detected with real-time quantitative PCR (qPCR). RT–qPCR was performed with the PowerUp™ SYBR® Green Master Mix (A25742; Thermo Fisher) in a 20 μL reaction containing 1 ng of cDNA as the template, in a CFX96 thermal cycler, under the following cycling conditions: 50°C for 2 min; 95°C for 2 min; and 40 cycles of 95°C for 15 s, 60°C for 15 s, and 72°C for 60 s. The other sample was stained with anti-N protein mAb (diluted 1:1,000) for immunohistochemical (IHC) examination.

Statistical Analysis

The numerical data are expressed as means ± standard deviations (SD), and all data were analyzed with the GraphPad Prism software (version 5.02 for Windows; GraphPad Software Inc.).

RESULTS

PEDV Detection and Phylogenetic Analysis Based on the S Gene

As shown in **Table 4**, of the 375 feces and small -intestine samples tested between 2015 and 2018, 177 were positive for PEDV (47.20%). The positivity rates in 2015, 2016, 2017, and 2018 were 48.57% (34 positive samples and 70 test samples), 67.14%% (47 positive samples and 70 test samples), 53.33% (32 positive samples and 60 test samples), and 36.57% (64 positive samples and 175 test samples), respectively. The positive rate was highest in 2016 and lowest in 2018. A sequence alignment showed that these strains shared 92.9–100% nucleotide homology and 91–100% amino acid identity. They also shared 93.1–96.8% nucleotide homology and 91.5–96.8% amino acid identity with reference strain CV777, and 93.8–99% nucleotide homology and 92.5–98.9% amino acid identity with the reference strains isolated from China.

Sixty-two S genes from the test strains and representative strains downloaded from GenBank were analyzed with a phylogenetic tree. As shown in **Figure 1**, the phylogenetic analysis divided these strains into two groups, GI and GII, based on whether the S gene contained the S-INDEL (23). GI included the classical strains (CV777 and SM98) and some isolates from China, the USA, and Japan collected after 2010. Therefore, GI was further divided into three subgroups: GI-a, GI-b. GI-a contained classical S-INDEL strains. GI-b contained a new S-INDEL strain. GII contained non-S-INDEL strains and was also divided into two subgroups, GII-a and GII-b, which consisted of a number of extremely virulent strains from all over the world, isolated since 2010. The strains isolated in the present study belonged to GI-a, GI-b, GII-a, and GII-b. GDjm18-2, was categorized as subtype GI-a, which also included the classical vaccine strains CV777-attenuated and JS2008. GDjm17-1 was categorized in GI-b cluster. The other strains identified in the present study formed eight clusters. Of these strains, 25 isolates from Guangdong, three isolates from Fujian, and one isolate from Jiangxi formed three clusters and belonged to GII-b, with strong similarity to GD-A and CH-GXNN-2012. The other 34 isolates formed five clusters and belonged to GII-a. Among these 34 strains, JXyc15 was closely related to the C4 cluster (North American strains), whereas the other strains showed closer identity to CH-ZMDZ-11, CH-HNAY-2015, and CH-HNCDE-2016L. As shown in **Table 5**, all the strains isolated in 2015 belonged to GII-a (100%). In 2016 and 2017, 46.15% and 43.75% of the isolated strains belonged to GII-a, respectively. Compared with GII-a, the rate slightly increased, and in 2016 and 2017, 53.84 and 50% of the isolated strains belonged to GII-b, respectively. However, in 2018, 72.22% of the isolated strains belonged to GII-b, which was much higher than the proportion that belonged to GII-a in 2017 (22.22%). The comparison result show: Variation of PEDV S gene is continuously occurring and GII-b strains may be the dominant strains in China in the future.

Amino Acid Sequence Analysis of Neutralizing Epitopes in the S Protein

Neutralizing antibodies play an important role in the prevention and control of viral infections. Therefore, it is important to identify and analyze the amino acid sequences of the neutralizing epitopes in viral proteins. To analyze the genetic characteristics of the South China PEDV strains, the deduced amino acid sequences of the S proteins detected in our study were aligned and compared with those of representative

TABLE 3 | Information of the representative strains.

Virus strain	Countries	Year	Accession no.	Virus strain	Countries	Year	Accession no.
CV777	Belgium	2001	AF353511	83P-5	Japan	2013	AB548618
JS-2004-2	China	2004	AY653204	OKN-1-JPN-2013	Japan	2013	LC063836
DX-S	China	2007	EU031893	CH-LXC-2014	China	2014	KT388418
LZC	China	2007	EF185992	PEDV-14	China	2014	KM609207
DR13/virulent	Korea	2007	DQ862099	CH-HNQX-3-14	China	2014	KR095279
JS2008	China	2008	KC109141	CH-HNYF-14	China	2014	KP890336
BJ-2011-1	China	2011	JN825712	CH-GD-22-2014	China	2014	KP870132
CH-JLCC-2011	China	2011	JQ638920	USA-Minnesota271-2014	USA	2014	KR265813
CH-S	China	2011	JN547228	MEX-124-2014	USA	2014	KJ645700
CH-FJND-1-2011	China	2011	JN543367	OH851	USA	2014	KJ399978
SM98	Korea	2011	GU937797	USA-Ohio126-2014	USA	2014	KJ645702
CH-GXNN-2012	China	2012	JX018179	AOM-2-JPN-2014	Japan	2014	LC063837
GD-A	China	2012	JX112709	AOM-3-JPN-2014	Japan	2014	LC063833
GD-B	China	2012	JX088695	KCH-2-JPN-2014	Japan	2014	LC063845
CH-SDDZ-2012	China	2012	KU133240	KPEDV-9	Korea	2014	KF898124
AH2012	China	2012	KC210145	KNU-1310	Korea	2014	KJ451045
JS-HZ2012	China	2012	KC210147	KNU-1401	Korea	2014	KJ451047
CH-ZJCX-1-2012	China	2012	KF840537	KNU-1406-1	Korea	2014	KM403155
CH9-FJ	China	2012	JQ979287	L00721-GER-2014	Germany	2014	LM645057
CV777/attenuated	China	2012	JN599150	FR-001-2014	France	2014	KR011756
CH7	China	2012	JQ239435	PEDV-WS	China	2015	KM609213
CH-HBXX2-11	China	2013	JX501319	CH-XBC-01-2015	China	2015	KR296677
CH-ZMDZY-11	China	2013	KC196276	CH-YGC-01-2015	China	2015	KR296678
CH-SBC-03-2013	China	2013	KC787542	CH-ZWBZa-01-2015	China	2015	KR296680
CH-YNKM-8-2013	China	2013	KF761675	CH-HNAY-2015	China	2015	KR809885
CH-JX-1-2013	China	2013	KF760557	CH-JPYC-02-2015	China	2015	JN547228
CH-HBQX-10	China	2013	JX501318	TW-Pingtung-63	China	2015	KP276250
USA-Indiana-17846-2013	USA	2013	KF452323	CBR2	Thailand	2015	KR610994
USA-Iowa-16465-2013	USA	2013	KF452322	HUA-PED47	Korea	2015	KP455314
USA-Minnesota90-2013	USA	2013	KJ645682	HUA-PED45	Korea	2015	KP455313
MN	USA	2013	KF468752	HUA-PED67	Korea	2015	KP455319
IA1	USA	2013	KF468753	15V010-BEL-2015	Belgium	2015	KR003452
IA2	USA	2013	KF468754	CH-HNCD-2016	China	2016	MF152600
NPL-PEDV-2013	USA	2013	KJ778615	HUA-14PED96	Korea	2016	KT941120
USA-Colorado-2013	USA	2013	KF272920	14JM-226	Japan	2018	KY619763
NK	Japan	2013	AB548623	14JM-126	Japan	2018	KY619740
MK	Japan	2013	AB548624	13JM-291	Japan	2018	KY619768

PEDV strains, including strains from GI-a (CV777 and DR13 virulent), GI-b (OH851 and CH-ZWZBa-01-2015), GII-a (CH-HNQX-3-14, CH-HNAY-2015, CH-ZMDZY-11), and GII-b (CH-GXNN-2012, CD-A). As shown in **Figure 2**, compared with strain CV777, the GI-a strain GDjm18-2 had three amino acid substitutions in the COE domain and one amino acid substitution in epitope SS6. The GII-a strains had amino acid substitutions at 35 positions in the COE domain, at two positions in epitope SS2, and at five positions in epitope SS6. Many new amino acid substitutions were detected in the COE regions of the GII-a strains, at positions 502 (S→ P), 507 (P→ M), 510 (N→ S), 516 (N→ D), 522 (S→ A), 527 (S→ G), 533 (A→ V), 535 (D→ E), 547 (D→ E), 559 (V→ I or A), 562 (S→ D), 567 (S→ A), 568 (K→ T or N), 570 (Q→ H), 571 (D→ N or Y), 575 (P→ L), 580 (S→ A), 588 (S→ G), 594 (T→ R or C), 608 (Y→ H), 613 (S→ I or G), 614 (G→ V), 626 (K→ E or S), and 637 (L→ F or S). Epitope 2C10 was conserved in all GII-a strains. Among the GII-a strains, GDhz16 had four continuous amino acid mutations in epitope SS6, which differed from the epitope sequence in the other strains and the reference strains. Compared with strain CV777, the GII-b strains had amino acid substitutions at 17 positions in the COE domain, and amino acid substitutions at one position in three epitopes (SS2, SS6, and 2C10). As well as the common amino acid mutations that were similar to those in the GII-b reference strains, there were novel amino acid substitutions at

TABLE 4 | The PEDV positive prevalence of different of tested strains in our study.

Year	Province	Positive samples	Total samples	Positive prevalence
2015	Fujian	3	7	42.86%
	Guangdong	26	58	44.83%
	Guangxi	1	1	100%
	Guizhou	1	1	100%
	Hubei	1	1	100%
	Jiangxi	2	2	100%
Total		34	70	48.57%
2016	Fujian	1	1	100%
	Guangdong	45	61	73.77%
	Hunan	1	1	100%
	Guangxi	0	3	0
	Jiangxi	0	4	0
Total		47	70	67.14%
2017	Fujian	4	7	57.14%
	Guangdong	18	34	52.94%
	Hu'nan	3	4	75%
	Guangxi	6	12	50%
	Jiangxi	1	3	33.33%
Total		32	60	53.33%
2018	Fujian	3	3	100%
	Guangdong	52	144	36.11%
	Guangxi	1	10	10%
	Jiangxi	3	10	30%
	Shandong	1	2	50%
	Hu'nan	0	2	0
	Hainan	4	4	100%
Total		64	175	36.57%
All total		177	375	47.20%

TABLE 5 | The PEDV positive prevalence of different groups of tested strains in our study.

Group	2015	2016	2017	2018
GI-a	0	0	0	5.56%
GI-b	0	0	6.25%	0
GII-a	100%	46.15%	43.75%	22.22%
GII-b	0	53.84%	50%	72.22%

eight positions in the COE region: 504 (V→ L), 510 (N→ D), 535 (D→ H), 542 (S→ H), 567 (S→ Y), 614 (G→ V), 626 (K→ T), and 637 (L→ V). These amino acid sequences demonstrate that the neutralizing epitopes of the PEDV S protein are constantly mutating. This phenomenon increases the difficulty of preventing and controlling PEDV infections because existing vaccines cannot effectively protect against PEDV. However, these finding may facilitate the development of effective novel vaccines in the future.

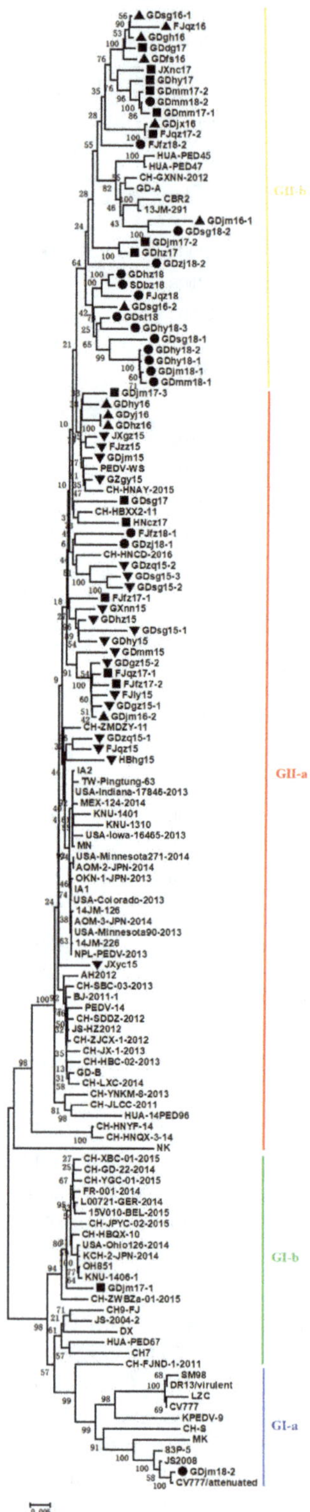

FIGURE 1 | Phylogenetic tree based on the complete S genes of 62 Chinese PEDV strains identified in this study and other global reference strains. The tree was constructed with the neighbor-joining method in the MEGA V.6.0 program. The Chinese PEDV strains isolated in this study are marked with black triangles, black squares, or solid circles.

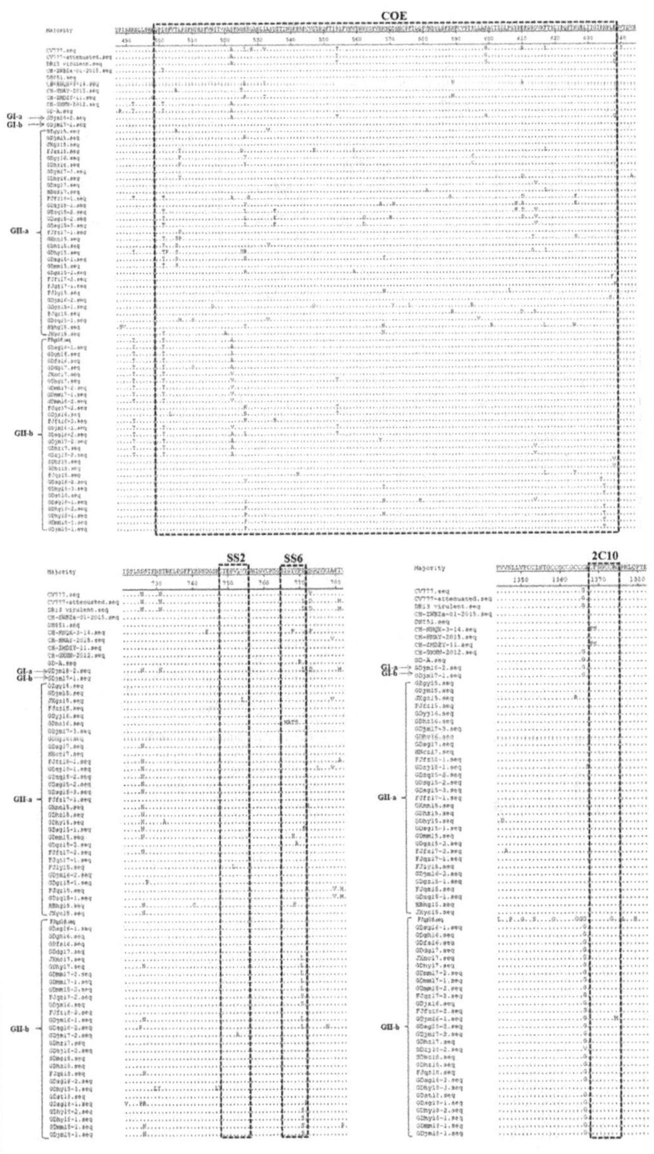

FIGURE 2 | Amino acid sequence analysis of the neutralizing epitopes of the S protein. Amino acid sequence alignment of the neutralizing epitopes of the S proteins of the isolated strains and reference strains, constructed with the Clustal W method.

Numbers of Mutated Amino Acid in Different Domains of the S Protein

To further analyze the amino acid mutations in the different domains of the S protein in these isolates, the different domains of the S protein were aligned with those of CV777, and the average number of amino acid mutations present in each year was calculated. The S protein can be divided into the S1 protein and the S2 protein. The S1 protein contains four domains: SP (amino acids 1–18), S1-NTD (amino acids 19–233), COE and RBD (amino acids 501–629), whereas the S2 protein contains five domains: SS6 (amino acids 764–771), HR1 (amino acids 978–1117), HR2 (amino acids 1274–1313), TM (amino acids 1324–1346), and 2C10 (amino acids 1368–1374). Previous data have indicated that 2C10 is conserved, so we did not analyze the 2C10 domain. As shown in **Figure 3**, in these strains, the S1 sequence had more amino acid mutations than the S2 sequence. From 2015 to 2018, the number of mutated amino acids in S1 remained at a high level, whereas that in S2 decreased. Furthermore, the numbers of mutated amino acids in SP (amino acids 1–18) and S1-NTD (amino acids 19–233) increased slightly, whereas the numbers of mutated amino acids in the COE and RBD domains decreased. SS6, HR1, HR2, and TM in the S2 protein did not change obviously from 2015 to 2018.

Pathogenicity of GDgh16

Because the samples of GDgh16 came from a scale pig farm that had experienced high mortality, and it displayed a high viral titer in Vero cells, we investigated its pathogenicity *in vivo*. As shown in **Figure 4A**, PEDV-infected cells showed a characteristic green color, indicating that PEDV was isolated successfully. The viral proliferation curve indicated that the titer of strain GDgh16 increased to $10^{6.33}$ $TCID_{50}$/mL at 36 hpi but decreased to $10^{4.99}$ $TCID_{50}$/mL at 96 hpi (**Figure 4B**). Six piglets were divided into two groups; one group was challenged orally with GDgh16 and the other group was inoculated with cell culture medium. All the challenged piglets showed classical clinical signs, including vomiting, watery diarrhea, and dehydration, at 16 hpi. The challenged piglets began to die at 24 hpi, and all had died by 48 hpi (**Figure 5A**). The control pigs remained healthy, with no detectable PEDV shedding. The control piglets were euthanized and necropsy was performed on all the piglets. The viral copy numbers in different parts of the intestine were determined with RT–qPCR. The duodenum, jejunum, ileum, cecum, and colon had higher viral copy numbers than the rectum (**Figure 5B**). The duodenums, jejunums, and ileums of the piglets were subjected to an IHC assay. As shown in **Figure 5C**, the tissues from the piglets in the challenged group showed remarkable levels of viral antigens compared to those in the control group. The results of GDgh16 challenge test indicate that the variant strains are a large threat to the pig industry and that the control of PEDV spread has become a critical issue.

DISCUSSION

PEDV has become an important diarrhea virus, causing extensive damage to pig farms worldwide. Because there is no effective vaccine against the emerging prevalent strains in China, the variant PEDV strains occur frequently on many farms in different areas (24). Because there are extensive viral variants and the protection afforded by commercial vaccines is limited, it is necessary to fully understand the genetic variations and epidemiology of PEDV to facilitate the development of next-generation vaccines.

In the present study, the genetic variations in PEDV in parts of China in 2015–2018 were analyzed.

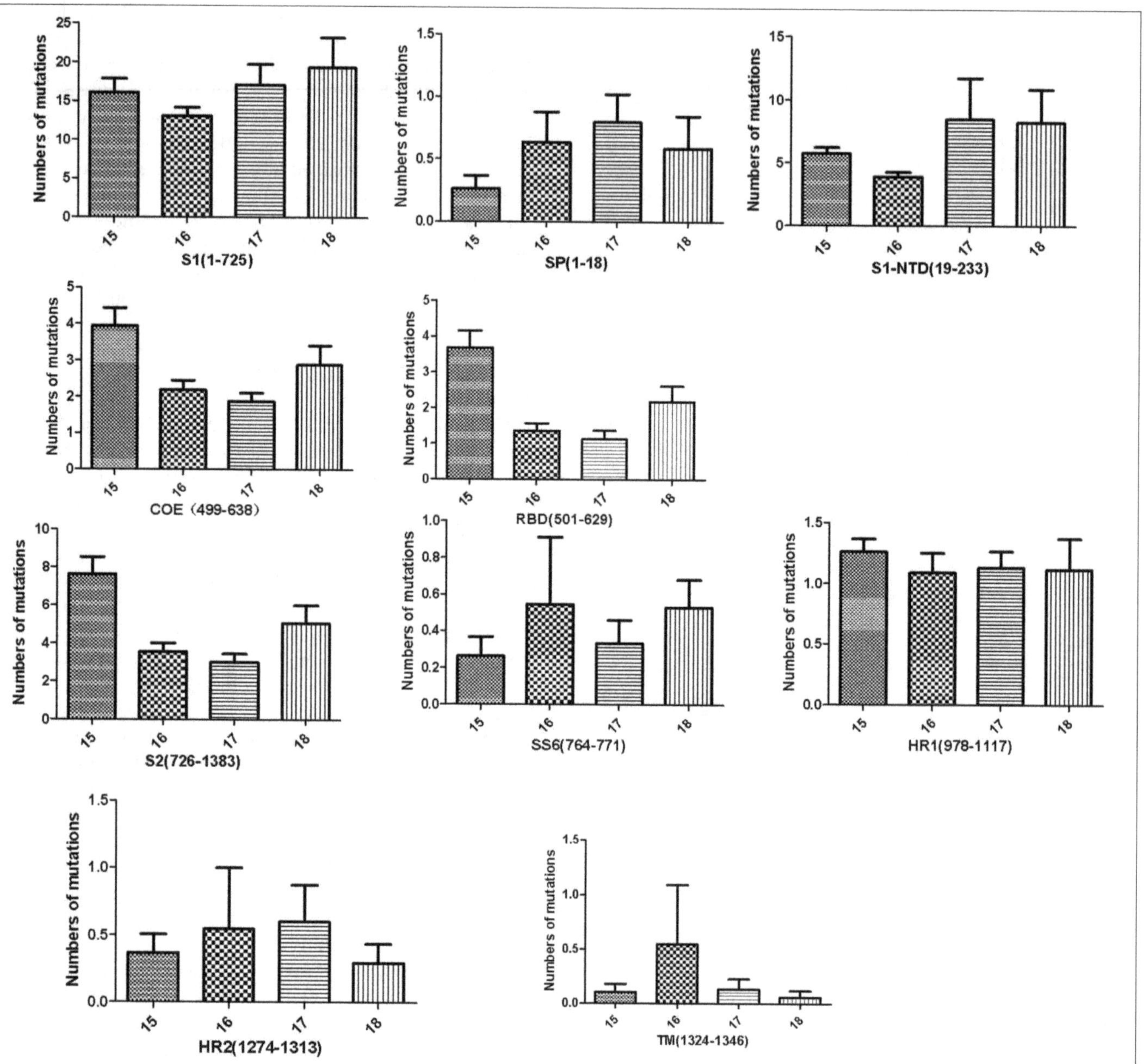

FIGURE 3 | Numbers of amino acid mutations in different domains of the S protein, including the S1 subunit (residues 1–725), S2 subunit (residues 726–1383), signal peptide (SP, residues 1–18), N-terminal domain of S1 (S1-NTD, residues 19–233), the neutralizing epitopes (COE, residues 499–638; SS2, residues 748–755; SS6, residues 764–771; 2C10, residues 1368–1374), two heptad repeat regions (HR1, residues 978–1117, and HR2, residues 1274–1313), and the transmembrane domain (TM, residues 1324–1346).

The S gene encodes the largest structural protein of PEDV and stimulates the host body to produce neutralizing antibodies against the virus. Because its variants are extensive, the S gene is commonly used as the target gene in studies of the genomic characteristics of PEDV (25). A phylogenetic analysis showed that strains from four subgroups of PEDV were present from 2015 to 2018, and that GII-a and GII-b were the two most prevalent subgroups in China at that time. From 2015 to 2018, eight strains belonging to four subgroups (GI-a, GI-b, GII-a, and GII-b) were epidemic in Jiangmen (Guangdong), which suggests that PEDV had mutated widely and the PEDV epidemic was becoming more complex. These results are consistent with those of Wen et al. (26). In 2015, all the isolated strains belonged to GII-a, whereas in 2018, 72.22% of strains belonged to GII-b, and only 22.22% of strains belonged to GII-a. Interestingly, unlike GII-a, which includes strains from other countries, such as America, South Korea, and Japan, the GII-b subgroup only contains Chinese-isolated

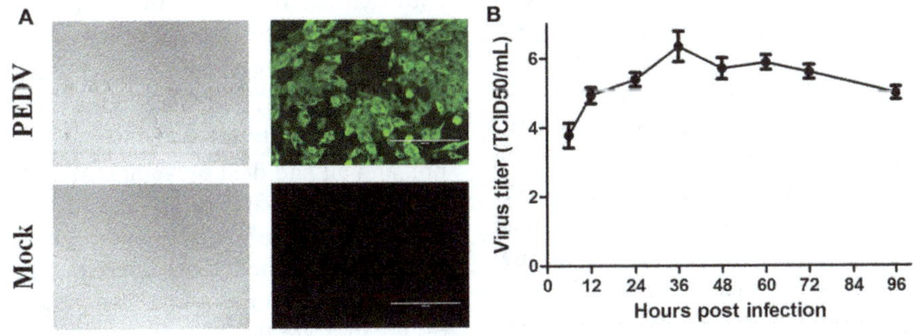

FIGURE 4 | Detection and proliferation curve of PEDV strain GDgh16. **(A)** Identification of GDgh16 in Vero cells. CPE of GDgh16 was observed at 24 hpi under white light and was tested with IFA using a monoclonal antibody directed against the PEDV N protein. **(B)** Proliferation curve of PEDV strain GDgh16. Vero cells were infected with GDgh16 at a multiplicity of infection of 0.01. Cells and culture solution were collected at 6, 12, 24, 36, 48, 60, and 72 hpi, frozen, thawed, and centrifuged. The supernatant was collected and $TCID_{50}$ determined.

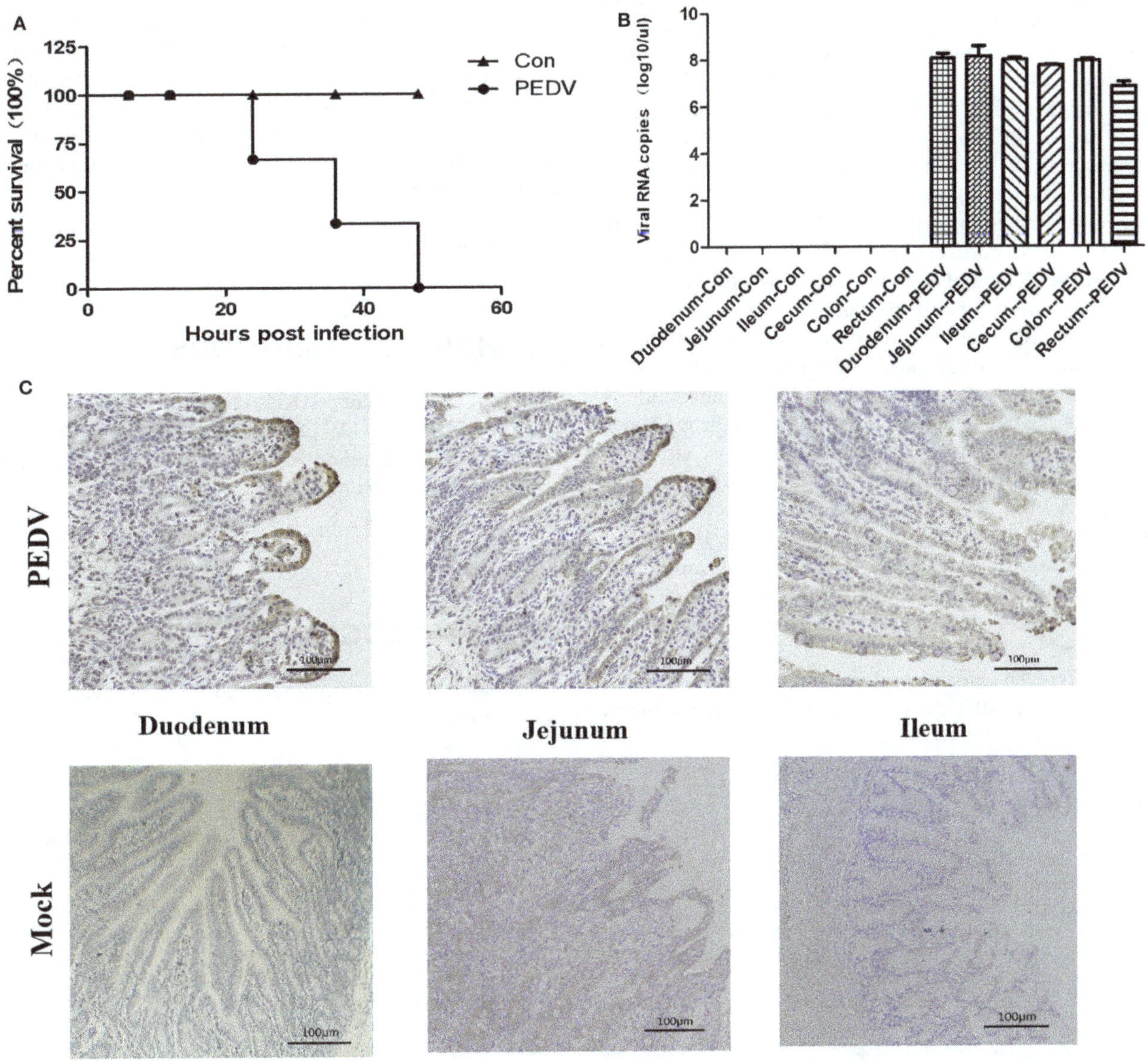

FIGURE 5 | Pathogenicity analysis of GDgh16. **(A)** Survival rate of piglets in each group. **(B)** Quantification of the viral loads in different parts of the intestine. Different parts of the intestine were isolated and the viral load was quantified with TaqMan real-time RT-PCR targeting the PEDV N gene. **(C)** Immunohistochemical analysis of intestines. Duodenum, jejunum, and ileum tissues from each group were stained with monoclonal antibody directed against PEDV N protein (diluted 1:100).

strains. Combined with previous studies, these results suggest that GII-b strains may be the dominant strains in China in the future (27, 28).

The S protein is highly variable, and many studies have shown that amino acid changes in the S protein can affect the virulence and pathogenicity of PEDV. Our study has shown that the numbers of amino acid mutations in the SP1 and S1-NTD domains of PEDV increased in 2017 and 2018. It had been suggested that S1-NTD is a vital domain related to viral virulence (29, 30) and that conformational changes in S1-NTD are related to the high pathogenicity of PEDV strain FJzz1 (18, 27). Increasing numbers of more-virulent PEDV strains have recently emerged (18, 27, 31). Whether the mutations identified in this study alter the major conformation and thus the pathogenicity of these strains will be investigated further in the future. Our data show that the PEDV positivity rate in the provinces tested increased from 2015 to 2016, but decreased from 2016 to 2018, which might be attributable to improvements in disease prevention and control strategies. Many pig farms use the "feed-back" mode to ensure sow immunity to PEDV and to protect piglets against PEDV infection. This is an effective measure to prevent PED, but there is also a risk of virus dispersal, which is responsible for the many GI-b strains reported to date (19, 20, 32–34).

Four neutralizing epitopes of the PEDV S protein have been determined: the COE domain (499–638), epitope SS2 (748–755), epitope SS6 (764–771), and epitope 2C10 (1368–1374) (15, 16). In the present study, we detected amino acid changes at 35 positions in the COE domain. Moreover, one strain, GDhz16, had four continuous amino acid mutations in epitope SS6. Epitopes SS2 and 2C10 also contained amino acid substitutions. The antigenicity, pathogenicity, and neutralization properties of isolated strains are altered by such mutations, especially some insertions and deletions in the S protein (35, 36). Therefore, the vaccine derived from prototype strain CV777 protects against the disease induced by classical strains but not the disease caused by variant strains (24, 37). Whether these amino acid changes affect the antigenicity and neutralization properties of the four neutralizing epitopes warrants investigation in future studies.

Based on previous epidemiological and clinical observations of field strains since 2010, the emerging GII strains are highly pathogenic (38). To investigate the pathogenicity of the isolated variant strains, three piglets were infected orally with GDgh16. The piglets in the infected group began to show clinical signs of diarrhea at 12 h, and developed the typical symptoms of PED at 16 h. Morbidity reached 100%. The piglets began to die at 24 hpi, and all had died by 48 hpi. Moreover, their small intestines contained high viral copies and many viral antigens, indicating that GDgh16 was a highly pathogenic strain. Other researchers have demonstrated that different types of pigs infected with variant PEDV strains shared consistent outcomes (39–42). These results indicate that the variant strains are a large threat to the pig industry, and that the control of PEDV spread has become a critical issue.

In conclusion, the PEDV strains circulating in parts of China between 2015 and 2018 clustered into four subgroups: GI-a, GI-b, GII-a, and GII-b. The GII-b strains became dominant in 2018. Compared with previous strains, these strains displayed multiple variations in the SP and S1-NTD domains and the neutralizing epitopes of the S protein. We successfully isolated and identified a new virulent GII-b strain, GDgh16, which is well-adapted to Vero cells and causes a high mortality rate in piglets. Our study provides insight into the genetic characteristics of the prevalent PEDV strains in parts of China, and suggests that the development of effective novel vaccines is both necessary and urgent.

AUTHOR CONTRIBUTIONS

LY, YL, JD, and CS conceived and designed the experiments. LY, YL, SW, LZ, PL, and LW performed the experiments. LY, JD, and CS analyzed the data and wrote the paper. All authors read and approved the final manuscript.

ACKNOWLEDGMENTS

This manuscript has been released as a pre-print at Research Square (43).

REFERENCES

1. Pensaert MB, de Bouck P. A new coronavirus-like particle associated with diarrhea in swine. *Arch Virol.* (1978) 58:243–7. doi: 10.1007/bf01317606
2. Boniotti MB, Papetti A, Lavazza A, Alborali G, Sozzi E, Chiapponi C, et al. Porcine epidemic diarrhea virus and discovery of a recombinant swine enteric coronavirus, Italy. *Emerg Infect Dis.* (2016) 22:83–7. doi: 10.3201/eid2201.150544
3. Kim YK, Cho YY, An BH, Lim SI, Lim JA, Cho IS, et al. Molecular characterization of the spike and ORF3 genes of porcine epidemic diarrhea virus in the Philippines. *Arch Virol.* (2016) 161:1323–8. doi: 10.1007/s00705-016-2758-2
4. Pasick J, Berhane Y, Ojkic D, Maxie G, Embury-Hyatt C, Swekla K, et al. Investigation into the role of potentially contaminated feed as a source of the first-detected outbreaks of porcine epidemic diarrhea in Canada. *Transbound Emerg Dis.* (2014) 61:397–410. doi: 10.1111/tbed.12269
5. Steinrigl A, Fernandez SR, Stoiber F, Pikalo J, Sattler T, Schmoll F. First detection, clinical presentation and phylogenetic characterization of Porcine epidemic diarrhea virus in Austria. *Bmc Vet Res.* (2015) 11:310. doi: 10.1186/s12917-015-0624-1
6. Sun RQ, Cai RJ, Chen YQ, Liang PS, Chen DK, Song CX. Outbreak of porcine epidemic diarrhea in suckling piglets, China. *Emerg Infect Dis.* (2012) 18:161–3. doi: 10.3201/eid1801.111259
7. Tian Y, Yu Z, Cheng K, Liu Y, Huang J, Xin Y, et al. Molecular characterization and phylogenetic analysis of new variants of the porcine epidemic diarrhea virus in Gansu, China in 2012. *Viruses.* (2013) 5:1991–2004. doi: 10.3390/v5081991
8. Sung MH, Deng MC, Chung YH, Huang YL, Chang CY, Lan YC, et al. Evolutionary characterization of the emerging porcine epidemic diarrhea virus worldwide and 2014 epidemic in Taiwan. *Infect Genet Evol.* (2015) 36:108–15. doi: 10.1016/j.meegid.2015.09.011
9. Stevenson GW, Hoang H, Schwartz KJ, Burrough ER, Sun D, Madson D,

et al. Emergence of Porcine epidemic diarrhea virus in the United States: clinical signs, lesions, and viral genomic sequences. *J Vet Diagn Invest.* (2013) 25:649–54. doi: 10.1177/1040638713501675

10. Jung K, Saif LJ. Porcine epidemic diarrhea virus infection: etiology, epidemiology, pathogenesis and immunoprophylaxis. *Vet J.* (2015) 204:134–43. doi: 10.1016/j.tvjl.2015.02.017
11. Mesquita JR, Hakze-van DHR, Almeida A, Lourenco M, van der Poel WH, Nascimento MS. Outbreak of porcine epidemic diarrhea virus in Portugal, 2015. *Transbound Emerg Dis.* (2015) 62:586–8. doi: 10.1111/tbed.12409
12. Wang L, Byrum B, Zhang Y. New variant of porcine epidemic diarrhea virus, United States, 2014. *Emerg Infect Dis.* (2014) 20:917–9. doi: 10.3201/eid2005.140195
13. Jarvis MC, Lam HC, Zhang Y, Wang L, Hesse RA, Hause BM, et al. Genomic and evolutionary inferences between American and global strains of porcine epidemic diarrhea virus. *Prev Vet Med.* (2016) 123:175–84. doi: 10.1016/j.prevetmed.2015.10.020
14. Wang D, Ge X, Chen D, Li J, Cai Y, Deng J, et al. The S gene is necessary but not sufficient for the virulence of porcine epidemic diarrhea virus novel variant strain BJ2011C. *J Virol.* (2018) 92:e00603-18. doi: 10.1128/JVI.00603-18
15. Chang SH, Bae JL, Kang TJ, Kim J, Chung GH, Lim CW, et al. Identification of the epitope region capable of inducing neutralizing antibodies against the porcine epidemic diarrhea virus. *Mol Cells.* (2002) 14:295–9.
16. Sun D, Feng L, Shi H, Chen J, Cui X, Chen H, et al. Identification of two novel B cell epitopes on porcine epidemic diarrhea virus spike protein. *Vet Microbiol.* (2008) 131:73–81. doi: 10.1016/j.vetmic.2008.02.022
17. Zhang Q, Liu X, Fang Y, Zhou P, Wang Y, Zhang Y. Detection and phylogenetic analyses of spike genes in porcine epidemic diarrhea virus strains circulating in China in 2016-2017. *Virol J.* (2017) 14:194. doi: 10.1186/s12985-017-0860-z
18. Liu X, Zhang Q, Zhang L, Zhou P, Yang J, Fang Y, et al. A newly isolated Chinese virulent genotype GIIb porcine epidemic diarrhea virus strain: biological characteristics, pathogenicity and immune protective effects as an inactivated vaccine candidate. *Virus Res.* (2019) 259:18–27. doi: 10.1016/j.virusres.2018.10.012
19. Wang P, Zhu J, Liu X, Guo J, Gu X, Ruan W. Isolation and recombinant analysis of variants of porcine epidemic diarrhea virus strains from Beijing, China. *Virus Dis.* (2019) 30:294–301. doi: 10.1007/s13337-019-00513-w
20. Chen N, Li S, Zhou R, Zhu M, He S, Ye M, et al. Two novel porcine epidemic diarrhea virus (PEDV) recombinants from a natural recombinant and distinct subtypes of PEDV variants. *Virus Res.* (2017) 242:90–5. doi: 10.1016/j.virusres.2017.09.013
21. Wang X, Niu B, Yan H, Gao D, Yang X, Chen L, et al. Genetic properties of endemic Chinese porcine epidemic diarrhea virus strains isolated since 2010. *Arch Virol.* (2013) 158:2487–94. doi: 10.1007/s00705-013-1767-7
22. Kumar S, Stecher G, Li M, Knyaz C, Tamura K. MEGA X: molecular evolutionary genetics analysis across computing platforms. *Mol Biol Evol.* (2018) 35:1547–9. doi: 10.1093/molbev/msy096
23. Wang D, Fang L, Xiao S. Porcine epidemic diarrhea in China. *Virus Res.* (2016) 226:7–13. doi: 10.1016/j.virusres.2016.05.026
24. Li W, Li H, Liu Y, Pan Y, Deng F, Song Y, et al. New variants of porcine epidemic diarrhea virus, China, 2011. *Emerg Infect Dis.* (2012) 18:1350–3. doi: 10.3201/eid1808.120002
25. Chen J, Liu X, Shi D, Shi H, Zhang X, Li C, et al. Detection and molecular diversity of spike gene of porcine epidemic diarrhea virus in China. *Viruses.* (2013) 5:2601–13. doi: 10.3390/v5102601
26. Wen Z, Li J, Zhang Y, Zhou Q, Gong L, Xue C, et al. Genetic epidemiology of porcine epidemic diarrhoea virus circulating in China in 2012-2017 based on spike gene. *Transbound Emerg Dis.* (2018) 65:883–9. doi: 10.1111/tbed.12825
27. Chen P, Wang K, Hou Y, Li H, Li X, Yu L, et al. Genetic evolution analysis and pathogenicity assessment of porcine epidemic diarrhea virus strains circulating in part of China during 2011-2017. *Infect Genet Evol.* (2019) 69:153–65. doi: 10.1016/j.meegid.2019.01.022
28. Yu J, Chai X, Cheng Y, Xing G, Liao A, Du L, et al. Molecular characteristics of the spike gene of porcine epidemic diarrhoea virus strains in Eastern China in 2016. *Virus Res.* (2018) 247:47–54. doi: 10.1016/j.virusres.2018.01.013
29. Hou Y, Lin CM, Yokoyama M, Yount BL, Marthaler D, Douglas AL, et al. Deletion of a 197-amino-acid region in the N-terminal domain of spike protein attenuates porcine epidemic diarrhea virus in piglets. *J Virol.* (2017) 91:e00227-17. doi: 10.1128/JVI.00227-17
30. Su Y, Hou Y, Prarat M, Zhang Y, Wang Q. New variants of porcine epidemic diarrhea virus with large deletions in the spike protein, identified in the United States, 2016-2017. *Arch Virol.* (2018) 163:2485–9. doi: 10.1007/s00705-018-3874-y
31. Zhang L, Liu X, Zhang Q, Zhou P, Fang Y, Dong Z, et al. Biological characterization and pathogenicity of a newly isolated Chinese highly virulent genotype GIIa porcine epidemic diarrhea virus strain. *Arch Virol.* (2019) 164:1287–95. doi: 10.1007/s00705-019-04167-3
32. Li B, Liu H, He K, Guo R, Ni Y, Du L, et al. Complete genome sequence of a recombinant porcine epidemic diarrhea virus strain from eastern china. *Genome Announc.* (2013) 1:e10513. doi: 10.1128/genomeA.00105-13
33. Li K, Song D, Zhang F, Gong W, Guo N, Li A, et al. Complete genome sequence of a recombinant porcine epidemic diarrhea virus strain, CH/JXJA/2017, isolated in jiangxi, China, in 2017. *Genome Announc.* (2018) 6:e01590-17. doi: 10.1128/genomeA.01590-17
34. Li R, Qiao S, Yang Y, Guo J, Xie S, Zhou E, et al. Genome sequencing and analysis of a novel recombinant porcine epidemic diarrhea virus strain from Henan, China. *Virus Genes.* (2016) 52:91–8. doi: 10.1007/s11262-015-1254-1
35. Park S, Kim S, Song D, Park B. Novel porcine epidemic diarrhea virus variant with large genomic deletion, South Korea. *Emerg Infect Dis.* (2014) 20:2089–92. doi: 10.3201/eid2012.131642
36. Zhang X, Pan Y, Wang D, Tian X, Song Y, Cao Y. Identification and pathogenicity of a variant porcine epidemic diarrhea virus field strain with reduced virulence. *Virol J.* (2015) 12:88. doi: 10.1186/s12985-015-0314-4
37. Puranaveja S, Poolperm P, Lertwatcharasarakul P, Kesdaengsakonwut S, Boonsoongnern A, Urairong K, et al. Chinese-like strain of porcine epidemic diarrhea virus, Thailand. *Emerg Infect Dis.* (2009) 15:1112–5. doi: 10.3201/eid1507.081256
38. Lin CM, Saif LJ, Marthaler D, Wang Q. Evolution, antigenicity and pathogenicity of global porcine epidemic diarrhea virus strains. *Virus Res.* (2016) 226:20–39. doi: 10.1016/j.virusres.2016.05.023
39. Madson DM, Arruda PH, Magstadt DR, Burrough ER, Hoang H, Sun D, et al. Characterization of porcine epidemic diarrhea virus isolate US/Iowa/18984/2013 infection in 1-day-old cesarean-derived colostrum-deprived piglets. *Vet Pathol.* (2016) 53:44–52. doi: 10.1177/0300985815591080
40. Chen Q, Gauger PC, Stafne MR, Thomas JT, Madson DM, Huang H, et al. Pathogenesis comparison between the United States porcine epidemic diarrhoea virus prototype and S-INDEL-variant strains in conventional neonatal piglets. *J Gen Virol.* (2016) 97:1107–21. doi: 10.1099/jgv.0.000419
41. Lin CM, Annamalai T, Liu X, Gao X, Lu Z, El-Tholoth M, et al. Experimental infection of a US spike-insertion deletion porcine epidemic diarrhea virus in conventional nursing piglets and cross-protection to the original US PEDV infection. *Vet Res.* (2015) 46:134. doi: 10.1186/s13567-015-0278-9
42. Thomas JT, Chen Q, Gauger PC, Gimenez-Lirola LG, Sinha A, Harmon KM, et al. Effect of porcine epidemic diarrhea virus infectious doses on infection outcomes in naive conventional neonatal and weaned pigs. *PLoS ONE.* (2015) 10:e139266. doi: 10.1371/journal.pone.0139266
43. Yu L, Liu Y, Wang S, Zhang L, Liang P, Wang L, et al. Molecular characteristics and pathogenicity of porcine epidemic diarrhea virus in some areas of China from 2015 to 2018. *Res Square.* (2020). doi: 10.21203/rs.3.rs-41418/v1

12

Transport of Moving Duck Flocks in Indonesia and Vietnam: Management Practices that Potentially Impact Avian Pathogen Dissemination

Shan Wen Stacy Khaw[1], *Le Tri Vu*[2], *Didik Yulianto*[3], *Joanne Meers*[1*] *and Joerg Henning*[1]

[1] *School of Veterinary Science, The University of Queensland, Gatton, QLD, Australia,* [2] *Regional Animal Health Centre VI, Ho Chi Minh City, Vietnam,* [3] *Disease Investigation Centre, Wates, Indonesia*

Correspondence:
Joanne Meers
j.meers@uq.edu.au

Highly pathogenic avian influenza (HPAI) virus is endemic in Indonesia and Vietnam, where "moving" duck production is commonly practiced. Questionnaire surveys were conducted with transporters of "moving" duck flocks in Indonesia ($N = 55$) and Vietnam ($N = 43$). The main purpose of transportation was to transport duck flocks between rice paddies used for scavenging. Trucks were commonly utilized for transport in both countries (Indonesia: 98.2%, 54/55; Vietnam: 37.2%, 16/43), while boats were only used in Vietnam (62.8%, 27/43). Transporters in Vietnam moved larger flocks and traveled over longer distances. Deaths of ducks due to diseases were reported in both countries (Indonesia: 16.4%, 9/55; Vietnam: 4.7%, 2/43; $p = 0.11$). Throwing away of carcasses was the primary method of disposal of dead birds in Indonesia (60.0%, 33/55), but was not practiced in Vietnam ($p < 0.001$), while more transporters in Vietnam (34.9%, 15/43) buried carcasses compared to Indonesia (6.8%, 4/55; $p = 0.001$). Consumption of carcasses (20.9%, 9/43), sale of dead ducks (14.0%, 6/43) and processing of ducks for fish feed (9.3%, 4/43) was conducted in Vietnam, but not in Indonesia. Vehicles were predominantly cleaned in rivers and stored outside in Vietnam, while cleaning and storage was usually conducted in houses/garages in Indonesia. In conclusion, we identified management practices that potentially impact transmission of avian pathogens, such as HPAI virus. In Indonesia, unsafe management practices were related to multipurpose usage of transport vehicles and disposal of birds in the environment, while in Vietnam, they were related to the mixing of birds during transport, the processing of dead carcasses and the storage and cleaning of transport vehicles.

Keywords: avian influenza, transport, moving ducks, biosecurity, virus transmission, Indonesia, Vietnam

INTRODUCTION

Highly Pathogenic Avian Influenza (HPAI) H5N1 virus is endemic in Vietnam and Indonesia and has caused substantial human and poultry losses (1, 2). From 2003 to September 2018, 454 human fatalities were reported out of 860 HPAI human cases worldwide, representing a case-fatality rate of 52.8% (3). At 84.0% (168/200), Indonesia has the highest human case fatality rate globally (3). Vietnam has experienced 64 deaths out of 127 human cases, representing a case fatality rate of 50.4% (3).

From 2004 to 2019, 22.5 and 20.0% of the global HPAI outbreaks in poultry occurred in Indonesia and Vietnam, respectively (4). Since 2003, more than 150 million domestic birds died or were culled as a result of H5N1 outbreaks in Indonesia (5, 6), while in Vietnam more than 52 million poultry losses occurred since 2003, with 86.5% of the domestic poultry population being culled in 2003-04 alone at an estimated cost of about US$205 million (7).

Duck farming is an important sector of the poultry industry in Indonesia and Vietnam. Duck management is classified into "stationary" and "moving" duck production, with stationary flocks allowed to graze around the village vicinity and secured at night near village houses, while moving flocks are moved between areas of recent rice harvests and kept in confinement overnight close to the daytime scavenging locations (8–10). Moving duck flocks are suspected to contribute toward the maintenance and circulation of HPAI viruses (11–14) and research had highlighted that road characteristics (e.g., road density; road length), human and poultry densities and long distance movement might facilitate the spread of HPAI viruses (15–19). Meyer et al. (20) described the actors involved in duck production, providing an overarching description of the poultry value chain system of Vietnam, while Henning et al. (9) described the structure of the moving duck flock network in Indonesia. However, specific transport practices that influence the dissemination of H5N1 virus have yet to be identified.

The objectives of this study were to (1) identify management factors during transport of moving duck flocks in Indonesia and Vietnam that could potentially be associated with an increased risk of avian pathogen dissemination (e.g., HPAI virus), and to (2) compare and contrast differences in movement, management and biosecurity practices implemented by duck flock transporters in Indonesia and Vietnam.

MATERIALS AND METHODS

Study Design

Previous research conducted with moving duck flock owners in Indonesia and Vietnam in 2008 and 2009 described the HPAI H5N1 infection status of ducks and the movements elected by owners for their duck flocks (8, 9). During this research, information about the transport provider used by moving duck farmers was collected. These data comprised the initial dataset of transporters to be contacted. As no register of transporters existed in either country, we used snowball sampling by asking identified transport providers about contact details of additional potential transporters working in the same region. Transporters were identified in six districts of Central Java (Pemalang, Batang, Klaten, Purworejo, Brebes, and Kendal) in Indonesia and in four provinces of the Mekong Delta in Vietnam (Ben Tre, Dong Thap, Tien Gian, and Vinh Long). The aim was to interview about 10 transporters per district or province.

Data collection was conducted in Indonesia by veterinarians from the Disease Investigation Centre (DIC) in Wates, Yogjakarta and in Vietnam by veterinarians from The Regional Animal Health Centre VI, Ho Chi Minh City using an interview process using local languages. All interviewers were trained in data collection.

The study design for this research was reviewed and approved in Indonesia by the Disease Investigation Centre (DIC) in Wates, Yogjakarta; and in Vietnam by the Regional Animal Health Centre VI, Ho Chi Minh City. Data collection for this study was conducted in accordance with the accepted survey guidelines for surveillance activities of both organizations.

Questionnaire

Questionnaires were developed in English and later translated into the national languages (Bahasa, Vietnamese) in order to capture potential associated risk factors associated with spread of avian pathogens such as HPAI virus during the transport of duck flocks: type of transport utilized; number of flocks (and ducks) transported per time period; age of ducks transported; number of duck flocks combined in a transport load; other poultry species transported; number of farms visited to obtain one transport load; cleaning and disinfection before and after transport; location where the transport vehicles were stored, cleaned and disinfected; distance and duration of transport; management of ducks before departure, during transport and after arrival in scavenging area; contact of transported ducks with other poultry and other animals; frequency of transporting ducks; raising of ducks at home by people loading and transporting poultry; transport of items (e.g., chickens, other animals, feed, and eggs) together with ducks; experiences of sickness or deaths of ducks during transport; disposal of dead ducks; and occurrence of health problem in people loading and transporting ducks. Thus, the questionnaires included a mixture of closed and open-ended questions. Copies of the questionnaires are provided in the **Supplementary Material (Data Sheets 1, 2)**.

Pilot testing of the questionnaires was performed with two transporters in both countries before conducting the main survey to identify any problems, misunderstandings or to discover additional risk factors of interest that should be surveyed. The questionnaires were updated accordingly. The total number of questions in the questionnaire was 39, with identical questions being used in Indonesia and Vietnam.

Data analysis was conducted in SPSS (IBM Corp, Release 2019, IBM SPSS Statistics for Windows, Version 26.0) and STATA (StataCorp, College Station, TX, 2019, Stata Statistical Software: Release 16). Descriptive analysis included the calculation of frequencies, means, medians and range values. The command -*tabplot*- in Stata was used to visualize the frequency of responses provided on a 4-point Likert scale. The total number of survey responses for each response category were compared between Indonesia and Vietnam using the Fisher's exact test. To facilitate the utilization of the Fisher's Exact Test for data analysis, Likert scale groups "very important" and "important" were combined into a category "importantly" and Likert scale groups "not important" and "not conducted" were combined into a category "not importantly." Similarly, Likert scale groups "common" and "sometimes" were combined into a category "commonly" and Likert scale groups "seldom" and "not conducted" were combined to a category "infrequently." The non-parametric Mann–Whitney U-test was used to compare ordinal and not normally distributed continuous variables between Indonesia and Vietnam.

RESULTS

A total of 114 transporters of moving duck flocks were interviewed, with 16 transporters being excluded from the analysis as they provided incomplete information in the questionnaire. Thus, 98 transporters provided completed responses to all questions and were analyzed in detail, consisting of 55 transporters from Indonesia and 43 from Vietnam (**Supplementary Table 1 - Data Sheet 3**).

Importance of Transport Activities for Income Generation

As expected, the transport of ducks to scavenging locations was the main activity for transporters (**Figure 1A**) in both countries (Indonesia: 98.2%, 54/55, Vietnam: 95.3%, 41/43; $p = 0.58$). Although not statistically significant, transporting of ducks to markets was less common in Indonesia (Indonesia: 9.3%, 4/43; Vietnam: 16.4%, 9/55; $p = 0.38$), while transport of ducklings to and from hatcheries was more common in Indonesia. Items transported together with ducks include chickens, other birds, feed, and eggs (**Figure 1B**). About 45.5% of transporters from Indonesia indicated that they "commonly" transport duck feed together with ducks compared to only 28.0% of transporters from Vietnam ($p = 0.09$). Additionally, 40.0% of transporters from Indonesia indicated that they "commonly" transport eggs together with ducks, but this was either seldom or not practiced in Vietnam ($p < 0.001$) (**Figure 1B**).

In general, transporters from Indonesia also used their transport vehicles more frequently to transport other items for income generation. This included the transport of feed (Indonesia: 25.5%, 14/55; Vietnam: 2.3%, 1/43; $p = 0.0014$), and transport of non-animal related items (Indonesia: 49.1%, 27/55; Vietnam: 9.5%, 4/42; $p < 0.001$), with the most common items transported being building materials (**Figure 1A**). More Indonesian transporters relied on additional income sources not related to transport (Indonesia: 58.2% 32/55; Vietnam: 23.3%, 10/43; $p < 0.001$), with farming being the most common activity in both countries (**Figure 1A**).

Transport Types Used, Volume of Transport and Distance Traveled

Trucks, boats and motorbikes were used for transportation (**Supplementary Figure 1 - Data Sheet 3**). Trucks were the most common transport type in Indonesia (Indonesia: 98.2%, 54/55; Vietnam: 37.2%, 16/43; $p < 0.001$), while boats were the most common mode of transport in Vietnam (62.8%, 27/43), but were not utilized in Indonesia ($p < 0.001$). Motorbikes were used by one transporter in each country. Almost all transporters (99.0%) utilized only one type of transport.

Of the 70 transporters, who provided data on truck designs, 95.7% (67/70) of trucks were not covered or closed. Trucks had between 1 and 4 levels, with the majority of them (58.6%, 41/70) having three levels. Boats were generally open (82.1%, 23/28) and had between 1 and 3 levels, with 85.7% (24/28) of them having three levels. Neither of the two motorbikes was covered.

Respondents from Vietnam were more likely to store their transport vehicles outside (60.5%, 26/43) compared to Indonesia (16.4%, 9/55; $p < 0.001$). Vietnamese transporters indicated more frequent exposure of their vehicles to wild birds compared to Indonesian transporters [23.3% (10/43) vs. 5.5% (3/55); $p = 0.015$].

The volume of transport and distance traveled in Indonesia and Vietnam are shown in **Table 1**. In Vietnam, transporters using trucks transported more duck flocks per year, over larger distances per year and with a larger number of ducks per flock compared to Indonesia. Individual journeys were ~25% longer in Vietnam compared to Indonesia, although this was not significant ($p = 0.13$).

Transport of Moving Duck Flocks to and From Scavenging Locations

The locations from where ducks were collected from and transported to by transporters are shown in **Supplementary Figure 2 (Data Sheet 3)**. As expected, the majority of transporters from both countries collected ducks from rice paddies as these represent the main scavenging locations. However, 78.2% (43/55) of transporters in Indonesia collected ducks and 63.0% (34/54) delivered ducks to farms, compared to only 23.3% (10/43) and 20.9% (9/43) from Vietnam ($p < 0.001$ and $p < 0.001$, respectively). About 34.5% (19/55) of transporters in Indonesia collected and 53.7% (29/54) delivered moving ducks to village areas compared to 58.1% (25/43) and 65.1% (28/43) in Vietnam ($p = 0.025$ and $p = 0.30$, respectively), highlighting that within-village scavenging areas are more common in Vietnam.

Collection and delivery of ducks to markets was uncommon for both Indonesia and Vietnam, with about 11% and <5% of transporters in Indonesia and Vietnam, respectively, "commonly" conducting this practice.

Characteristics of return journeys are outlined in **Supplementary Figure 3 (Data Sheet 3)**. Although usually transporters from both countries returned "empty" after delivering ducks, 34.9% (15/43) of transporters in Vietnam and 20.4% (11/54) of transporters from Indonesia ($p = 0.17$) did "commonly" return with other ducks.

A higher proportion of transporters in Vietnam compared to Indonesia provided care to birds during transport. In Indonesia, water and feed was provided to ducks by 13.0% (7/54) and 7.4% (4/54) of transporters, respectively, compared to 88.4% (38/43) and 65.1% (28/43) of transporters, respectively, in Vietnam. Spraying of birds with water was conducted by 5.6% (4/54) of transporters in Indonesia and 32.6% (14/43) of transporters in Vietnam, while rest stops for ducks were provided by 11.1% (6/54) of transporters in Indonesia and 18.6% (28/43) of transporters in Vietnam.

Duck Deaths and Disposal of Carcasses

Out of 41 transporters providing information on the number of duck deaths per truck load in Indonesia, the mean number (median, range) of duck deaths per load was 2.4 (2, 0.5–10), while

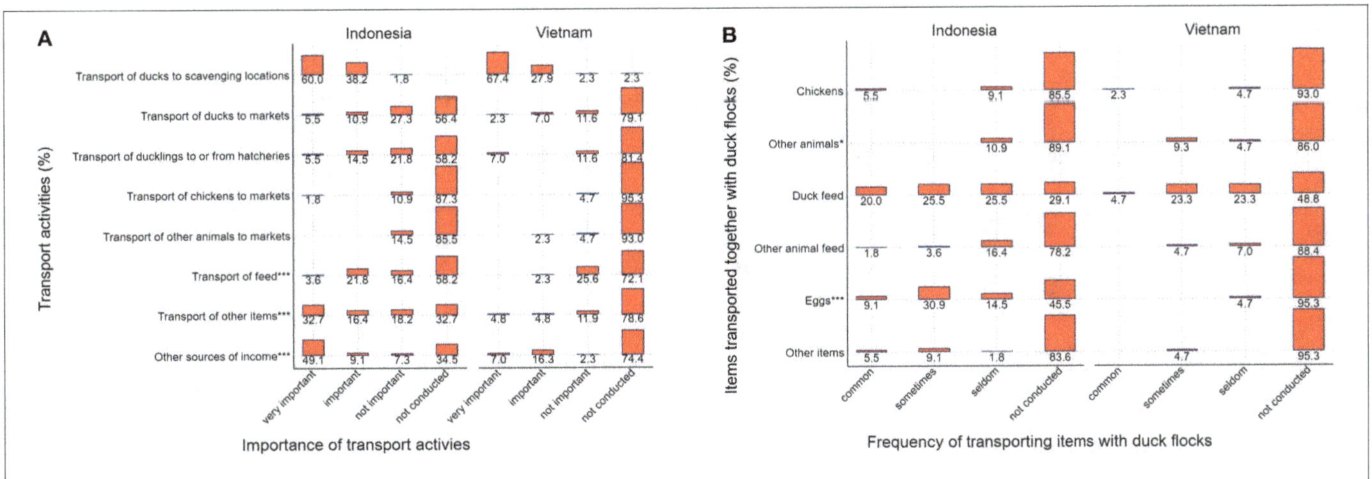

FIGURE 1 | (A) Importance of transport activities for transporters of moving duck flocks in Indonesia ($N = 55$) and Vietnam ($N = 43$), with percent of respondents by importance category. **(B)** Items transported together with ducks to scavenging locations for Indonesia ($N = 55$) and Vietnam ($N = 43$), with percent of respondents by frequency category. *P*-values for comparisons between countries for each category are presented as follows: * for $P \leq 0.05$, *** for $P \leq 0.001$.

TABLE 1 | Volume of transport and distance traveled by transporters of moving duck flocks in Indonesia.

	Transport by truck			Transport by boat
	Indonesia	**Vietnam**	***p*-value**	**Vietnam**
Number of scavenging duck flocks transported per year	44 (48; 2–270) ($N = 45$)	123 (110; 50–220) ($N = 14$)	<0.001	113 (120; 40–250) ($N = 28$)
Number of ducks transported in a single load	431 (450; 100–800) ($N = 51$)	4,792 (750; 300–25,000) ($N = 13$)	<0.001	18,527 (12,000; 800–80,000) ($N = 26$)
Distance traveled per year (in km) to scavenging locations	1,831 (800; 80–20,000) ($N = 37$)	9,483 (10,000; 900–35,000) ($N = 15$)	<0.001	10,450 (6,000; 50–55,000) ($N = 26$)
Distance traveled per journey (in km) to scavenging locations	68 (60; 10–200) ($N = 45$)	94 (80; 25–200) ($N = 16$)	0.13	97 (80; 10–300) ($N = 26$)

Mean (median; minimum - maximum) is shown with number of respondents in brackets. P-value refers to the comparison between Indonesia and Vietnam.

for Vietnam, out of 16 transporters providing information, the mean number (median, range) of duck deaths per truck load was 3.4 (3, 1–10). For 26 transporters with boats from Vietnam who provided data, the mean number (median, range) of duck deaths per load was 2.6 (2, 1–5).

Transporters reported the causes of death as "disease," "dehydration," "injury," "other," and "unknown." Deaths of ducks during transport due to diseases were observed by transporters in both countries at similar frequencies (**Figure 2A**, $p = 0.11$). Injuries occurred in similar frequencies during transport in Indonesia and Vietnam ($p = 0.84$). In contrast, transporters from Vietnam more frequently experienced death of ducks due to dehydration (Vietnam: 72.1%, 31/43; Indonesia: 30.9%, 17/55; $p < 0.001$).

There were considerable differences in how transporters disposed of ducks that died during transport (**Figure 2B**). Throwing away carcasses in the environment was most common in Indonesia (60.0%, 33/55), but not practiced in Vietnam ($p < 0.001$). Sale of dead ducks ($p = 0.006$), processing of ducks for fish feed ($p = 0.034$), giving ducks to neighbors ($p < 0.001$), and household consumption of ducks ($p < 0.001$) were all practiced in Vietnam, but not in Indonesia (**Figure 2B**).

In Indonesia, two transporters specified as "other" management practice that duck carcasses were returned to duck owners (3.6%, 2/55). For Vietnam, "other" management practices also included return of carcasses to duck owners (20.9%, 9/43), while 9.3% (4/43) of transporters provided carcasses to para-veterinarians.

Cleaning and Disinfection of Transport Vehicles

Cleaning and disinfection of transport vehicles in the water of nearby rivers was common in both countries (Vietnam: 67.4%, 29/43; Indonesia: 49.1%, 27/55; $p = 0.10$). However, the most common location for cleaning transport vehicles in Indonesia was inside houses or garages (67.3%, 37/55), but this was less common in Vietnam (25.6%, 11/43; $p < 0.001$). Car washes were more utilized by Indonesian transporters compared to Vietnamese transporters (27.3%, 15/55 vs. 9.3%, 4/43; $p = 0.038$).

The most common cleaning practices, i.e., removing feces from loading surfaces and washing loading surfaces with water

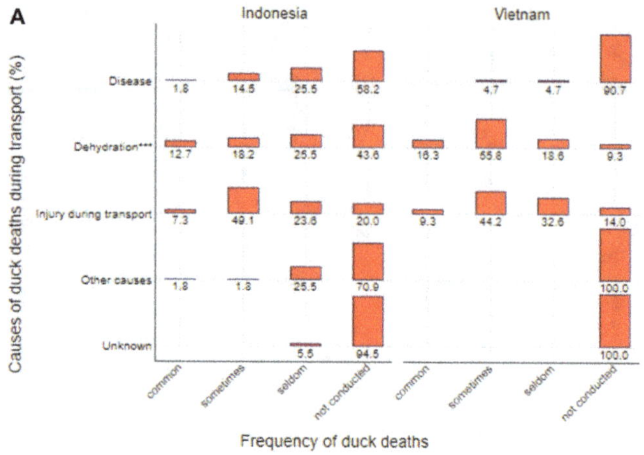

B

Management Strategies	Indonesia	Vietnam	p-value
	% (N)	% (N)	
Burned	0.0 (0)	25.6 (11)	<0.001
Sold	0.0 (0)	14.0 (6)	0.006
Processed for fish feed	0.0 (0)	9.3 (4)	0.034
Given to neighbours	0.0 (0)	25.6 (11)	<0.001
Buried	6.8 (4)	34.9 (15)	0.001
Household consumption	0.0 (0)	20.9 (9)	<0.001
Thrown away	60.0 (33)	0.0 (0)	<0.001
Others	3.6 (2)	30.2 (13)	<0.001

FIGURE 2 | (A) Causes of death ducks during transport in Indonesia ($N = 55$) and Vietnam ($N = 43$) with percent of respondents by frequency category. *P*-values for comparisons between countries for each category are presented as follows: *** for $P \leq 0.001$. **(B)** Disposal of ducks that died during transport in Indonesia and Vietnam.

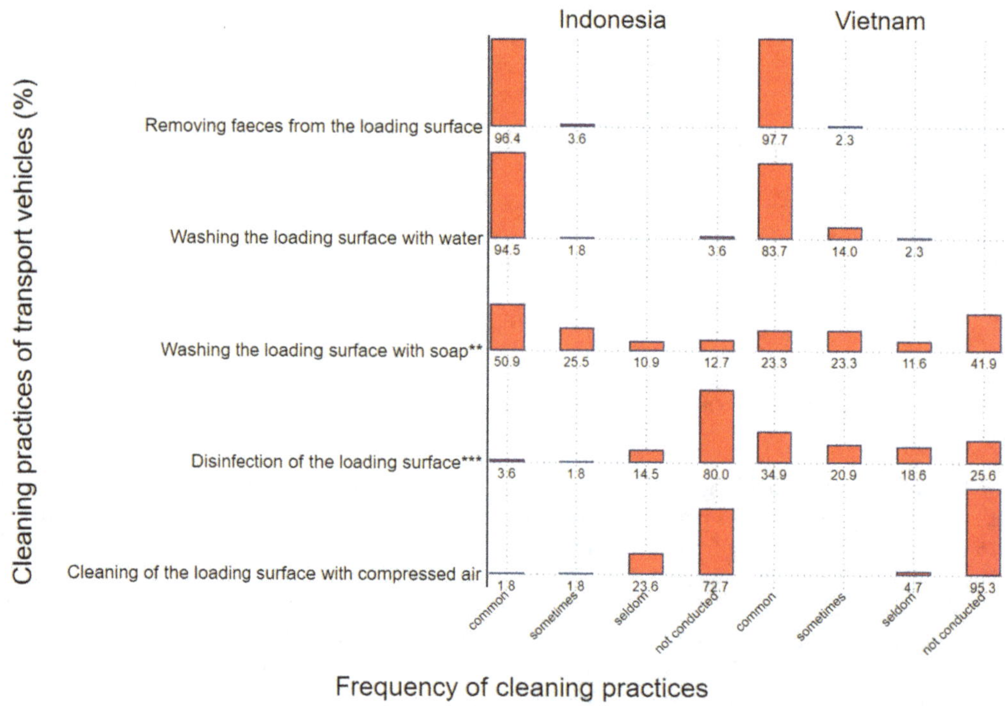

FIGURE 3 | Cleaning practices conducted on transport vehicles in Indonesia ($N = 55$) and Vietnam ($N = 43$) with percent of respondents by frequency category. *P*-values for comparisons between countries for each category are presented as follows: ** for $P \leq 0.01$, *** for $P \leq 0.001$.

were similar for both countries ($p = 1$; and $p = 0.10$, respectively) (**Figure 3**). However, the use of soap to wash loading surfaces was more common in Indonesia compared to Vietnam ($p = 0.0067$), while transporters from Vietnam more "commonly" used disinfectant on loading surfaces compared to Indonesia ($p < 0.001$).

Health of Transporters

Information was also obtained about whether transporters had experienced health problems while loading and transporting ducks. Almost all of transporter respondents from Indonesia (98.2%; $N = 54$) and Vietnam (95.3%; $N = 41$) indicated that they did not experience any health problems ($p = 0.58$).

DISCUSSION

This study investigated factors involved in the transportation of moving duck flocks in Vietnam and Indonesia that might facilitate the transmission of avian pathogens such as HPAI virus, and compared the magnitude of these factors between the two countries. While many practices were common to both countries, there were significant differences between the occurrence of some factors, which might help to identify strategies to reduce HPAI transmission during the transport of ducks in each country.

Compared to Vietnamese transporters, Indonesian transporters had more varied sources of income that contributed to a substantial portion of their financial needs and they were more likely to travel to many different locations, such as markets and hatcheries. The more frequent use of transport vehicles for different purposes may have implications for direct (if ducks are transported at the same time with ducks from other farms or other animal species) or indirect (if cleaning is not conducted properly between transports session) spread of HPAI virus (16, 17, 20). Also, considerably more transporters from Indonesia engaged in buying/selling of ducks in markets as an additional income source. This is a concern because wet markets facilitate interspecies transmission of HPAI virus and are considered to be the most likely source for HPAI outbreaks (16, 18, 21, 22). In contrast, transporters in Vietnam mainly specialized in transporting ducks between scavenging locations and did not generally use transport vehicles for other purposes. Although distances traveled per journey with trucks were similar between both countries, the total distance traveled per year was six times larger in Vietnam and more duck flocks and more ducks per load were transported in Vietnam. Compared to Indonesian transporters, Vietnamese transporters more frequently transported other duck flocks on their return journeys (although not significant at $p < 0.05$), thus proving potential opportunities for dissemination of avian pathogens if surface areas of transport vehicles were not properly cleaned and disinfected (16, 17, 23). Adding to this is the fact that transport vehicles were more commonly stored and left open during transport in Vietnam which suggests a higher likelihood for transport vehicles and duck flocks to be exposed to wild birds which could be harboring or excreting avian pathogens such as HPAI virus (15, 23, 24).

In general, collection and delivery of ducks to markets was not very common for transporters in either Indonesia or Vietnam. This indicates that the collection of ducks and delivery to markets is not in their domain, and is more likely conducted by middle men or traders, who have their own vehicles and collect moving ducks from scavenging areas or from farms. Similar observations were made by Meyer et al. (10) and Meyer et al. (20), who surveyed duck farmers in Vietnam.

Differing from the findings of Henning et al. (9) and Meyer et al. (10), our study found that an overwhelming majority of transporters from Indonesia and Vietnam clean their vehicles regularly after each journey, although both previous studies focussed on duck farmers and not directly on transporters of moving duck flocks. Almost all transporter respondents from both Indonesia and Vietnam removed feces and washed the vehicle loading surfaces, with transporters in Vietnam also commonly using disinfectant. This indicates that transporters recognize to a certain extent, the importance of biosecurity practices to prevent the spread of avian pathogens such as HPAI virus. However, further education to increase the biosecurity awareness among actors within the poultry industry is needed, in particular in HPAI endemically infected countries (25–28).

Transporters from Indonesia more frequently experienced deaths of ducks due to disease during the journeys, while transporters from Vietnam more frequently experience deaths of ducks due to dehydration. This difference may be explained by the fact that Indonesian transporters had more opportunities of direct and indirect contact between ducks as birds were sourced and delivered to a wider range of locations; while transporters from Vietnam generally traveled longer distances resulting in potentially longer stressful periods for ducks.

With regards to the disposal of duck carcasses, guidelines from international organizations recommend burial, composting, incineration, rendering or landfill disposal as they are effective in mitigating virus spread and minimizes public health and environmental effects (25, 29, 30). However, despite education campaigns conducted in Indonesia (25), the preferred method of carcass disposal by Indonesian transporters, was to throw carcasses into the environment (in particular into rivers), which has been described previously (31). This increases the likelihood of direct contact of other birds with the carcasses (31) or that scavengers such as roaming dogs open up carcasses and potentially increase virus exposure in the environment (when carcasses are infectious).

Additionally, it also presents a public health risk if untreated river water is consumed by people, especially given that around 4% of households in Indonesia rely on rivers as their main water supply (32–34). Interestingly, a substantial percentage of transporters from Vietnam indicated appropriate methods of disposal including incineration and burial. However, a sizeable proportion of respondents indicated that they prefer to give away the carcasses that died during transport to neighbors (the carcasses may eventually be consumed by the neighbors) or keep them for consumption within their own household. Corroborating with Manabe et al. (28), this suggests that despite a reasonably high awareness of H5N1 infection, Vietnamese transporters adhered to traditional habits. This may be due to insufficient knowledge about the risks of HPAI virus infection, compounded by financial hardships.

None of the transporters involved in this study was using Personal Protective Equipment (PPE), during handling of ducks or cleaning of transport vehicles. Previous research highlighted that lack of awareness and training, but also that low income influences the under-use of protective equipment in developing countries (35).

Data Limitations

It is difficult to determine if the cohort of transporters recruited into the study is representative of the spatio-temporal distribution of transporters in both countries. This is due to limited literature describing nationwide spatio-temporal distribution of moving duck flocks in both Indonesia and Vietnam and the non-existence of a sampling frame of transporters for both countries. Government lists of moving duck farmers, let alone transporters of moving duck flocks do not exist in either country. The snowball sampling strategy used in this study was the only methodology that allowed us to overcome this problem. It has been previously noted that duck farming is widespread in West and Central Java in Indonesia; and highly concentrated around the Mekong Delta region in Vietnam (10, 17, 36, 37). Therefore, the use of Central Java and the Mekong Delta regions provided a good representation in terms of concentration of duck farming activities in those countries.

The use of survey questionnaires introduced biasness of various forms: recall bias, as the journeys may have been conducted many months earlier resulting in errors in recording journey characteristics and parameters; and social desirability bias, such as that transporters may be unwilling to disclose past experiences of ill-health after handling ducks; and that they may erroneously reported a greater frequency of disinfecting their transport vehicles than in reality. However, we used well-trained interviewers in this study and we are confident that the information we collected is reliable.

Finally, the data summarized here were collected in 2009. Some might argue that there could be changes to the duck industry since then. However, based on the value chain analysis elucidated by Meyer et al. (20) and further described by Kasim et al. (38), our description of the relationship between duck farmers and transporters appears to be a system that exists till this day.

CONCLUSION

In conclusion, while HPAI is endemic in both Indonesia and Vietnam, known risk factors that perpetuate HPAI in duck farming differ in importance between the two countries. This is due to dissimilarities in the duck farming industries between the two countries that impact the mode of transport used, movement patterns, disposal methods, and cleaning and disinfection approaches. While practices associated with higher biosecurity risk in Indonesia are related to the multipurpose usage of transport vehicles and the disposal of birds in the environment, unsafe practices in Vietnam relate to the potential mixing of birds during transport, the processing of dead carcasses and the storage and cleaning of transport vehicles.

ETHICS STATEMENT

Ethical approval for interviews with human participants in this study was not provided because the study design for this research was reviewed and approved in accordance with local legislation and institutional requirements in Indonesia and Vietnam. In Indonesia, this was conducted by the Disease Investigation Centre (DIC) in Wates, Yogjakarta; and in Vietnam by the Regional Animal Health Centre VI, Ho Chi Minh City. Data collection for this study was conducted in accordance with the accepted survey guidelines for surveillance activities of both organizations. Written informed consent for participation was not required for this study in accordance with the national legislation and the institutional requirements.

AUTHOR CONTRIBUTIONS

JH, JM, LTV, and DY: design of the research study. JH, LTV, and DY: data collection. SWSK and JH: data analysis. SWSK, JH, and JM: development of manuscript. All authors contributed to the manuscript and approved the submitted version.

ACKNOWLEDGMENTS

We thank all transporters who were involved in this research project.

REFERENCES

1. Otte J, Hinrichs J, Rushton J, Roland-Holst D, Zilberman D. Impacts of avian influenza virus on animal production in developing countries Introduction and Context. *CAB Rev.* (2009) 3:1–18. doi: 10.1079/PAVSNNR2008 3080
2. Pongcharoensuk P, Adisasmito W, Sat LM, Silkavute P, Muchlisoh L, Cong Hoat P, et al. Avian and pandemic human influenza policy in South-East Asia: the interface between economic and public health imperatives. *Health Policy Plan.* (2012) 27:374–83. doi: 10.1093/heapol/czr056
3. World Health Organisation. *Cumulative Number of Confirmed Human Cases for Avian Influenza A(H5N1) Reported to WHO, 2003–2018.* (2018). Available online at: https://www.who.int/influenza/human_animal_interface/2018_03_02_tableH5N1.pdf (accessed February 25, 2021).
4. Food and Agriculture Organization of the United Nations. *EMPRES-i - Global Animal Disease Information System.* (2019). Available online at: http://empres-i.fao.org/eipws3g/ (accessed February 25, 2021).
5. Forster P. *The Political Economy of Avian Influenza in Indonesia.* (2009). Available online at: www.steps-centre.org/publications (accessed February 25, 2021).
6. Ministry of Agriculture, National Coordination Meeting for Avian Influenza Control, Indonesia. *Evaluasi Pengendalian Avian Influenza Tahun 2006.* Surabaya (2006).
7. Pfeiffer DU, Minh PQ, Martin V, Epprecht M, Otte MJ. An analysis of the spatial and temporal patterns of highly pathogenic avian influenza occurrence in Vietnam using national surveillance data. *Vet J.* (2007) 174:302–9. doi: 10.1016/j.tvjl.2007.05.010

8. Henning J, Henning KA, Long NT, Ha NT, Vu LT, Meers J. Characteristics of two duck farming systems in the Mekong Delta of Viet Nam: stationary flocks and moving flocks, and their potential relevance to the spread of highly pathogenic avian influenza. *Trop Anim Health Prod.* (2013) 45:837–48. doi: 10.1007/s11250-012-0296-9
9. Henning J, Pfeiffer DU, Stevenson M, Yulianto D, Priyono W, Meers J. Who is spreading avian influenza in the moving duck flock farming network of Indonesia? *PLoS ONE.* (2016) 11:e0152123. doi: 10.1371/journal.pone.0152123
10. Meyer A, Dinh TX, Nhu TV, Pham LT, Newman S, Nguyen TTT, et al. Movement and contact patterns of long-distance free-grazing ducks and avian influenza persistence in Vietnam. *PLoS ONE.* (2017) 12:e0178241. doi: 10.1371/journal.pone.0178241
11. Gilbert M, Chaitaweesub P, Parakamawongsa T, Premashthira S, Tiensin T, Kalpravidh W, et al. Free-grazing ducks and highly pathogenic avian influenza, Thailand. *Emerg Infect Dis.* (2006) 12:227–34. doi: 10.3201/eid1202.050640
12. McLeod A, Kobayashi M, Gilman J, Siagian A, Young M. The use of poultry value chain mapping in developing HPAI control programmes. *Worlds Poult Sci J.* (2009) 65:217–23. doi: 10.1017/S0043933909000166
13. Songserm T, Jam-On R, Sae-Heng N, Meemak N, Hulse-Post DJ, Sturm-Ramirez KM, et al. Domestic ducks and H5N1 influenza epidemic, Thailand. *Emerg Infect Dis.* (2006) 12:575–81. doi: 10.3201/eid1204.051614
14. Sturm-Ramirez KM, Hulse-Post DJ, Govorkova EA, Humberd J, Seiler P, Puthavathana P, et al. Are ducks contributing to the endemicity of highly pathogenic H5N1 influenza virus in Asia? *J Virol.* (2005) 79:11269–79. doi: 10.1128/JVI.79.17.11269-11279.2005
15. Loth L, Gilbert M, Osmani MG, Kalam AM, Xiao X. Risk factors and clusters of highly pathogenic avian influenza H5N1 outbreaks in Bangladesh. *Prev Vet Med.* (2010) 96:104–13. doi: 10.1016/j.prevetmed.2010.05.013
16. Paul M, Tavornpanich S, Abrial D, Gasqui P, Charras-Garrido M, Thanapongtharm W, et al. Anthropogenic factors and the risk of highly pathogenic avian influenza H5N1: prospects from a spatial-based model. *Vet Res.* (2010) 41:2009076. doi: 10.1051/vetres/2009076
17. Stevens KB, Gilbert M, Pfeiffer DU. Modeling habitat suitability for occurrence of highly pathogenic avian influenza virus H5N1 in domestic poultry in Asia: a spatial multicriteria decision analysis approach. *Spat Spatiotemporal Epidemiol.* (2013) 4:1–14. doi: 10.1016/j.sste.2012.11.002
18. Yupiana Y, de Vlas SJ, Adnan NM, Richardus JH. Risk factors of poultry outbreaks and human cases of H5N1 avian influenza virus infection in West Java Province, Indonesia. *Int J Infect Dis.* (2010) 14:e800–5. doi: 10.1016/j.ijid.2010.03.014
19. Chen H, Smith GJD, Li KS, Wang J, Fan XH, Rayner JM, et al. Establishment of multiple sublineages of H5N1 influenza virus in Asia: implications for pandemic control. *Proc Natl Acad Sci USA.* (2006) 103:2845–50. doi: 10.1073/pnas.0511120103
20. Meyer A, Dinh TX, Han TA, Do DV, Nhu TV, Pham LT, et al. Trade patterns facilitating highly pathogenic avian influenza virus dissemination in the free-grazing layer duck system in Vietnam. *Transbound Emerg Dis.* (2018) 65:408–19. doi: 10.1111/tbed.12697
21. Si Y, de Boer WF, Gong P. Different environmental drivers of highly pathogenic avian influenza H5N1 outbreaks in poultry and wild birds. *PLoS ONE.* (2013) 8:e53362. doi: 10.1371/journal.pone.0053362
22. Zhang J, Jing W, Zhang W, Jin Z. Avian influenza A (H7N9) model based on poultry transport network in China. *Comput Math Methods Med.* (2018) 2018:7383170. doi: 10.1155/2018/7383170
23. Martin V, Forman A, Lubroth J. *FAO Animal Production and Health manual: Preparing for Highly Pathogenic Avian Influenza.* (2009). Available online at: http://www.fao.org/3/i0808e/i0808e.pdf (accessed February 25, 2021).
24. Bui CM, Adam DC, Njoto E, Scotch M, MacIntyre CR. Characterising routes of H5N1 and H7N9 spread in China using Bayesian phylogeographical analysis. *Emerg Microbes Infect.* (2018) 7:1–8. doi: 10.1038/s41426-018-0185-z
25. FAO. *Avian Influenza Control Programme in Indonesia - Annual Report 2010.* (2010). Available online at: http://www.fao.org/3/be823e/be823e.pdf (accessed February 25, 2021).
26. Kurscheid J, Millar J, Abdurrahman M, Ambarawati IGAA, Suadnya W, Yusuf RP, et al. Knowledge and perceptions of highly pathogenic avian influenza (HPAI) among poultry traders in live bird markets in Bali and Lombok, Indonesia. *PLoS ONE.* (2015) 10:e0139917. doi: 10.1371/journal.pone.0139917
27. Liao Q, Lam WWT, Bich TH, Dang VT, Fielding R. Comparison of behaviors regarding live poultry exposure among rural residents in Vietnam and Thailand. *J Infect Dev Ctries.* (2014) 8:526–34. doi: 10.3855/jidc.3545
28. Manabe T, Hanh TT, Lam DM, Van DTH, Thuy PTP, Thi Thanh Huyen D, et al. Knowledge, attitudes, practices and emotional reactions among residents of avian influenza (H5N1) hit communities in Vietnam. *PLoS ONE.* (2012) 7:e47560. doi: 10.1371/journal.pone.0047560
29. Brglez B, Hahn J. *Methods for Disposal of Poultry Carcasses. In: Avian Influenza.* Oxford, UK: Blackwell Publishing Ltd. (2009).
30. United States Environmental Protection Agency. *Carcass Management During Avian Influenza Outbreaks.* (2021). Available online at: https://www.epa.gov/homeland-security-waste/carcass-management-during-avian-influenza-outbreaks (accessed February 25, 2021).
31. US Agency for International Development Project. *Operational Research in Indonesia for More Effective Control of Highly Pathogenic Avian Influenza.* (2011). Available online at: https://cgspace.cgiar.org/bitstream/handle/10568/35218/ORI%20HPAI-FinalProjectReport.pdf?sequence=1&isAllowed=y (accessed February 25, 2021).
32. de Jong MD, Cam B Van, Qui PT, Hien VM, Thanh TT, Hue NB, et al. Fatal avian influenza A (H5N1) in a child presenting with diarrhea followed by coma. *N Engl J Med.* (2005) 352:686–91. doi: 10.1056/NEJMoa044307
33. Glanville W de, Idris S, Costard S, Unger F, Pfeiffer D. *A Quantitative Risk Assessment for the Onward Transmission of Highly Pathogenic Avian Influenza H5N1 From an Infected Small-Scale Broiler Farm in Bogor, West Java, Indonesia. Africa/Indonesia Team Working Paper.* (2010) p. 137. Report No.:23. Available online at: http://ebrary.ifpri.org/utils/getfile/collection/p15738coll2/id/8468/filename/8469.pdf (accessed November 6, 2019).
34. Rand Corporation. *Indonesian Family Life Survey (IFLS4) Survey Description.* (2007). Available online at: https://www.rand.org/well-being/social-and-behavioral-policy/data/FLS/IFLS/ifls4.html (accessed February 25, 2021).
35. Migheli M. Income, wealth and use of personal protectionequipment in the Mekong Delta. *Environ Sci Pollut Res.* (2021). 21:13449. doi: 10.1007/s11356-021-13449-w
36. Center for Indonesian Veterinary Analytical Studies. *A Review of Free Range Duck Farming Systems in Indonesia and Assessment of their Implication in the Spreading of the Highly Pathogenic (H5N1) Strain of Avian Influenza (HPAI).* (2006). Available online at: http://civas.net/2006/12/01/a-review-of-free-range-duck-farming-systems-in-indonesia-and-assessment-of-their-implication-in-the-spreading-of-the-highly-pathogenic-h5n1-strain-of-avian-influenza-hpai/?lang=en (accessed February 25, 2021).
37. Nguyen VL. *The Epidemiology of Avian Influenza in the Mekong River Delta of Viet Nam.* (PhD thesis). Massey University, Palmerston North, New Zealand. (2013). Available online at: https://www.massey.ac.nz/massey/fms/Colleges/College%20of%20Sciences/epicentre/Nguyen_Long_PhD_thesis.pdf?CF3E4C6A4FDFAA5604747A47F836AF9C (accessed February 25, 2021).
38. Kasim K, Salman D, Siregar AR, Nadja RA, Ahmad A. Vulnerability and adaptive strategies on duck breeder in Pinrang District, Indonesia. In: *IOP Conference Series: Earth and Environmental Science.* Pinrang (2019). p. 012046. doi: 10.1088/1755-1315/235/1/012046

Genetic Diversity of Bovine Pestiviruses Detected in Backyard Cattle Farms between 2014 and 2019 in Henan Province

Hongfei Shi [1], Huan Li [1], Yang Zhang [1], Lulu Yang [1], Yun Hu [1], Zhicheng Wang [1], Lisha Duan [1], Chaoliang Leng [1], Baolong Yan [2]* and Lunguang Yao [3]**

[1] Henan Provincial Engineering Laboratory of Insects Bio-reactor, Henan Provincal Engineering and Technology Center of Health Products for Livestock and Poultry, China-UK-NYNU-RRes Joint Library of Insect Biology, Nanyang Normal University, Nanyang, China, [2] Department of Parasitology, School of Basic Medical Sciences, Wenzhou Medical University, Wenzhou, China, [3] Henan Provincal Engineering and Technology Center of Health Products for Livestock and Poultry, Key Laboratory of Ecological Security and Collaborative Innovation Centre of Water Security for Water Source Region of Mid-line of South-to-North Diversion Project of Henan Province, School of Agricultural Engineering, Nanyang Normal University, Nanyang, China

***Correspondence:**
Hongfei Shi
kcn1@163.com;
504239031@qq.com
Baolong Yan
1982ybllog@163.com
Lunguang Yao
lunguangyao@163.com

Bovine pestiviruses include *Pestivirus A* (BVDV-1), *Pestivirus B* (BVDV-2), and *Pestivirus H*, which was originally called *HoBi-like pestivirus*. We conducted an epidemiological investigation for pestiviruses circulating in backyard cattle farms in central China. RT-PCR assays and sequences analysis were conducted on 54 nasal swabs, 26 serum samples, and three lung samples from cattle with respiratory infections and identified 29 pestivirus strains, including 24 *Pestivirus A* and five *Pestivirus H* strains. Phylogenetic analysis based on partial 5′-UTR and Npro sequences showed that the genotypes of 24 *Pestivirus A* strains included *Pestivirus A* 1b (six isolates), *Pestivirus A* 1m (six isolates), *Pestivirus A* 1q (two isolates), *Pestivirus A* 1u (one isolates), and *Pestivirus A* 1o (nine isolates, a putative new sub-genotype). In addition, a single *Pestivirus H* agenotype included all five *Pestivirus H* strains. This study revealed extensive genetic variations within bovine pestivirus isolates derived from cattle in backyard farms in Central China, and this epidemiological information improves our understanding of the epidemics of bovine Pestiviruses, as well as will be useful in designing and evaluating diagnostic methods and developing more effective vaccines.

Keywords: ***Pestivirus A*, *Pestivirus H*, cattle, genotype, China**

INTRODUCTION

Pestiviruses are single-stranded, positive-sense, enveloped RNA viruses with a genome of ~12.3 kb, which belong to the family *Flaviviridae*, genus *Pestivirus*. According to the proposed revision to its taxonomy, the *Pestivirus* genus includes 11 species, namely *Pestivirus A* (*bovine viral diarrhea virus 1*, BVDV-1), *Pestivirus B* (*bovine viral diarrhea virus 2*, BVDV-2), *Pestivirus C* (*classical swine fever virus*, CSFV) and *Pestivirus D* (*border disease virus*, BDV), *Pestivirus E* (*pronghorn pestivirus*), *Pestivirus F* (*Bungowannah virus*), *Pestivirus G* (*giraffe pestivirus*), *Pestivirus H* (*Hobi-like pestivirus*), *Pestivirus I* (*Aydin-like pestivirus*), *Pestivirus J* (*rat pestivirus*), and *Pestivirus K* (*atypical porcine pestivirus*) (1). Among these species, *Pestivirus A*, *Pestivirus B*, and *Pestivirus*

H aroused great concern because these cause significant economic losses in the cattle industry worldwide (2–4). *Pestivirus A* and *Pestivirus B* are major viruses associated with a number of clinical manifestations that range from mild to severe in feedlot cattle, including respiratory disease, digestive disease, and/or reproductive system disturbances and suppression of the immune system (5–7). Natural infections in cattle involving *Pestivirus H* showed similar clinical signs as those of *Pestivirus A* or *Pestivirus B* infections (8–11).

To date, at least 23 genotypes of *Pestivirus A* (12–16) and six genotypes (17) of *Pestivirus B* have been classified based on sequence comparison analyses and the palindromic nucleotide substitutions (PNS) genotyping method (18, 19). *Pestivirus H*, first isolated from fetal calf serum (20), has spread to different continents, including North America, South America, Europe, and Asia (21–26). In China, nine genotypes of *Pestivirus A* (1a,1b, 1c,1d, 1m, 1o, 1p,1q, and 1u) (27–30), two genotypes (2a, 2b) of *Pestivirus B* (31–33), and *Pestivirus H* (24, 34) have been reported. Cattle production by backyard farming is a widespread cattle-keeping pattern in developing countries. In central China, which includes Henan Province, more than 3,720,000 cattle have been raised (35), and previous data showed that over 20% of cattle were kept in small farms (cattle number <10), including a large number of backyard farms in China (36), especially in the southern region of Henan Province, where free-range cattle farms are key economic sectors (35). However, the limited biosecurity measures in these farms usually lead to the introduction and spread of exotic or endemic disease (37–39). Furthermore, in backyard cattle farms in China, most of the animals graze in the wilderness, and thus come into contact with infected cattle. To our knowledge, information on the epidemiology of pestiviruses in cattle in backyard farms in China is limited. The aim of this study was to investigate the distribution of pestiviruses that are associated with respiratory disease from backyard farms in Henan Province, China.

MATERIALS AND METHODS

Samples

From November 2014 to April 2019, a total of 54 nasal swabs and 26 serum samples were collected from different cattle in 41 backyard farms in Henan Province in Central China; these animals had never been vaccinated against *Pestivirus A* and were diagnosed with respiratory infections by rural veterinarians and treated with antibiotics for days, resulting in slow recovery. In addition, three lungs of deceased calves were collected in 2015, 2016, and 2018. All samples were stored at −80°C until analysis.

Primer Selection

The nested RT-PCR primers for genotyping bovine pestiviruses, including *Pestivirus A*, *Pestivirus B*, and *Pestivirus H* (40) were used to detect the pestivirus genome in the samples. For phylogenetic analysis, the BVDV-positive samples were further subjected to 5′-UTR and Npro RT-PCR using primers 324/326 (41) and BD1/BD2 (42), respectively. Because the sequences of *Pestivirus H*-positive samples were most closely related to the HN1507 strain (43), the positive samples further subjected to RT-PCR covering a partial 5′-UTR fragment and the entire Npro region with the primers HN-F (sense; 5′-CCTTCAGTAGGACGAGCATAA-3′) and HN-R (antisense; 5′- AGACGGGCTATACCACAATAA-3′), corresponding to nt 109–1,107 of *Pestivirus H* strain HN1507 (GenBank accession number: KU563155).

RNA Extraction, Amplification, and Sequencing

The three lung samples were first homogenized, then RNA was extracted from the lung homogenates, nasal swabs, and serum samples using an EasyPure Viral DNA/RNA Kit (Transgen Biotech, China) according to the manufacturer's instructions. The RNA was resuspended in DEPC-treated water and kept until analysis. cDNA was synthesized from RNA using Easyscript Reverse Transcriptase kit (Transgen Biotech, China) using random 9-mers as reverse transcription primer.

nRT-PCR to detect the pestivirus genome was performed as described elsewhere (40). Then, the BVDV-positive samples were further subjected to 5′-UTR and Npro RT-PCR earlier described (41, 42). The *Pestivirus H*-positive samples were subjected to RT-PCR in a 50-μL reaction mixture similar to the *Pestivirus A* reaction mixture according using the following conditions: reverse transcription at 50°C for 60 min, then denaturation at 93°C for 3 min; followed by 30 cycles of 94°C for 45 s, 56°C for 45 s, and 72°C for 1 min; and a final extension at 72°C for 10 min. Then the amplified products were recovered from the agarose gel using a gel extraction kit (Omega Bio-Tek, China), and the purified amplicons were directly sequenced in both directions using an ABI automated A373 sequencer (ABI, USA). Lastly, all of the sequences were compared to the NCBI databases using a BLAST search.

Phylogenetic Analysis

The nucleotide regions of the 5′-UTR were compared and aligned using CLUSTAL W program. Molecular Evolutionary Genetics Analysis version 6 (MEGA6) (44) was used for phylogeny inference according to the neighbor-joining criterion and the Kimura 2-parameter model. The robustness of the hypothesis was tested with 1000 non-parametric bootstrap analyses.

Following strains were used for 5′-UTR Phylogenetic analysis: NADL [M31182] and Singer [L32875] are the references for the Pestivirus A 1a genotype, strains Osloss [M96687], and Draper [L32880] are the references for the Pestivirus A 1b genotype and strains Europa [AB000898], and F [AF298065] are the reference for the Pestivirus A 1.3 genotype. Strains 438/02 [AY159540], PT42-03 [AY944293], 23-15 [AF298059], so CP/75 [AB042661], Shitara-02-06 [LC089876], IS25CP/01 [AB359931], AQGN96B15 [AB300691], Bega [AF049221], Manasi [EU159702], KM [AF298068], G [AF298066], SD0803 [JN400273], isolate 6 [JX276543], 10-84 [AF298054], 3186V6 [AF298062], 11207/98 [AJ304390], 22146/81 [AJ304376], 2561 [JQ920287], 17P [AF244954], KS86-1ncp [AB042713], Deer [AB040132], TR70 [MG670547], TR75 [MG670549], ZM-95[AF526381], TJ0801 [GU120255], BJ1305 [KF925505], XZ-24 [KJ578918], TR-2007-Gu-175454-4695 [EU716150], TR16 [MG670548], TR72 [MG670546], J [AF298067], W [AF298073],

BJ0702 [GU120248], BJ0703 [GU120249], A [AF298064], L [AF298069], CH-01-08 [EU180024], 71-03 [KF205294], PG/13a/07 [not deposited], GXBH-EB34 [KJ578813], GXLZ-BB4 [KJ578814], 130/15-4215 [KY085998], 130/15-5364 [KY085999], Rebe [AF299317], SuwaCp [AF117699], SuwaNcp [AF117700], CH-05-b1 [EU180030], and S153 [KF006964] are references for the Pestivirus A 1.4 to Pestivirus A 1.23.

Following strains were used for Npro Phylogenetic analysis: NADL [M31182], Oregon C24V [AF091605] and SD-1 [M96751] are the references for the Pestivirus A 1a genotype, strain Osloss [M96687] is the reference for the Pestivirus A 1b genotype. Strains F [AF287284], 10JJSKR [KC757383], 23/15 [AF287279], 58-1 [KF023454], 2541 [JQ920342], so CP/75 [AB105590] are references for the Pestivirus A 1.3, 1.5 and 1.6 genotypes. Strains IS25CP/01 [AB359931], IS26NCP/01 [AB359932], Bega [AF049221], 519 [AF144464], Deer-NZ1 [U80903], G [AF287285], CH-SM09/20 [AY895007], SD0803 [JN400273], isolate 6 [KC207072], 3186V6 [AF287282] and 26-V639 [AF287282] are references for the Pestivirus A 1.7 to Pestivirus A 1.11 genotypes. Strains Deer-GB1 [U80902] and KS86-1ncp [AB078950] are references for the genotypes Pestivirus A 1.13. Strains TR70 [KF154779], TR73 [KF154777] and TR75 [KF154778], reported as genotype R (Yesilbag et al., 2014), are references for genotype 1.14. Strains BJ1305 [KF925522], TJ0801 [GU120262] and ZM-95 [AF526381] are references for the genotype Pestivirus A 1.15. Strains TR16 [EU163964], TR27 [EU163975], TR29 [EU163977] and TR72 [KF154776] are references for the genotype Pestivirus A 1.16. Strains J [AF287286], W [AF287290], BJ0701 [GU120259], BJ0702 [GU120260], BJ0703 [GU120261], A [AF287283], L [AF287287], CH-01-08 [EU180033], 71-03 [KF205326], M31182 [JQ799141], 441/09 [KY040435], CH-Bohni [AY894997] and CH-Suwa [AY894998] are references for the Pestivirus A 1.17 to Pestivirus A 1.22 genotypes.

RESULTS

Using first-round nRT-PCR to identify bovine pestivirus by amplification of a 1,013-bp fragment, 83 samples were screened and the pestivirus genome was detected in 17 out of the 54 nasal swab samples, 10 out of the 26 serum samples, and two out of three lung samples. The results of the second-round nRT-PCR showed that in 17 positive nasal swab samples, 14 were positive for *Pestivirus A* and the other three were positive for *Pestivirus H*; in the 10 positive serum samples, nine were positive for *Pestivirus A* and one was positive for *Pestivirus H*; in the two positive lung samples, one was positive for *Pestivirus A* and the other was positive for *Pestivirus H*; no *Pestivirus B*-positive samples were detected. The 29 pestivirus-positive samples are presented in **Figure 1**.

The sequences detected by 5′-UTR and Npro RT-PCR in 24 BVDV-positive samples were deposited in GenBank under accession numbers: MN442360–MN442383 and MN442389–MN442412. Sequence alignment of the 5′-UTR and Npro region of the 24 samples using CLUSTAL W indicated a sequence identity within the range 82.0–100% and 70.0–99.8%, respectively. BLAST analysis of the 5′-UTR and Npro sequences showed that all 24 BVDV-positive isolates belonged to *Pestivirus A*. The comparative analysis among Henan isolates and the reference strains of *Pestivirus A* (NADL, VEDEVAC) shared a 5′-UTR and Npro region sequence identity within the range 82.9–98.8%, 72.2–97.6%, respectively.

The sequences detected by 5′-UTR and Npro RT-PCR in the five *Pestivirus H*-positive samples were deposited in GenBank as accession numbers MN442384–MN442388 and MN442413–MN442417. Sequence alignment using CLUSTAL W program of the five samples revealed a 5′-UTR and Npro region respective sequence identity within the range 95.8–99.5% and 98.4–99.6%. BLAST analysis of the 5′-UTR and Npro sequences showed that all five *Pestivirus H*-positive isolates belonged to *Pestivirus H*. Comparative analysis of the 5′-UTR and Npro region of the Henan isolates and the reference strains of *Pestivirus H* (TH/04_KhonKaen, HN1507) revealed a sequence identity within the range of 87.5–99.5% and 90.3.2–99.4%, respectively. In particular, the nucleotide homologies between these isolates and the other strain (HN1507) (24, 43) isolated from goat in the same area were 97.9±1.6% and 98.6 ± 0.4% in the above two regions.

All 24 isolates from the BVDV-positive samples were classified as *Pestivirus A*, and on the basis of phylogenetic analysis of 5′-UTR and Npro genes (**Figure 2**) further classified into five genotypes: *Pestivirus A* 1b (six isolates), *Pestivirus A* 1m (six isolates), *Pestivirus A* 1q (two isolates), *Pestivirus A* 1u (one isolate), and the other nine *Pestivirus A* isolates cluster in the same genotype with Chinese strain XH-2 which was assigned as *Pestivirus A* 1o, but phylogenetic analysis showed this cluster of isolates were under different cluster from other *Pestivirus A* 1o strains, further analyzed by the PNS software which available at www.pns-software.com (45), these cluster should be members of a new sub-genotype (1.7.2) within the genotype 1o (1.7). In addition, five isolates from *Pestivirus H*-positive samples were classified as *Pestivirus H*, and all further were classified into genotype "*Pestivirus H* a" based on the results of phylogenetic analysis of the 5′-UTR and Npro genes (46) (**Figure 2**).

DISCUSSION

China is one of the countries that have the largest domesticated ruminant population in the world, including a large number of backyard farms (35). In 2017, commercial *Pestivirus A or Pestivirus B* vaccines were released to the market. However, vaccination is not mandatory, and awareness of the importance of immunization to prevent Pestivirus infections among backyard farm keepers is rare, despite the occurrence of pestivirus epidemics in large-scale farms in China in recent years (27–29, 47). It is thus essential to investigate the genetic diversity of pestiviruses in backyard farms. Furthermore, the new genotype pestivirus might result in the immune failure of pestivirus vaccine (48). For these above reasons, the genetic diversity of 29 pestivirus-positive samples derived from infected calves in backyard farms from central China was investigated by phylogenetic analysis of the 5′-UTR and Npro partial genomic regions.

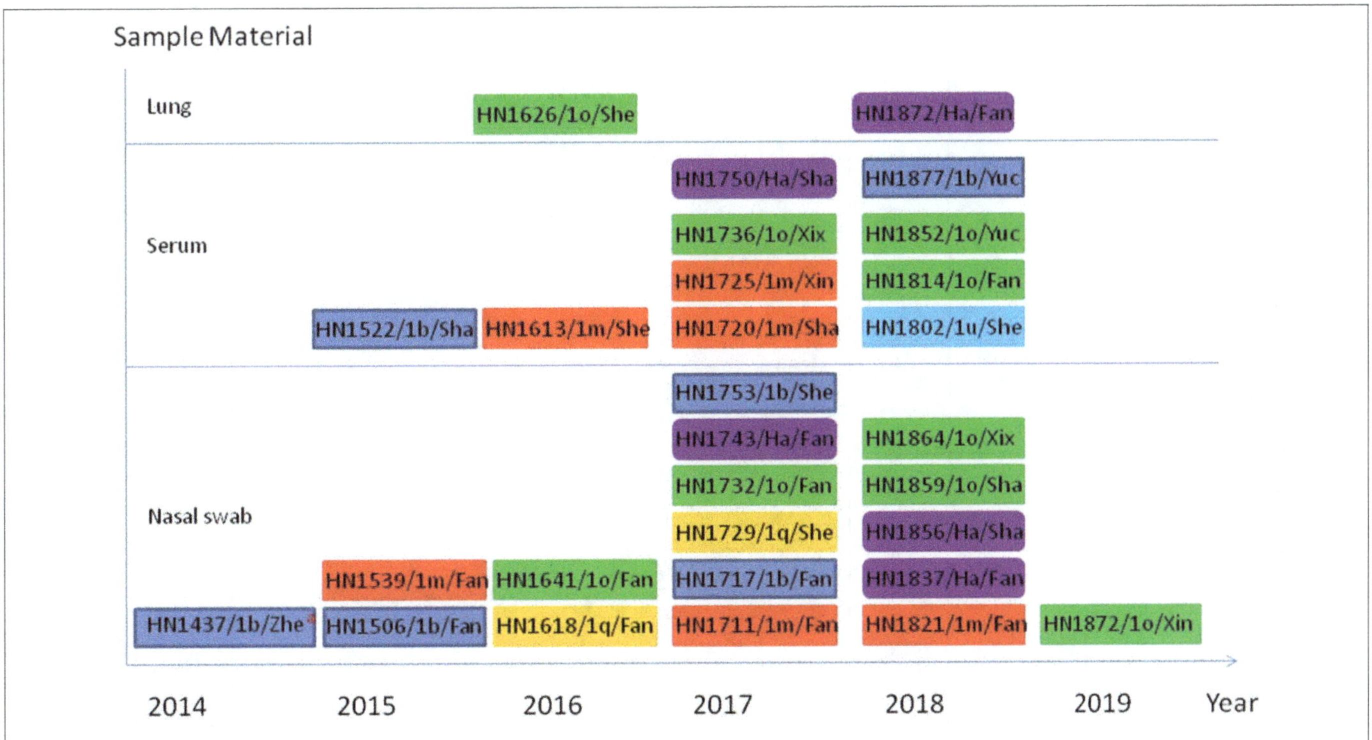

FIGURE 1 | Schematic representation of 29 bovine *Pestivirus* positive in this work. [a]indicate the information of sample including sample number/genotype/county. The county names: Zhe, Zhenping; Fan, Fangcheng; Sha, Shangcai; She, Sheqi; Xin, Xinye; Xix, Xixia; Yuc, Yucheng. The blue rectangle represents *Peativirus A* 1b genotype; the red rectangle represents *Peativirus A* 1m genotype; the yellow rectangle represents *Peativirus A* 1q genotype; the green rectangle represents *Peativirus A* 1o genotype; the light blue rectangle represents *Peativirus A* 1u genotype; the purple rounded rectangle represents *Peativirus H* a genotype.

The results of phylogenetic analysis showed that *Pestivirus A*−1o, *Pestivirus A*−1b, and *Pestivirus A*−1m were the predominant genotypes in our samples, followed by *Pestivirus A*−1q and *Pestivirus A*−1u. Furthermore, among these three predominant genotypes, *Pestivirus A*−1b and *Pestivirus A*−1m are frequently reported in China (27–30, 49, 50) the *Pestivirus A* 1a found in Henan province (51) was not detected in this work.

Six isolates of the *Pestivirus A* 1b genotype were detected in Zhenping, Fangcheng, Shangcai, Sheqi, and Yucheng in this study (**Figures 1, 2**). This widespread distribution of *Pestivirus A* is not surprising, as the first genotype of *Pestivirus A* was isolated in China in 1983. Subsequently, *Pestivirus A*−1b was later detected in most of the provinces, including Henan Province and the neighboring provinces numerous reports (27–29, 47, 49, 52–55). Meanwhile, a recent study has shown that 31.6% (2193:6939) of the corresponding *Pestivirus A* isolates around the world were *Pestivirus A*−1b (16). These reports indicate the strong spreading ability of *Pestivirus A*−1b among large-scale farms, and the high detection rate (6/24) in our study also suggests that *Pestivirus A*−1b is a predominant genotype among backyard farms.

Six isolates of the *Pestivirus A* 1m genotype were detected in Fangcheng, Sheqi, Shangcai, and Xinye in this study (**Figures 1, 2**). The first *Pestivirus A*−1m strain ZM-95 in China was isolated from pigs in 1995 (56). Subsequent reports revealed that *Pestivirus A*−1m is emerging in most of provinces and is considered to be a predominant *Pestivirus A* genotype in herds (27, 30, 50, 54, 57), and also detected in Henan province and neighbor province (29). In addition, sequences of *Pestivirus A*−1m strains in different regions showed high-nucleotide homology, indicating that these strains share the same origin (27, 49). Recently, other surveys on goats uncovered that the *Pestivirus A*−1m could infect goats naturally and cause diarrhea (58). In this study, *Pestivirus A* 1m strains were detected in different backyard farms that shared grassland with goats, this feeding method provided more chances for interspecies transmission of BVDV-1m, further accelerating the evolution of these viruses and more widely spreading disease.

The other nine *Pestivirus A* isolates shared the highest sequence identities (97–98%) in strains such as XH-6, XH-5, XH-1, XH-2, and BJ09 that were isolated from other provinces in China which was assigned as *Pestivirus A* 1o. Furthermore, the Npro sequences of these strains were not found in GenBank, and thus, confirmation could not be done based on the Npro phylogenetic tree analysis. The Npro sequences of the 21 isolates were also analyzed by BLAST, and the highest identities (86–91%) were observed in strain IS26/01ncp from Japan, and BJ0703, BJ0702, BJ0701, and JS12/02 that were isolated from other provinces including the Jiangsu province near to the Henan province in China and were classified as BVDV-1o or BVDV-1p (27, 58, 59). Then the PNS method was used to analyze the existing strain such as XH-2, then the genotype *Pestivirus A* 1.7 (1o) was verified, but the cluster in phylogenetic tree this cluster

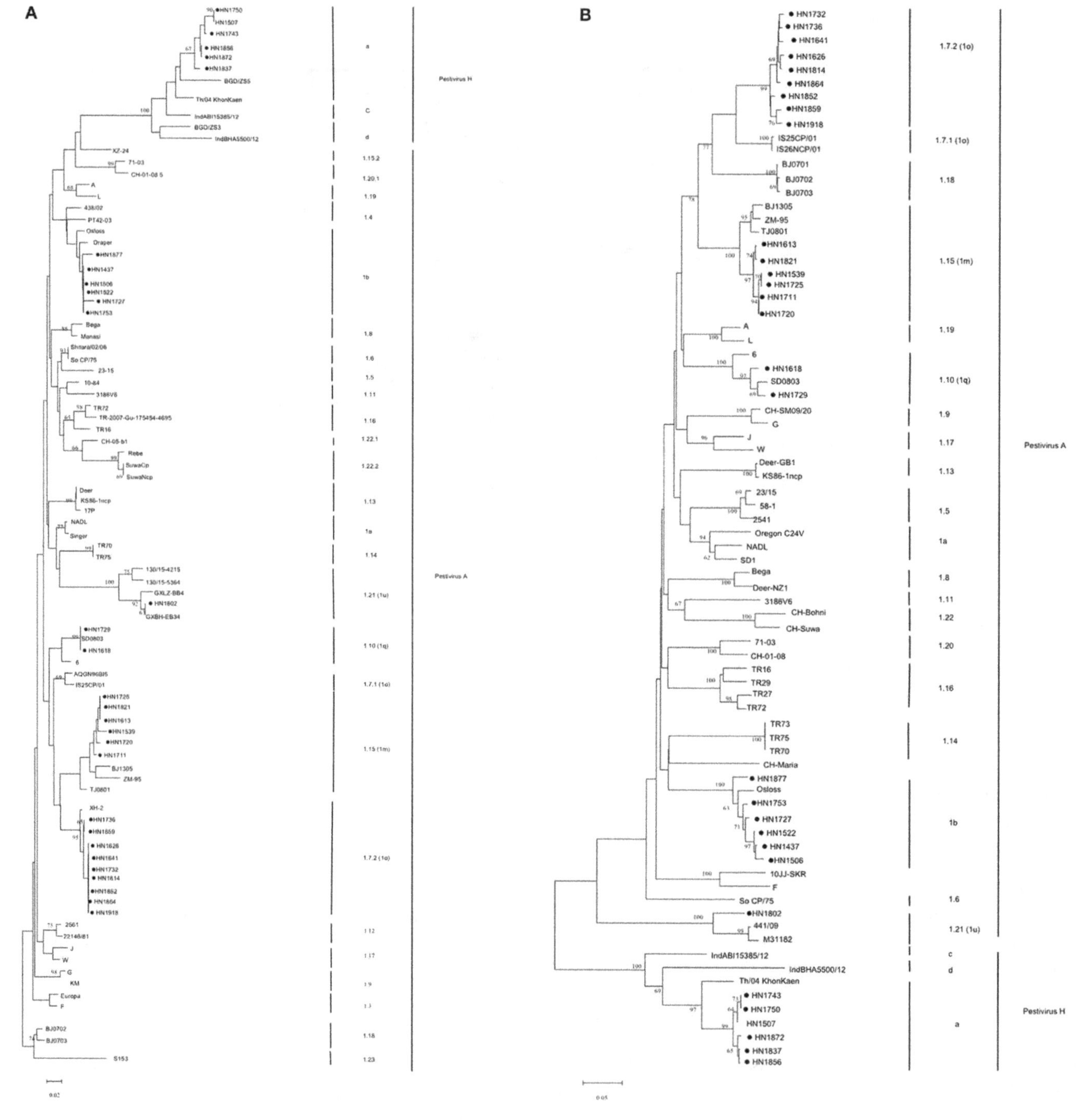

FIGURE 2 | Phylogenetic analysis of bovine *Pestivirus* from cattle in backyard farms in Central China, and reference strains using the 5′-UTR **(A)** and Npro **(B)** sequences. Bootstrap analyses that were supported by >60% of 1,000 replicates are indicated in nodes. Henan pestivirus isolates in this work are highlighted with a symbol (•).

was in different cluster from other *Pestivirus A* 1.7 (1o) strains, this result indicated these strains form a new sub-genotype (1.7.2). (**Figures 2A,B**). *Pestivirus A* 1o was first isolated from a calf that developed a mucosal disease and from PI calves in Japan (60), and has been detected in camels, goats, and pigs in China (30, 50, 58). In this study the new sub-genotype *Pestivirus A* 1o were detected in different backyard farms in a few of counties, and the *Pestivirus A* 1o could infect goats and sheep, it is in need that necessary measures should be taken to avoid this new sub-genotype *Pestivirus A* 1o spread in other hosts.

Five isolates of the *Pestivirus H* "a" genotype were detected in Fangcheng and Shangcai in this study (**Figures 1, 2**). Before this research, Pestivirus H has been previously detected in goats and sheep in Fangcheng (24), and phylogenetic analysis showed that these five isolates were closely related to the HN1507 strain isolated from goat (43). These results indicated that these isolates shared the same origin. Furthermore, considering that these strains were all isolated from animals raised in backyard farms where livestock commonly grazed in the mix, this specific feeding method provides a convenient route for interspecies transmission of *Pestivirus H*. To date, in China, *Pestivirus H* has been reported in contaminated cells, commercial FCS, goats, and sheep (24, 34, 61). This study showed that *Pestivirus H* could be detected in cattle immediately after being detected in goats and sheep in Central China (24).

Bovine pestivirus isolates in backyard farms exhibited a high level of genetic diversity, as indicated in the novel epidemic genotypes of *Pestivirus A* and *Pestivirus H* first emerging in cattle in China. These results indicate that backyard cattle farms could be a special reservoir for the evolution of bovine Pestivirus and provide an important complement to understand the epidemics of bovine Pestivirus. Furthermore, this study will be useful in designing and evaluating diagnostic methods and in developing more effective vaccines.

CONCLUSION

Several genotypes of *Pestivirus A* and *Pestivirus H* infections were identified in cattle with respiratory diseases and kept in backyard farms by RT-PCR, sequencing, and phylogenetic analysis. This is the first report on the molecular evidences on natural infections of *Pestivirus H* in cattle in China.

AUTHOR CONTRIBUTIONS

HS participated in the design of the study, and drafted the main parts of the manuscript. HL, YZ, and LYan participated in the sample collection and PCR detection. YH, ZW, LD, and CL participated in the data analyzing. BY and LYao participated in revised the manuscript and supervised the project.

ACKNOWLEDGMENTS

We thank LetPub (www.letpub.com) for its linguistic assistance during the preparation of this manuscript.

REFERENCES

1. Smith DB, Meyers G, Bukh J, Gould EA, Monath T, Scott Muerhoff A, et al. Proposed revision to the taxonomy of the genus pestivirus, family flaviviridae. *J Gen Virol.* (2017) 98:2106–12. doi: 10.1099/jgv.0.000873
2. Decaro N, Lucente MS, Losurdo M, Larocca V, Elia G, Occhiogrosso L, et al. HoBi-like pestivirus and its impact on cattle productivity. *Transbound Emerg Dis.* (2016) 63:469–73. doi: 10.1111/tbed.12529
3. Gates MC, Humphry RW, Gunn GJ, Woolhouse ME. Not all cows are epidemiologically equal: quantifying the risks of bovine viral diarrhoea virus (BVDV) transmission through cattle movements. *Vet Res.* (2014) 45:110. doi: 10.1186/s13567-014-0110-y
4. Pinior B, Firth CL, Richter V, Lebl K, Trauffler M, Dzieciol M, et al. A systematic review of financial and economic assessments of bovine viral diarrhea virus (BVDV) prevention and mitigation activities worldwide. *Prev Vet Med.* (2017) 137(Pt. A):77–92. doi: 10.1016/j.prevetmed.2016.12.014
5. Scharnbock B, Roch FF, Richter V, Funke C, Firth CL. A meta-analysis of Bovine Viral Diarrhoea Virus (BVDV) prevalences in the global cattle population. *Sci Rep.* (2018) 8:14420. doi: 10.1038/s41598-018-32831-2
6. Obritzhauser W, Baumgartner W, Kasbohrer A, Pinior B, Hancock AS, Younis PJ, et al. Infectious reproductive disease pathogens in dairy herd bulls. *Sci Rep.* (2015) 93:349–53. doi: 10.1038/s41598-018-32831-210.1111/avj.12369
7. Silveira S, Weber MN, Mosena AC, da Silva MS, Streck AF, Pescador CA, et al. Genetic diversity of brazilian bovine pestiviruses detected between 1995 and 2014. *Transbound Emerg Dis.* (2017) 64:613–23. doi: 10.1111/tbed.12427
8. Decaro N, Lanave G, Lucente MS, Mari V, Varello K, Losurdo M, et al. Mucosal disease-like syndrome in a calf persistently infected by Hobi-like pestivirus. *J Clin Microbiol.* (2014) 52:2946–54. doi: 10.1128/JCM.00986-14
9. Decaro N, Mari V, Pinto P, Lucente MS, Sciarretta R, Cirone F, et al. Hobi-like pestivirus: both biotypes isolated from a diseased animal. *J Gen Virol.* (2012) 93:1976–83. doi: 10.1099/vir.0.044552-0
10. Decaro N, Lucente MS, Mari V, Sciarretta R, Pinto P, Buonavoglia D, et al. Hobi-like pestivirus in aborted bovine fetuses. *J Clin Microbiol.* (2012) 50:509–12. doi: 10.1128/JCM.05887-11
11. Decaro N, Lucente MS, Mari V, Cirone F, Cordioli P, Camero M, et al. A typical pestivirus and severe respiratory disease in calves, Europe. *Emerg Infect Dis.* (2011) 17:1549–52. doi: 10.3201/eid1708.101447
12. Booth RE, Thomas CJ, El-Attar LM, Gunn G, Brownlie J. A phylogenetic analysis of Bovine Viral Diarrhoea Virus (BVDV) isolates from six different regions of the UK and links to animal movement data. *Vet Res.* (2013) 44:43. doi: 10.1186/1297-9716-44-43
13. Giangaspero M, Yesilbag K, Apicella C. Who's who in the Bovine viral diarrhea virus type 1 species: genotypes L and R. *Virus Res.* (2018) 256:50–75. doi: 10.1016/j.virusres.2018.07.009
14. Vilcek S, Durkovic B, Kolesarova M, Paton DJ. Genetic diversity of BVDV: consequences for classification and molecular epidemiology. *Prev Vet Med.* (2005) 72:31–5. doi: 10.1016/j.prevetmed.2005.08.004
15. Vilcek S, Paton DJ, Durkovic B, Strojny L, Ibata G, Moussa A, et al. Bovine viral diarrhoea virus genotype 1 can be separated into at least eleven genetic groups. *Arch Virol.* (2001) 146:99–115. doi: 10.1007/s007050170194
16. Yesilbag K, Alpay G, Becher P. Variability and global distribution of subgenotypes of bovine viral diarrhea virus. *Viruses.* (2017) 9:128. doi: 10.3390/v9060128
17. Giangaspero M, Decaro N, Turno P, Apicella C, Gargano P, Buonavoglia C. Pathogen spread and globalization: the case of pestivirus heterogeneity in southern Italy. *Res Vet Sci.* (2019) 125:100–12. doi: 10.1016/j.rvsc.2019.05.017
18. Harasawa R, Giangaspero M. A novel method for pestivirus genotyping based on palindromic nucleotide substitutions in the 5'-untranslated region. *J Virol Methods.* (1998) 70:225–30. doi: 10.1016/s0166-0934(97)00180-8
19. Giangaspero M, Harasawa R. Numerical taxonomy of the genus pestivirus based on palindromic nucleotide substitutions in the 5' untranslated region. *J Virol Methods.* (2007) 146:375–88. doi: 10.1016/j.jviromet.2007.07.009
20. Schirrmeier H, Strebelow G, Depner K, Hoffmann B, Beer M. Genetic and antigenic characterization of an atypical pestivirus isolate, a putative member of a novel pestivirus species. *J Gen Virol.* (2004) 85:3647–52. doi: 10.1099/vir.0.80238-0
21. Silveira S, Falkenberg SM, Elderbrook MJ, Sondgeroth KS, Dassanayake RP, Neill JD, et al. Serological survey for antibodies against pestiviruses in Wyoming domestic sheep. *Vet Microbiol.* (2018) 219:96–9. doi: 10.1016/j.vetmic.2018.04.019
22. Flores EF, Cargnelutti JF, Monteiro FL, Bauermann FV, Ridpath JF, Weiblen R. A genetic profile of bovine pestiviruses circulating in Brazil (1998–2018). *Anim Health Res Rev.* (2018) 19:134–41. doi: 10.1017/s1466252318000130

23. Lanave G, Decaro N, Lucente MS, Guercio A, Cavaliere N, Purpari G, et al. Circulation of multiple subtypes of bovine viral diarrhoea virus type 1 with no evidence for HoBi-like pestivirus in cattle herds of southern Italy. *Infect Genet Evol.* (2017) 50:1–6. doi: 10.1016/j.meegid.2017.02.009
24. Shi H, Kan Y, Yao L, Leng C, Tang Q, Ji J, et al. Identification of natural infections in sheep/Goats with HoBi-like pestiviruses in China. *Transbound Emerg Dis.* (2016) 63:480–4. doi: 10.1111/tbed.12551
25. Mishra N, Rajukumar K, Pateriya A, Kumar M, Dubey P, Behera SP, et al. Identification and molecular characterization of novel and divergent HoBi-like pestiviruses from naturally infected cattle in India. *Vet Microbiol.* (2014) 174:239–46. doi: 10.1016/j.vetmic.2014.09.017
26. Decaro N, Mari V, Lucente MS, Sciarretta R, Elia G, Ridpath JF, et al. Detection of a Hobi-like virus in archival samples suggests circulation of this emerging pestivirus species in Europe prior to (2007). *Vet Microbiol.* (2013) 167:307–13. doi: 10.1016/j.vetmic.2013.09.006
27. Xue F, Zhu YM, Li J, Zhu LC, Ren XG, Feng JK, et al. Genotyping of bovine viral diarrhea viruses from cattle in China between 2005 and (2008). *Vet Microbiol.* (2010) 143:379–83. doi: 10.1016/j.vetmic.2009.11.010
28. Gong X, Liu L, Zheng F, Chen Q, Li Z, Cao X, et al. Molecular investigation of bovine viral diarrhea virus infection in yaks (*Bos gruniens*) from Qinghai, China. *Virol J.* (2014) 11:29. doi: 10.1186/1743-422x-11-67
29. Deng M, Ji S, Fei W, Raza S, He C, Chen Y, et al. Prevalence study and genetic typing of bovine viral diarrhea virus (BVDV) in four bovine species in China. *PLoS ONE.* (2015) 10:e0121718. doi: 10.1371/journal.pone.0121718
30. Gao S, Luo J, Du J, Lang Y, Cong G, Shao J, et al. Serological and molecular evidence for natural infection of Bactrian camels with multiple subgenotypes of bovine viral diarrhea virus in Western China. *Vet Microbiol.* (2013) 163:172–6. doi: 10.1016/j.vetmic.2012.12.015
31. Zhu LQ, Lin YQ, Ding XY, Ren M, Tao J, Wang JY, et al. Genomic sequencing and characterization of a Chinese isolate of Bovine viral diarrhea virus 2. *Acta Virol.* (2009) 53:197–202. doi: 10.4149/av_2009_03_197
32. Tao J, Wang Y, Wang J, Wang JY, Zhu GQ. Identification and genetic characterization of new bovine viral diarrhea virus genotype 2 strains in pigs isolated in China. *Virus Genes.* (2013) 46:81–7. doi: 10.1007/s11262-012-0837-3
33. Zhu LQ, Ren M, Lin YQ, Ding XY, Zhang GP, Zhao X, et al. Identification of a bovine viral diarrhea virus 2 isolated from cattle in China. *Acta Virol.* (2009) 53:131–4. doi: 10.4149/av_2009_02_131
34. Mao L, Li W, Zhang W, Yang L, Jiang J. Genome sequence of a novel Hobi-like pestivirus in China. *Virol J.* (2012) 86:12444. doi: 10.1128/JVI.02159-12
35. N. National Bureau of statistics of China. *No. of Livestock and Poultry.* (2017). Available online at: http://data.stats.gov.cn/easyquery.htm?cn=E0103
36. A. Agricultural Commodity Production Cost and Return Data. *Agricultural Commodity Production Cost and Return Data.* Beijing: China Statistical Publisher (2009).
37. Pires FA, Peterson A, Baron JN, Adams R, Martinez-Lopez B, Moore D. Small-scale and backyard livestock owners needs assessment in the western United States. *PLoS ONE.* (2019) 14:e0212372. doi: 10.1371/journal.pone.0212372
38. Hernandez-Jover M, Schembri N, Holyoake PK, Toribio JL, Martin PA. A comparative assessment of the risks of introduction and spread of foot-and-mouth disease among different pig sectors in Australia. *Front Vet Sci.* (2016) 3:85. doi: 10.3389/fvets.2016.00085
39. Kuster K, Cousin ME, Jemmi T, Schupbach-Regula G, Magouras I. Expert opinion on the perceived effectiveness and importance of on-farm biosecurity measures for cattle and swine farms in Switzerland. *PLoS ONE.* (2015) 10:e0144533. doi: 10.1371/journal.pone.0144533
40. Decaro N, Sciarretta R, Lucente MS, Mari V, Amorisco F, Colaianni ML, et al. A nested PCR approach for unambiguous typing of pestiviruses infecting cattle. *Mol Cell Probes.* (2012) 26:42–6. doi: 10.1016/j.mcp.2011.11.003
41. Vilcek S, Herring AJ, Herring JA, Nettleton PF, Lowings JP, Paton DJ. Pestiviruses isolated from pigs, cattle and sheep can be allocated into at least three genogroups using polymerase chain reaction and restriction endonuclease analysis. *Arch Virol.* (1994) 136:309–23.
42. Vilcek S, Nettleton PF, Paton DJ, Belak S. Molecular characterization of ovine pestiviruses. *J Gen Virol.* (1997) 78:725–35. doi: 10.1099/0022-1317-78-4-725
43. Shi H, Leng C, Xu Q, Shi H, Sun S, Kan Y, et al. Characterization of a pestivirus H isolate originating from goats. *Virus Genes.* (2018) 54:603–7. doi: 10.1007/s11262-018-1579-7
44. Tamura K, Stecher G, Peterson D, Filipski A, Kumar S. MEGA6: Molecular Evolutionary Genetics Analysis version 6.0. *Mol Biol Evol.* (2013) 30:2725–9. doi: 10.1093/molbev/mst197
45. Giangaspero M, Apicella C, Harasawa R. Numerical taxonomy of the genus pestivirus: new software for genotyping based on the palindromic nucleotide substitutions method. *J Virol Methods.* (2013) 192:59–67. doi: 10.1016/j.jviromet.2013.04.023
46. Silveira S, Baumbach LF, Weber MN, A.Mosena CS, da Silva MS, Cibulski SP, et al. HoBi-like is the most prevalent ruminant pestivirus in Northeastern Brazil. *Transbound Emerg Dis.* (2018) 65:e113–20. doi: 10.1111/tbed.12689
47. Gong X, Cao X, Zheng F, Chen Q, Zhou J, Yin H, et al. Identification and characterization of a novel subgenotype of bovine viral diarrhea virus isolated from dairy cattle in Northwestern China. *Virus Genes.* (2013) 46:375–6. doi: 10.1007/s11262-012-0861-3
48. Ridpath JF. Bovine viral diarrhea virus: global status. *Vet Clin North Am Food Anim Pract.* (2010) 26:105–21. doi: 10.1016/j.cvfa.2009.10.007
49. Weng XG, Song QJ, Wu Q, Liu MC, Wang ML, Wang JF. Genetic characterization of bovine viral diarrhea virus strains in Beijing, China and innate immune responses of peripheral blood mononuclear cells in persistently infected dairy cattle. *J Vet Sci.* (2015) 16:491–500. doi: 10.4142/jvs.2015.16.4.491
50. Deng Y, Sun CQ, Cao SJ, Lin T, Yuan SS, Zhang HB, et al. High prevalence of bovine viral diarrhea virus 1 in Chinese swine herds. *Vet Microbiol.* (2012) 159:490–3. doi: 10.1016/j.vetmic.2012.04.023
51. Wang W, Shi X, Tong Q, Wu Y, Xia MQ, Ji Y, et al. A bovine viral diarrhea virus type 1a strain in China: isolation, identification, and experimental infection in calves. *Virol J.* (2014) 11:8. doi: 10.1186/1743-422x-11-8
52. Zhang S, Tan B, Ding Y, Wang F, Guo L, Wen Y, et al. Complete genome sequence and pathogenesis of bovine viral diarrhea virus JL-1 isolate from cattle in China. *BioMed Res Int.* (2014) 11:67. doi: 10.1155/2014/147145/10.1186/1743-422x-11-67
53. Xie Z, Fan Q, Xie Z, Liu J, Pang Y, Deng X, et al. Complete genome sequence of a bovine viral diarrhea virus strain isolated in southern china. *Genome Announc.* (2014) 2:e00512–14. doi: 10.1128/genomeA.00512-14
54. Zhong F, Li N, Huang X, Guo Y, Chen H, Wang X, et al. Genetic typing and epidemiologic observation of bovine viral diarrhea virus in Western China. *Virus Genes.* (2011) 42:204–7. doi: 10.1007/s11262-010-0558-4
55. Wang L, Wu X, Wang C, Song C, Bao J, Du J. Origin and transmission of bovine viral diarrhea virus type 1 in China revealed by phylodynamic analysis. *Res Vet Sci.* (2020) 128:162–9. doi: 10.1016/j.rvsc.2019.11.015
56. Wang X, Tu C, Li H, Jin K, Xuan H, Chang G, et al. Detection and isolation of bovine viral diarrhea virus from classical swine fever suspected pigs. *Chinese J Vet Sci.* (1996) 16:341–5.
57. Zhu L, Lu H, Cao Y, Gai X, Guo C, Liu Y, et al. Molecular characterization of a novel Bovine viral diarrhea virus isolate SD-15. *PLoS ONE.* (2016) 11:e0165044. doi: 10.1371/journal.pone.0165044
58. Mao L, Li W, Yang L, Wang J, Cheng S, Wei Y, et al. Primary surveys on molecular epidemiology of bovine viral diarrhea virus 1 infecting goats in Jiangsu province, China. *BMC Vet Res.* (2016) 12:181. doi: 10.1186/s12917-016-0820-7
59. Sato A, Tateishi K, Shinohara M, Naoi Y, Shiokawa M, Aoki H, et al. Complete genome sequencing of bovine viral diarrhea virus 1, subgenotypes 1n and 1o. *Genome Announc.* (2016) 4:e01744–15. doi: 10.1128/genomeA.01744-15
60. Nagai M, Hayashi M, Itou M, Fukutomi T, Akashi H, Kida H, et al. Identification of new genetic subtypes of bovine viral diarrhea virus genotype 1 isolated in Japan. *Virus Genes.* (2008) 36:135–9. doi: 10.1007/s11262-007-0190-0
61. Gao S, Du J, Tian Z, Xing S, Chang H, Liu G, et al. Genome analysis of an atypical bovine pestivirus from fetal bovine serum. *Virus Genes.* (2016) 52:561–3. doi: 10.1007/s11262-016-1321-2

14

The Distribution and Localization of Collagen Triple Helix Repeat Containing-1 in Naturally and Experimentally Avian Leukosis Virus Subgroup J-Infected Chickens

Yu Pang [1], Defang Zhou [1], Jing Zhou [1], Jingwen Xue [1], Yiya Wang [2] and Ziqiang Cheng [1]**

[1] *College of Veterinary Medicine, Shandong Agricultural University, Tai'an, China,* [2] *School of Life Sciences, Qilu Normal University, Jinan, China*

***Correspondence:**
Ziqiang Cheng
czqsd@126.com
Yiya Wang
wangyiyaxwz@126.com*

Collagen triple helix repeat containing-1 (CTHRC1) has recently been identified as avian leukosis virus subgroup J (ALV-J) replication-dependent factor that remarkably facilitates ALV-J replication via interaction with the envelope glycoprotein (SU) of ALV-J. However, the dynamic distribution and localization of CTHRC1 in various tissues upon ALV-J infection are still unknown. In this study, data revealed that the levels of CTHRC1 were significantly increased in various tissues and that the protein was mainly located in the cytoplasm and nucleus of parenchymal cells in tissues of chickens that were infected by ALV-J naturally and experimentally. Interestingly, CTHRC1 was also observed in leukocytes other than erythrocytes in congested veins of ALV-J-infected tissues. Consequently, the positive cells in these veins were confirmed as lymphocytes by laser confocal microscopy. Taken together, these results conclude that the CTHRC1 is an inducible protein and exhibited ubiquitous expression in ALV-J-infected chickens, which may provide basic information for in-depth study of ALV-J infection and replication mechanisms.

Keywords: ALV-J, Cthrc1, IHC, Myelocytomas, Poultry

INTRODUCTION

Avian leukosis virus subgroups (ALVs) belonging to type C *retroviruses* are generally divided into seven subgroups (A–E, J, and K) (1–3). It is noteworthy that since isolation of the first strain (HPRS-103) from meat-type chickens in the United Kingdom in the late 1980s, more attention has been focused on the J subgroup of ALV (ALV-J), which caused high mortality, wide host ranges, and strong tumorigenicity (4, 5). Thus, it is absolutely imperative that the strategies should be implemented to prevent and control ALV-J infection in poultry industry. Attributed to the implementation of ALV-J eradication program (6), there were rarely reports of ALV-J or myelocytomatosis in China after 2013. Nevertheless, there were another intensive reports about ALV-J breakout almost simultaneously in six provinces of China in 2018, which attracted our attention (7). It is rather remarkable that there were extensive medullary-like tumor cells in the bone marrow, liver, and kidney, and all of the neoplasms were myelocytomas (7).

In recent years, a variety of studies have explored that collagen triple helix repeat containing-1 (CTHRC1) highly related to collagen synthesis was remarkably up-regulated in solid tumors (8–10), including hepatocellular carcinoma (11, 12), oral squamous cell carcinoma (13, 14), gastric carcinogenesis (9, 15), ductal carcinoma (16), and colorectal cancer (17–19), and that the expression abundance of CTHRC1 was significant low in normal tissues. CTHRC1 is a highly conserved cancer-secreted glycosylated protein; human CTHRC1 shares 80% sequence identity with the *Gallus* homolog, which was discovered in a screening for differentially expressed genes in a rat model of balloon-injured vasculature (15, 20–22). Thus far, the studies of CTHRC1 focus on the field of oncology; there is rare coverage on the role of CTHRC1 in the field of viral replication. Recently, we have firstly reported that CTHRC1 facilitates ALV-J replication through interaction with the SU protein of ALV-J, which indicates that CTHRC1 plays a crucial role in regulating ALV-J replication (23). These studies may provide new enlightenment to the study of interaction between host protein(s) and ALV-J, and these expand the biological function of CTHRC1 in the field of virus replication (23). However, the distribution and expression of CTHRC1 in chicken tissues upon ALV-J infection are still unknown, which may provide a theoretical basis for the subsequent research of ALV-J and CTHRC1.

In the study, we investigated for the first time the expression and distribution of CTHRC1 in chickens that were infected with ALV-J naturally and experimentally. Interestingly, we found that ALV-J could infect with lymphocytes and activate the expression of CTHRC1 in the lymphocytes.

MATERIALS AND METHODS

Virus, Antibodies, and Experimental Animals

ALV-J strain GM0209 was isolated from a broiler breeder maintained in our laboratory (7). Monoclonal antibody directed against ALV-J SU protein was produced as described previously (23, 24). Rabbit polyclonal antibody against CTHRC1 was purchased from Absin Corporation (Shanghai, China). Specific pathogen free (SPF) chick embryos were acquired from the SPAFAS Corporation (Jinan, China; a joint venture with Charles River Lab, Wilmington, MA, USA). Chick embryos were incubated in an SPF environment at the Laboratory Animal and Resources Facility, Shandong Agricultural University. Chick embryos were inoculated with ALV-J (GM0209 strain) via allantoic cavity at the sixth embryonic age, with the titer of $10^{3.8}$ tissue culture infective dose ($TCID_{50}$)/0.1 ml. Chicks then were euthanized at 15, 22, and 35 days post-infection. Chick heart, liver, kidney, spleen, lung, brain, duodenum, proventriculus, and bone marrow (thymus and bursa of Fabricius will not be discussed in this article) were collected and fixed in 4% formaldehyde solution. Animal experimental protocols were approved by the Shandong Agricultural University Animal Care and Use Committee (permit No. SDAU 19-098; July 8, 2019).

Tissue Information of Natural Avian Leukosis Virus Subgroup J-Infected Chickens

ALV-J infection broke out in Jiangsu, Shandong, Henan, Hebei, Heilongjiang, and Guangdong provinces of China in February 2018 (7). On-site, a total of 19,500 Ross broiler breeder chickens aged 15–20 weeks suffered from depression, paralysis, and weight loss. Tissues samples including the liver, kidney, and bone marrow were collected from broiler breeder flocks in Gaomi and Binzhou. Samples were verified that the case was only ALV-J infection by performing hematoxylin and eosin (HE) staining and PCR (7).

Immunohistochemistry Staining

The tissue microarray glass slides were prepared using the tissues of naturally and experimentally ALV-J-infected chickens and normal chickens. Then, the tissue microarray glass slides were dried at 60°C for 30 min and then deparaffinized gradually through xylene, 50% xylene, and gradient concentrations of ethanol until being immersed in water (25). Chicken tissue sections were blocked for peroxidase activity with 0.3% hydrogen peroxide for 40 min. Antigen retrieval was performed through boiling in 10 mmol/L citrate buffer (pH 6.0) for 25 min. Then the tissues were incubated with anti-CTHRC1 antibody (1:100 dilution) at 4°C for 12 h. The tissues were washed with phosphate-buffered saline (PBS) for three times and incubated with horseradish peroxidase (HRP)-labeled anti-rabbit secondary antibody (1:500 dilution) for 70 min at 37°C. Immunostaining was performed by using diaminobenzidine substrate chromogen method. Tissues were immersed in hematoxylin for cell nuclear staining. The slides were then dehydrated via gradient concentrations of ethanol, cleared with xylene, and cover slipped with neutral balsam (Shenggong, Shanghai, China) (26).

Immunofluorescence Staining

Lymphocytes and erythrocytes were separated from the peripheral blood of ALV-J-infected and normal chickens. Lymphocytes and erythrocytes were fixed with 4% paraformaldehyde and then permeabilized with methanol for 20 min prior to the addition of primary antibody (anti-mouse ALV-J SU protein and anti-rabbit CTHRC1) and incubation at 37°C for 60 min. These two types of cells then were washed in Tris-buffered saline-Tween 20, followed by incubation with Alexa Fluor 488-conjugated donkey anti-rabbit or 594-conjugated donkey anti-mouse antibodies. Cell nuclei were stained with 4′,6-diamidino-2-phenylindole (DAPI). Finally, lymphocytes and erythrocytes were mixed in a 1:1 ratio. Fluorescent images were obtained with a confocal laser scanning microscope (Leica SP8).

Reverse Transcription and Quantitative Real-Time PCR and PCR

Total RNA was extracted from cells according to manufacturer instructions (Qiagen), and RNA concentration was measured using a spectrophotometer (Qiagen). We used 1 μg of total RNA as a template to synthesize cDNA using a

TABLE 1 | Primer used for real-time PCR.

Name	Sequence (5′-3′)	Reference or GenBank
GAPDH	F: GAACATCATCCCAGCGTCCA	(23)
	R: CGGCAGGTCAGGTCAACAAC	
CTHRC1	F: ACGCTG GCTTGGTGGA	(23)
	R: CAGTTCTTCAATGATGATACGG	
ALV-A	F: GATGTTCACTTACTCGAGC	GenBank: MF926337.1
	R: CGTTTACGTCTTATACCTG	
ALV-B	F: ATGTCCACTTACTCGAGCA	GenBank: KC282901.1
	R: TCGTTTGCGTCTTATACCTG	
ALV-J	F: AACAGGTTACATCTGAGCAAGC	GenBank: DQ115805.1
	R: TGTTCCATTGTCATCGCTAACG	
ALV-K	F: CTCGAGCAGCCAGGGAAC	GenBank: KY581580.1
	R: CTTCGTTTACGTCTTATACC	
MDV	F: GCCTTTTATACACAAGAGCCGAG	(27)
	R: TTTATCGCGGTTGTGGGTCATG′	
REV	F: CATACTGGAGCCAATGGTT	(28)
	R: AATGTTGTAGCGAAGTACT	

reverse transcriptase kit (TaKaRa, Shiga, Japan) according to manufacturer instructions. A SYBR Green I kit (TaKaRa) was used for cDNA amplification in a total volume of 20 μl. CTHRC1-specific primers and glyceraldehyde 3-phosphate dehydrogenase (GAPDH), a housekeeping gene, are shown in **Table 1**. A LightCycler 96 system (Roche, Basel, Switzerland) was used for qPCR with the following cycling conditions: denaturation at 95°C for 30 s, followed by 40 cycles at 95°C for 5 s, and 60°C for 34 s. A melting curve was generated at 95°C for 10 s, 65°C for 60 s, and 97°C for 1 s. CTHRC1 levels were analyzed using the $2^{-\Delta\Delta Ct}$ method. Total RNA was extracted from clinical case, and then RNA is reverse transcribed into cDNA. PCR was performed according to the manufacturer's instructions of PrimeSTAR HS DNA Polymerase with GC Buffer (Takara, Japan) (PCR primer is shown in **Table 1**).

ELISA

Virus isolated from clinical cases was inoculated into DF-1 cells, where are a continuous chicken embryonic fibroblast cell line that exhibits normal fibroblastic morphology and is free of endogenous sequences related to leukosis viruses and avian sarcoma (29). Importantly, DF-1 cells are capable of sustaining ALV-J replication, and the cell supernatant was collected at different time points. ELISA kits (SenBeiJia, Nanjing, China) (http://www.sbjbio.com/Products/P1.html) were used to measure CTHRC1 levels in cell supernatant, according to manufacturer instructions. Each experiment included three biological replicates.

Statistical Analysis

All data are reported as the mean ± standard error of the mean (SEM). Prism 7.0 software (GraphPad Software, San Diego, CA, USA) was used to determine statistically significant differences by performing a two-tailed unpaired Student's *t*-test. Differences between groups were considered statistically significant when the *p*-value was less than 0.05 ($^{*}p < 0.05$; $^{**}p < 0.01$; $^{***}p < 0.001$).

RESULTS

The Expression of Collagen Triple Helix Repeat Containing-1 Is Increased in Naturally and Experimentally Avian Leukosis Virus Subgroup J-Infected Chickens

Data obtained from previous studies of our lab indicated that the chickens from farms were only infected with ALV-J (7). According to Zhou et al. (7), the virus was isolated from the samples of kidneys of tumor-bearing chickens from farms (29). In order to detect the purity of the virus that we isolated, PCR was performed. The results of PCR indicated that all tumor-bearing chickens forming a clinical case were positive for ALV-J and negative for ALV-A, ALV-B, ALV-K, REV, and MDV (**Supplementary Figures 1A–F**) (7).

The expression of CTHRC1 is low in normal tissues, which can be activated with the stimulation of certain pathogens (30, 31). Then, we detected the expression of CTHRC1 in the liver, kidney, and bone marrow of naturally ALV-J-infected chickens. As shown in **Figure 1A**, the levels of CTHRC1 were remarkably up-regulated in the tissues of naturally ALV-J-infected chickens, and the expression of CTHRC1 was mainly and widely distributed with the parenchymal parts of organs, compared with the normal tissues of the same age of SPF chickens. CTHRC1 is widely expressed in the tissues of clinical cases infected with ALV-J. In order to further clarify that CTHRC1 is an inducible protein upon ALV-J infection, we inoculated the virus of isolated into DF-1 cells and then tested whether ALV-J up-regulated the expression of CTHRC1. The results showed that CTHRC1 was elevated upon ALV-J infection (**Figures 1B,C**).

In order to accurately clarify the dynamic distribution of CTHRC1 in various organs upon ALV-J infection and the expression of CTHRC1 with the extension of infection time, SPF chick embryos were inoculated with ALV-J in the allantoic cavity on the 6th day of incubation, and then chicks were euthanized at 15, 22, and 35 days post-infection. As shown in **Figure 1D**, the levels of CTHRC1 were obviously raised upon ALV-J infection than those of normal SPF chickens. Meanwhile, we found that CTHRC1 was mainly expressed in the parenchymal cells of the tissues than those of the interstitial cells of tissues. It was worth noting that the expression of CTHRC1 was lower in the spleen than those of other organs, such as the heart, liver, kidney, lung, brain, duodenum, the proventriculus; and the expression of CTHRC1 featured high intensity in the Purkinje cells of the brain tissue.

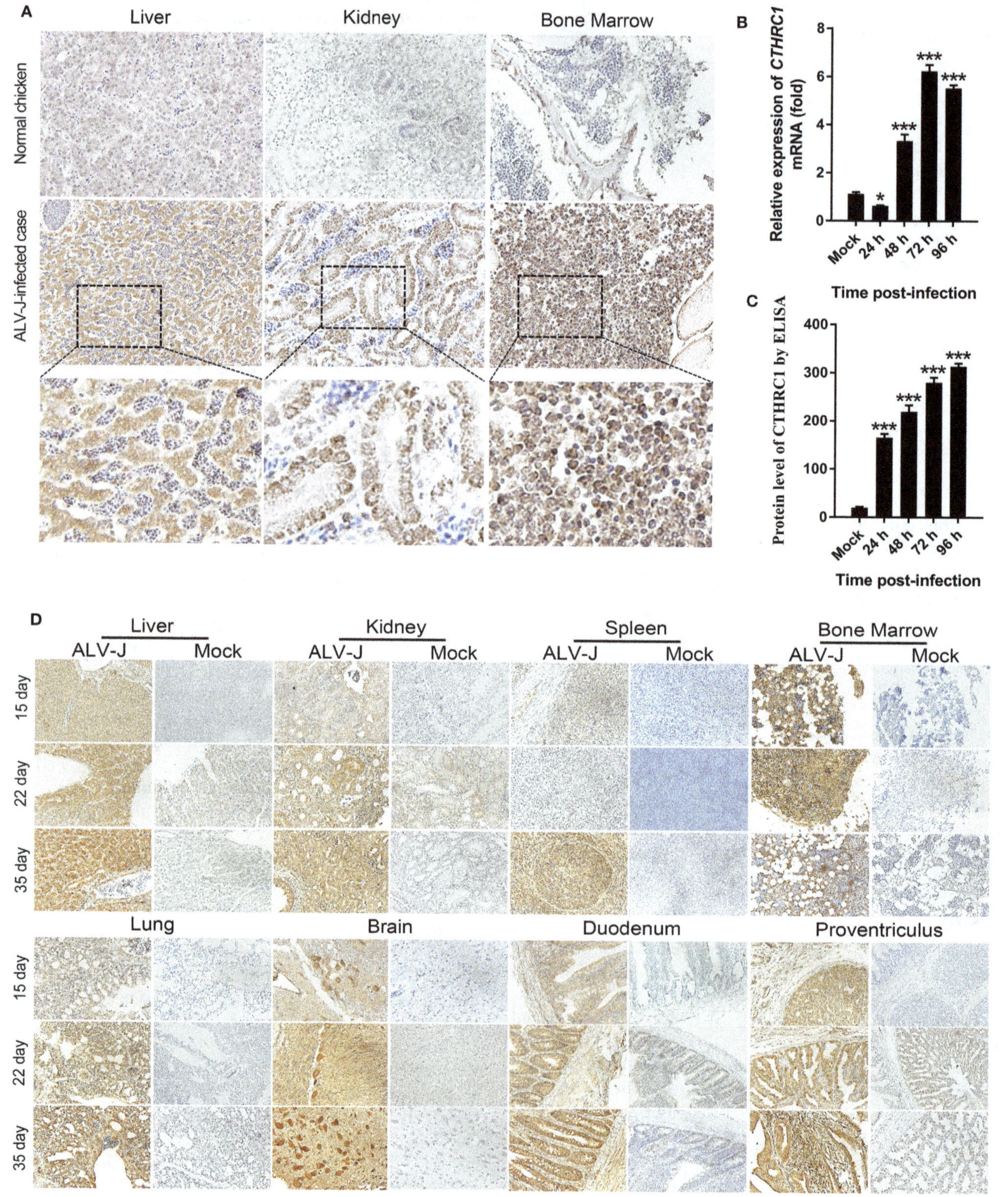

FIGURE 1 | Avian leukosis virus subgroup J (ALV-J) infection facilitates collagen triple helix repeat containing-1 (CTHRC1) expression *in vivo*. Immunohistochemical staining of tissues of naturally **(A)** and experimentally **(D)** ALV-J-infected chickens with the CTHRC1 antibody. The CTHRC1 protein was weakly stained in normal tissues. In contrast, CTHRC1 staining was moderate to strong in ALV-J-infected tissues. Original magnification, 400×. **(B)** Total RNA was extracted from ALV-J-infected and uninfected DF-1 cells. CTHRC1 mRNA was measured by qPCR. **(C)** CTHRC1 protein levels were measured by ELISA in supernatant from ALV-J infected and uninfected DF-1 cells. $^{*}p < 0.05$; $^{***}p < 0.001$.

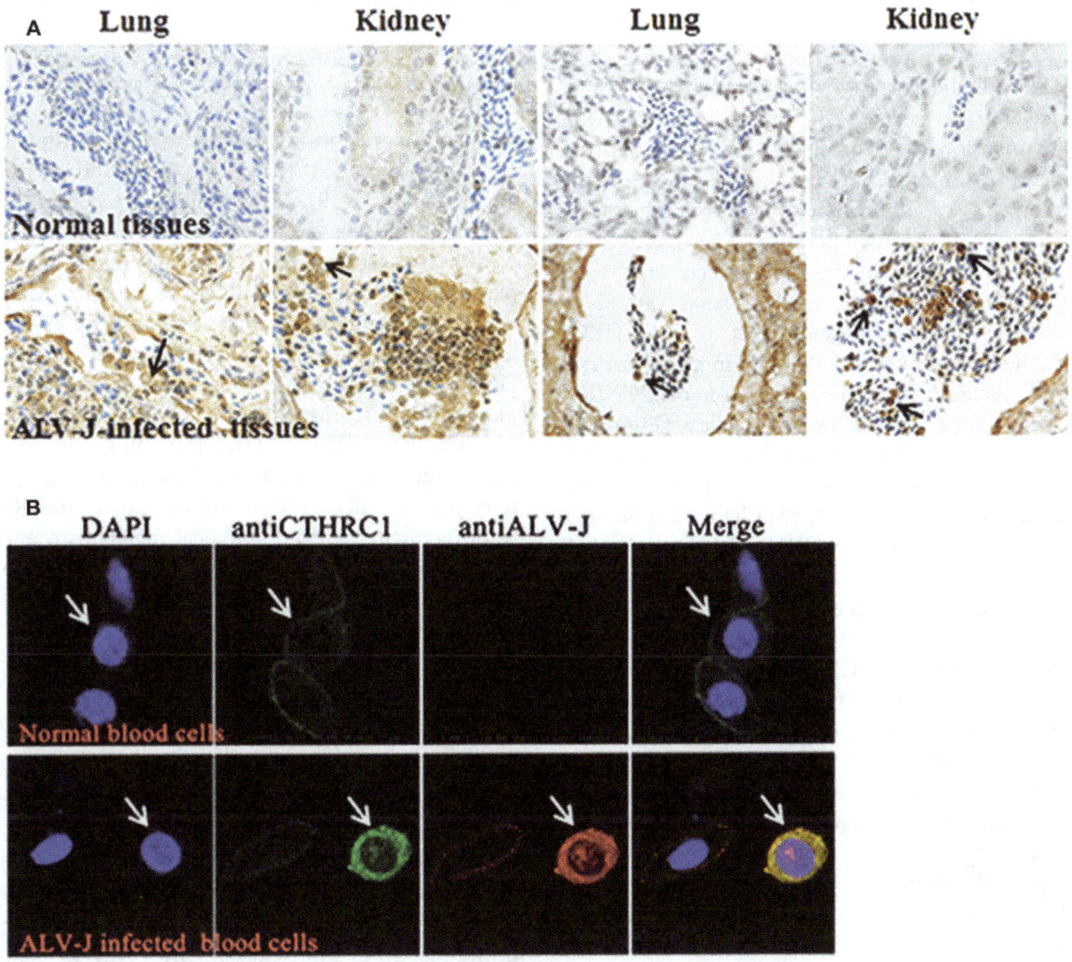

FIGURE 2 | Avian leukosis virus subgroup J (ALV-J) activates the expression of collagen triple helix repeat containing-1 (CTHRC1) in blood lymphocytes **(A)**. The CTHRC1 protein was strongly stained in certain blood cells tested by the immunohistochemistry (IHC) assay. (The lungs and kidneys are derived from different ALV-J-infected chickens.) **(B)** Lymphocytes and erythrocytes isolated from the blood of ALV-J-infected chicken. Cells were fixed for an immunofluorescence assay to detect ALV-J (red) and CTHRC1 (green) with primary antibodies. Nuclei were counterstained with 4′,6-diamidino-2-phenylindole (DAPI) (blue). Fluorescent images were acquired with a confocal laser scanning microscope (Leica SP8). White arrows indicate lymphocytes.

Collagen Triple Helix Repeat Containing-1 Is Activated in Blood Lymphocytes of Avian Leukosis Virus Subgroup J-Infected Chickens

Interestingly, during immunohistochemistry (IHC), we found that CTHRC1 was stained in certain blood cells of congested veins and that erythrocytes were not stained. Thus, we speculated that the stained cells were lymphocytes according to cell morphology (**Figure 2A**). To further identify the stained blood cells, lymphocytes, and erythrocytes were isolated from blood of ALV-J-infected chickens and normal chickens to exactly explore the phenomenon by laser confocal assay. As shown in **Figure 2B**, CTHRC1 was mainly located in the cytoplasm and was activated in the blood lymphocytes of ALV-J infected chickens than those of normal chickens. CTHRC1 was interacted with ALV-J SU protein and co-localized in the cytoplasm (23), which was in line with our results obtained in **Figure 2B** that CTHRC1 and ALV-J were co-located in the cytoplasm of lymphocytes. Meanwhile, according to Cui et al. (1999), ALV-J was not infected with erythrocytes of blood, which only transport ALV-J, but it can infect lymphocytes of blood (32). In our study, we found that ALV-J was only located in the cell membrane of erythrocytes (**Figure 2B**), which was coincident with results obtained in previous studies.

DISCUSSION

CTHRC1, as a host-cell protein, plays a significant role in facilitating ALV-J infection (23). Here, we explored the distribution and localization of CTHRC1 in tissues of chickens that were infected with ALV-J naturally and experimentally. Meanwhile, utilizing IHC and laser confocal assay, we found that

CTHRC1 was activated in blood lymphocytes of ALV-J infection, which meant that ALV-J can infect lymphocytes.

In this study, we found that the expression of CTHRC1 gradually elevated with the extensive infection of ALV-J tested by the IHC assay. Furthermore, ALV-J-infected samples with deeper depths of invasion showed higher levels of CTHRC1, illustrating that CTHRC1 may have an irreplaceable role in ALV-J pathogenicity. It was important to note that the result was further substantiated through *in vitro* experiments (23). Therefore, CTHRC1, a candidate tumor marker, may be a potential metastasis-related gene in myelocytomas caused by ALV-J. Moreover, it was a remarkable fact that CTHRC1 staining in ALV-J-infected tissues was strongly intensely located in cytoplasm and nucleus, while the expression of CTHRC1 in normal chicken tissues was of weak intensity (**Figure 1**). CTHRC1 is a secreted-extracellular protein (9). Pyagay et al. (33) found that CTHRC1 may experience proteolytic process, which could acquire the activity of the molecule (31). Thus, it is possible that the secreted form of CTHRC1 overproduced through ALV-J-infection may act on the surrounding microenvironment, including the stromal cells and extracellular matrix (ECM), which elevates tumor invasion and migration. Previous studies have described that the level of CTHRC1 was very low in normal tissues, which was consistent with results obtained in **Figure 1**.

For young animals, the bone marrow in the marrow cavity is mainly red bone marrow, whose main function is to produce hematopoietic stem cells. The red bone marrow in the marrow cavity is gradually replaced with age by yellow bone marrow, whose main component is fat that is not stained by IHC (34). As shown in **Figure 2B**, after 35 days of ALV-J infection, the staining of CTHRC1 was slightly decreased, which may be because the red bone marrow in the marrow cavity is gradually replaced by the yellow bone marrow. Nowadays, effort has mainly been concentrated on the tumorigenic mechanism of ALV-J (7, 35).

As shown in **Figure 1**, compared with other structures of the kidney, the renal tubule is highly colored, which shows that the renal tubule highly expresses CTHRC1 after being infected with ALV-J. Enhanced expression of CTHRC1 could restrict collagen type I and III deposition (33, 36). Meanwhile, the inhibition of the expression of collagen types I and III could alter the host membrane permeability, which could promote viral replication (37). It is well-known that the kidney is the main target organ of ALV-J. It is newly revealed that the high expression of CTHRC1 in renal tubules is caused by ALV-J infection.

ALV-J belonging to an avian C type *retrovirus* can integrate into the host genome to induce tumor and immunological tolerance by impairment in the effect of host lymphocytes, which was consistent with results obtained in **Figure 2B** (32, 38). It can be observed that ALV-J could activate CTHRC1 in blood lymphocytes, but not in erythrocytes (**Figures 2A,B**), which indicated that CTHRC1 might be involved in immunological tolerance induced by ALV-J by impairing lymphocyte function. Here, CTHRC1 was found in the blood lymphocytes of ALV-J-infected SPF chickens, which revealed that it may be a potential key factor influencing ALV-J infection and production.

CTHRC1 was widely up-regulated in multiple human tumors, such as cancers of the liver, pancreas, and gastrointestinal tract and melanoma (39). Meanwhile, the recombinant of CTHRC1 protein could elevate the capacities of invasion and migration of primary gastrointestinal stromal tumors (40). Thus, CTHRC1 plays a vital role in the fields of human tumor (21). ALV-J, MDV, and REV, as the three major neoplastic diseases, cause huge economic losses to the poultry industry every year (35). However, how to prevent and control these three diseases still plague many workers. Our research found that CTHRC1 was activated upon ALV-J (23), MDV, and REV infection through proteomic analysis (data not shown), and we speculated that it may play a crucial role in ALV-J, MDV, and REV replication, tumorigenicity, and pathological mechanism and that it might also become a common target for the prevention and control of ALV-J, MDV, and REV infection. Additionally, CTHRC1 may serve as a common effective biomarker for evaluating the poor clinical pathological characteristics of ALV-J, MDV, and REV infection. In the future, we will investigate the effect of CTHRC1 on ALV-J, MDV, and REV replication, tumorigenicity, and pathological mechanism.

In conclusion, our current study revealed that CTHRC1, as an invasion-driving protein, was widely activated in the parenchymal cells of tissues of ALV-J-infected natural and experimental cases. CTHRC1 was up-regulated in blood lymphocytes, which may be associated with the immunosuppression caused by ALV-J. Thus, combined with previous studies, this research may provide precise information for in-depth study of ALV-J infection and replication mechanisms.

AUTHOR CONTRIBUTIONS

ZC and YP conceived and designed the experiments. YP performed the experiments. YP, DZ, JX, and JZ analyzed the data. ZC, YW, and YP wrote the paper. All authors contributed to the article and approved the submitted version.

ACKNOWLEDGMENTS

We are grateful to the teacher of Li Zhang for providing the necessary infrastructure facilities for the study.

REFERENCES

1. Fan Z, Hu X, Zhang Y, Yu C, Qian K, Qin A. Proteomics of DF-1 cells infected with avian leukosis virus subgroup J. *Virus Res.* (2012) 167:314–21. doi: 10.1016/j.virusres.2012.05.016
2. Sun Y, Chen X, Zhang L, Liu H, Liu S, Yu H, et al. The antiviral property of Sargassum fusiforme polysaccharide for avian leukosis virus subgroup J *in vitro* and *in vivo*. *Int J Biol Macromol.* (2019) 138:70–8. doi: 10.1016/j.ijbiomac.2019.07.073
3. Li X, Lin W, Chang S, Zhao P, Zhang X, Liu Y, et al. Isolation, identification and evolution analysis of a novel subgroup of avian leukosis virus isolated from a local Chinese yellow broiler in South China. *Arch Virol.* (2016) 161:2717–25. doi: 10.1007/s00705-016-2965-x
4. Payne LN, Howes K, Gillespie AM, Smith LM. Host range of Rous sarcoma virus pseudotype RSV (HPRS-103) in 12 avian species: support for a new avian retrovirus envelope subgroup, designated J. *J Gen Virol.* (1992) 73 (Pt 11):2995–7. doi: 10.1099/0022-1317-73-11-2995
5. Payne LN, Brown SR, Bumstead N, Howes K, Frazier JA, Thouless ME. A novel subgroup of exogenous avian leukosis virus in chickens. *J Gen Virol.* (1991) 72 (Pt 4):801–7. doi: 10.1099/0022-1317-72-4-801
6. Li Y, Cui S, Li W, Wang Y, Cui Z, Zhao P, et al. Vertical transmission of avian leukosis virus subgroup J (ALV-J) from hens infected through artificial insemination with ALV-J infected semen. *BMC Vet Res.* (2017) 13:204. doi: 10.1186/s12917-017-1122-4
7. Zhou D, Xue J, Zhang Y, Wang G, Feng Y, Hu L, et al. Outbreak of myelocytomatosis caused by mutational avian leukosis virus subgroup J in China, 2018. (2019) 66:622–6. doi: 10.1111/tbed.13096
8. Ma Z, Chao F, Wang S, Song Z, Zhuo Z, Zhang J, et al. CTHRC1 affects malignant tumor cell behavior and is regulated by miR-30e-5p in human prostate cancer. *Biochem Biophys Res Commun.* (2020) 525:418–24. doi: 10.1016/j.bbrc.2020.02.098
9. Wang P, Wang YC, Chen XY, Shen ZY, Cao H, Zhang YJ, et al. CTHRC1 is upregulated by promoter demethylation and transforming growth factor-β 1 and may be associated with metastasis in human gastric cancer. *Cancer Sci.* (2012) 103:1327–33. doi: 10.1111/j.1349-7006.2012.02292.x
10. Liu Y, Abulimiti N, Wang C. Collagen triple helix repeat containing 1 expression in osteosarcoma: a new predictor of prognosis. *Ann Clin Lab Sci.* (2018) 48:338–44. Available online at: http://www.annclinlabsci.org/content/48/3/338.full
11. Zhang R, Cao Y, Bai L, Zhu C, Li R, He H, et al. The collagen triple helix repeat containing 1 facilitates hepatitis B virus-associated hepatocellular carcinoma progression by regulating multiple cellular factors and signal cascades. *Mol Carcinog.* (2015) 54:1554–66. doi: 10.1002/mc.22229
12. Tameda M, Sugimoto K, Shiraki K, Yamamoto N, Okamoto R, Usui M, et al. Collagen triple helix repeat containing 1 is overexpressed in hepatocellular carcinoma and promotes cell proliferation and motility. *Int J Oncol.* (2014) 45:541–8. doi: 10.3892/ijo.2014.2445
13. Liu G, Sengupta PK, Jamal B, Yang HY, Bouchie MP, Lindner V, et al. N-glycosylation induces the CTHRC1 protein and drives oral cancer cell migration. *J Biol Chem.* (2013) 288:20217–27. doi: 10.1074/jbc.M113.473785
14. Lee CE, Vincent-Chong VK, Ramanathan A, Kallarakkal TG, Karen-Ng LP, Ghani WM, et al. Collagen triple helix repeat containing-1 (CTHRC1) expression in oral squamous cell carcinoma (OSCC): prognostic value and clinico-pathological implications. *Int J Med Sci.* (2015) 12:937–45. doi: 10.7150/ijms.11605
15. Yu J, Feng J, Zhi X, Tang J, Li Z, Xu Y, et al. Let-7b inhibits cell proliferation, migration, and invasion through targeting Cthrc1 in gastric cancer. *Tumour Biol.* (2015) 36:3221–9. doi: 10.1007/s13277-014-2950-5
16. Kim JH, Baek TH, Yim HS, Kim KH, Jeong SH, Kang HB, et al. Collagen triple helix repeat containing-1 (CTHRC1) expression in invasive ductal carcinoma of the breast: the impact on prognosis and correlation to clinicopathologic features. *Pathol Oncol Res.* (2013) 19:731–7. doi: 10.1007/s12253-013-9636-y
17. Tan F, Liu F, Liu H, Hu Y, Liu D, Li G. CTHRC1 is associated with peritoneal carcinomatosis in colorectal cancer: a new predictor for prognosis. *Med Oncol.* (2013) 30:473. doi: 10.1007/s12032-013-0473-3
18. Ni S, Ren F, Xu M, Tan C, Weng W, Huang Z, et al. CTHRC1 overexpression predicts poor survival and enhances epithelial-mesenchymal transition in colorectal cancer. *Cancer Med.* (2018) 7:5643–54. doi: 10.1002/cam4.1807
19. Yang XM, You HY, Li Q, Ma H, Wang YH, Zhang YL, et al. CTHRC1 promotes human colorectal cancer cell proliferation and invasiveness by activating Wnt/PCP signaling. *Int J Clin Exp Pathol.* (2015) 8:12793–801.
20. Bian Z, Miao Q, Zhong W, Zhang H, Wang Q, Peng Y, et al. Treatment of cholestatic fibrosis by altering gene expression of Cthrc1: implications for autoimmune and non-autoimmune liver disease. *J Autoimmun.* (2015) 63:76–87. doi: 10.1016/j.jaut.2015.07.010
21. Bai L, Zhang W, Tan L, Yang H, Ge M, Zhu C, et al. Hepatitis B virus hijacks CTHRC1 to evade host immunity and maintain replication. *J Mol Cell Biol.* (2015) 7:543–56. doi: 10.1093/jmcb/mjv048
22. Li Y, Zhou J, Wang J, Chen X, Zhu Y, Chen Y. Mir-30b-3p affects the migration and invasion function of ovarian cancer cells by targeting the CTHRC1 gene. *Biol Res.* (2020) 53:10. doi: 10.1186/s40659-020-00277-4
23. Pang Y, Zhou D, Xue J, Zhou J, Zhang Y, Zheng G, et al. Interplay between CTHRC1 and the SU protein of avian leukosis virus subgroup J (ALV-J) facilitates viral replication. *Virus Res.* (2019) 264:32–9. doi: 10.1016/j.virusres.2019.02.014
24. Zhou D, Xue J, He S, Du X, Zhou J, Li C, et al. Reticuloendotheliosis virus and avian leukosis virus subgroup J synergistically increase the accumulation of exosomal miRNAs. *Retrovirology.* (2018) 15:45. doi: 10.1186/s12977-018-0427-0
25. Maity B, Sheff D, Fisher RA. Immunostaining: detection of signaling protein location in tissues, cells and subcellular compartments. *Methods Cell Biol.* (2013) 113:81–105. doi: 10.1016/B978-0-12-407239-8.00005-7
26. Miller RT. Avoiding pitfalls in diagnostic immunohistochemistry-important technical aspects that every pathologist should know. *Semin Diagn Pathol.* (2019) 36:312–35. doi: 10.1053/j.semdp.2019.05.002
27. Silva RF. Differentiation of pathogenic and non-pathogenic serotype 1 Marek's disease viruses (MDVs) by the polymerase chain reaction amplification of the tandem direct repeats within the MDV genome. *Avian Dis.* (1992) 36:521–8. doi: 10.2307/1591744
28. Aly MM, Smith EJ, Fadly AM. Detection of reticuloendotheliosis virus infection using the polymerase chain reaction. *Avian Pathol.* (1993) 22:543–54. doi: 10.1080/03079459308418942
29. Himly M, Foster DN, Bottoli I, Iacovoni JS, Vogt PK. The DF-1 chicken fibroblast cell line: transformation induced by diverse oncogenes and cell death resulting from infection by avian leukosis viruses. *Virology.* (1998) 248:295–304. doi: 10.1006/viro.1998.9290
30. Tano K, Mizuno R, Okada T, Rakwal R, Shibato J, Masuo Y, et al. MALAT-1 enhances cell motility of lung adenocarcinoma cells by influencing the expression of motility-related genes. *FEBS Lett.* (2010) 584:4575–80. doi: 10.1016/j.febslet.2010.10.008
31. Wu Q, Yang Q, Sun H. Role of collagen triple helix repeat containing-1 in tumor and inflammatory diseases. *J Cancer Res Ther.* (2017) 13:621–4. doi: 10.4103/jcrt.JCRT_410_17
32. Dai M, Li S, Shi K, Liao J, Sun H, Liao M. Systematic identification of host immune key factors influencing viral infection in PBL of ALV-J infected SPF chicken. *Viruses.* (2020) 12:114. doi: 10.3390/v12010114
33. Pyagay P, Heroult M, Wang Q, Lehnert W, Belden J, Liaw L, et al. Collagen triple helix repeat containing 1, a novel secreted protein in injured and diseased arteries, inhibits collagen expression and promotes cell migration. *Circ Res.* (2005) 96:261–8. doi: 10.1161/01.RES.0000154262.07264.12
34. Vishnyakov A, Udavliev D, Timofeev D, Kvan O. Evaluation of bone marrow hemopoiesis and the elemental status of the red bone marrow of chickens under introduction of copper to the organism. *Environ Sci Pollut Res Int.* (2020) 27:17393–400. doi: 10.1007/s11356-020-08161-0
35. Li H, Wang P. The emergence of the infection of subgroup J avian leucosis virus escalated the tumour incidence in commercial Yellow chickens in Southern China in recent years. *Transbound Emerg Dis.* (2019) 66:312–6. doi: 10.1111/tbed.13023
36. Shekhani MT, Forde TS, Adilbayeva A, Ramez M, Myngbay A, Bexeitov Y, et al. Collagen triple helix repeat containing 1 is a new promigratory marker of arthritic pannus. *Arthritis Res Ther.* (2016) 18:171. doi: 10.1186/s13075-016-1067-1

37. Martinez-Gil L, Bano-Polo M, Redondo N, Sanchez-Martinez S, Nieva JL, Carrasco L, et al. Membrane integration of poliovirus 2B viroporin. *J Virol.* (2011) 85:11315–24. doi: 10.1128/JVI.05421-11
38. Ye F, Wang Y, He Q, Cui C, Yu H, Lu Y, et al. Exosomes transmit viral genetic information and immune signals may cause immunosuppression and immune tolerance in ALV-J infected HD11 cells. *Int J Biol Sci.* (2020) 16:904–20. doi: 10.7150/ijbs.35839
39. Tang L, Dai DL, Su M, Martinka M, Li G, Zhou Y. Aberrant expression of collagen triple helix repeat containing 1 in human solid cancers. *Clin Cancer Res.* (2006) 12:3716–22. doi: 10.1158/1078-0432.CCR-06-0030
40. Ma MZ, Zhuang C, Yang XM, Zhang ZZ, Ma H, Zhang WM, et al. CTHRC1 acts as a prognostic factor and promotes invasiveness of gastrointestinal stromal tumors by activating Wnt/PCP-Rho signaling. *Neoplasia (New York, NY).* (2014) 16:265–78.e1–13. doi: 10.1016/j.neo.2014.03.001

15

A Pilot Study to Investigate the Feasibility of a Multiple Locus Variable Number Tandem Repeat Analysis to Understand the Epidemiology of *Dichelobacter nodosus* in Ovine Footrot

Katharina Giebel[1,2], Laura E. Green[3†] and Kevin J. Purdy[1†]*

[1] School of Life Sciences, University of Warwick, Coventry, United Kingdom, [2] School of Agriculture, Food and the Environment, Royal Agricultural University, Gloucestershire, United Kingdom, [3] College of Life and Environmental Sciences, Institute for Microbiology and Infection, University of Birmingham, Birmingham, United Kingdom

***Correspondence:**
Katharina Giebel
Katharina.Giebel@rau.ac.uk

† These authors have contributed equally to this work

Dichelobacter nodosus is the essential pathogen in ovine footrot, an important cause of lameness in sheep that reduces productivity and welfare. The aim of this study was to investigate the feasibility of using multiple locus variable number tandem repeat analysis (MLVA) developed to investigate isolates to understand the molecular epidemiology of *Dichelobacter nodosus* in ovine footrot by investigation of communities of strains. MLVA sensitivity was improved by optimizing PCR conditions to 100% specificity for *D. nodosus.* The improved MLVA scheme was used to investigate non-cultured DNA purified from swabs (swab DNA) and cultured DNA from isolates (isolate DNA) from 152 foot and 38 gingival swab samples from 10 sheep sampled on four occasions in a longitudinal study. Isolate DNA was obtained from 6/152 (3.9%) feet and 5/6 yielded complete MLVA profiles, three strains were detected. Two of the three isolate strains were also detected in isolate DNA from 2 gingival crevice cultures. Complete MLVA profiles were obtained from swab DNA from 39 (25.7%) feet. There were 22 *D. nodosus* community types that were comprised of 7 single strain and 15 multi-strain communities. Six community types were detected more than once and three of these were detected on the same four sheep and the same two feet over time. There were a minimum of 17 and a maximum of 25 strain types of *D. nodosus* in the study. The three isolate strain types were also the most frequently detected strain types in swab DNA. We conclude that the MLVA from swab DNA detects the same strains as culture, is much more sensitive and can be used to describe and differentiate communities and strains on sheep, feet and over time. It is therefore a sensitive molecular tool to study *D. nodosus* strains directly from DNA without culture.

Keywords: *Dichelobacter nodosus*, footrot, sheep, MLVA, veterinary epidemiology, bacteriology, PCR

INTRODUCTION

Footrot (FR) is the most common cause of lameness in sheep in the UK and it is a health and welfare concern in sheep flocks globally (1–4). Footrot reduces productivity and sustainability of sheep farming (5, 6), costing the UK industry £20–£80 million per annum (6, 7).

There are two clinical presentations of footrot, interdigital dermatitis (ID), characterized by inflammation of the interdigital skin, and severe footrot (SFR), characterized by separation of the hoof horn from underlying tissues (8). The essential pathogen in footrot is the fastidious gram negative, aerotolerant, anaerobic bacterium *Dichelobacter nodosus* (9, 10) which is key in initiation of ID and in progression to SFR (11–13). *D. nodosus* is present in >90% of UK sheep flocks and causes ~70 % of lameness (4).

In cross-sectional studies, *D. nodosus* has been detected on healthy and diseased feet (11, 14–18), and in the gingival cavity (19).

Russell et al. (20) developed an MLVA assay as a strain-typing tool for cultured *D. nodosus* isolates based on four polymorphic loci (DNTR02, 09, 10, and 19). The assay was used by Smith et al. (21) to investigate within-flock population dynamics of strains of *D. nodosus*. They reported that *D. nodosus* strains clustered within sheep and were transmitted between ewes over time. *D. nodosus* isolation is challenging and time consuming, because of the organism's fastidious and anaerobic nature and direct PCR from swab DNA is more sensitive than culture (15, 22).

Muzafar et al. (23) used the MLVA developed by Russell et al. (20) to analyse *D. nodosus* directly from DNA extracted from interdigital skin swabs of healthy and footrot affected feet using only DNTR10 and DNTR19. They did not use DNTR09 due to poor amplification nor DNTR02 due to non-specific amplification.

Therefore, the aim of this study was to optimize and validate the full *Dichelobacter nodosus* MLVA for isolate DNA and community DNA and investigate its value in a pilot longitudinal study of persistence of *D. nodosus* in sheep.

MATERIALS AND METHODS

Sample Collection

In 2014, swab samples were collected in a longitudinal study of 10 sheep (5 ewes, 5 lambs) from a UK flock with footrot. All sheep were sampled on four occasions at 2-week intervals from May to June. On each occasion, all four feet and the gingival crevice were swabbed with two swabs each, one for DNA analysis and one for culture. In addition, foot lesions were scored for ID and SFR using two 5-point scales (15). A total of 152 foot and 38 mouth swabs were collected.

Isolation and Detection of *Dichelobacter nodosus*

Swabs for culture were inoculated onto 4% hoof agar (HA) followed by subculture onto a 2% HA (15). Plates were incubated under anaerobic conditions at 30°C for 4–5 days (MACS-MG-1000 anaerobic workstation, Don Whitley Scientific, Shipley, UK, 80% N_2, 10% CO_2, 10% H_2). Isolate DNA was extracted with a DNeasy Blood and Tissue Kit (Qiagen Ltd., Manchester,

TABLE 1 | Input and recovery of MLVA PCR amplicons and peak sizes in *Dichelobacter nodosus* isolates and model communities.

D.nodosus isolates	Size (bp)	Peak size (RFU)*		Size (bp)	Peak size (RFU)		Size (bp)	Peak size (RFU)		Size (bp)	Peak size (RFU)	
		DNTR02			DNTR09			DNTR10			DNTR19	
		Individ	Comm		Individ	Comm		Individ	Comm		Individ	Comm
Community 1												
VCS 1703A	545	15,530	209**	985	11,722	2,323**	693	9,795	182**	851	7,855	219**
JIR3918	610	8,091	2,950	768	28,924	16,045	835	22,117	483**	1,019	3,692	1,621
JIR3919	650	13,779	2,681	876	18,892	11,636	646	10,793	101**	1,019	2,078	1,621
JIR3350	560	16,543	4,975	985	23,681	12,323	505	25,910	8,144	932	6,326	1,178
Community 1 (diluted)												
VCS 1703A (1:5)	545	13,092	85**	985	11,812	1,205**	693	5,382	138**	851	8,624	372**
JIR3918	610	8,091	4,034	768	28,924	16,045	835	22,117	1,158	1,019	3,692	3,384
JIR3919	650	37,779	4,501	876	18,892	11,363	646	10,793	3,786	1,019	2,078	3,384
JIR3350	560	16,543	1,597	985	23,681	1,205**	505	25,910	3,030	932	6,326	242**
Community 2												
VCS 1703A	545	15,530	150**	985	11,812	5,194	693	5,382	339**	851	8,627	129**
JIR3918	610	8,091	1,874	786	28,924	10,421	835	22,117	2,322	1,019	3,692	872
4303 LBV	635	9,853	705**	985	19,638	5,194	788	/***	687	1,019	2,714	872
BS8	555	18,255	4,529	985	9,345	5,194	835	3,475	2,322	933	5,191	1,814

**Peak size (RFU), the size of the peak observed in relative fluorescent units; Individ, peak size for a single strain; Comm, Peak size of the strain in a mixed model community. **Recovered products that fall below the established threshold, ***No PCR product detected.*

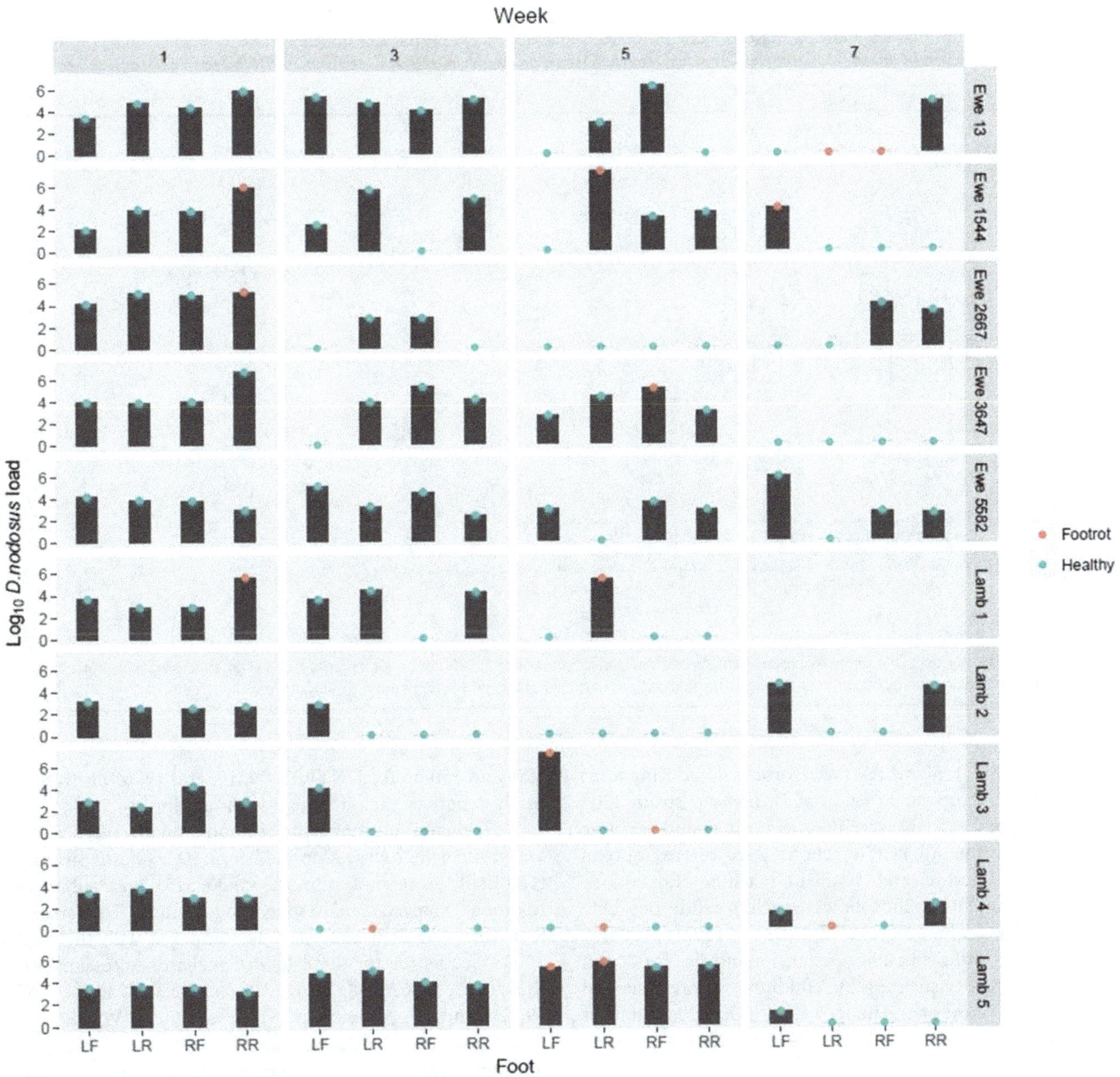

FIGURE 1 | Log_{10} *Dichelobacter nodosus* load on DNA swabs from feet from weeks 1, 3, 5, and 7. Green dots: Healthy foot (Interdigital dermatitis score 0 or 1, footrot score 0) Red dots: Foot classed as diseased with footrot (Interdigital dermatitis score >1 and/or footrot score >0) LF, Left front; LR, left rear; RF, Right front; RR, Right Rear.

United Kingdom) according to the manufacturer's instructions with a lysis time of 1 h. DNA was extracted directly from swabs using the hydroxyapatite spin-column method (24) using only 0.5 ml of the sodium phosphate extraction buffers. *D. nodosus* was detected in DNA extracted from the foot and mouth swabs using a *D. nodosus*-specific *rpoD*-targeted qPCR (25).

MLVA Optimization and Protocol

The sensitivity of the MLVA primers (**Supplementary Table 1**) was determined using DNA from *D. nodosus* isolates and swab samples. Improvements in sensitivity were made by changing the PCR Master mix (From Promega x2 PCR Master Mix to Bioline MyTaq™ Red Mix), increasing primer concentration (from 10 pmoles of each primer in a 50 μl reaction to 10 pmoles of each primer in a 25 μl reaction), DNA template concentration (from 1 μl/50 μl reactions to 1 μl/25 μl reactions) and the number of PCR cycles (from 30 to 40 cycles). The final protocol was, in 25 μl reactions; 12.5 μl MyTaq™ Red Mix (Bioline, London, United Kingdom), 1 μl of each primer (10 μM stock concentration; **Supplementary Table 1**), 1 μl bovine serum

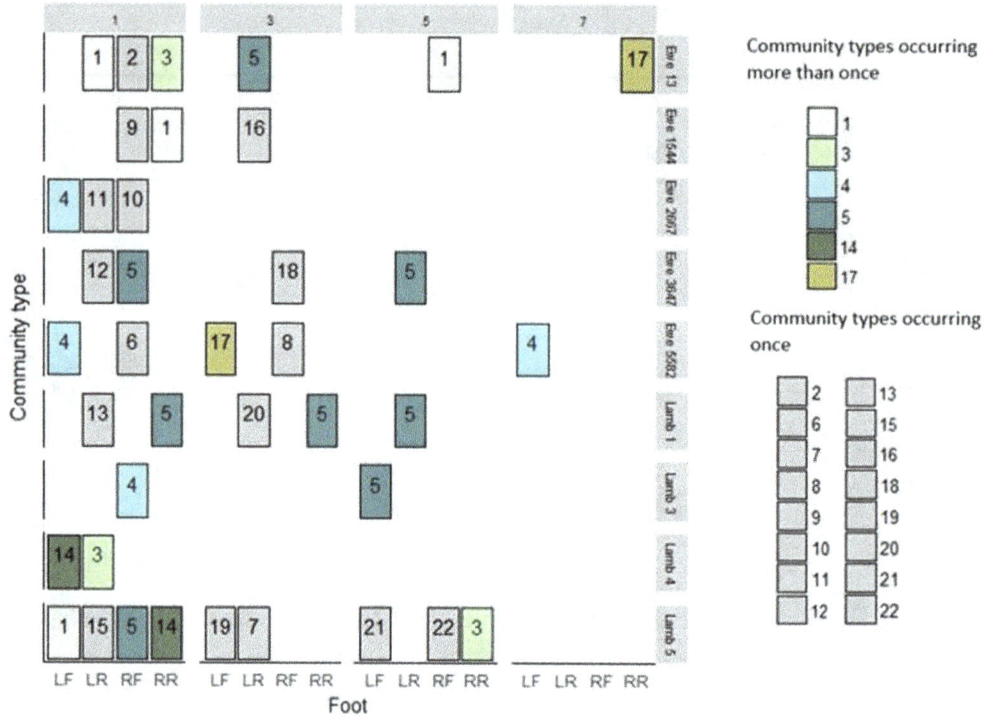

FIGURE 2 | *Dichelobacter nodosus* community profiles from 39 feet of 9 sheep from weeks 1, 3, 5, and 7. Community types in green shades were detected repeatedly. Community types in gray occurred only once in the study. LF, Left front; LR, left rear; RF, Right front; RR, Right Rear.

albumin (20 mg ml^{-1}) (Sigma Aldrich, Dorset, United Kingdom) and 1 μl of DNA template. DNA from *D. nodosus* strain 4303 LBV and nuclease free H_2O were used as positive and negative controls, respectively. All PCR reactions were carried out on an Eppendorf Mastercycler ep gradient machine (Eppendorf, Hamburg, Germany) using the following cycling conditions: One cycle of 95°C for 2 min, 40 cycles of 95°C for 1 min, 59°C for 30 s and 72°C for 1 min with a final extension of 72°C for 2 min. PCR products were visualized by ethidium bromide-stained agarose gel electrophoresis and imaged using a Gene Flash imager (Syngene Bio Imaging, Cambridge, United Kingdom).

Determination of VNTR Amplicon Size Using Fragment Analysis

MLVA amplicon size was determined using fragment analysis. Forward primers for the four loci were labeled with different fluorescent dyes (**Supplementary Table 1**) and amplicons for each locus were submitted separately for fragment analysis (DNA Sequencing and Services, University of Dundee, Scotland). PCR products from *D. nodosus* isolates were diluted 1:100 and products originating from swabs were diluted either 1:20 or 1:100 depending in the PCR band intensity seen on agarose gel. 1200 Liz dye (Applied Biosystems, Warrington, United Kingdom) was used as a size standard and data were analyzed using Peak Scanner? Software (Applied Biosystems, Warrington, United Kingdom). The bin range was set to 4bp (fragment size ± 2 bp) and minimum fragment length cut off values 500, 500, 400, and 550 bp for DNTR02, 09, 10, and 19, respectively, based on the length of each fragment without repeats.

To provide additional information on the accuracy of the assay, the 4 loci were amplified from *D. nodosus* strain 1703A (GenBank Accession number CP000513) and submitted for fragment analysis and Sanger sequencing. The size of the loci from fragment analysis was compared with the published 1703A sequences for the 4 loci (Genebank Accession numbers KC676717, KC676718, KC676719, and KC676720 for DNTR02, 09, 10, and 19, respectively). The sequenced VNTR loci from *D. nodosus* strain 1703A were analyzed using tandem repeat (TR) finding software (26) to determine the numbers of repeats in the sequence.

MLVA analysis of two isolates resulted in a primary peak and a number of small secondary peaks ≤ 20% the height of the primary peak at expected TR intervals (**Supplementary Figure 1**). To investigate secondary peaks, 14 more *D. nodosus* isolates were analyzed (**Supplementary Table 2**). Secondary peaks were observed in some, but not all, isolates. The secondary peaks might have been due to non-axenic *D. nodosus* cultures. However, this is unlikely because multiple peaks were detected at all 4 loci (**Supplementary Figure 1**) which would indicate many isolate strains in each culture. Other explanations for secondary peaks might be rapid, minor, within-strain variation or an artifact in the PCR process. It was not possible to adjust the PCR to prevent the formation of these small secondary peaks, therefore it was

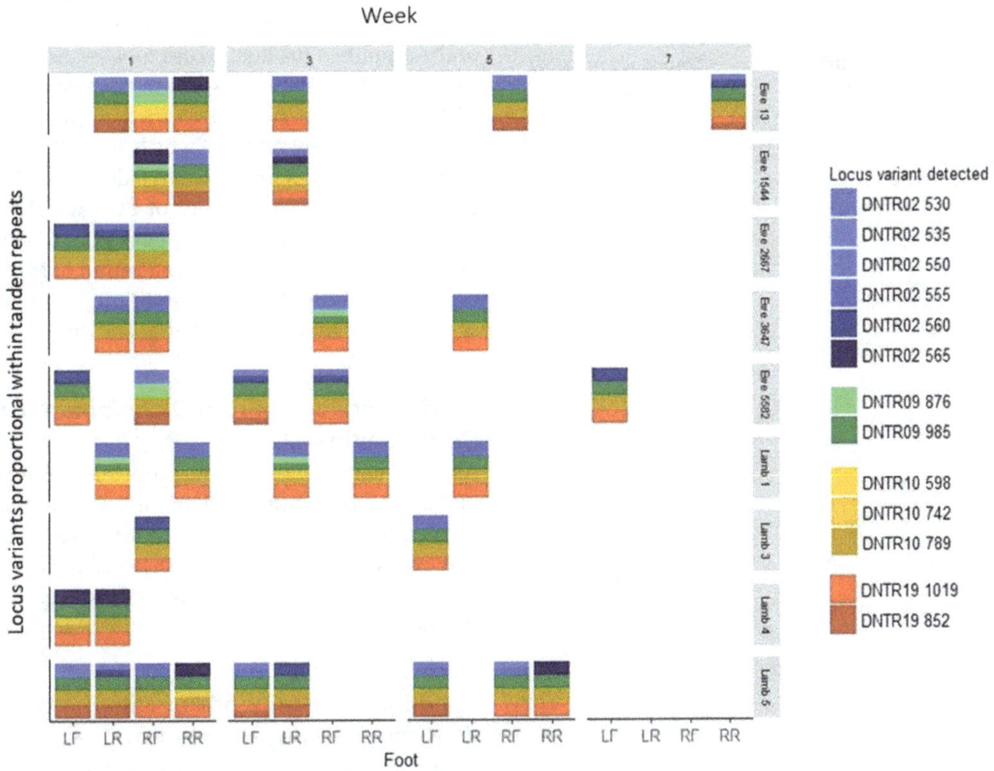

FIGURE 3 | *D. nodosus* MLVA DNTR = *D. nodosus* tandem repeat 02, 09, 10, 19, variants proportional within TR from DNA from swab samples from 39 feet from 9 sheep in weeks 1, 3, 5, and 7. LF, Left front; LR, left rear; RF, Right front; RR, Right rear. Four colors, each of one shade, indicates a single strain.

decided to consider secondary peaks $\leq$ 20% the height of the primary peak as artifacts (**Supplementary Figure 2**).

Validation of the MLVA PCR and Testing on Model Communities

Primer specificity was tested by MLVA analysis of DNA from non-target organisms previously detected on sheep feet or present in soil or feces. These were *Streptococcus uberis, Staphylococcus epidermis, Staphylococcus intermedius, Staphylococcus aureus, Staphylococcus hyicus, Staphylococcus chromogenis, Streptococcus dysgalactidae, Streptococcus agalactidae, Mannheimia spp., Fusobacterium necrophorum, Pseudomonas aeruginosa, Escherichia coli,* and *Mycobacterium tuberculosis.*

To confirm specificity PCR products from 10 *D. nodosus* positive samples from foot swabs and 1 gingival swab were analyzed using MLVA and the resulting VNTR amplicons were submitted for Sanger sequencing (GATC Biotech AG, Cologne, Germany). Sequences were assessed for quality using CodonCode Aligner version 6.0.2. and analyzed using BLAST (27).

MLVA sensitivity was investigated by assessing its limit of detection of *D. nodosus* load. *D. nodosus* strain 4303 LBV was incubated on Eugon Agar (28) for 5 days. After incubation 1 ml of PBS, pH 7.4, was added to the *D. nodosus* plates, creating a cell suspension. Suspended cells were quantified using a Petroff-Hausser counting chamber (Hausser Scientific, PA, USA) and serially diluted. Sterile swabs were spiked with 50 μl of the serially diluted cell suspension resulting in 1.07×10^6 to 1.07 *D. nodosus* cells per swab (equivalent to *rpoD* copies per sample). DNA was extracted from these swabs as above. Samples were then screened for *D. nodosus* using the MLVA assay. To test whether detection could be improved further, all samples were submitted to a second round of the MLVA PCR assay using the same cycling conditions.

The feasibility of using MLVA to analyse multistrain communities was investigated using model communities created from eight *D. nodosus* isolates with different MLVA profiles. Two model communities (1 and 2) were created, each with 4 isolates (**Table 1**). DNA from each isolate was standardized to a concentration of 15 ng/μl and 5 μl of DNA from each isolate mixed in a 1:1:1:1 ratio. A third model community was created with the isolates in community 1, with one isolate (*D. nodosus* 1703A) diluted 5-fold to investigate whether non-dominant isolates could be detected. These model communities were amplified and analyzed using the MLVA protocol above.

Assessment of the MLVA Assay on DNA Extracted From Foot and Gingival Swab Samples

Swab DNA and isolate DNA from feet and gingivae from the longitudinal study that were positive for *D. nodosus* by

TABLE 2 | MLVA *Dichelobacter nodosus* strain types from swab DNA from the feet of sheep by definitely and possibly present.

MLVA strain type	Frequency definitely present	Frequency possibly present
A	4	2
B	1	2
C*	10	12
D*	7	9
E*	8	5
F	2	5
G	2	8
H	5	10
I	1	4
J	1	1
K	0	1
L	0	1
M	1	2
N	1	1
O	1	1
P	0	1
Q	1	2
R	1	1
S	0	1
T	0	1
U	0	1
V	0	2
W	1	2
X	0	1
Y	1	1

*Strain also detected in culture isolates.

rpoD qPCR were analyzed using MLVA and fragment analysis. Secondary peaks $\leq$ 20% the height of the primary peak were excluded (**Supplementary Figure 2**). Distinct community fingerprints were obtained that could be compared visually (**Figure 1**). In addition, strain types within a community could be defined as "definitely present" when a community had only one variant at each locus or when more than 1 variant was detected at one locus only and one variant at the other three loci. When there were 2 or more variants at 2 or more loci strains were defined as "possibly present." The minimum and maximum number of strain types in a community were calculated using the formulae:

$$\begin{aligned}&\textit{Minimum number of strains}\\&\quad= \textit{number of variants at the most variable locus}\\&\textit{Maximum number of strains}\\&\quad= \textit{product of the number of variants at each locus}\end{aligned}$$

RESULTS

Validation and Optimisation of the MLVA Scheme

The number of TRs at the four loci for strain 1703A was the same as reported by Russell et al. (20). The MLVA assay was specific for *D. nodosus* with no amplification in any of the 4 loci in non-target species (**Supplementary Figure 3**). DNA sequencing of the amplified products from foot swabs were 99–100% similar to their target sequences confirming specificity of the MLVA PCR. The mouth swab DNA yielded products for three MLVA loci, DNTR02, 09 and 10, which were 96–97% similar to their target sequence. The improved detection limit of the MLVA protocol after a single round of PCR was 10^2,10^3, 10^2, and 10^3 copies μl^{-1} DNA template for DNTR02, DNTR09, DNTR10, and DNTR19, respectively. A second round of MLVA PCR resulted in non-specific amplification and diluting samples did not improve specificity or sensitivity (data not shown).

VNTR Amplicons From *Dichelobacter nodosus* Model Communities

All *D. nodosus* strains in the model communities were detected, including community 3 where one strain was at 5 fold dilution; 17/48 secondary peaks were $\leq$ 20% the height of the primary peak and excluded (**Table 1**); 11 of these 17 were from the VCS strain, which was only detected correctly once, suggesting that this laboratory strain is particularly difficult to detect using MLVA.

Longitudinal Study of Persistence of *D. nodosus* in the Epidemiology of Footrot

FR was detected at least once on the feet of 8/10 sheep (**Figure 1**). *D. nodosus* was detected by qPCR in 97/152 (63.8%) foot swab DNA samples. It was detected on both healthy and diseased feet and on all sheep, but not all weeks (**Figure 1**).

Out of the 97 *D. nodosus* positive foot swab DNA samples, 53 (54.6%) amplified all 4 MLVA loci and in 39/53 (73.6%) samples complete MLVA profiles were obtained (**Figure 2**). The 39 complete profiles had a total of 156 loci with 75/156 (48.1%) with secondary peaks. The total number of peaks in these 156 loci was 220. After application of the $\leq$ 20% threshold (**Supplementary Figure 2**) 106/220 (48.2%) peaks were excluded from further analysis. DNTR02 was the most variable locus with 6 TRs and DNTRs 09 and 10 were the least variable with only 2 TRs (**Figure 3**).

D. nodosus was detected by qPCR in 8/38 (21.1%) gingival swab DNA samples, however, no complete MLVA profiles were obtained. Three loci were amplified in one sample and these matched loci in community types 3 and 4.

Dichelobacter nodosus Community Profiles From Foot Swab DNA

There were more MLVA positive feet in week 1, and detections declined over the 4 visits (**Figure 3**). There were 22 *D. nodosus* community types in total; seven were single strains and fifteen were multistrain; six community types were detected more than once, three of these were detected on the same four sheep and the same two feet over time (**Figure 2**). Community type 5, a single strain community, was most frequently detected (8/39 feet) (**Figure 2**). The results indicate that the MLVA differentiated *D. nodosus* communities spatially between feet, sheep, and over time.

TABLE 3 | MLVA profile of *Dichelobacter nodosus. nodosus* from isolate DNA compared with swab DNA.

Sample origin	Sheep ID	Week of study	Locus fragment size/number of repeats				Isolate DNA strain type	Swab DNA strain types
Foot			DNTR02	DNTR09	DNTR10	DNTR19		
RR	13	1	565/10	985/5	789/8	1,019/5	C	C
LR	3,647	1	555/8	985/5	789/8	1,019/5	C	E, C**
RF	3,647	1	555/8	985/5	789/8	1,019/5	E	E
LF	5,582	1	560/9	985/5	789/8	1,019/5	D	D
RR	13	3	565/10	985/5	789/8	1,019/5	C	NS
LR	13	3	555/8	985/5	789/8	/	E*	E
Mouth	13	3	560,565/9–10	985/5	789/8	1,019/5	C, D	NS
Mouth	3	3	560,565/9–10	985/5	789/8	1,019/5	C, D	∧

*RR, Right rear; RF, Right front; LR, Left rear; LF, Left front. *DNTR19 did not amplify, but strain type E present in corresponding swab. **E, C = both strain types are definitely present, NS, no swab data for all 4 loci, ∧DNTR19 did not amplify, other VNTR's identical.*

Dichelobacter nodosus Strain Type Analysis From Foot Swab DNA

There were 17 strains definitely present and a further 8 possibly present in the 22 *D. nodosus* community types in foot DNA (**Table 2**). Seven strains were, definitely or possibly, present on more than 4 occasions and the remaining 18 strains were present on 1 to 3 occasions. The three most frequently detected single strains were C, D and E (**Table 2**), these were the single strain community types 3, 4, 5 (**Figure 2**).

Dichelobacter nodosus Strains and Communities From Isolate DNA

D. nodosus was cultured from 6/152 (3.9%) foot swabs from 3 sheep in weeks 1, 3, and 5, with 5 complete and 1 partial MLVA profile obtained from these isolates. The three most frequently detected strains, C, D, and E (**Table 2**), were also detected in swab DNA from the same foot at the same time (**Table 3**). Complete MLVA profiles were obtained from 2 isolates from the gingival crevice and *D. nodosus* strains C and D (Community types 3 and 4) were detected in both samples (**Table 3**).

DISCUSSION

The optimized *D. nodosus* MLVA (20) was developed and used successfully to investigate *D. nodosus* isolates and communities from DNA extracted directly from swab samples. The variability in loci and community types in the longitudinal study indicate that the improved MLVA scheme is more sensitive than previous studies (21, 23) and can be used to improve understanding of the epidemiology of communities of *D. nodosus* on feet over time.

Smith et al. (21) investigated transmission and persistence of *D. nodosus* strains on sheep's feet over a 10 months period using the original assay (20) on isolates of *D. nodosus*. They reported 45 animal-level repeat *D. nodosus* isolation events, 47% of those were isolation events of the same strain from the same foot over time. In addition, they detected and isolated the population dominant strain. In this, albeit shorter study, we obtained similar results with 4 animal-level repeat detection of *D. nodosus* communities and one dominant single strain community (community 5) that was detected on the same foot consecutively.

There was a high level of variability in *D. nodosus* communities in our study, with most variation occurring in week 1. This is possibly attributable to rainfall on and preceding the day of sampling as wet weather facilitates persistence of *D. nodosus* (29). A high level of *D. nodosus* variability was also reported by Smith et al. (21) who isolated 87 MLVA types over 10 weeks, which suggest that a large number of strains are present in footrot affected flocks and suggest that our findings represent true variability.

Our optimized MLVA was used in a subsequent longitudinal study to investigate persistence of *D. nodosus* strains on feet; this demonstrated that *D. nodosus* strains persist on the feet of diseased sheep, but not on the feet of healthy sheep (29).

Only 6 isolates were cultured in this study using published *D. nodosus* isolation techniques, however, the strain types from culture isolates were a subset of the strains detected from the non-culture DNA (**Table 3**) at the same site and time, indicating that MLVA analysis of non-cultured DNA is more sensitive than DNA from culture, as reported by others for other bacterial species (30–32). This indicates that previous studies that have compared relationships between *D. nodosus* using MLVA profiles of isolates (21) are incomplete and analysis would have been improved using MLVA from DNA directly.

The MLVA scheme had a limit of detection of $\sim 10^3$ genome copies μl^{-1} of extracted DNA and so there were a number of samples that were positive for *D. nodosus* by qPCR and negative by MLVA. Therefore, even the MLVA is not 100% sensitive. Despite this, the ability to use MLVA on non-cultured DNA to identify strains as definitely and possibly present and to produce fingerprint profiles is novel and adds to the value of MLVA as a tool to investigate strains of *D. nodosus* on feet over time.

This is the first occasion that a *D. nodosus* strain profile has been obtained from the gingival crevice, although complete strain profiles were detected from isolates and only incomplete strain profiles were obtained directly from swab DNA. Strain types C and D were present in mouths and were also among the strains most frequently detected on feet (**Table 3**).

The presence of regular secondary peaks in fragment analysis when testing isolate DNA has not been reported previously, although artifactual DNA extension during PCR has been reported but usually only for short sequences (33, 34). Further investigation of the secondary peaks was outside the scope of the current study and so a conservative threshold was applied to decrease the probability of artificially increasing the number of loci in a sample. As a consequence, it is possible that some non-dominant strains that were present at low abundance were classified as artifacts.

CONCLUSIONS

A sensitive and specific *D. nodosus* MLVA assay using four VNTR loci was validated and optimized for use on non-culture DNA. The strain types detected from isolate DNA from the same site were a subsample of those detected from swab DNA, but many more strains were present in swab DNA, indicating that it is more sensitive to analyse *D. nodosus* from DNA directly rather than via culture. Because the MLVA can be used to identify communities of *D. nodosus* on the feet of sheep over time it can be used to investigate persistence and transmission of communities of *D. nodosus* and so improve epidemiological understanding of *D. nodosus*. Other MLVA schemes may be developed for use in the non-culture based study other bacterial species.

AUTHOR CONTRIBUTIONS

The work presented in this article was conducted by the KG. LG and KP supervised the research. All authors contributed to the article and approved the submitted version.

ACKNOWLEDGMENTS

We thank Dr Ruth Kennan, Monash University for providing isolates of *D. nodosus* and Drs Ed Smith, Emma Monaghan, Rachel Clifton, and Jessica Taylor for their assistance with collection of samples from sheep and laboratory support.

REFERENCES

1. Gurung RB, Tshering P, Dhungyel OP, Egerton JR. Distribution and prevalence of footrot in Bhutan. *Vet J.* (2006) 171:346–51. doi: 10.1016/j.tvjl.2004.11.012
2. Gilhuus M, Kvitle B, L'Abee-Lund TM, Vatn S, Jorgensen HJ. A recently introduced *Dichelobacter nodosus* strain caused an outbreak of footrot in Norway. *Acta Vet Scand.* (2014) 56:29. doi: 10.1186/1751-0147-56-29
3. Sreenivasulu D, Vijayalakshmi S, Raniprameela D, Karthik A, Wani SA. Prevalence of ovine footrot in in the tropical climate of southern India and isolation and characterization of *Dichelobacter nodosus*. *Rev Sci Tech OIE.* (2013) 32:869–77. doi: 10.20506/rst.32.2.2209
4. Winter JR, Kaler J, Ferguson E, KilBride AL, Green LE. Changes in prevalence of, and risk factors for, lameness in random samples of english sheep flocks: 2004-2013. *Prev Vet Med.* (2015) 122:121–8. doi: 10.1016/j.prevetmed.2015.09.014
5. Marshall DJ, Walker RI, Cullis BR, Luff MF. The effect of footrot on body-weight and wool growth of sheep. *Aust Vet J.* (1991) 68:45–9. doi: 10.1111/j.1751-0813.1991.tb03126.x
6. Wassink GJ, King EM, Grogono-Thomas R, Brown JC, Moore LJ, Green LE. A within farm clinical trial to compare two treatments (parenteral antibacterials and hoof trimming) for sheep lame with footrot. *Prev Vet Med.* (2010) 96:93–103. doi: 10.1016/j.prevetmed.2010.05.006
7. Nieuwhof GJ, Bishop SC. Costs of the major endemic diseased in sheep in Great Britain and the potential benefits of reduction in disease impact. *J of Anim Sci.* (2005) 81:23–9. doi: 10.1079/ASC41010023
8. Green L, Clifton R. Diagnosing and managing footrot in sheep: an update. *Practice.* (2018) 40:17–26. doi: 10.1136/inp.j4575
9. Beveridge WIB. Footrot in sheep: a transmissible disease due to infection with *Fusiformis nodosus*. Studies on its cause, epidemiology and control. *CSIR.* (1941) 140:1–56.
10. Kennan RM, Han X, Porter CJ, Rood JI. The pathogenesis of ovine footrot. *Vet Microbiol.* (2011) 153:59–66. doi: 10.1016/j.vetmic.2011.04.005
11. Witcomb LA, Green LE, Kaler J, Ul-Hassan A, Calvo-Bado LA, Medley GF, et al. A longitudinal study of the role of *Dichelobacter nodosus* and *Fusobacterium necrophorum* load in initiation and severity of footrot in sheep. *Prev Vet Med.* (2014) 115:48–55. doi: 10.1016/j.prevetmed.2014.03.004
12. Witcomb LA, Green LE, Calvo-Bado LA, Russell CL, Smith EM, Grogono-Thomas R, et al. First study of pathogen load and localisation of ovine footrot using fluorescence *in situ* hybridisation (FISH). *Vet Microbiol.* (2015) 176:321–32. doi: 10.1016/j.vetmic.2015.01.022
13. Atia J, Monaghan E, Kaler J, Purdy K, Green L, Keeling M. Mathematical modeling of ovine footrot in thye UK: the effect of *Dichelobacter nodosus* and *Fusobacterium necrophorum* on the disease dynamics. *Epidemics.* (2017) 21:13–20. doi: 10.1016/j.epidem.2017.04.001
14. Bennett G, Hickford J, Sedcole R, Zhou H. *Dichelobacter nodosus, Fusobacterium necrophorum* and the epidemiology of footrot. *Anaerobe.* (2009) 15:173–6. doi: 10.1016/j.anaerobe.2009.02.002
15. Moore LJ, Wassink GJ, Green LE, Grogono-Thomas R. The detection and characterisation of *Dichelobacter nodosus* from cases of ovine footrot in England and Wales. *Vet Microbiol.* (2005) 108:57–67. doi: 10.1016/j.vetmic.2005.01.029
16. Stäuble A, Steiner A, Frey J, Kuhnert P. Simultaneous detection and discrimination of virulent and benign *Dichelobacter nodosus* in sheep of flocks affected by footrot and in clinically healthy flocks by competitive real-Time PCR. *J Clin Microbiol.* (2014) 52:1228–31. doi: 10.1128/JCM.03485-13
17. Maboni G, Frosth S, Aspan A, Totemeyer S. Ovine footrot: new insights into bacterial colonisation. *Vet Record.* (2016) 176:228. doi: 10.1136/vr.103610
18. Kraft AF, Strobel H, Hilke J, Steiner A, Kuhnert O. The prevalence of *Dichelobacter nodosus* in clinically footrot-free sheep flocks: comparative field study on elimination strategies. *BMC Vet Res.* (2020) 16:21. doi: 10.1186/s12917-020-2243-8
19. Witcomb LA. *The in Situ Analysis of the Microbial Community Associated in Sheep.* (PhD thesis), University of Warwick, Coventry (2012).
20. Russell CL, Smith EM, Calvo-Bado LA, Green LE, Wellington EMH, Medley GF, et al. Multiple locus VNTR analysis highlights that geographical clustering and distribution of *Dichelobacter nodosus*, the causal agent of footrot in sheep, correlates with inter-country movements. *Infect Genet Evol.* (2014) 22:273–9. doi: 10.1016/j.meegid.2013.05.026
21. Smith EM, Gilbert A, Russell CL, Purdy KJ, Medley GF, Muzafar M, et al. Within-flock population dynamics of *Dichelobacter nodosus*. *Front Vet Sci.* (2017) 4:58. doi: 10.3389/fvets.2017.00058
22. McPherson AS, Dhungyel OP, Whittington RJ. Detection and Serogrouping of *Dichelobacter nodosus* infection by use of direct PCR from lesion swabs to support outbreak-specific vaccination for virulent footrot in sheep. *J Clin Microbiol.* (2018) 56:e01730–17. doi: 10.1128/JCM.01730-17
23. Muzafar M, Calvo-Bado LA, Green LE, Smith EM, Russell CL, Grogono-Thomas R, et al. The role of the environment in transmission of *Dichelobacter nodosus* between ewes and their lambs. *Vet Microbiol.* (2015) 179:53–9. doi: 10.1016/j.vetmic.2015.04.010
24. Purdy KJ. Nucleic acid recovery from complex environmental samples.

Method Enzymol. (2005) 397:271–92. doi: 10.1016/S0076-6879(05)97016-X

25. Calvo-Bado LA, Oakley BB, Dowd SE, Green LE, Medley GF, Ul-Hassan A, et al. Ovine pedomics: the first study of the ovine foot 16S rRNA-based microbiome. *ISME J.* (2011) 5:1426–37. doi: 10.1038/ismej.2011.25
26. Benson G. Tandem repeats finder: a program to analyze DNA sequences. *Nucleic Acids Res.* (1999) 27:573–80. doi: 10.1093/nar/27.2.573
27. Altschul SF, Gish W, Miller W, Myers EW, Lipman DJ. Basic local alignment search tool. *J Mol Biol.* (1990) 215:403–10. doi: 10.1016/S0022-2836(05)80360-2
28. Cagatay IT, Hickford JGH. Update on ovine footrot in New Zealand: isolation, identification, and characterization of *Dichelobacter nodosus* strains. *Vet Microbiol.* (2005) 111:171–80. doi: 10.1016/j.vetmic.2005.09.010
29. Clifton R, Giebel K, Liu NLBH, Purdy KJ, Green LE. Sites of persistence of *Fusobacterium necrophorum* and *Dichelobacter nodosus*: a paradigm shift in understanding the epidemiology of footrot in sheep. *Sci Rep.* (2019) 9:14429. doi: 10.1038/s41598-019-50822-9
30. Vranckx K, Maes D, Calus D, Villarreal I, Pasmans F, Haesebrouck F. Multiple-locus variable-number tandem-repeat analysis is a suitable tool for differentiation of *Mycoplasma hyopneumoniae* strains without cultivation. *J Clin Microbiol.* (2011) 49:2020–3. doi: 10.1128/JCM.00125-11
31. Ceglie L, Guerrini E, Rampazzo E, Barberio A, Tilburg J, Hagen F, et al. Molecular characterization by MLVA of *Coxiella burnetii* strains infecting dairy cows and goats of north-eastern Italy. *Microb Infect.* (2015) 17:776–81. doi: 10.1016/j.micinf.2015.09.029
32. Sannö X, Jacobson M, Sterner S, Thisted-Lambertz S, Aspán A. The development of a screening protocol for *Salmonella spp.* and enteropathogenic Yersinia spp. in samples from wild boar (Sus scrofa) also generating MLVA-data for *Y. enterocolitica* and *Y. pseudotuberculosis. J Microbiol Methods.* (2018) 150:32 8. doi: 10.1016/j.mimet.2018.05.014
33. Tuntiwechapikul W, Salazar M. Mechanism of *in vitro* expansion of long DNA repeats: Effect of temperature, repeat length, repeat sequence, and DNA polymerases. *Biochemistry.* (2002) 41:854–60. doi: 10.1021/bi0110950
34. Vondrušková J, Parízková N, Kypr J. Factors influencing DNA expansion in the course of polymerase chain reaction. *Nucleos Nucleot Nucl.* (2007) 26:65–82. doi: 10.1080/15257770601052299

16

Non-Antibiotic Approaches for Disease Prevention and Control in Nursery Pigs

Lee V. Wisener[1,2*], *Jan M. Sargeant*[1,2], *Terri L. O'Sullivan*[1], *Annette M. O'Connor*[3†], *Scott A. McEwen*[1], *Mark Reist*[1] and *Katheryn J. Churchill*[1]

[1] Department of Population Medicine, Ontario Veterinary College, University of Guelph, Guelph, ON, Canada, [2] Centre for Public Health and Zoonoses, University of Guelph, Guelph, ON, Canada, [3] Department of Large Animal Clinical Sciences, College of Veterinary Medicine, Michigan State University, East Lansing, MI, United States

Correspondence:
Lee V. Wisener
lwisener@uoguelph.ca

†ORCID:
Annette O'Connor
orcid.org/0000-0003-0604-7822

Swine producers are encouraged to practice antibiotic stewardship by reducing their use of antibiotics belonging to classes of medical importance to humans. We conducted a scoping review of non-antibiotic approaches in the form of products or management practices that might prevent or control disease and thus reduce the need for antibiotics in nursery pigs. Our objectives were to systematically describe the research on this broad topic for the North American context, identify specific topics that could feasibly support systematic reviews, and identify knowledge gaps. A search of multiple databases identified 11,316 articles and proceedings for relevance screening. From these, 441 eligible clinical trials and observational studies were charted. The majority were clinical trials (94%). Study results from EU countries were mostly communicated through journal articles, whereas study results from the USA were mostly communicated through conference proceedings. Interventions and health outcomes were diverse. The two most frequent intervention categories were feed additives and piglet vaccines. The three most frequent outcomes reported were diarrhea, mortality, and indices of vaccine immunity. There were 13 specific topics comprising various feed additives and vaccines that might feasibly support systematic reviews. There were relatively few studies in which interventions were compared with antibiotic comparison groups and relatively few studies evaluating management practices.

Keywords: antibiotic stewardship, disease control, disease prevention, non-antibioic approaches, nursery pigs, scoping review

INTRODUCTION

Antimicrobial resistance (AMR) poses a serious threat to advances in modern human medicine, livestock health and production, and animal welfare (1, 2). There are limited or few alternative treatment options in patients infected with pathogens resistant to medically important antibiotics, particularly those with resistance to critically important antibiotics (3). The World Health Organization (WHO), the World Organization for Animal Health (OIE), and the Food and Agriculture Organization of the United Nations (FAO) regard antimicrobial use (AMU) in as a significant driver of AMR in humans and animals alike (2, 4, 5). In a tripartite "One Health" approach, these major global institutions have called for a worldwide effort to reduce inappropriate and unnecessary AMU in all sectors (2, 4, 5). The WHO and the OIE have categorized antibiotic classes according to their importance for human and animal health, respectively

(3, 6). Categorization of antibiotic classes is useful for prioritization of strategies to limit AMR, such as antibiotic stewardship. To help achieve this goal, the WHO has published guidelines recommending certain restrictions on the use of medically important antibiotics in non-human sectors (7). Food production sectors use antibiotics of importance to humans that are the same or belong to the same antibiotic class as those used in human medicine for animal disease treatment or prevention in vulnerable individuals or groups (3, 5, 8).

Worldwide, nations are heeding the call for reduced antibiotic use in food production through regulation and industry guidelines. For example, in the USA, the US Food and Drug Administration Center for Veterinary Medicine promotes prudent use of livestock antibiotics belonging to classes of importance to humans by requiring they be administered with veterinary oversight and be limited to the purpose of assuring animal health. The use of medically important antibiotics in healthy animals for growth promotion was prohibited by 2017 in the USA (9). In Canada, similar regulations enacted by December 2018 eliminated the over-the-counter use of antibiotics belonging to classes of medical importance to humans by requiring veterinary oversight for administration of these antibiotics by injection or by addition to feed or water (10). In the European Union (EU), the use of antibiotics in feeds for growth promotion has been banned since 2006 (11). In their systematic review of antibiotic use in swine production from 2000 to 2017, Lekagul et al. (12) reported that there was geographical variation in antibiotic use by types of diseases. Choice of antibiotic was dependent upon the common pathogens associated with age-specific diseases and upon route of administration, typically oral in-feed medication in nursery pigs. Lekagul et al. (12) concluded that medically important antibiotics are still commonly used worldwide for disease prevention and control in swine production, particularly in modern commercial swine production during the suckling piglet and nursery pig stages.

Scoping review methodology is used to systematically map the literature with regard to the extent, range, and nature of existing research of a particular topic area (13, 14). Scoping reviews are also useful as preliminary "reconnaissance" to assess the feasibility of undertaking a full systematic review of a specific topic and to identify gaps in the existing research (13, 14). While scoping reviews are descriptive and broad in nature, systematic reviews aim to address a specific research question by using explicit systematic methods to collate all the evidence that fits pre-specified eligibility criteria while minimizing bias (13, 15). To help inform antibiotic stewardship goals, a scoping review of non-antibiotic approaches to nursery pig health could help researchers advance the knowledge of alternative approaches by indicating topics that could be subject to formal systematic reviews or merit further research. In addition, a scoping review could illuminate current gaps in research on non-antibiotic approaches to nursery pig health for swine industry professionals, swine researchers, and research funding agencies.

The objectives of this scoping review were three-fold: (i) to examine and describe the volume, range, and nature of research on non-antibiotic approaches for disease prevention and control in commercial nursery pig production; (ii) to identify specific topics where available research literature may support systematic reviews; (iii) to identify knowledge gaps in the primary literature on the effectiveness of various non-antibiotic approaches. Summarizing the literature regarding intervention effectiveness was not an objective for this scoping review.

MATERIALS AND METHODS

This scoping review followed the framework for scoping reviews as outlined by Arksey and O'Malley (13) using the PRISMA-ScR (i.e., Preferred Reporting Items for Systematic Reviews and Meta-Analyses Extension for Scoping Reviews) guidelines for reporting scoping reviews (16). The registered protocol can be located through UoG Atrium https://atrium.lib.uoguelph.ca/xmlui/handle/10214/12929.

Our review question was as follows: What are the volume and nature of the primary research literature published between 2000 and 2018 that evaluated non-antibiotic interventions (i.e., products such as vaccines or feed additives and management practices such as weaning methods or biosecurity) to prevent or control bacterial and viral illnesses in nursery pig production in North America and regions or countries with similar production conditions? Viral illnesses were included because we presumed that preventing viral infections may reduce secondary bacterial illnesses.

Expert Stakeholder Engagement

As the volume of literature on the broad topic of non-antibiotic approaches for nursery pig health was potentially very extensive, we sought expert opinion to refine our research question and help to inform our search strategy and study eligibility criteria. More specifically, the stakeholder engagement served six objectives: (i) to identify the countries or regions with similar commercial swine production practices to those of North America, (ii) to select the swine production stage(s) for which non-antibiotic approaches could most effectively reduce total AMU in swine production, (iii) to solicit opinions on the importance of various antimicrobial types to antimicrobial stewardship in the swine industry (e.g., antibiotics belonging to medically important classes used to prevent or control swine diseases, anticoccidials, and anthelmintics), (iv) to identify the health and production outcomes of greatest importance to swine producers, (v) to identify the most important non-antibiotic interventions in the form of specific products (e.g., vaccines, feed additives, medications, or supplements) or specific management practices (e.g., weaning practices, biosecurity, housing, feed type, and restricted feeding); and (vi) to identity any additional outcomes or interventions that we had not included on our initial lists. We also asked the stakeholders to recommend other experts who should be consulted.

The expert opinion was gathered through an anonymous online survey (Qualtrics XM). The respondents selected and ranked options from a list for a particular question and/or responded in an open-ended format. Expert stakeholders who were consulted included representatives within provincial or national Canadian swine industry associations, representatives

TABLE 1 | Data platform and database information sources used in the scoping review search on non-antibiotic approaches to reduce the need for antibiotics in nursery pig production.

Data platform	Databases
ProQuest	Agricultural and environmental science AGRICOLA and TOXLINE
	Biological science database (MEDLINE and TOXLINE), dissertations and theses Guelph, ProQuest dissertations and theses
ProQuest	AGRICOLA
PubMed	PubMed (not MEDLINE)
Web of science	Science citation index, conference proceedings citation index–science
Web of science	MEDLINE
AASV	Annual meeting proceedings
AASV	International pig veterinary congress (biannual meetings) proceedings

in provincial agriculture departments, and Canadian scientists engaged in swine agriculture and/or swine veterinary research. We assumed that the responses from stakeholders of Canadian institutions would be representative of experts from the USA and other countries with commercial swine production. Stakeholders' most common responses and suggested additional responses were used to inform the parameters of the search, eligibility criteria, and data items. Ethics approval for this survey was not required, as the results were used strictly to inform the review process and not reported as a finding of the review.

Eligibility Criteria

Eligible information sources were from North America, EU countries, Australia, and New Zealand, available since 2000, as these sources of evidence were most likely to reflect current commercial swine production systems most similar to those of North America. Eligible publication types included English-language journal articles, conference proceedings, theses, and technical reports. In addition to electronic databases, proceedings were sourced from the American Association of Swine Veterinarians (AASV) Annual Meeting and Pre-conference seminar from 2000 to 2018 and the International Pig Veterinary Society Congress biannual meetings from 2000 to 2016. We included research reports that reported a challenge trial, a clinical trial (i.e., a controlled trial), or observational study of a modifiable intervention, and we reported a health or production outcome in nursery pigs. For purposes of this review, "interventions" also included modifiable risk factors. Consistent with our stakeholder engagement results, interventions related to breed or genetic improvement were not included. Our stakeholder engagement also informed our *a priori* selected outcomes of interest. These included health outcomes of bacterial or viral infections significant to swine health in North America, treatment costs, and measures of performance. Studies evaluating toxicities or parasitic infections were excluded. Non-English information sources were excluded. Quasi-experimental intervention studies designed as "before period" vs. "after period" of the intervention application were excluded.

Information Sources

To aid in the development and validation of the search, we checked that 25 known relevant citations are included. The primary reviewer (LW) performed the database search from March 27, 2018, to April 19, 2018, using multiple databases hosted by the data platforms of ProQuest, Web of Science, and PubMed (**Table 1**). Though the database CAB Direct was originally targeted for inclusion, due to technical difficulties, it was not used. The search for proceedings was conducted manually by the primary reviewer and a second reviewer working independently subsequent to obtaining access to the online AASV Swine Information Library through a membership, September 20, 2018.

Search

The database search was filtered by language (English), date of publication (published between 2000 and date of search in 2018), and by location filters for eligible countries if available. Additional filters were applied as were allowable within the data platform. These included source and document type (i.e., article, proceedings paper, meeting abstract, and thesis), subject or research areas, and Medical Subject Headings (MeSH) or qualifiers. The search terms were limited to the title or abstract in the PubMed and Web of Science platforms or "anywhere except full text" for the ProQuest platform databases. Management of the identified citations was as follows: first, they were imported into the reference manager software EndNote (Clarivate Analytics, Philadelphia, United States); second, they underwent exact match deduplication in EndNote; and third, they were imported into the systematic review software DistillerSR (Evidence Partners, Ottawa, Canada) where they underwent further deduplication based on close matches.

The database search strategy included a string of the population term groupings (e.g., weanling, nursery pig, and starter pig), one of two intervention term groupings, and an outcome term grouping (e.g., health, diarrhea, or growth) with each grouping connected by the Boolean operator "AND" (**Table 2**). There were two intervention term groupings, one for interventions of interest in the form of a product (e.g., vaccine, feed supplement, or plant extract) and another for interventions in the form of a management practice (e.g., antibiotic-free and late weaning as defined by the study authors, or disinfection). Within each term grouping, terms were combined by the use of the Boolean operator "OR." The search was conducted by the primary reviewer (LW) in consultation with a University of Guelph research librarian.

The online proceedings identified as being potentially relevant based on subject headings and titles were entered onto a Microsoft Excel (2010) spreadsheet for tracking of further screening decisions. Relevant full-text proceedings were entered into the DistillerSR database. Proceedings that were duplicates of journal articles were removed.

Selection of Sources of Evidence

Our review team consisted of veterinary epidemiologists, one of whom acted as the primary reviewer, a topic expert in swine research (TOS), and two trained MSc epidemiologists who acted

TABLE 2 | Search terms for non-antibiotic approaches to reduce the need for antibiotics in nursery pig production.

Groupings	Search terms
Population terms	(Piglet* OR weaner* OR "weaning pig*" OR "weanling pig*" OR "weaner pig*" OR "weaned pig*" OR "weaner stage" OR "weaner phase" OR "nursery pig*" OR "young pig*" OR "younger pig*" OR "early-weaned pig*" OR "late-weaned pig*" OR "nursery-age*" OR "naïve pig*" OR "starter pig*" OR "neonate pig*" OR "neonatal pig*" OR "suckling pig*")
Product intervention terms	(Antibiotic* OR antimicrobial* OR vaccin* OR immunization OR "sow vacc*" OR "dam vacc*" OR "gilt vacc*" OR "sow immunization" OR "dam immunization" OR "gilt immunization" OR "trace mineral*" OR "essential mineral*" OR "mineral source*" OR "mineral form*" OR Zinc*OR vitamin* OR "dietary acid*" OR "organic acid*" OR "dietary fatty acid*" OR "medium chain fatty acid*" OR acidif* OR "feed enzyme*" OR fermentable OR fermented OR "plant extract*" OR herbal OR seaweed OR spice OR phytogenic OR "dietary lysine" OR "dietary tryptophan" OR lactoferrin OR lysozyme OR L-glutamine OR nutraceutical* OR neutraceutical* OR supplemental OR "dietary supplement*" OR "diet supplement*" OR "feed supplement*" OR "dietary additive*" OR "diet additive*" OR inulin OR oligosaccharide* OR polysaccharide* OR mannan* OR B-glucan* OR probiotic* OR prebiotic* OR synbiotic* OR "direct-fed microbial*" OR "competitive exclusion" OR yeast OR "Saccharomyces cerevisiae" OR "essential oil*" OR "fish meal" OR "blood meal" OR "spray-dried" OR immunoprophylaxis OR immunotherapeutic* OR "egg-yolk antibod*" OR "IgY antibod*" OR bacteriophages OR "antimicrobial peptide*" OR "bovine colostrum" OR "epidermal growth factor*" OR "rare earth" OR clay OR "natural alternative*" OR homeopath*)
Management intervention terms	("natural pig*" OR "organic swine" OR "organic pig*" OR "natural conditions" OR "non-conventional" OR "antibiotic-free" OR "weaning practice*" OR "weaning method*" OR "weaning procedure*" OR "weaning regime*" OR "weaning system" OR "conventional weaning" OR "weaning age" OR "early weaning" OR "late wean*" OR "age at weaning" OR "creep feed*" OR "stocking" OR crowding OR overcrowding OR "floor space" OR "feeder space" OR "housing system*" OR "housing design*" OR "housing environment*" OR "housing type" OR ventilation OR "air quality" OR co-mingling OR "mingl*" OR "mixed litter" OR mixing OR "batch system" OR "batch management" OR biosecurity OR "sanit*" OR "disinfect*" OR "cleaning" OR hygiene OR "all-in-all-out" OR "pig flow" OR "disease eradication" OR "disease control*" OR "multi-site" OR "liquid feed" OR "liquid diet*" OR "pellet*" OR "low protein" OR "decreased protein" OR "restricted protein" OR "protein restrict*" OR "protein nutrition" OR "protein level" OR "protein source" OR "dietary protein" OR "restricted feed*" OR "feed restrict*" OR "control fed" OR "quality assurance" OR education)
Outcome terms	(health OR immun* OR diarrhea OR diarrhea OR scours OR "colibacillosis" OR "fecal score" OR "clinical response*" OR "clinical parameters" OR "fecal shedding" OR "fecal shedding" OR morbidity OR mortality OR performance OR growth OR "daily weight gain" OR "average daily gain" OR "G:F" OR "gain-to-feed" OR "feed conversion" OR "feed intake" OR "ADG" OR ADFI OR "lightweight gain" OR productivity)

A search string included the population terms and either the product intervention terms, or the management intervention terms plus the outcome terms connected by the Boolean operator "AND".

as second reviewers. Pre-testing of the relevance screening form was conducted on 100 citations based on title and abstracts. Pre-testing of the data charting was conducted on 25 full-text articles. Using forms created in DistillerSR, two independent reviewers screened and charted the data. Any disagreements were resolved by consensus or a third reviewer. After pre-testing, the level 1 relevance screening form did not change.

However, due to the large volume of literature identified after the first level of relevance screening, three additional relevance screening levels were applied to the titles and abstracts to refine the selection of relevant citations to the literature that was most pertinent to our research question (**Appendix 1**, level 1–4 relevance screening forms). Level 2 screened by eligible countries or regions by first author address. Level 3 screened by study type and information regarding the challenge pathogen or antigen that was collected, but then challenge trials were excluded from further screening and data charting. Level 3 also screened by pig type (i.e., included only conventional or specific pathogen-free pigs). Level 4 screened by intent of the intervention (i.e., included non-antibiotic interventions for viral or bacterial infections, excluded interventions for mycotoxins and soy allergens) and by eligible diseases (i.e., excluded reportable or rare diseases such as classic swine fever, Aujeszky's disease and foot and mouth disease, and outcomes only of public health impact such as swine hepatitis E virus and methicillin-resistant *Staphylococcus aureus*). At level 4, the articles that only reported a performance outcome without any health outcomes of interest were excluded from data charting. Health outcomes of interest were defined *a priori* and included clinical outcomes [i.e., mortality all-cause, diarrhea, respiratory disease and non-specific morbidity defined as non-diarrheal, non-respiratory non-specific morbidity (e.g., pyrexia, removals, or unthriftiness), or other morbidities such as lameness], surrogate health outcomes such as shedding of clinically important pathogens [i.e., *Salmonella* spp., *Campylobacter* spp., enterotoxigenic *Escherichia coli* (ETEC *E. coli*)], and measures of specific and non-specific immunity to vaccines or bacterins (**Table 3**). In summary, articles that were selected for data charting reported research on non-antibiotic approaches to improve health outcomes of important viral and/or bacterial infections in conventional or specific pathogen-free nursery pigs in North America, EU countries, the UK, New Zealand, or Australia. The additional relevance screening levels 2–4 were a protocol deviation intended to focus the data charting on studies that addressed our research question.

Data Charting Process

Data charting of full-text articles (i.e., journal articles, technical reports, theses, and conference proceedings) was conducted by both the primary reviewer and a second reviewer working independently using a form in DistillerSR (**Appendix 2**, Data charting form). Any disagreements were resolved by consensus or a third reviewer. Data were charted at the individual study level.

TABLE 3 | Description of data charting items for relevant journal articles, technical reports, proceedings, or theses.

Variable	Description of items
General study characteristics	
Study design	Clinical trial (i.e., experimental or field-based trial under conditions of natural exposure), challenge trial (i.e., deliberate exposure to a pathogen or antigen under the control of the investigator), observational study
Study location	Country and region where the study was conducted as stated in the article or if not stated, first author address
Year of publication	Year of publication or year of proceeding
Farm setting	Population farm setting (i.e., experimental research farm, commercial farm, or unclear)
Detailed trial or observational study characteristics	
Specific pig population in which the intervention was given	Specific population based on production stage included dams, suckling piglets, nursery pigs
Purpose[a] of the intervention as stated in the title or objective statement	Disease prevention (i.e., no pre-existing health problems or known exposures), disease treatment (i.e., individual pigs or groups in whole or part or the farm were known to have clinical disease or exposure to viral or bacterial pathogens. In addition, some studies included performance (e.g., feed intake, growth or body weight, feed efficiency)
Non-antibiotic interventions in the form of a product or management practice or risk factor studied	*Products*: Piglet vaccines, maternal vaccination, non-antibiotic feed or water additive including the addition of specific dietary components, non-antibiotic medication (e.g., any medication, vitamin, mineral, antibodies, etc. administered directly to an individual). Combination products used as interventions that contained both an antibiotic [e.g., Zinc Oxide (ZnO) plus an antibiotic] were excluded. *Management:* Feeding regime as amount or schedule (e.g., protein level, creep feeding, restricted feeding); diet type or format (e.g., pelleted vs. mash, fermented feeds, complexity of feeds); weaning method or weaning stage as defined by the authors (e.g., early vs. late); biosecurity (e.g., comingling, mixing, introductions, animal movements); housing, flooring or feeders (e.g., animal density, feed troughs and water supply factors, flooring); air quality; producer education
Comparison groups	No treatment or conventional practice comparison, placebo or sham, different level or form of treatment, antibiotic and/or ZnO[b]
Health outcomes of interest reported	Mortality (i.e., piglet deaths in absolute terms, deaths per time period, excess deaths, or other metric); clinical diarrhea (e.g., scours, fecal consistency, or fecal score); clinical respiratory disease; non-diarrheal, non-respiratory non-specific morbidity (e.g., fever, removals or unthriftiness) or other morbidities such as lameness; treatment for illnesses or antibiotic use; pathology or lesions; fecal shedding of specific swine pathogens; measures of specific and non-specific immunity and infection (i.e., serology, cell mediated immunity, viremia, PCR, immune markers such as acute-phase proteins, or tumor necrosis factor (TNF)
Other outcomes measured	None, performance outcomes (i.e., feed intake, growth or body weight, or feed efficiency), farm economics or treatment costs, diet digestibility, gastrointestinal microflora, gastrointestinal morphology
Study size	Number of study subjects in each study at the hierarchical level of the analysis (e.g., individual, pen or group, herd or farm)

[a]*Studies in which the purpose included both prevention and treatment were counted as disease control in results.*
[b]*Some studies compared a non-antibiotic intervention group to a zinc oxide comparison group while other studies compared a zinc oxide treatment group to a no-treatment control group, antibiotic or other treatment comparison group.*

We focused the data charting on clinical trials and observational studies that reported a health outcome of interest in the nursery stage of production. However, for studies that reported a health outcome of interest, additional data charting related to other health outcomes and non-health outcomes was completed. A further protocol deviation included an additional question regarding the stage of production at which the intervention was applied (e.g., reproduction, suckling, or nursery).

Data Items

We charted data for the publication type and for the following study characteristics: study design, study location and year of publication or conference year, study size, and farm settings of the study population (i.e., experimental farm vs. commercial farm). In addition, we charted data for the following: production stage(s) of animals receiving the intervention, purpose of intervention as disease prevention, and/or treatment, and/or performance; specific intervention evaluated; comparison group(s); health outcomes of interest reported; other outcomes reported; and study size and the hierarchical level at which the outcome was measured (i.e., individual, group/pen, or herd/farm) (**Table 3**). Data were charted using preselected response options with an added text box for additional responses or clarification for the interventions, comparator groups, and outcomes reported (**Appendix 2**).

In this review, interventions such as non-antibiotic medication, vitamin, mineral, or antibody given directly to individual animals *via* injection or oral bolus were charted as a "medication," whereas the same intervention given to groups of animals *via* feed was charted as a "feed additive." There were two data charting options related to measures of immunity as an outcome, one specifically for vaccine immunity and another for non-vaccine immunity.

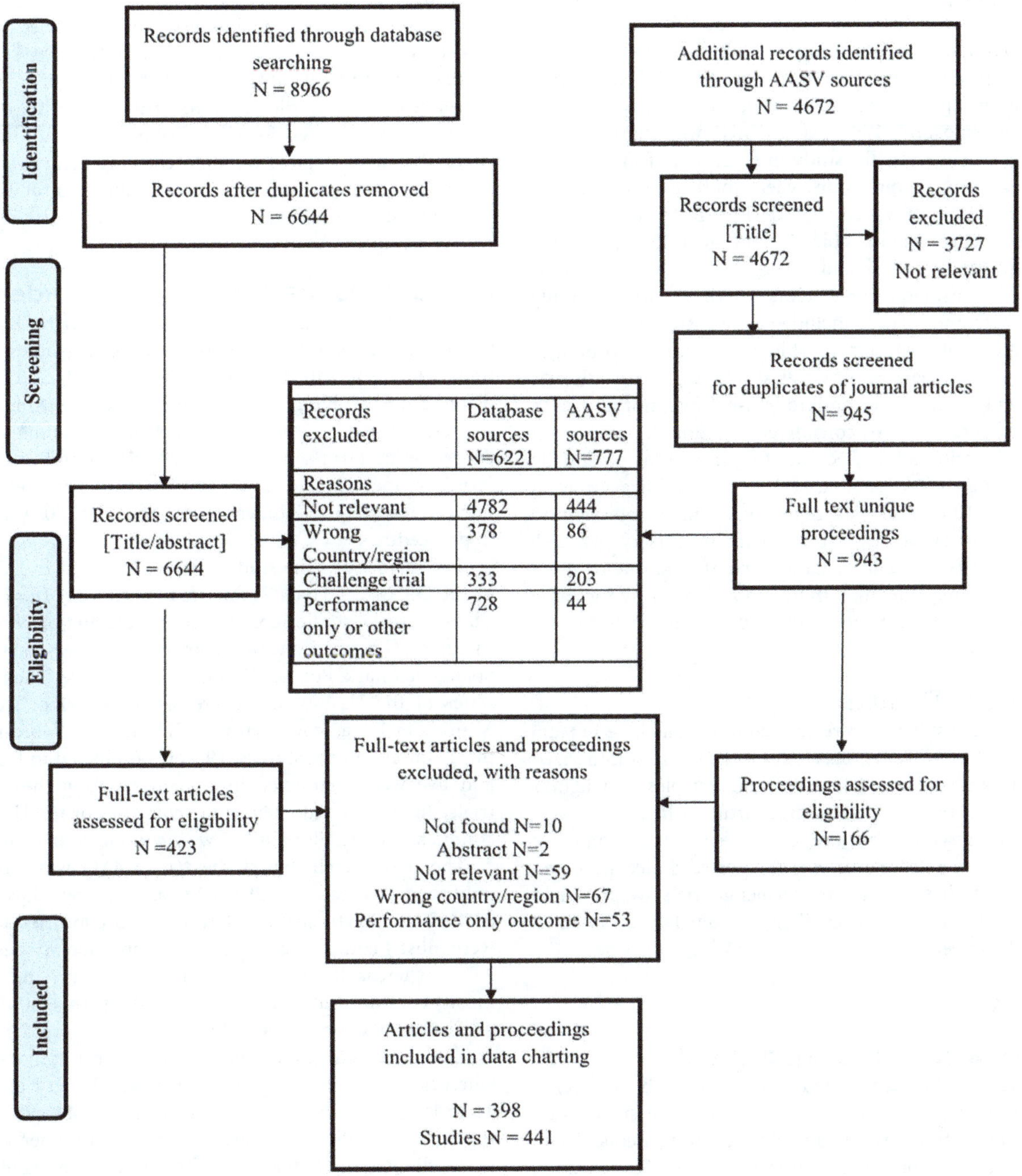

FIGURE 1 | Preferred Reporting Items for Systematic Reviews and Meta-Analyses (PRISMA) flow diagram of citations from literature search through to relevance screening and data extraction.

Data charted regarding the purpose(s) of the intervention were based on information in the title or objective statement. Prevention was selected if the herd or group of pigs showed no clinical or subclinical evidence of disease or infection, whereas treatment was selected if the pigs as individuals or groups in part or whole showed evidence of infection, or were known to be exposed. Although we charted data for disease prevention and/or treatment, in the results, we reported disease control for those studies that described an intervention given for both purposes, treatment and prevention (i.e., the intervention was given to groups of pigs assumed to comprise both healthy and clinically or subclinically affected or exposed pigs). Definitions for disease prevention, treatment, control, and pig performance were based on those provided by the United States Government Accountability Office (GAO) (17) and the American Veterinary Medical Association (18).

Comparison groups that were not clearly stated as "no treatment" or "conventional practice" were charted as comparison groups that received a "different form or level" of the intervention or exposure. Studies could be charted with multiple types of comparison groups (i.e., both a "no treatment" control group and "different form or level" if additional comparison groups received various levels or forms of the treatment or exposure). Zinc oxide (ZnO) was charted as an intervention when it was the study intervention of interest and charted as a comparison group when another non-antibiotic intervention of interest was compared with zinc treatment.

To meet our second objective of identifying specific intervention topics that could be combined for systematic reviews, we considered only clinical trials with clinically important outcomes. These included mortality; non-diarrheal, non-respiratory non-specific morbidity, or other morbidities such as lameness; diarrhea or fecal score; respiratory disease; and treatment for illness or antibiotic use. Thus, not all health outcomes of interest were considered as clinically important outcomes. The criteria for selection of topic areas as potentially extensive enough for systematic reviews were arbitrarily set at a minimum of 10 clinical trials reporting a similar intervention in the same population (e.g., amino acids in nursery pig feed, specific piglet vaccines, and/or dam vaccines) and one or more clinically important outcomes, though not necessarily the same clinically important outcome among all clinical trials for the specific topic area.

Synthesis of Results

Data charted in DistillerSR were entered into a database in Stata 15.1 (College Station, Texas, USA). These data were summarized descriptively and presented in the form of tables and figures in accordance with our stated data charting scheme. So as to emphasize the research with the highest evidentiary value, we present detailed results for articles that reported clinical trials and observational studies (19). For the challenge trials, we presented only details of the types of challenges evaluated as obtained during level 3 screening.

RESULTS

Expert Stakeholder Engagement

A total of 73 experts were invited to respond to the survey, of which 33 responded (45%). We incorporated the stakeholder input into our search strategy and data charting items. There were no suggested publications that were not identified through our search.

Selection of Sources of Evidence

There were 11,316 unique citations screened for eligibility: 6,644 were from the database search and 4,672 were from the gray literature proceedings of the AASV Swine Information Library sources (**Figure 1**). Two proceedings that were duplicates of journal articles were removed (**Figure 1**). A total of 536 challenge trials were identified at level 3 screening of database sources and at full-text screening of proceedings. A description of the types of challenge agents is presented in **Appendix 3**. A total of 772 journal articles and proceedings that described clinical trials or observational studies but only reported a performance outcome or other outcome without reporting any health outcome of interest were excluded at level 4 screening of the database sources and full-text screening of proceedings. In total, 589 citations (5%) describing clinical trials or observational studies and reporting a health outcome of interest were screened for eligibility based on full text. Among these, 398 were eligible for data charting. Thirty-four eligible articles (8.5%) described one or more studies; in total, there were 441 relevant clinical trial or observational studies included for data charting.

Characteristics of Sources of Evidence

The majority of eligible studies were clinical trials (n = 414, 94%). The remainder were observational studies (n = 27, 6%). The observational studies were conducted exclusively using animals living in commercial farm settings, whereas the clinical trials were conducted using animals living in experimental farm settings (n = 206, 50%) and in commercial farm settings (n = 182, 44%). The farm settings were unclear for 26 (6%) clinical trials, of which 20 were reported in proceedings.

The majority of the studies were conducted in EU countries or the UK (n = 284, 64%) followed by the USA (n = 110, 25%). There were 17 studies conducted in Australia or New Zealand. The five EU countries with the greatest numbers of studies were Spain, Denmark, Poland, Germany, and France. The five specific states of the USA with the greatest numbers of studies were Minnesota, Iowa, North Carolina, Illinois, and Nebraska. Among the 27 observational studies, 19 were conducted in EU countries and five were conducted in Canada. Among the 414 clinical trials, 265 were conducted in EU countries or the UK, 108 were conducted in the USA, and 25 were conducted in Canada.

The body of eligible studies (n = 441) was composed of published articles (n = 297, 67%) and proceedings (n = 144, 33%). The 284 studies reported from EU countries and the UK were mostly communicated through published articles (n = 212, 75%), whereas the 110 studies reported from the USA were mostly communicated through proceedings (n = 60, 55%).

The annual number of included studies reported in published articles increased in an approximately linear trend since 2000, whereas the number of proceedings varied every other year in accordance with the alternate year schedule of the International Pig Veterinary Society Congress and the number of accepted proceedings at the congress and the Annual Meeting of the AASV (**Figure 2**).

Synthesis of Results for Clinical Trials and Observational Studies

The stated purpose(s) of the intervention as disease prevention, disease control, and/or performance varied according to the farm settings among the 414 clinical trials and 27 observational studies. There were no studies that evaluated an intervention for the clearly stated purpose of treatment of individual sick pigs.

Studies where the purpose of the intervention was for disease control (n = 134) were conducted primarily on commercial farms (n = 122, 91%), whereas when the purpose of the intervention as prevention (n = 250), studies were conducted on both

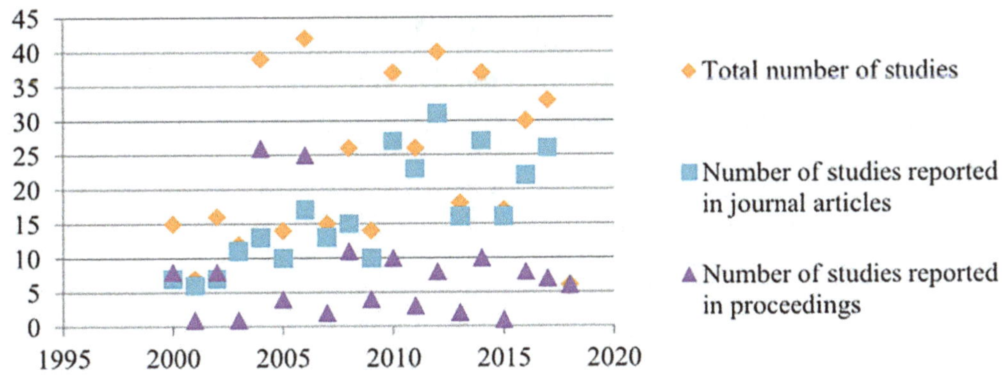

FIGURE 2 | Annual number of included studies by study type from journal articles from 2000 to 2017 and proceedings from 2000 to 2018.

commercial farms ($n = 75$, 30%) and research farms ($n = 153$, 61%). Among the 414 clinical trials, 238 (57%) evaluated an intervention for the purpose of prevention of which the majority were an evaluation of vaccines in piglets and/or dams ($n = 167$, 70%). Although all included studies ($n = 441$) reported a health outcome of interest in nursery pigs, many clinical trials ($n = 238$, 57%) and some observational studies ($n = 5$, 19%) also reported performance as a purpose of the intervention.

Non-antibiotic Interventions or Risk Factors

All eligible studies measured a health outcome in nursery pigs; however, interventions were applied to one or more specific populations based on production stage comprising dams, suckling piglets, or nursery pigs. Some studies reported the application of the intervention to more than one population. Among the total populations described in the eligible studies ($n = 553$), interventions were most commonly applied to nursery pigs ($n = 406$, 73%), followed by suckling piglets ($n = 86$, 16%), and dams ($n = 61$, 11%). Some studies reported the application of the intervention to all three populations ($n = 27$).

We charted data for 11 different categories of interventions or risk factors (**Figure 3**). Among the 414 clinical trial studies, there were 495 interventions described (**Appendix 4**). The two categories of interventions most frequently reported were feed additives ($n = 179$) and nursery or suckling piglet vaccination ($n = 160$) (**Figure 3**). Together, these two categories accounted for 68% of all interventions. The least common categories were air quality ($n = 3$) and producer education ($n = 4$). Details of all specific interventions for clinical trials are presented in **Appendix 4**; and further details for these specific interventions regarding comparison groups and health outcomes reported are available upon request. Among the 27 observational studies, there were 84 interventions or risk factors described (**Table 4**). The two categories that were most frequently studied were biosecurity ($n = 19$) and vaccinations of dams ($n = 14$).

Interventions Evaluated as Comparison Groups

Among the clinical trials and the observational studies, there were 672 comparison groups described. The most frequently reported comparison group was "different form or level" of the intervention or exposure ($n = 328$, 49%), followed by a no treatment control group ($n = 221$, 33%). The clinical trials also described comparison groups that received placebo ($n = 84$, 13%), antibiotics ($n = 24$, 4%), ZnO ($n = 8$, 1%), or a combination product containing an antibiotic and ZnO ($n = 3$, <1%). Note that some studies compared a non-antibiotic intervention group with a ZnO comparison group, whereas other studies compared a ZnO treatment group with a no treatment control group, or antibiotic or other treatment comparison group.

Among the 27 clinical trials that included an antibiotic comparison group, 21 investigated various feed additives, three investigated vaccinations to control *Mycoplasma hyopneumoniae*, one investigated a feed type, one investigated housing at the time of weaning, and one investigated producer education in the form of individual pig care training vs. standard metaphylactic antibiotic use in cases of nursery pig morbidities (20) (**Appendix 4**). Among the 179 clinical trials that investigated feed additives, 10 included a ZnO comparison group (**Appendix 4**).

Outcomes Measured

We charted data for nine health outcomes of interest. Among the clinical trials and observational studies, there were 729 reported outcomes (**Figure 4**). The three most commonly reported outcomes included clinical diarrhea ($n = 188$, 26%), mortality ($n = 158$, 22%), and vaccine immunity ($n = 140$, 19%). Immunity to vaccines included measures of specific immunity ($n = 140$) (e.g., serology and/or pathogen recovery or identification with PCR, and cell-mediated immunity) and in five studies also included non-specific immunity. Reporting of measures of immunity to a vaccine, with or without reporting other outcomes, was common among vaccine clinical trials ($n = 118$). A total of 43 (36%) vaccine clinical trials only reported measures of immunity without reporting any clinically important outcomes. These trials were conducted on research farms ($n = 18$), commercial farms ($n = 20$), and farm settings in which it was unclear ($n = 5$). Other outcomes reported included treatment for illness or antibiotic use ($n = 60$, 8%). Antibiotic treatments were typically

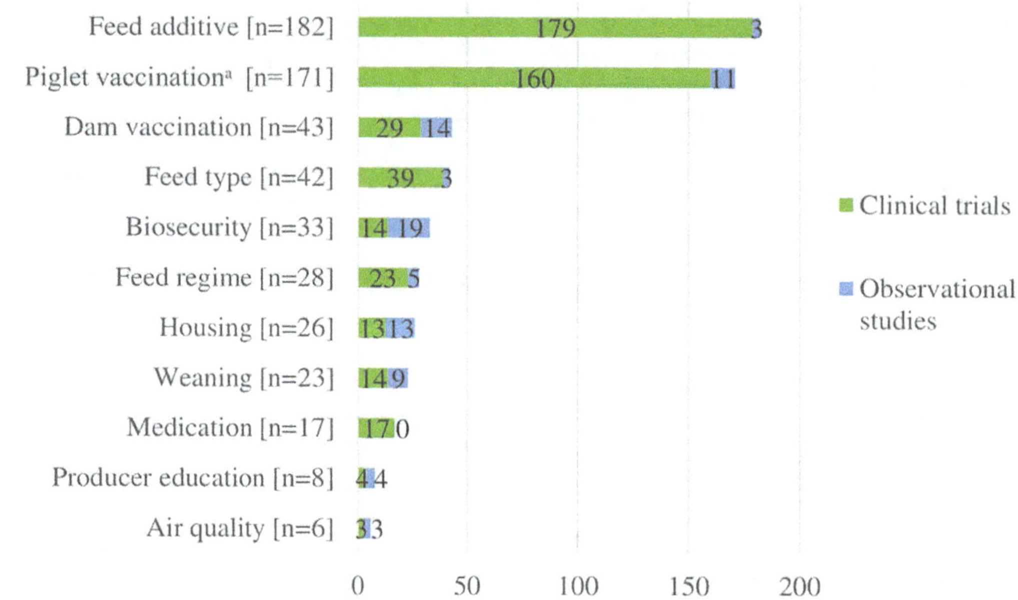

FIGURE 3 | Number of interventions or risk factors ($n = 579$) described in clinical trials ($n = 414$) and observational studies ($n = 27$).

TABLE 4 | Risk factors described in observational studies ($n = 27$).

Risk factors[a] ($n = 84$)	Risk factor details
Biosecurity ($n = 19$)	All-in-all-out vs. continuous flow ($n = 7$), mixing/cross fostering ($n = 5$), internal and external biosecurity ($n = 5$), air space separation ($n = 2$), piglet movement between stages ($n = 3$), infection control ($n = 4$), dead pig removal ($n = 1$)
Vaccination of dams ($n = 14$)	Porcine reproductive and respiratory syndrome virus (PRRSV) ($n = 4$), Porcine Circovirus type 2 (PCV2) ($n = 3$), Enterotoxigenic *Escherichia coli* (ETEC) ($n = 3$), rotavirus ($n = 1$), not clear or unspecified ($n = 3$)
Housing ($n = 13$)	Pen floor type ($n = 4$), space allowance/pig density ($n = 4$), use of bedding ($n = 2$), drinker type ($n = 2$), climatic and temperature conditions ($n = 3$), age of buildings ($n = 1$), indoors vs. outdoors ($n = 1$)
Vaccination of piglets[b] ($n = 11$)	PRRSV ($n = 4$), PCV2 ($n = 4$), not clear, or unspecified ($n = 5$)
Weaning ($n = 9$)	Weaning age ($n = 8$), mixing at weaning or weaning management ($n = 3$)
Feed regime ($n = 5$)	Restricted feeding ($n = 4$), creep feeding ($n = 3$), starter diet protein content restriction ($n = 1$)
Producer education ($n =4$)	Experience level of manager/producer/worker ($n = 3$), Education level of manager/producer/worker ($n = 2$)
Feed type ($n = 3$)	Pelleted nursery feed ($n = 1$), feed composition quality ($n = 1$), level of soybean and canola ($n = 1$)
Feed additive ($n = 3$)	Zinc product (e.g., ZnO) ($n = 3$)
Air quality ($n = 3$)	Ventilation ($n = 3$)

Categories of risk factors presented in order of decreasing frequency.
[a] *Risk factors included modifiable exposures regardless of the positive or negative impact of the exposure on an outcome.*
[b] *Piglet vaccination includes suckling piglet or nursery pig vaccination.*

for diarrhea when specified. The metric used for treatment for illness or antibiotic use varied (e.g., number of treatments, percent treated animals, treatment incidence calculated on an animal daily dose basis, and farm-level antibiotic use). Less commonly reported outcomes included non-diarrheal, non-respiratory, non-specific morbidity (e.g., fever, removals, or unthriftiness) or other morbidities such as lameness ($n = 55$, 8%) and pathogen shedding ($n = 54$, 7%). The remainder of the reported health outcomes of interest included non-vaccine immunity ($n = 32$, 4%), which comprised studies that measured specific immunity ($n = 21$), non-specific immunity ($n = 10$), or both ($n = 1$). Presence of pathological lesions (e.g., lung lesions at necropsy or injection site lesions) ($n = 26$, 3.5%) and clinical respiratory disease ($n = 16$, 2%) also were reported (**Appendix 4**).

Among the 441 included clinical trials and observational studies, all of which reported a health outcome of interest, the most commonly reported additional outcomes included performance outcomes such as growth ($n = 297$, 67%), feed efficiency ($n = 197$, 45%), and feed intake ($n = 186$, 42%).

Study Size

Among both clinical trials and observational studies, the study size varied widely from the smallest study using six individuals to evaluate an autogenous vaccine (21) to the largest

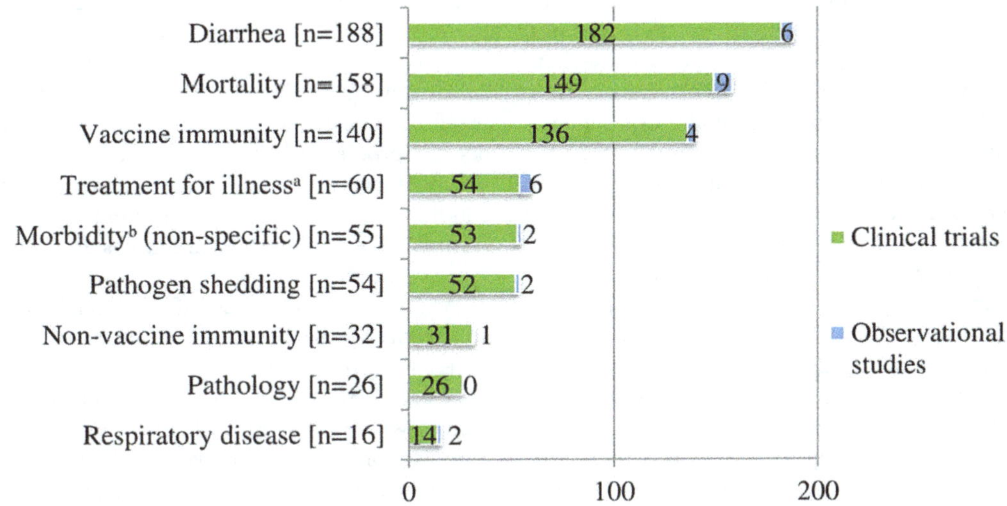

FIGURE 4 | Number of health outcomes of interest[a] ($n = 729$) described in clinical trials ($n = 414$) and observational studies ($n = 27$).

TABLE 5 | Study size[a] of clinical trials and observational studies at the hierarchical level of the data analysis.

	Number of studies	Range of study sizes	Experimental settings	Commercial settings	Unclear settings
Individual	405	9–3,31,592	200	179	26
Group/pen/room	113	2–653	63	45	5
Herd	37	3–1,513	0	37	0

[a]Study size was the number of study subjects included in the analyses.
Some studies measured outcomes at multiple levels.
For some studies some outcomes were measured at the individual level but performance was measured at the pen level.

study using 331,592 individual pigs to evaluate the impact of a producer education program on nursery pig mortality (22) (**Table 5**). Some studies measured health outcomes at the individual level but performance outcomes at the pen level. Most studies measured outcomes at the individual level regardless of the level of intervention allocation (**Table 5**). Among the observational studies alone, studies varied from 160 to 3,736 individuals.

Material for Potential Systematic Review Questions

There were 13 interventions evaluated in clinical trials that met our inclusion criteria for studies that could feasibly support systematic reviews; these included feed additives (e.g., amino acids, diet acidification, organic acids, fiber, phytobiotics, pre-biotics, probiotics, egg yolk antibodies, and ZnO), vaccination of piglets [e.g., porcine circovirus 2 (PCV2), porcine reproductive and respiratory syndrome virus (PRRSV), and *M. hyopneumoniae*], and vaccination of dams (e.g., PCV2) (**Appendix 4**).

Knowledge Gaps

The selection of knowledge gaps identified discretionary items based on the authors' opinions. We found that there were relatively few studies in which a non-antibiotic intervention was compared directly with an antibiotic comparison group. Among the vaccine clinical trials, approximately one third failed to report a clinically important outcome.

DISCUSSION

This scoping review of non-antibiotic approaches for disease prevention or control that may reduce the need for antibiotics in nursery pigs relevant to the North American context identified a large body of literature with considerable breadth and depth. Since most of the studies described in this ScR were conducted in the EU or the UK, we may have not captured a body of knowledge on this broad topic for the North American context. The breadth of this literature was reflected in the diversity of interventions or risk factors evaluated, whereas the depth of this literature was reflected in the number of specific topic areas with similar studies that might feasibly support systematic reviews.

Clinical and policy decisions are generally regarded as best guided by the interpretation of findings of multiple studies evaluating the same research question rather than the findings of a single study, which is a random event from a distribution of possible results (23). A summary of multiple relevant studies in the form of a systematic review can provide a credible summary of the primary literature (23). However, a third of the literature included in this scoping review was sourced from proceedings that present at least three challenges to systematic reviews. First, proceedings obtained through the AASV Swine Information Library were available exclusively to members and thus would not be available to review teams through database searches. Second, these proceedings databases were not searchable through word string searches, which are an efficient method to search the literature on a specific topic. Third, these proceedings were not peer-reviewed and often were short; thus, the quality of research reporting in proceedings may be insufficient for inclusion into systematic reviews. Brace et al. (24), in an evaluation of the quality of reporting of vaccine trials at veterinary conferences, concluded that it would be difficult to assess validity from the information provided in most conference proceedings. Although there was apparently considerable depth in this body of literature, without the inclusion of proceedings, the depth may actually be considerably less. Interestingly, the majority of research from the USA on this broad topic was available only through proceedings. Similarly, Brace et al. (24) reported that only 6% of 89 proceedings presented on swine vaccines at the AASV annual conference from 1988 to 2003 were later published as full articles. Although assessing the proceedings-to-publication ratio from AASV conferences was not our objective, our findings of only two duplicate journal articles with conference proceedings suggest the ratio is still low. This may represent a lost opportunity for the communication of research.

We chose to focus our data charting on controlled clinical trials. We did not include quasi-experimental trial design (i.e., before and after intervention comparisons), as this design does not provide an equal evidentiary value to clinical trials (19). Though challenge trials serve an important purpose in providing proof of concept prior to field trials under natural exposures, challenge trials tend to report more favorable outcomes compared with clinical trials of the same intervention (25). We found that the body of literature in this review was dominated by clinical trials with comparatively few observational studies. This may reflect the comparative ease of conducting and study design appropriateness of clinical trials vs. observational studies on swine farms.

This scoping review identified a wide variety of vaccines and feed additives, which together comprised the majority of interventions evaluated in clinical trials. There was a dearth of clinical trials that evaluated management interventions such as biosecurity and infection control, feed or nutrient restrictions, housing, and weaning. This may reflect the difficulty of evaluating these types of interventions in clinical trial settings and/or the difficulty in sourcing funding for trials of these interventions (26). Biosecurity was the most frequently studied intervention among the relatively low number of observational studies identified by this scoping review. Thus, the depth of research available for synthesis on management practices was far less than for other interventions.

Despite the approximately equal number of studies conducted on research farms vs. commercial farms, there was a strong predominance of research with the purpose of preventing disease on research farms, whereas research with the purpose of disease control was predominately conducted on commercial farms. Variables that may impact the outcome of a trial, such as prior disease-free status, could potentially be better controlled on research farms than commercial farms, whereas the field conditions of commercial farms, such as an existing disease problem, provides a better setting to truly test the effectiveness of an intervention under "natural commercial" conditions (27). However, it is unknown to what extent the research vs. commercial farm settings impact external validity in swine research.

Among the studies identified through this scoping review, approximately half reported a comparison group that was a different form or level of the intervention itself. Traditional systematic reviews and meta-analyses are not just based on studies with similar interventions, populations, and outcomes but also on similar comparison groups. In the absence of sufficient studies with similar comparison groups, combining studies with the same outcome through network meta-analysis may prove useful. Network meta-analysis allows comparisons of interventions that may not have been directly compared in head-to-head trials by mathematically evaluating both direct and indirect comparison evidence of multiple interventions and comparisons (28). If we had restricted our scoping review to studies that compared a non-antibiotic intervention group with an antibiotic intervention group, our review would have been very limited: first, because most of these studies evaluated a feed additive intervention, and second, because there were relatively few feed additive intervention studies with an antibiotic comparison group. In a body of literature that describes non-antibiotic approaches to improve the health of nursery pigs, this lack of comparisons with antibiotics may represent a knowledge gap for decisions about antibiotic alternatives. Where it may be appropriate to use an antibiotic comparison group, the results could potentially demonstrate the superiority or at least the non-inferiority of a non-antibiotic intervention.

Approximately one third of vaccine clinical trials did not report a clinically important outcome, though they did report measures of immunity. The lack of reporting clinically important outcomes when they could have been measured reduces our opportunity to build a body of evidence best suited for clinical decision making. Clinically important outcomes as determined by guidelines, clinicians, patients, or the researcher provide the best evidence for inclusion in systematic reviews, whereas indirect outcomes such as measures of immunity provide a lower quality of evidence (29–33). To enhance research efficiency, future vaccine clinical trials should report clinically important outcomes.

Beyond describing the body of literature pertaining to non-antibiotic approaches that may reduce the need for antibiotics for disease prevention or control in nursery pigs, an additional objective of this review was to identify specific topic areas where there may be sufficient literature to support systematic reviews. We identified 13 specific topic areas with a minimum of 10 clinical trials that may feasibly support systematic reviews. These topic areas were composed of various vaccines and feed additives. Although we listed the ZnO as an intervention for which there may be sufficient material to support an SR, we do not recommend knowledge synthesis for this intervention given that concerns regarding AMR co-selection with the use of ZnO in swine (34). Though this scoping review identified numerous specific topic areas that might be feasibly combined in systematic reviews, similarity among comparison groups and choice of outcome would need to be carefully considered. Nevertheless, systematic reviews of these topic areas for nursery pigs, if not already conducted, could provide a useful synthesis of existing knowledge. Some systematic reviews of related topics have been conducted (35–39); however, none of these systematic reviews pertained exclusively to health outcomes in nursery pigs.

In determining the specific topic areas with sufficient similar studies to support systematic reviews, we used an arbitrary number of 10 similar clinical trials with some commonality of the intervention and population. Technically, a minimum of two studies are all that is needed for combination in a meta-analysis if those studies are similar enough to combine in a meaningful way (40). However, having additional studies provides an opportunity to explore between-study variability, which in turn impacts the interpretation and meaning of the meta-analysis (40), (41).

There were potential limitations that may have impacted the comprehensiveness of this scoping review. First, we may have missed some articles if we did not include all possible terms for each of the many non-antibiotic interventions included in the search. Systematic reviews for specific interventions should maximize comprehensiveness by including all possible terms. Second, we may have overlooked some interventions or outcomes if they did not appear in the title or abstract. Third, we accessed bibliographic sources available through the University of Guelph data platforms and two conference proceedings available through the AASV library. We may have missed additional published articles available through other databases, and unpublished studies generated by companies testing products or proceedings from other conferences. Fourth, our search using the CAB Direct platform was unsuccessful due to technical difficulties. Without the additional studies identified through that platform, our search may not have been as comprehensive as we had intended. The coverage provided by CAB Abstracts was found to be excellent in a comparison of nine databases for veterinary journals (42), so it is possible that the CAB platform contained relevant articles that our search did not identify. Finally, due to limited resources, we could not include all possibly relevant sources of gray literature such as symposia proceedings. We chose to focus on the gray literature of North America.

include all possibly relevant sources of gray literature such as symposia proceedings. We chose to focus on the gray literature of North America.

In addition to limitations to comprehensiveness, this review may have two additional limitations. First, we may have misclassified the purpose of the intervention for disease control by including in this category pig herds or groups that also had a known exposure to an infection and not solely groups that contained clinically ill or infected pigs as defined by AVMA and GAO reports. Finally, we did not assess inherent biases of included studies such as lack of appropriate randomization of clinical trials, lack of concealment or blinding, loss to follow-up, or selective outcome reporting. Any systematic reviews of non-antibiotic approaches that may reduce the need for antibiotic prevention or control in nursery pig production should include a risk of bias assessment (43).

AUTHOR CONTRIBUTIONS

LW coordinated the project, acted as the primary reviewer for relevance screening and data charting, analyzed data, interpreted the results, and wrote the manuscript drafts. JS oversaw the work, piloted the relevance screening and data charting forms, assisted with the interpretation of results, reviewed manuscript drafts, and approved the final manuscript. AO'C and SM provided guidance for interpretation of the results, commented on the manuscript drafts, and approved the final manuscript. TO'S provided guidance for the stakeholder survey and interpretation of the results, commented on the manuscript drafts, and approved the final manuscript. MR and KC conducted relevance screening and data charting as a second reviewer, commented on manuscript drafts, and approved the final manuscript version. All authors contributed to the article and approved the submitted version.

ACKNOWLEDGMENTS

We thank our stakeholders for their invaluable guidance. We also thank our research librarian, Ms. Ali Versluis, for her help.

REFERENCES

1. Laxminarayan R, Duse A, Wattal C, Zaidi AKM, Wertheim HFL, Sumpradit N, et al. Antibiotic resistance-the need for global solutions. *Lancet Infect Dis.* (2014) 13:1057–98. doi: 10.1016/S1473-3099(13)70318-9
2. World Organization for Animal Health (OIE). *The OIE Strategy on Antimicrobial Resistance and the Prudent Use of Antimicrobials.* (2016). p. 4–6. Available online at: http://www.oie.int/fileadmin/Home/eng/Media_Center/docs/pdf/PortailAMR/EN_OIE-AMRstrategy.pdf (accessed July 6, 2018).
3. World Health Organization (WHO). *Critically Important Antimicrobials for Human Medicine*, 6th Revision Geneva (CH): WHO Press (2018). p. 1–13.
4. World Health Organization (WHO). The Evolving Threat of Antimicrobial Resistance. Options for action. Geneva (CH): WHO Press (2012). p. 8–9. Available online: http://whqlibdoc.who.int/publications/2012/9789241503181_eng.pdf (accessed July 6, 2018).
5. Food and Agriculture Organization of the United Nations (FAO). *The FAO Action Plan on Antimicrobial Resistance 2016-2020.* (2016). p. 1–12. Available

online at: http://www.fao.org/publications or http://www.fao.org/3/a-i5996e.pdf (accessed July 6, 2018).

6. World Organization for Animal Health (OIE). *List of Antimicrobial Agents of Veterinary Importance.* (2015). p. 1–9. Available online at: https://rr-africa.oie.int/wp-content/uploads/2019/09/eng_oie_list_antimicrobials_may2015.pdf (accessed June 14, 2019).
7. World Health Organization (WHO). WHO Guidelines on Use of Medically Important Antimicrobials in Food-Producing Animals. Geneva (CH): WHO Press (2017). p. 18–22. Available online at: https://www.who.int/foodsafety/areas_work/antimicrobial-resistance/cia_guidelines/en/ (accessed June 14, 2019).
8. Gelband H, Miller-Petrie M, Pant S, Gandra S, Levinson J, Barter D, et al. *State of the World's Antibiotics 2015.* Washington, DC: Centre for Disease Dynamics, Economics and Policy 2015. p. 38. Available online at: https://cddep.org/publications/state_worlds_antibiotics_2015/ (accessed August 23, 2018).
9. U.S. Food and Drug Administration. *Veterinary Feed Directive Final Rule and Next Steps.* (2019). Fact Sheet. Available online at: https://www.fda.gov/animal-veterinary/development-approval-process/fact-sheet-veterinary-feed-directive-final-rule-and-next-steps (accessed June 17, 2019).
10. Government of Canada (CA). *Responsible Use of Medically Important Antimicrobials in Animals.* (2018). Available online at: https://www.canada.ca/en/public-health/services/antibiotic-antimicrobial-resistance/animals/actions/responsible-use-antimicrobials.html (accessed March 7, 2019).
11. European Parliament and Council (EU). *Regulation (EC) No1831/2003 of the European Parliament and Council. Official Journal of the European Union L268/29.* (2003). Available online at: https://eur-lex.europa.eu/legal-content/EN/TXT/PDF/?uri=CELEX:32003R1831&from=EN) (accessed November 25, 2019).
12. Lekagul A, Tangcharoensathien V, Yeung S. Patterns of antibiotic use in global pig production. *Vet Anim Sci.* (2019) 100058:1–12. doi: 10.1016/j.vas.2019.100058
13. Arksey H, O'Malley L. Scoping studies: towards a methodological framework. *Int J Soc Res Methodol.* (2005) 8:19–32. doi: 10.1080/1364557032000119616
14. Levac D, Colquhoun H, O'Brien KK. Scoping studies: advancing the methodology. *Implement Sci.* (2010) 5:69. doi: 10.1186/1748-5908-5-69
15. Tricco AC, Lillie E, Zarin W, O'Brien K, Colquhoun H, Kastner M, et al. A scoping review on the conduct and reporting of scoping reviews. *BMC Med Res Methodol.* (2016) 16:15. doi: 10.1186/s12874-016-0116-4
16. Tricco AC, Lillie E, Zarin W, O'Brien KK, Colquhoun H, Levac D, et al. PRISMA extension for scoping reviews (PRISMA-ScR): checklist and explanation. *Ann Intern Med.* (2018) 169:467–73. doi: 10.7326/M18-0850
17. United States Government Accountability Office (GAO). *Report GAO-11-801, September 2011 Antibiotic Resistance.* Available online at: https://www.gao.gov/new.items/d11801.pdf (accessed November 08, 2011).
18. American Veterinary Medical Association (internet). *AVMA Definitions for Disease Prevention, Control and Treatment US.* (2019). Available online at: https://www.avma.org/KB/Policies/Pages/AVMA-Definitions-of-Antimicrobial-Use-for-Treatment-Control-and-Prevention.aspx (accessed November 8, 2019).
19. Sargeant JM, Kelton DF, O'Connor AM. Study designs and systematic review of interventions: building evidence across study designs. *Zoon Public Health.* (2014) 61:10–7. doi: 10.1111/zph.12127
20. Pineiro C, Morales J, Dereu A, Wuyts N, Azlor O, Vizcaino E, et al. Individual pig care program improves productive performance. *J Swine Health Prod.* (2014) 22:296–9.
21. Lapointe L, D'Allaire S, Lebrun A, Lacouture S, Gottschalk M. Antibody response to an autogenous vaccine and serological profile for Streptococcus suis capsular type 1/2. *Can J Vet Res.* (2002) 66:8–14.
22. Pantoja LG, Kuhn M, Hoover T, Amodie D, Weigel D, Dice C, et al. Impact of a husbandry education program on nursery pig productivity. In: *22nd International Pig Veterinary Society Congress (IPVS)* (Jeju: WO-116) (2012).
23. Garg AX, Hackam D, Tonelli M. Systematic review and meta-analysis: when one study is just not enough. *Clin J Am Soc Nephrol.* (2008) 3:253–60. doi: 10.2215/CJN.01430307
24. Brace S, Taylor D, O'Connor AM. The quality of reporting and publication status of vaccine trials presented at veterinary conferences from 1988 to 2003. *Vaccine.* (2010) 28:5306–14. doi: 10.1016/j.vaccine.2010.05.041
25. Wisener LV, Sargeant JM, O'Connor AM, Faires MC, Glass-Kaastra SK. The evidentiary value of challenge trials for three pre-harvest food safety topics: a systematic assessment. *Zoon Public Health.* (2014) 61:449–76. doi: 10.1111/zph.12083
26. Ribble CS, Stitt T, Iwasawa S, Toews L, Stephen C. *A Review of Alternative Practices to Antimicrobial Use for Disease Control in the Commercial Feedlot.* Winnipeg, SK: National Collaborating Centre for Infectious Diseases (2010). p. 2–5.
27. Johnston LJ, Renteria A, Hannon MR. Commentary, improving validity of on-farm research. *J Swine Health Prod.* (2003) 11:240–6.
28. Li T, Puhan MA, Vedula AA, Singh S, Dickersin K. Commentary, Network meta-analysis-highly attractive but more methodological research is needed. *BMC Medicine.* (2011) 9:79. doi: 10.1186/1741-7015-9-79
29. Guyatt GH, Oxman AD, Kunz R, Atkins D, Brozek J, Vist G, et al. GRADE guidelines: 2. Framing the question and deciding on important outcomes. *J Clin Epidemiol.* (2011) 64:395–400. doi: 10.1016/j.jclinepi.2010.09.012
30. Guyatt GH, Oxman AD, Kunz R, Woodcock J, Brozek J, Helfand M, et al. GRADE Working Group. GRADE guidelines: 8. Rating the quality of evidence-indirectness. *J Clin Epidemiol.* (2011) 64:1303–10. doi: 10.1016/j.jclinepi.2011.04.014
31. Fleming TR, Powers JH. Biomarkers and surrogate endpoints in clinical trials. *Stat Med.* (2012) 31:2973–84. doi: 10.1002/sim.5403
32. O'Connor AM, Anderson KM, Goodell CK, Sargeant JM. Conducting systematic reviews of intervention questions I: writing the review protocol, formulating the question and searching the literature. *Zoon Public Health.* (2014) 61:28–38. doi: 10.1111/zph.12125
33. Ryan R, Santesso N, Hill S. *Preparing Summary of Findings (SoF) Tables.* Cochrane Consumers and Communication Group [Online] (2016). Available online at: http://cccrg.cochrane.org/author-resources (accessed June 21, 2019).
34. Cheng G, Ning J, Ahmed S, Huang J, Ullah R, An B, et al. Selection and dissemination of antimicrobial resistance in Agri-food production. *Antimicrob Resist Infect Control.* (2019) 8:158. doi: 10.1186/s13756-019-0623-2
35. Diraviyam T, Zhao B, Wang Y, Schade R, Michael A, Zhang X. Effect of chicken egg yolk antibodies (IgY) against diarrhea in domesticated animals: a systematic review and meta-analysis. *PLoS ONE.* (2014) 9:e97716. doi: 10.1371/journal.pone.0097716
36. da Silva N, Carriquiry A, O'Neill K, Opriessnig T, O'Connor AM. Mixed treatment comparison meta-analysis of porcine circovirus type 2 (PCV2) vaccines used in piglets. *Prev Vet Med.* (2014) 117:413–24. doi: 10.1016/j.prevetmed.2014.10.006
37. Mathie RT, Clausen J. Veterinary homeopathy: systematic review of medical conditions studied by randomized trials controlled by other than placebo. *BMC Vet Res.* (2015) 11:236. doi: 10.1186/s12917-015-0542-2
38. Ayrle H, Mevissen M, Kaske M, Nathues H, Gruetzner N, Melzig M, et al. Medicinal plants—prophylactic and therapeutic options for gastrointestinal and respiratory diseases in calves and piglets? A systematic review. *BMC Vet Res.* (2016) 12:1–31. doi: 10.1186/s12917-016-0714-8
39. Sargeant J, Bergevin M, Bhumika D, Churchill K, Dawkins K, Dunn J, et al. Efficacy of bacterial vaccines to prevent respiratory disease in swine: a systematic review and network meta-analysis. *Anim Health Res Rev.* (2019) 20:274–90. doi: 10.1017/S1466252319000173
40. Borenstein M, Hedges LV, Higgins JPT, Rothstein HR. *Introduction to Meta-Analysis.* West Sussex: John Wiley and Sons Ltd. (2009). p. 363–4.
41. Ioannidis J, Patsopoulos N, Rothstein H. Reasons or excuses for avoiding meta-analysis in forest plots. *BMJ Res Methodol.* (2008) 336:1413–5. doi: 10.1136/bmj.a117
42. Grindlay DJ, Brennan ML, Dean RS. Searching the veterinary literature: a comparison of the coverage of veterinary journals by nine bibliographic databases. *J Vet Med Educ.* (2012) 39:404–12. doi: 10.3179/jjmu.39.404
43. Higgins JPT, Thomas J, Chandler J, Cumpston M, Li T, Page MJ, et al., editors. *Cochrane Handbook for Systematic Reviews of Interventions Version 6.0.* (2019). Available online at: www.training.cochrane.org/handbook (accessed December 17, 2019).

17

Spatial Distribution of Trypanosomes in Cattle

Velma Kivali[1,2*]*, Alice N. Kiyong'a*[1]*, Jenna Fyfe*[2]*, Philip Toye*[1]*, Eric M. Fèvre*[1,3] *and Elizabeth A. J. Cook*[1,3*]

[1] *International Livestock Research Institute, Nairobi, Kenya,* [2] *Biomedical Sciences, Edinburgh Medical School, University of Edinburgh, Edinburgh, United Kingdom,* [3] *Institute of Infection, Veterinary and Ecological Sciences, University of Liverpool, Liverpool, United Kingdom*

Correspondence:
Velma Kivali
velmakivali@gmail.com
Elizabeth A. J. Cook
e.cook@cgiar.org

African Animal Trypanosomiasis (AAT) is a tsetse-transmitted protozoan disease endemic in "the tsetse belt" of Africa. Past studies investigating the epidemiology of the disease rarely focused on spatial distribution when reporting the prevalence. The challenge of understanding the spatial epidemiology of the disease is further confounded by low-sensitive parasitological techniques used in field investigations. This study aimed to identify trypanosome species in cattle and their spatial distribution in western Kenya. Low-sensitive microscopic analysis and highly-sensitive polymerase chain reaction (PCR) techniques were also compared to better understand the epidemiology of *Trypanosoma* infections by use of the geographical information system (GIS). Blood samples from 888 cattle, collected between August 2010 and July 2012, were examined for *Trypanosoma* parasites by light microscopy and PCR. The spatial distribution of *Trypanosoma* positive cases by species were mapped and overlaid on the map for tsetse distribution. The estimated prevalence was 4.17% by PCR compared to 2.48% by microscopy. Trypanosomes were detected in tsetse free areas. *Trypanosoma vivax* and *Trypanosoma b. brucei* were identified, but not the zoonotic *Trypanosoma b. rhodesiense*. This study demonstrated the importance of geospatial data analysis to understand the epidemiology of the parasite, to inform future research and formulate control strategies.

Keywords: trypanosomiasis, tsetse, cattle, Kenya, spatial distribution

INTRODUCTION

Trypanosomiasis is a disease of humans and animals caused by protozoan parasites of the genus *Trypanasoma* and is transmitted by tsetse flies of the genus *Glossina.* It is endemic in 38 countries in sub-Saharan Africa (1). The disease exists in two forms; Human African Trypanosomiasis (HAT), a neglected tropical disease that is fatal if left untreated (2) and African Animal Trypanosomiasis (AAT). AAT is associated with substantial economic losses to farmers and is a major constraint in the fight against poverty in the affected countries (3). *Trypanasoma* species that affect cattle are *Trypanasoma vivax, Trypanasoma congolense*, and *Trypanasoma brucei.* Trypanosomiasis has a zoonotic aspect whose etiological agents are *Trypanasoma b. rhodesiense* and *Trypanasoma b. gambiense.* Cattle and other domestic animals are the reservoirs for these zoonotic trypanosomes which are transmitted cyclically between humans and animals by tsetse flies (4).

Diagnosis of trypanosomiasis can be clinical, parasitological, serological, or by use of molecular techniques (5). Control of trypanosomiasis is through the combination of both vector control, to reduce the tsetse fly population, and prophylactic chemotherapy (6). Trypanocidal drugs are also used to treat clinical cases of bovine trypanosomiasis (7).

Kenya lies partially within the tsetse belt of sub-Saharan Africa. According to Machila et al. (8) trypanosomiasis is endemic to the western and coastal regions of Kenya. Epidemiological studies of both HAT and AAT have been conducted in different parts of the country (8–11).

Previous studies have shown that AAT is a major constraint to cattle production in western Kenya (10). Epidemiological studies in this area in 2004 estimated a prevalence of 20.1% of trypanosomiasis in cattle, 8.4 and 17.4% in pigs from two different sites in the region and a prevalence of <5% in small ruminants (11). A study conducted in Teso and Suba Districts in western Kenya in 2006 investigated the spatial distribution of AAT and showed the majority of *Trypanasoma* infections were caused by *T. vivax* outside the tsetse belt (12).

This study aimed to identify the different trypanosome species infecting cattle in Busia county and surrounding areas and map their distribution. Additionally, it sought to establish whether human infective *T. brucei*, i.e., *T. b. rhodesiense* was present in cattle in this region.

MATERIALS AND METHODS

Cattle samples used in this study were collected between August 2010 and July 2012 as part of a cross-sectional study conducted in Busia region of the former Western province of Kenya (13). Sampling was conducted within a 45 km radius of Busia town spreading into the current Siaya, Kakamega, and Bungoma Counties. The sample size was determined and adjusted using the Survey package in the R program version 3.1.1 (http://cran.r-project.org/) and the study design powered by an estimated lowest prevalence of 5% of disease in cattle with a standard error of 2%. The primary sampling unit was a homestead defined as the place where family members shared an evening meal. Eight hundred and eighty eight cattle samples were collected from 416 randomly selected homesteads. These were apparently healthy animals on farms included in a cross-sectional survey of zoonotic infections. Sampling was done after seeking consent from the head of all eligible homesteads.

Structured questionnaires were administered prior to sampling to capture animal characteristics, such as age, sex, and breed. Venous blood was collected from the jugular vein of each animal into ethylenediaminetetraacetic acid (EDTA) coated tubes which were barcoded and labeled with the animal identity. The samples were transported in upright position to the project laboratory in Busia and stored at −40°C, before being shipped to Nairobi for subsequent analysis. All samples were examined by both microscopy and PCR and the results interpreted in parallel.

Thin and thick blood smears were prepared in the field at the point of collection from the marginal ear veins of the study cattle. Microscopic diagnosis on thick and thin blood smears was used to determine presence or absence of the trypanosomes. Thick smears were examined using X10 objective lens and the number of parasites counted in each of 100 fields. Thin smears were also examined at X10 and then at X100 under oil immersion and number of parasites in every 100 fields was recorded. The results were interpreted as per the OIE recommendations, i.e., one parasite in 10 fields examined was interpreted as low, one parasite in 5 fields was interpreted as medium and more than one parasite in 1 field was interpreted as high.

DNA was extracted from all EDTA blood samples using the MagNa Pure LC DNA Isolation Kit I (Cat. No. 03 003 990 001) and the MagNa Pure LC 2.0 Instrument (Roche Applied Science, Mannheim, Germany). Conventional species specific PCR testing was performed on extracted DNA for detection of *T. b. brucei*, *T. congolense*, *T. vivax*. All *T. b. brucei* positive samples were further analyzed to determine if they were zoonotic, i.e., *T. b. rhodesiense*. Previously described PCR protocols (14–16) were used for:

- *T. b. brucei*

forward primer sequence GAATATTAAACAATGCGCAG
reverse primer CCATTTATTAGCTTTGTTGC,

- *T. congolense*

forward primer sequence CGAGAACGGGCACTTTGCGA
reverse primer GGACAAACAAATCCCGCACA,

- *T. vivax*

forward primer sequence CAGCTCGGCGAAGGCCACTTCG CTGGGGTG
reverse primer sequence TCGCTACCACAGTCGCAATCG TCGTCT CAAGG,

- *T. b. rhodesiense*

forward primer sequence ATAGTGACAAGATGCGTACTC AACGC
reverse primer sequence AATGTGTTCGAGTACTTCGGT CACGCT.

Annealing temperatures for the primers were determined using gradient PCR. Reaction volume for each sample consisted of 1X DreamTaq Green PCR Master Mix (ThermoFisher Scientific; Waltham, Massachusetts), 10 μM of forward and reverse species-specific primers, DNA and nuclease-free water. Thermocycling was done on the C1000 touch Thermo cycler (BIO-RAD, Hercules, California, United States) and amplicons were detected using gel electrophoresis.

Descriptive analysis was performed to determine the distribution of the results obtained based on age, sex, and breed of the animals. This was achieved using the "frequency" tool of IBM SPSS® version 20. A Cohen's Kappa test was run (17) to compare the level of agreement between microscopy and PCR.

ESRI ArcGIS 10.3.1 software was used to spatially map all the positive cases using the x and y coordinates. Additional data layers' describing the tsetse distribution in the study area was obtained from a GIS database available at the International Livestock Research Institute website (http://www.ilri.org/GIS). A positive case was defined as positive using either microscopy, PCR or both diagnostic techniques.

A spatial risk map was generated to identify areas with the greatest relative risk for trypanosome infection. The density of positive cases of trypanosomes was assessed using Kernel smoothing in the *spatstat* package (18) in R. This was done with a fixed bandwidth of 5 km and correlation for edge effects. The kernel intensity of positive homesteads was divided by the kernel intensity of the all homesteads in the study area creating a risk surface.

RESULTS

Out of the 888 cattle analyzed, 65.3% were female and almost all of them belonged to the shorthorn Zebu and Zebu breeds (**Supplementary Table**).

The estimated prevalence of trypanosome species detected by both microscopy and PCR was 4.17% (95% CI 3.931–4.409). Thirty four animals were infected with a single trypanosome species while three animals had mixed trypanosome infections of *T. vivax and T. b. brucei. T. congolense* constituted the smallest proportion of all trypanosomes found in cattle in the study site (**Table 1**).

Spatial Distribution and Relative Risk

The locations of all positive cases were mapped as shown in **Figure 1**. Most of the infected cattle were located in the western and south-western parts of the study area (**Figures 1A–C**). The addition of the tsetse fly distribution layer to the map revealed that there were trypanasome positive cattle in tsetse-free areas in the eastern part of the study area. The distribution of positive cattle was the same for both diagnostic tests used (**Figures 1A,B**).

Spatial relative risk maps (**Figure 2**) also demonstrated that areas of greatest relative risk for trypanosome infection were the south western parts of the study area around Lake Victoria.

Comparison of Microscopy and PCR

T. vivax was the most common infection detected by microscopy (**Figure 1A**) and *T. brucei* was the most common infection detected by PCR (**Figure 1B**). Only *T. vivax* results provided a statistically reasonable number of positives hence possible to determine the level of agreement between the PCR and microscopy results. A Cohen's Kappa test was run and the results revealed a moderate agreement between the two tests, i.e., K = 0.403 (95% CI 0.098–1.521), $p < 0.0005$.

TABLE 1 | Prevalence of trypanosoma species identified based on the test used.

Trypanosome species (Test used)	Positive/ sample size	Apparent prevalence (95% confidence interval)
All species tested	37/888	4.17 (3.931–4.409)
T. brucei (thick smears)	1/888	0.11 (0.131–0.089)
T. brucei (thin smears)	1/888	0.11 (0.089–0.131)
T. brucei (PCR)	8/888	0.90 (0.920–0.880)
T. congolense (thick smear)	4/888	0.45 (0.483–0.417)
T. congolense (thin smear)	2/888	0.23 (0.258–0.202)
T. congolense savannah (PCR)	0/888	0.00 (0.000–0.000)
T. vivax (thick smear)	13/888	1.46 (1.514–1.406)
T. vivax (thin smear)	13/888	1.46 (1.514–1.406)
T. vivax (PCR)	12/888	1.35 (0.468–0.332)

DISCUSSION

This study found a prevalence of 4.17% of *Trypanosoma* infection which is lower compared to earlier studies in cattle in the same region that established a prevalence of 41% and 29% in Suba and Teso regions of western Kenya, respectively in 2006 (12) and 20.1% in the former Busia district in 2004 (11). This might suggest the impact of improved control strategies against trypanasomiasis, improved local knowledge of the disease or a change in disease dynamics since the other studies were conducted. Between 1999 and 2012 different control strategies were implemented in the region with funding from the European Union for Farming in Tsetse Controlled Areas (FITCA) and Pan African Tsetse And Trypanosomiasis Eradication Council (PATTEC) projects. A study conducted in 2008 demonstrated that 61% of people in western Kenya were aware of tsetse and trypanosome control methods and bush clearing was recently used by almost half of respondents as a control method (19). These interventions might have greatly contributed to the decrease in prevalence of trypansomiasis. However, it is important to determine the current prevalence status as there has been less focus, support and funding for trypanosomiasis in recent years (20) and hence a possibility of an increase in prevalence.

Mapping the positive cases by microscopy (**Figure 1A**) and by PCR (**Figure 1B**) showed a similar geographical distribution of trypanasome infection with most cases located in the south western parts of the study area. Spatial mapping of the distribution of *Trypanasoma* species overlaid with the tsetse infested layer showed a number of trypanosomes in the tsetse-free areas which was previously demonstrated in the former Teso and Suba districts (12). Most infections in the tsetse-free areas were of *T. vivax*, which is known to be a mechanically-transmitted parasite by both biting flies and tsetse flies (12, 21). There is a need for further studies to establish whether this is due to mechanical transmission or a change in the distribution of tsetse flies resulting from land use changes due to habitat transformation, degradation and encroachment into the tsetse free areas. The geo-spatial data maps demonstrating the distribution of tsetse flies were developed in the year 1998, using data collected in 1973 (22). There is a likelihood that urbanization and changes in landuse could have modified and even interfered with the tsetse habitats and their distribution.

The risk of trypanasome infection in the study area is similar regardless of the diagnostic test used (**Figures 2A,B**). The spatially-smoothed risk maps showed the area with the highest risk of trypanasome infection to be the south western region of the study close to Lake Victoria. This may indicate a localized hot-spot for trypanosome transmission in this region which could be targeted for future control initiatives.

Microscopic analysis of trypanosomes is a cheap and simple technique and is easily employed in the field in the detection of trypanaomiasis. It has been shown to have low sensitivity (23). However, in this study microscopy provided an important pre-screening step and enabled comparative assessment of the results obtained. Earlier studies have shown that PCR has a

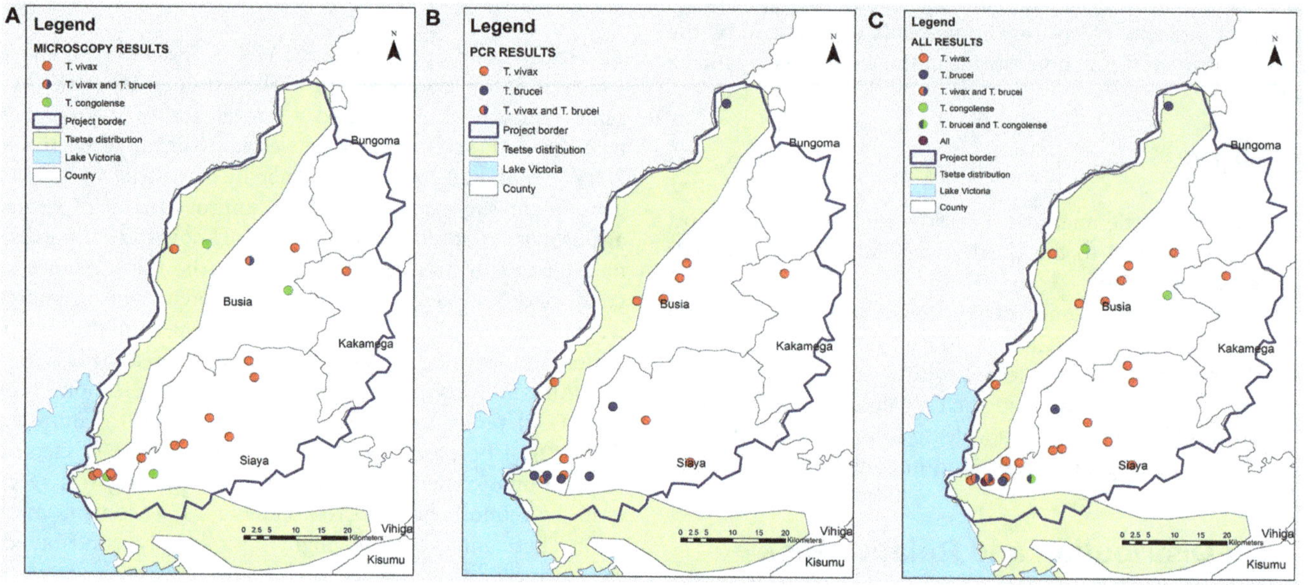

FIGURE 1 | Map of the distribution of homesteads with trypanosome positive cattle in Busia region detected by **(A)** Microscopy, **(B)** PCR, and **(C)** Microscopy and PCR.

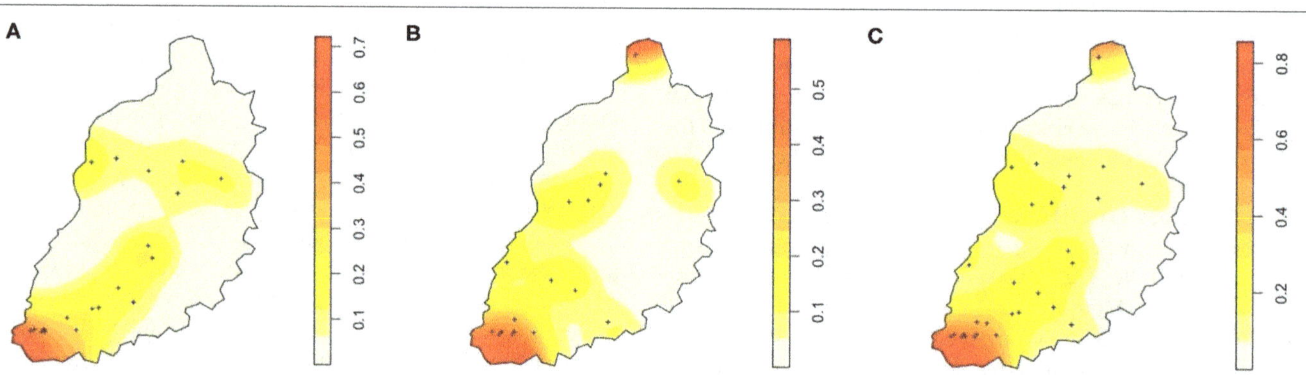

FIGURE 2 | Spatially-smoothed risk map for trypanosomes in cattle in Busia region detected by **(A)** Microscopy, **(B)** PCR, and **(C)** Microscopy and PCR. The points indicate locations of hometeads with positive trypanasome samples. Risk is measured as a ratio between 0 and 1 with results closest to 1 having the highest risk and demonstrated by increasing color intensity.

high specificity and sensitivity when diagnosing trypanosome infections (15, 24). Using PCR increased the number of total positive cases identified from 22 to 37 with the diagnosis of *T. brucei* cases being greatly improved as demonstrated in **Figure 1B**. The predominant *Trypanasoma* infection was *T. vivax* by both tests which agrees with a study conducted in other parts of western Kenya (former Teso and Suba district) (12). There were no positive *T. congolense* cases on PCR and this could be attributed to the primers used which were only specific for *T. congolense* savannah and hence there is a possibility that other sub-species of *T. congolense* could be present but were not detected.

It is important to note that PCR is a very sensitive technique for detecting parasite DNA and not every PCR-positive animal will be clinically ill. This must be considered when relating the prevalence recorded to impacts on animal health and production as these will not be directly proportional. We were not able to make conclusions regarding the clinical status of positive animals in this study. It has been suggested that asymptomatic carrier cattle may impact the success of control programmes targeting the treatment of symptomatic cattle (11).

Human infective *T. b. rhodesiense* infections were not detected even though this part of western Kenya has previously been reported to be a sleeping sickness focus with sporadic cases of HAT (11). Earlier studies reported the prevalence of *T. b. rhodensiense* in cattle to be 21.5% (11). However, the implementation of the PATTEC project in the Lake Victoria region from 2005 to 2012 may have reduced the prevalence of *T. b. rhodesiense* and Kenya has not reported a sleeping sickness case in more than 10 years (25).

CONCLUSION AND RECOMMENDATIONS

This study has demonstrated the crucial role that geospatial data analysis has in improving the understanding of disease status. This will greatly inform future research and policy formulation as it will provide evidence crucial in spearheading informed control strategies to mitigate this disease. The evidence of multiple species co-infections of trypanosomes warrants the need for change of research outlook from single-species to multiple-species investigations to better understand how the different pathogens co-exist in the targeted host. Additionally, it is crucial for continuous studies to be carried out to establish whether cattle in this region are reservoirs for zoonotic trypanosomes which is of great public health importance. This information may help Kenya with its move toward declaring the elimination of HAT as a public health problem.

AUTHOR CONTRIBUTIONS

VK and EF: conceptualization. VK and EC: formal analysis. EF: funding acquisition. VK and AK: investigation. EF, EC, and VK: methodology. EF and VK: project administration. EF, PT, and JF: supervision. VK, PT, and EC: writing-original draft. All authors: writing, review, and edit.

FUNDING

The Wellcome Trust (085308) supported the People, Animals and their Zoonoses (PAZ) project. Support was also received from the CGIAR Research Program on Agriculture for Nutrition and Health (A4NH), led by the International Food Policy Research Institute (IFPRI). We acknowledge the CGIAR Fund Donors (https://www.cgiar.org/funders/). This work was part-funded by the Global Challenges Research Fund (GCRF) One Health Regional Network for the Horn of Africa (HORN) Project, from UK Research and Innovation (UKRI) and Biotechnology and Biological Sciences Research Council (BBSRC) (project number BB/P027954/1).

ACKNOWLEDGMENTS

We were grateful to all the members of the PAZ field and laboratory teams in Busia in particular James Akoko, Omoto Lazarus, Maseno Cleophas, Jenipher Ambaka, Fredrick Amanya, Lorren Alumasa, Daniel Cheruiyot, George Omondi, John Mwaniki, Hannah Kariuki, and Lilian Achola.

REFERENCES

1. Van den Bossche P, Rocque S de La, Hendrickx G, Bouyer J. A changing environment and the epidemiology of tsetse-transmitted livestock trypanosomiasis. *Trends Parasitol.* (2010) 26:236–43. doi: 10.1016/j.pt.2010.02.010
2. Stich A, Abel PM, Krishna S. Clinical review: human African trypanosomiasis sickness presents. *Br Med J.* (2012) 325:203–6. doi: 10.1136/bmj.325.7357.203
3. Shaw APM, Cecchi G, Wint GRW, Mattioli RC, Robinson TP. Mapping the economic benefits to livestock keepers from intervening against bovine trypanosomosis in Eastern Africa. *Prev Vet Med.* (2014) 113:197–210. doi: 10.1016/j.prevetmed.2013.10.024
4. Simarro PP, Jannin J, Cattand P. Eliminating human African trypanosomiasis: where do we stand and what comes next? *PLoS Med.* (2008) 5:0174–80. doi: 10.1371/journal.pmed.0050055
5. Gadahi JA, Bhutto B, Javaid SB, Kashif J, Duchoan T, Sciences V. Diagnostic approach towards camel trypanosomiasis. *Int J Livest Res.* (2013) 4:41–5. doi: 10.5455/ijlr.20131207030112
6. Peterson C, Grinnage-Pulley T. Tsetse transmitted trypanosomiasis. In: Aiello SE, Moses M, editors. The Merck Veterinary Manual. Kenilworth, NJ: Merck & Co., Inc. (2015). Available online at: https://www.merckvetmanual.com/circulatory-system/blood-parasites/trypanosomiasis?query=tsetse%20transmitted%20trypanosomiasis (accessed December 1, 2019).
7. Geerts S, Holmes PH, Diall O, Eisler MC. African bovine trypanosomiasis: the problem of drug resistance. *Parasitol Today.* (2001) 17:25–8. doi: 10.1016/S0169-4758(00)01827-5
8. Machila N, Wanyangu SW, McDermott J, Welburn SC, Maudlin I, Eisler MC. Cattle owners' perceptions of African bovine trypanosomiasis and its control in Busia and Kwale Districts of Kenya. *Acta Trop.* (2003) 86:25–34. doi: 10.1016/S0001-706X(02)00288-7
9. Catley A, Irungu P, Simiyu K, Dadye J, Mwakio W, Kiragu J, et al. Participatory investigation of bovine trypanosomiasis in Tana river district, Kenya. *Med Vet Entomol.* (2002) 16:1–12. doi: 10.1046/j.0269-283x.2002.00346.x
10. Karanja SM. *Epidemiology and Importance of Trypanosomosis, Helminthosis and Tick-Borne Diseases on the Performance of Cattle in Busia district*, Kenya (Ph.D. Thesis). Freien Universität Berlin, Berlin, Germany (2006).
11. von Wissmann B, Machila N, Picozzi K, Fevre EM, dec Bronsvoort BM, Handel IG, et al. Factors associated with acquisition of human infective and animal infective trypanosome infections in domestic livestock in Western Kenya. *PLoS Negl Trop Dis.* (2011) 5:e941. doi: 10.1371/journal.pntd.0000941
12. Thumbi SM, Jung'a JO, Mosi RO, McOdimba FA. Spatial distribution of African Animal Trypanosomiasis in Suba and Teso districts in Western Kenya. *BMC Res Notes.* (2010) 3:6. doi: 10.1186/1756-0500-3-6
13. Fèvre EM, de Glanville WA, Thomas LF, Cook EAJ, Kariuki S, Wamae CN. An integrated study of human and animal infectious disease in the Lake Victoria crescent small-holder crop-livestock production system, Kenya. *BMC Infect Dis.* (2017) 17:457. doi: 10.1186/s12879-017-2559-6
14. Masake RA, Majiwa PAO, Moloo SK, Makau JM, Njuguna JT, Maina M, et al. Sensitive and specific detection of *Trypanosoma vivax* using the polymerase chain reaction. *Exp Parasitol.* (1997) 85:193–205. doi: 10.1006/expr.1996.4124
15. Masiga DK, Smyth AJ, Hayes P, Bromidge TJ, Gibson WC. Sensitive detection of trypanosomes in tsetse flies by DNA amplification. *Int J Parasitol.* (1992) 22:909–18. doi: 10.1016/0020-7519(92)90047-O
16. Radwanska M, Chamekh M, Vanhamme L, Claes F, Magez S, Magnus E, et al. The serum resistance-associated gene as a diagnostic tool for the detection of *Trypanosoma brucei* rhodesiense. *Am J Trop Med Hyg.* (2002) 67:684–90. doi: 10.4269/ajtmh.2002.67.684
17. Altman DG. *Practical Statistics for Medical Research.* New York, NY: Chapman Hall; CRC Press (1999).
18. Baddeley A, Rubak E, Turner R. *Spatial Point Patterns: Methodology and Applications With R.* London: Chapman and Hall; CRC (2015).

19. Rutto JJ, Osano O, Thuranira EG, Kurgat RK, Agab V. Socio-economic and cultural determinants of human African trypanosomiasis at the Kenya–Uganda transboundary. *PLoS Negl Trop Dis.* (2013) 7:e2186. doi: 10.1371/journal.pntd.0002186
20. Grant C, Anderson N, Machila N. Stakeholder narratives on trypanosomiasis, their effect on policy and the scope for one health. *PLoS Negl Trop Dis.* (2015) 9:e4241. doi: 10.1371/journal.pntd.0004241
21. Desquesnes M, Dia ML. Mechanical transmission of *Trypanosoma congolense* in cattle by the African tabanid *Atylotus agrestis*. *Exp Parasitol.* (2003) 105:226–31. doi: 10.1016/j.exppara.2003.12.014
22. Ford J, Katondo KM. Maps of tsetse fly (Glossina) distribution in Africa, 1973, according to sub-generic groups on a scale of 1:5,000,000. *Bull Anim Health Prod Afr.* (1977) 15:188–93.
23. Ng'ayo MO, Njiru ZK, Kenya EU, Muluvi GM, Osir EO, Masiga DK. Detection of trypanosomes in small ruminants and pigs in western Kenya: important reservoirs in the epidemiology of sleeping sickness? *Kinetoplastid Biol Dis.* (2005) 4:5. doi: 10.1186/1475-9292-4-5
24. Majiwa PA, Thatthi R, Moloo SK, Nyeko JH, Otieno LH, Maloo S. Detection of trypanosome infections in the saliva of tsetse flies and buffy-coat samples from antigenaemic but aparasitaemic cattle. *Parasitology.* (1994) 108:313–22. doi: 10.1017/S0031182000076150
25. WHO. Trypanosomiasis, Human African (Sleeping Sickness). WHO (2019). Available online at: https://www.who.int/health-topics/human-african-trypanosomiasis#tab=tab (accessed December 1, 2019).

18

Thermal Image Scanning for the Early Detection of Fever Induced by Highly Pathogenic Avian Influenza Virus Infection in Chickens and Ducks and its Application in Farms

Jin-Yong Noh[1], *Kyu-Jik Kim*[1], *Sun-Hak Lee*[2], *Jun-Beom Kim*[1], *Deok-Hwan Kim*[2], *Sungsu Youk*[2†], *Chang-Seon Song*[1,2] *and Sang-Soep Nahm*[3*]

[1] Konkuk Ctc bio Animal Vaccine KCAV Co. Ltd, Seoul, South Korea, [2] Department of Avian Disease, College of Veterinary Medicine, Konkuk University, Seoul, South Korea, [3] Department of Anatomy, College of Veterinary Medicine, Konkuk University, Seoul, South Korea

***Correspondence:**
Sang-Soep Nahm
ssnahm@konkuk.ac.kr

†Present address:
Sungsu Youk,
Southeast Poultry Research Laboratory, Agricultural Research Service, U.S. Department of Agriculture, U.S. National Poultry Research Center, Athens, GA, United States

Highly pathogenic avian influenza (HPAI) is considered as one of the most devastating poultry diseases. It is imperative to immediately report any known outbreaks to the World Organization for Animal Health. Early detection of infected birds is of paramount importance to control virus spread, thus minimizing the associated economic loss. In this study, thermal imaging camera devices were used to detect change in the maximum surface temperature (MST) of chickens ($n = 5$) and ducks ($n = 2$) as an early indicator of experimental HPAI infection. The MST of both chickens and ducks increased at least 24 h before the manifestation of clinical signs of HPAI infection, depending on the severity of the infection. The basal MST was recorded for broiler chickens housed under small pen and normal farm conditions without intentional infection. A threshold cutoff of MST was established based on the circadian rhythm of normal MST. This study suggests that thermal imaging of chickens and ducks is a promising tool to screen any potential HPAI-infected flock in order to expedite HPAI diagnosis.

Keywords: thermal imaging, highly pathogenic avian influenza, early detection, circadian rhythm, farm application

INTRODUCTION

Highly pathogenic avian influenza (HPAI) is considered as one of the most devastating poultry diseases (1). HPAI virus infection in gallinaceous birds is associated with high mortality, often without any apparent clinical signs, imposing difficulties in controlling virus transmission prior to viral detection (2). Since 2003, seven HPAI outbreaks involving different clades of the H5 HPAI virus have occurred in South Korea; these outbreaks have been controlled by enhanced biosecurity measures and stamping-out policies (3, 4). For better implementation of preemptive measures, early disease detection and the subsequent reporting system should precede the virus spread (5). To date, the diagnosis of HPAI infection has mostly relied on passive surveillance upon suspicion and reporting by farmers or veterinarians. However, the absence of apparent clinical signs before sudden death poses difficulties in discriminating HPAI-induced death from daily mortality at the early stage of HPAI infection (5, 6).

A network of sensors refers to a variety of wireless micro-sensors attached to, or installed near, target objects to collect behavioral, biological, or modal information of individuals or groups, followed by its transmission to a comprehensive analytic system for risk assessment (7). Many studies have demonstrated the application of sensors in the poultry industry to improve flock management through the detection of abnormal night vocalization (8), jumping and landing force in laying hens (9), and floor distribution of broilers (10) under laboratory conditions. A thermal imaging device (TID) comprises a network of sensors that detect radiant heat from single or multiple target objects. As a non-invasive tool, its potential use has been investigated in the human and veterinary fields and confirmed for the detection of fever induced by pathogen infections or an increase in maximum surface temperature (MST) caused by heat stress or ventilation problems (11–14).

In the present study, we examined the potential use of TID to detect changes in MST associated with HPAI infection in chickens and ducks before the manifestation of clinical signs. For practical application, the MST of broiler chickens was monitored by TID over 4 weeks to establish a threshold cutoff of MST during their housing in simulated small pen and real broiler farm conditions with no intentional infection. In addition, real-time data collection and analyses were performed with a central analytic system to activate an alarm system when the monitored MST of chickens exceeded the threshold setup as per the experimental infection data.

MATERIALS AND METHODS

Ethics Statement

All animal procedures performed in this study (permit number: KU18193) were reviewed, approved, and supervised by the Institutional Animal Care and Use Committee (IACUC) of Konkuk University.

Viruses

All experiments with viable virus were conducted in biosafety level 3 and animal biosafety level (BL) 3 facilities at the Konkuk University. The HPAI H5N6 A/duck/Korea/ES2/2016(H5N6) strain was provided by the Animal and Plant Quarantine Agency, Korea, and propagated in 9–11-day-old specific pathogen-free (SPF) embryonated chicken eggs and stored at −70°C until further use.

Thermal Imaging Analysis

Thermal video was recorded using an SM080TIP camera (Somo Energy & Technology Co., Ltd, Korea, Emissivity 0.98). Real-time changes in MST were monitored throughout the animal experiment. The MST was considered as one pixel representing the highest temperature among 80 × 60 pixels at each time point, regardless of the body part and number of animals. The MST of every 5 min was automatically transferred to a laptop via a network. The collected data of every 5 min were analyzed using the Argus viewer software program (Somo Energy & Technology Co., Ltd), and used for 3 h interval analyses (36 5-min time points for 3 h).

Temperature Measurement Setup Under Normal Condition

First, 6-week-old SPF chickens and 5-week-old ducks were tested negative for influenza A virus using enzyme-linked immunosorbent assay (ELISA). To examine the compatibility of the TID in the experimental setup, five chickens and one duck, respectively, were monitored with an infrared camera in the BL2 facility at Konkuk University. The thermal images were taken into consideration for analysis based on the following criteria: (1) Which body area was the site for the recognition of the highest temperature? (2) Was there any difference in temperature monitoring between individual animals and groups of animals? (3) How does the distance between the TID and photographed animal affect the measured temperature?

Temperature Measurement According to HPAI Infection

The five chickens used for the TID configuration were moved to negative pressure isolators in BL3. A thermal imaging camera was installed and fixed at the door of the isolator (0.3 m from the chickens) to minimize the effect of the distance between the camera and target object. MST was monitored at 5-min intervals. Basal MST was recorded from 24 h pre-challenge. The chickens were then intranasally challenged with 100 μL of H5N6 HPAI virus suspension (dose of $10^{6.0}$ EID_{50}/bird). Changes in MST were compared with those reported before virus inoculation. Clinical signs and mortality were recorded daily, and swab samples were obtained at 40 h post-infection (hpi) to evaluate viral shedding. The lights were turned on and off every 12 h.

In addition, a separated duck experiment similar to the chicken experiment was conducted using two ducks. The ducks used for the TID configuration were intranasally challenged with 100 μL of two different doses of HPAI H5N6 virus ($10^{8.0}$ EID_{50}/bird, high dose; $10^{4.0}$ EID_{50}/bird, low dose) to differentiate between the MST changes caused by higher and lower dose infection (15). MST was measured in the same way as that in chickens. Clinical signs and mortality were recorded daily, and swab samples were collected to quantify viral shedding at 2, 4, 7, 10, and 14 days post-infection (dpi). The temperature and relative humidity (20 ± 1°C and 50% humidity) of the animal facility were constantly maintained throughout the experiments.

Virus Detection and Quantification

To investigate the replication of the virus inoculated in chickens and ducks, oropharyngeal and cloacal swab samples were collected as section Temperature Measurement According to HPAI Infection and re-suspended in 1 mL of sterile phosphate buffer solution. The suspension was centrifuged at 15,000 × g, and 200 μL of the supernatant was used for RNA extraction using MagNA Pure 96 DNA and Viral NA Small Volume Kit on a MagNA Pure 96 instrument (Roche Applied Sciences, Germany), according to the manufacturer's instructions. The amount of viral RNA was measured by real-time reverse-transcription quantitative polymerase chain reaction (RT-qPCR) and expressed as the cycle threshold (Ct) value (16).

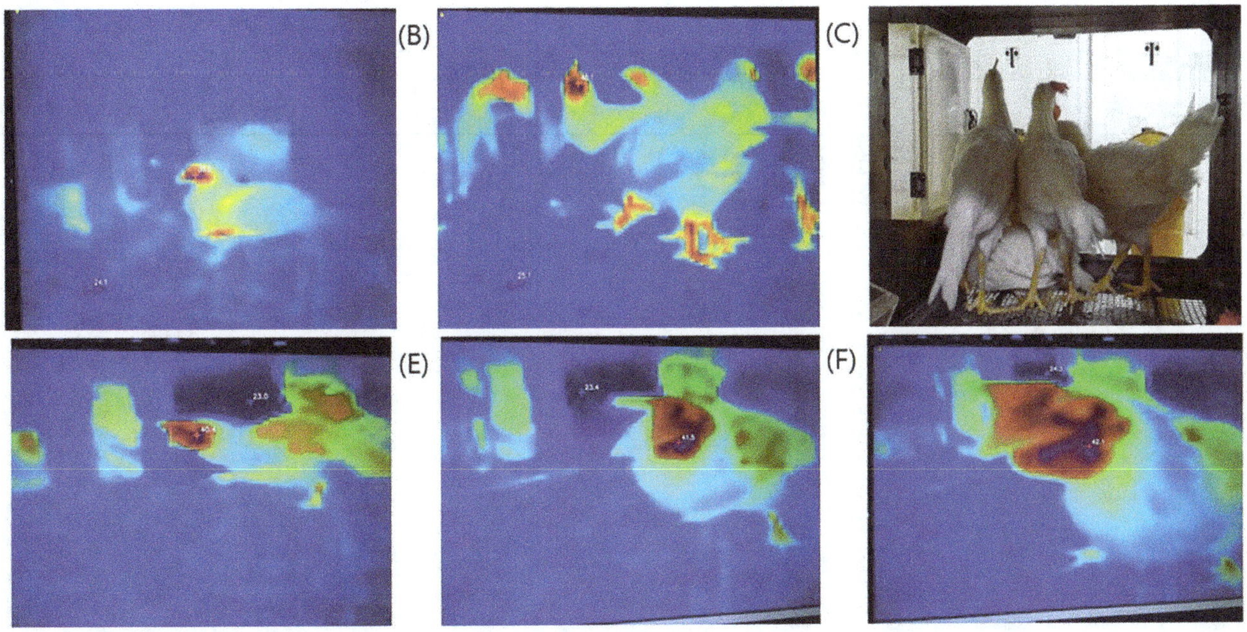

FIGURE 1 | Thermal images taken from different experimental set-ups. Top photos **(A–C)**: Temperature measurement site of one chicken or several chickens compared to the actual photographs. **(A)** One chicken; **(B)** several chickens; **(C)** actual photo. Bottom photos **(D–F)**: Differences in temperature measurement relative to distance. The shorter the distance, the higher was the measured temperature. **(D)** long distance, 40.4°C; **(E)** intermediate distance, 41.5°C; **(F)** short distance 42.1°C.

Maximum Surface Temperature Threshold Cut-Off Establishment in Actual Farm Setting

To establish a threshold cutoff for the MST in an actual farm setting, 30 1-day-old broiler chickens were raised in a 2 × 2 m pen for 4 weeks, thereby simulating a small-scale floor environment. For a larger scale environment, a broiler house with ~20,000 birds was monitored for the entire rearing period. Under simulated farm conditions, a thermal imaging camera was installed at a height of 2 m from the ground at a vertical shooting angle. In the broiler farm, a thermal imaging camera was installed at a height of 1.5 m from the ground near the farm door at a shooting angle of ~30° relative to the ground level (**Supplementary Figure 1**), unlike that in the case of the simulated farm. The temperature in a broiler house was changed from 33 to 23°C as per broiler growth and relative humidity was maintained at 50%. This monitoring was designed to set the threshold cutoff of the MST under farm conditions, considering environmental factors that affect MST, such as the circadian rhythm related to lighting.

Statistical Analysis

For the challenge study, the 24 h temporal temperature data before challenge were averaged to set the basal MST and compared to the average of temperatures recorded at 3 h intervals following infection using one-way analysis of variance (ANOVA) with a Bonferroni *post-hoc* test. Time points with asterisks denote statistically different time points after infection. $P < 0.05$ were considered statistically significant.

RESULTS

Temperature Measurement Under Normal Conditions

We investigated the possibility of temperature detection using a thermal imaging camera by monitoring chickens and ducks before they were subjected to virus challenge. The MST was detected at the head and legs of the chickens, and the beak, wings, and legs of the ducks (**Figure 1**, **Supplementary Figure 2**). There was no interference effect in MST monitoring upon examination of a single bird or multiple birds. In addition, it was confirmed that TID could successfully identify the highest temperature among multiple birds, although the only one pixel representing highest temperature was sent to the laptop.

Change in the Surface Temperature of Chickens After HPAI Virus Challenge

To determine the effect of viral infection on the MST of chickens, we monitored their MST starting from 24 h before virus inoculation. The basal MST before viral infection varied from 40.5 to 42.4°C at each time point, and the mean maximum surface temperature (MMST) over time for 24 h was 41.6°C (**Supplementary Figure 3**). After virus inoculation, the MST decreased by as low as 1.3°C until 24 hpi The MST started increasing from 26 hpi and peaked to 42.9°C from 27 to 36 hpi

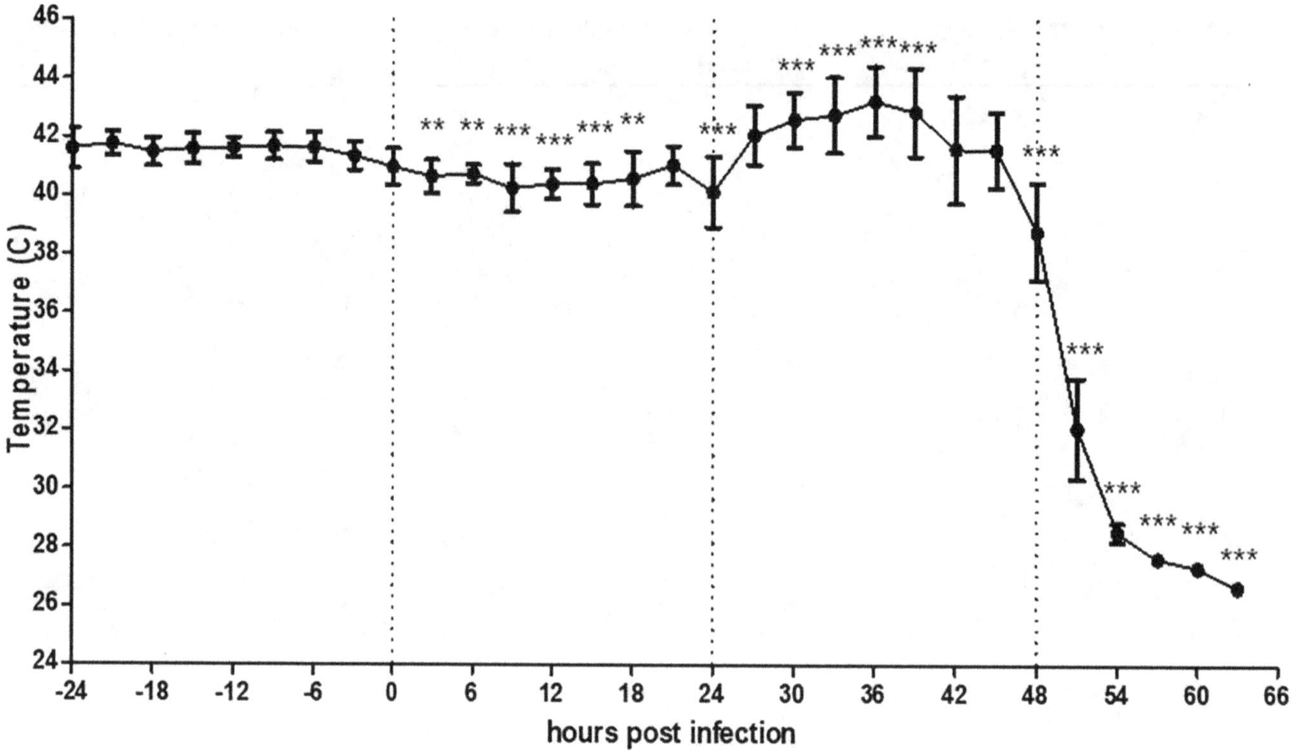

FIGURE 2 | Average temperature per 3 h interval before and after HPAI virus challenge in chickens ($n = 5$). Chickens were further monitored several more hours after death without removal. The error bars represent standard deviations of 36 5-min time points. Statistical significance was determined using ANOVA followed by Bonferroni *post-hoc* test. $^{***}P < 0.001$; $^{**}P < 0.01$.

(**Figure 2**), and suddenly decreased thereafter. This decrease in temperature was accompanied by lethargic behavior; the chickens finally died at 44 hpi. All chickens showed high viral shedding at 40 hpi from both the oropharynx (Ct = 25.7–30.5) and cloaca (Ct = 26.1–29.7).

Change in the Surface Temperature of Ducks After HPAI Virus Challenge

The recorded basal MST of the two ducks at 5 weeks of age varied from 36.6 to 39.9°C (MMST = 38.2°C) and 38.7 to 41.8°C (MMST = 40.2°C) at each time point (**Supplementary Figures 4, 5**). This difference was not calibrated to body temperature because it had no effect on the monitoring of infection-related changes in MST. To demonstrate MST changes caused by either lethal or non-lethal infection of HPAI H5N6 virus, two different doses ($10^{8.0}$ EID_{50}/bird, high dose; $10^{4.0}$ EID_{50}/bird, low dose) were used for the duck experiment.

The duck challenged with the high dose of the virus was found dead at 105 hpi. The dead duck showed a similar trend of increased MST as that observed in the chickens. After virus inoculation, the MST decreased by as low as 1.0°C until 27 hpi and started increasing from 40 hpi and peaked to 40.3°C from 80 to 86 hpi, which was 2.1°C higher than the MMST before viral challenge (**Figure 3**). The duck showed no obvious clinical signs before death, but viral shedding was detected in both oropharyngeal (Ct = 26.8 at 2 dpi and 30.8 at 4 dpi) and cloacal swabs (Ct = 31.2 at 2 dpi and undetermined at 4 dpi).

The duck challenged with the low viral dose showed a bimodal temperature increase (42.8°C and 41.4°C, which was 2.6°C and 1.2°C higher than the MMST before viral challenge) and maintained its temperature below the basal MST after 39 hpi (**Figure 4**). Although the surviving duck showed no specific clinical signs, viral shedding was observed in oropharyngeal swabs (Ct = 31.6 at 2 dpi and undetermined at 4 dpi); this indicated that, viral infection was successfully performed.

Chickens Housed Under Farm Conditions

In the small pen of the simulated floor farm conditions, the background temperature was too high to allow the recording of the MST of the chickens until the brooder was turned off. Therefore, the recording started once the heat lamp was turned off. It was confirmed that the MST of the chickens could be normally recorded even in a much wider environment than that of a small cage (**Figure 5, Supplementary Figure 6**). In addition, the circadian rhythm of MST was successfully detected using the thermal imaging camera by controlling the light at regular intervals. However, the recorded MST was lower than the actual MST and varied greatly from 28.0 to 38.0°C, thereby necessitating the calibration of image analysis.

In the actual broiler farm condition, it was possible to normally shoot videos even when the brooder was

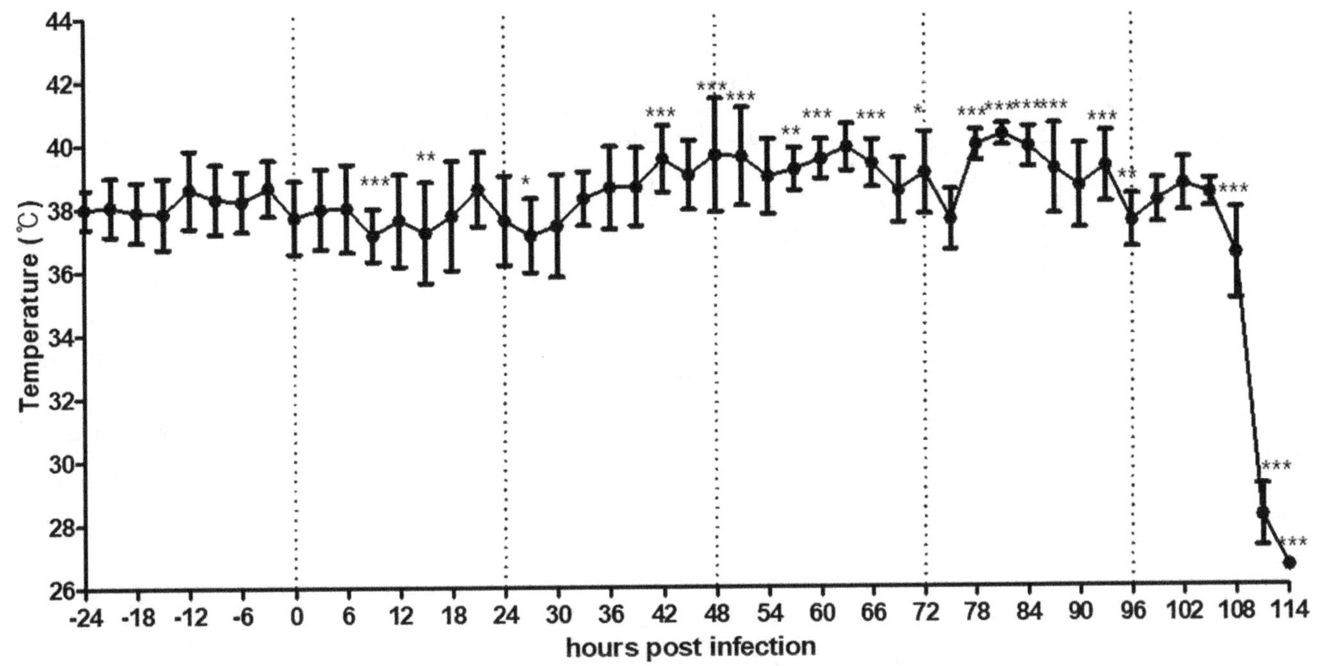

FIGURE 3 | Average temperature per 3 h interval before and after HPAI virus challenge in a duck intranasally exposed to the virus at a dose of $10^{8.0}$ EID_{50}/bird. Duck was further monitored several more hours after death without removal. The error bars represent standard deviations of 36 5-min time points. Statistical significance was determined using ANOVA followed by Bonferroni *post-hoc* test. ****P* < 0.001; ***P* < 0.01; **P* < 0.05.

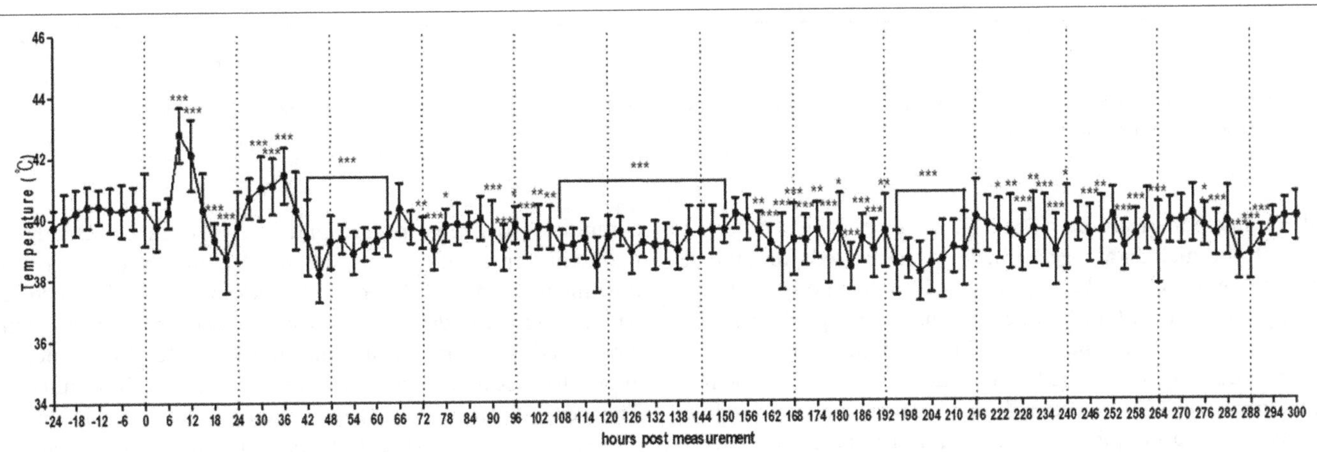

FIGURE 4 | Average temperature per 3 h interval before and after HPAI virus challenge in a duck intranasally challenged with virus at $10^{4.0}$ EID_{50}/bird dose. The error bars represent standard deviations of 36 5-min time points. Statistical significance was determined by ANOVA, followed by Bonferroni *post-hoc* test. ****P* < 0.001; ***P* < 0.01; **P* < 0.05.

turned on, as the brooder was installed on the ceiling and did not fall within the range of the thermal image. Consistent with the small pen simulation, the circadian rhythm of MST was observed under this actual broiler farm condition (**Figure 6**, **Supplementary Figure 7**). The temperature fluctuation was less than that in the small pen setting (39.0–42.0°C).

DISCUSSION

Thermal imaging cameras have been used for the screening of various infectious and non-infectious diseases in both human and veterinary fields, including the detection of severe acute respiratory syndrome (SARS) and coronavirus disease 2019 (COVID-19) (17, 18) in humans, bovine respiratory disease

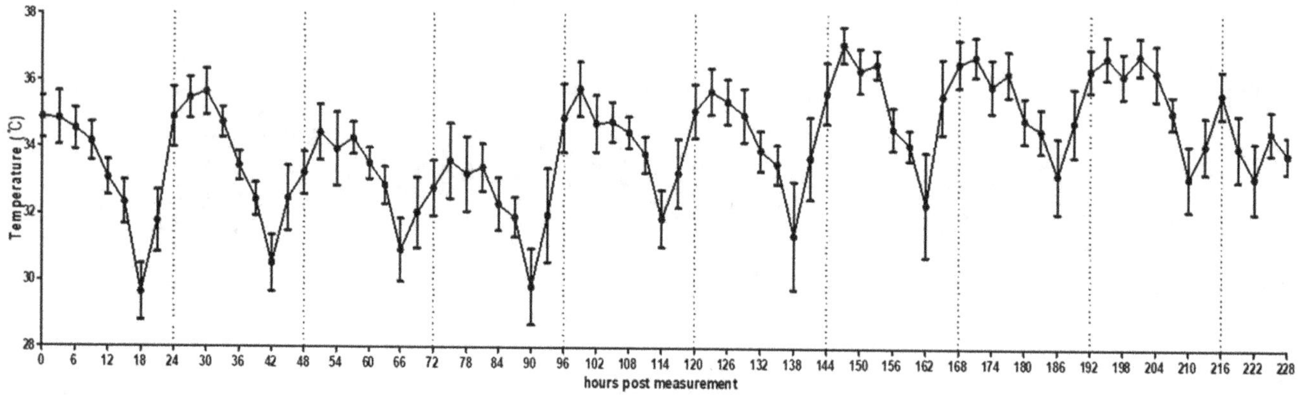

FIGURE 5 | Average temperature per 3 h interval of broilers ($n = 30$) housed in a small pen size (2 × 2 m). The error bars represent standard deviations of 36 5-min time points.

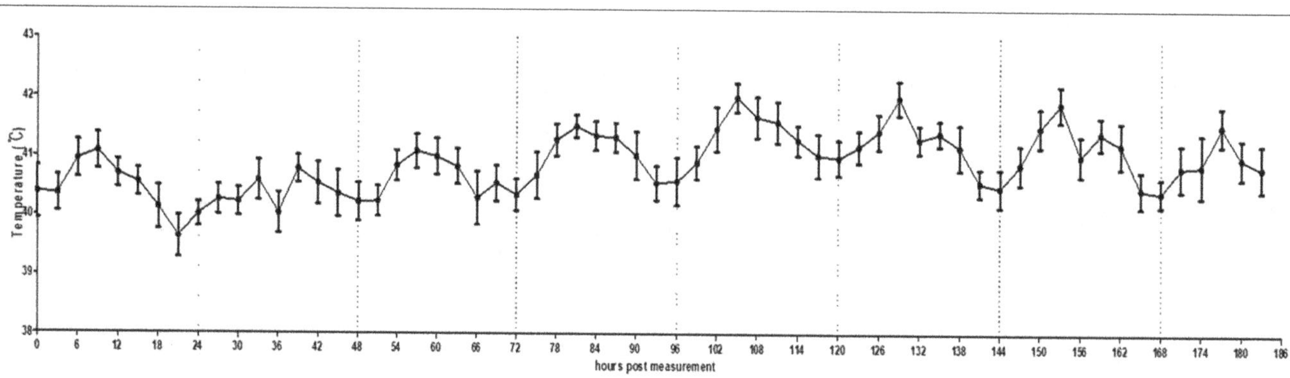

FIGURE 6 | Average temperature per 3 h interval of broilers housed in an actual farm. The error bars represent standard deviations of 36 5-min time points. Thermography was performed for 7 days.

and bumblefoot in animals (19–21). In general, two different types of thermal data loggers have been devised for animal use, one of which is directly attached to the body and the other, placed at a certain distance to sense or image the surface temperature. A study showed that the attached sensors were able to precisely detect HPAI infection under experimental setup conditions (22). However, limited battery capacity and low coverage of data sampling are the main hurdles associated with the practical use of this technique. On the other hand, thermal imaging cameras can measure the temperature at a distance. The measured temperature may vary depending on the distance and humidity because the temperature recognition method involves the analysis of the infrared rays emitted from the object. However, the camera-type sensor is easy to maintain, and the calibration of the actual temperature based on the distance from which the image is obtained, as a default step, could minimize the variations in measurements. In addition, the use of thermal imaging cameras would be beneficial for monitoring the level of population in terms of flock-based surveillance for chickens and ducks.

In the present study, thermal imaging cameras could successfully record the temperature of an individual or community of birds in cage and broiler farm conditions and maintain a track of the patterns in MST fluctuations. It is well-documented that the MST of both chickens and ducks inoculated with a range of HPAI virus rises and is accompanied with active virus shedding early during the infection (22, 23). Hence, we aimed to detect the increased MST following HPAI infection. The MST was measured at the heads and legs of chickens and ducks, presumably owing to the presence of relatively fewer hair over these areas. In addition, the detected temperature varied with the distance between the thermal imaging camera and the object (**Figure 1**). Therefore, we set the normal temperature standard by shooting at a fixed measurement position to take the image in a uniform distance from 24 h before viral challenge or by continuous temperature monitoring for the farm experiment.

Throughout the recording period, different patterns in MST change were observed depending on the species, dose of virus inoculation, and severity of clinical signs. At high viral doses, both chickens and ducks succumbed to infection and showed a slight decrease in MST, which is statistically significant increased thereafter. This effect may be attributed to the inability of the body to function normally after initial infection, followed by fever related to the immune response. However, chickens showed lethargy a few hours before their death, whereas ducks did not show any clinical signs. As recording with thermal imaging cameras can detect statistically significant increase in MST at least 24 h before the death of an animal that the farmers usually recognize the infection, these results indicate that thermal imaging could serve as a useful strategy to rapidly predict HPAI-induced fever and minimize the response time to diagnosis or related preemptive measures. However, subclinical infection of ducks with low viral doses showed a different pattern than that of the lethal infection and might not be recognized until the subsequent virus spreads.

In the present study, we also recorded the pattern of change in basic temperature without intentional infection under farm conditions. Throughout the monitoring process, MST was not only influenced by disease conditions that induce fever but also by the circadian rhythm in a large number of birds under simulated and normal farm conditions. These circadian rhythm results will serve as the baseline under normal conditions, thereby allowing the tracking of temperature deviations induced by HPAI-induced fever. Thus, the alarming deviation in MST should be set in consideration of the daylight time and local temperature that affects the circadian rhythm of specific animals. In addition, the difference between the maximum and minimum temperatures in the simulated farm and actual farm conditions was very high, probably owing to the difference in the percentage of space used or shooting angle. The changes in the camera setting may have affected actual amplitude of minimum/maximum temperature within 24 h. Further vigorous experiments on the distance effect should be carried out to understand effects of shooting distance. Therefore, preliminary testing under normal conditions is essential for optimal calibration (for example, by comparing body temperature and TID; using more than one TID to monitor birds from different angles and making "stereo view" to apply triangulation).

Thermal imaging alone is inadequate for the diagnosis of any specific disease. However, the present study shows that thermal imaging can be used as an early monitoring tool for diseases such as HPAI. As a part of smart animal agriculture methods, thermal imaging could be applied across a wider range of applications for disease monitoring and detection of heat stress or ventilation problems for flock-based management.

AUTHOR CONTRIBUTIONS

J-YN, K-JK, and S-HL gathered the data for the study and conducted the data analysis. J-YN prepared the manuscript. SY contributed to the interpretation of the results and manuscript preparation. J-BK contributed to the statistical analysis. D-HK coordinated the sample submission and testing. C-SS and S-SN conceived and supervised the study. S-SN reviewed, edited, and approved the manuscript. All authors contributed to the article and approved the submitted version.

ACKNOWLEDGMENTS

We thank SL solution Co., Ltd (Seoul, Korea) and Somo IR Co., Ltd (Seoul, Korea) for their assistance and technical contributions to this project.

REFERENCES

1. Lee DH, Criado MF, Swayne DE. Pathobiological origins and evolutionary history of highly pathogenic avian influenza viruses. *Cold Spring Harb Perspect Med.* (2020) 11:a038679. doi: 10.1101/cshperspect.a038679
2. Kelly TR, Hawkins MG, Sandrock CE, Boyce WM. A review of highly pathogenic avian influenza in birds, with an emphasis on Asian H5N1 and recommendations for prevention and control. *J Avian Med Surg.* (2008) 22:1-16. doi: 10.1647/2006-036R.1
3. Lee EK, Song BM, Lee YN, Heo GB, Bae YC, Joh SJ, et al. Multiple novel H5N6 highly pathogenic avian influenza viruses, South Korea, 2016. *Infect Genet Evol.* (2017) 51:21–3. doi: 10.1016/j.meegid.2017.03.005
4. Kwon JH, Jeong S, Lee DH, Swayne DE, Kim YJ, Lee SH, et al. New reassortant clade 2.3.4.4b avian influenza A(H5N6) virus in wild birds, South Korea, 2017-18. *Emerg Infect Dis.* (2018) 24:1953–5. doi: 10.3201/eid2410.180461
5. Mo IP, Bae YJ, Lee SB, Mo JS, Oh KH, Shin JH, et al. Review of avian influenza outbreaks in South Korea from 1996 to 2014. *Avian Dis.* (2016) 60:172–7. doi: 10.1637/11095-041715-Review
6. Golden NJ, Schlosser WD, Ebel ED. Risk assessment to estimate the probability of a chicken flock infected with H5N1 highly pathogenic avian influenza virus reaching slaughter undetected. *Foodborne Pathog Dis.* (2009) 6:827–35. doi: 10.1089/fpd.2008.0253
7. Halachmi I, Guarino M, Bewley J, Pastell M. Smart animal agriculture: application of real-time sensors to improve animal well-being and production. *Annu Rev Anim Biosci.* (2019) 7:403–25. doi: 10.1146/annurev-animal-020518-114851
8. Du X, Lao F, Teng G. A sound source localisation analytical method for monitoring the abnormal night vocalisations of poultry. *Sensors.* (2018) 18:2906. doi: 10.3390/s18092906
9. Banerjee D, Daigle CL, Dong B, Wurtz K, Newberry RC, Siegford JM, et al. Detection of jumping and landing force in laying hens using wireless wearable sensors. *Poult Sci.* (2014) 93:2724–33. doi: 10.3382/ps.2014-04006
10. Guo Y, Chai L, Aggrey SE, Oladeinde A, Johnson J, Zock G. A machine vision-based method for monitoring broiler chicken floor distribution. *Sensors.* (2020) 20:3179. doi: 10.3390/s20113179
11. Mahmoud AM, Dutta D, Lavery L, Stephens DN, Villanueva FS, Kim K. Noninvasive detection of lipids in atherosclerotic plaque using ultrasound thermal strain imaging: in vivo animal study. *J Am Coll Cardiol.* (2013) 62:1804–9. doi: 10.1016/j.jacc.2013.07.013
12. Perng CK, Ma H, Chiu YJ, Lin PH, Tsai CH. Detection of free flap pedicle thrombosis by infrared surface temperature imaging. *J Surg Res.* (2018) 229:169–76. doi: 10.1016/j.jss.2018.03.054
13. Duncan AE, Torgerson-White LL, Allard SM, Schneider T. An evaluation of infrared thermography for detection of bumblefoot (Pododermatitis) in penguins. *J Zoo Wildl Med.* (2016) 47:474–85. doi: 10.1638/2015-0199.1
14. Ximendes EC, Rocha U, Del Rosal B, Vaquero A, Sanz-Rodríguez F, Monge L, et al. *In vivo* ischemia detection by luminescent nanothermometers. *Adv Healthc Mater.* (2017) 6:10.1002/adhm.201601195. Epub 2016 Dec 23. doi: 10.1002/adhm.201601195

15. Kwon JH, Noh JY, Jeong JH, Jeong S, Lee SH, Kim YJ, et al. Different pathogenicity of two strains of clade 2.3.4.4c H5N6 highly pathogenic avian influenza viruses bearing different PA and NS gene in domestic ducks. *Virology.* (2019) 530:11–8. doi: 10.1016/j.virol.2019.01.016
16. Spackman E, Senne DA, Bulaga LL, Myers TJ, Perdue ML, Garber LP, et al. Development of real-time RT-PCR for the detection of avian influenza virus. *Avian Dis.* (2003) 47:1079–82. doi: 10.1637/0005-2086-47.s3.1079
17. Chiu WT, Lin PW, Chiou HY, Lee WS, Lee CN, Yang YY, et al. Infrared thermography to mass-screen suspected SARS patients with fever. *Asia Pac J Public Health.* (2005) 17:26–8. doi: 10.1177/101053950501700107
18. Manigandan S, Wu MT, Ponnusamy VK, Raghavendra VB, Pugazhendhi A, Brindhadevi K. A systematic review on recent trends in transmission, diagnosis, prevention and imaging features of COVID-19. *Process Biochem.* (2020) 98:233–40. doi: 10.1016/j.procbio.2020.08.016
19. Ring EF, McEvoy H, Jung A, Zuber J, Machin G. New standards for devices used for the measurement of human body temperature. *J Med Eng Technol.* (2010) 34:249–53. doi: 10.3109/03091901003663836
20. Schaefer AL, Cook NJ, Bench C, Chabot JB, Colyn J, Liu T, et al. The non-invasive and automated detection of bovine respiratory disease onset in receiver calves using infrared thermography. *Res Vet Sci.* (2012) 93:928–35. doi: 10.1016/j.rvsc.2011.09.021
21. Wilcox CS, Patterson J, Cheng HW. Use of thermography to screen for subclinical bumblefoot in poultry. *Poult Sci.* (2009) 88:1176–80. doi: 10.3382/ps.2008-00446
22. Suzuki K, Okada H, Itoh T, Tada T, Mase M, Nakamura K, et al. Association of increased pathogenicity of Asian H5N1 highly pathogenic avian influenza viruses in chickens with highly efficient viral replication accompanied by early destruction of innate immune responses. *J Virol.* (2009) 83:7475–86. doi: 10.1128/JVI.01434-08
23. Pantin-Jackwood MJ, Costa-Hurtado M, Shepherd E, DeJesus E, Smith D, Spackman E, et al. Pathogenicity and transmission of H5 and H7 highly pathogenic avian influenza viruses in mallards. *J Virol.* (2016) 90:9967–82. doi: 10.1128/JVI.01165-16

19

Evaluation of Antimicrobial or Non-Antimicrobial Treatments in Commercial Feedlot Cattle with Mild Bovine Respiratory Disease Based on a Refined Case-Definition

Jason Nickell[1]*, *Lonty Bryant*[2], *Kelly F. Lechtenberg*[3,4] *and Charley Cull*[3,4]

[1] *Allflex Livestock Intelligence, Madison, WI, United States,* [2] *Merck Animal Health, De Soto, KS, United States,* [3] *Midwest Veterinary Services, Oakland, NE, United States,* [4] *Veterinary and Biomedical Research Center, Manhattan, KS, United States*

Correspondence:
Jason Nickell
jason.nickell@merck.com

The study objective was to compare clinical and performance outcomes among feedlot steers treated for bovine respiratory disease (BRD) with tildipirosin (TIL), flunixin transdermal solution (FTS; topical application), or both, based on a refined BRD case-definition. Crossbred steer calves (N = 2,380) were enrolled based on a clinical illness score (CIS) of 1–3; a rectal temperature between >102.5° F and ≤103.9° F; and a Whisper Score (WS) = 1 or ≥2. Within each WS stratum, steers were randomly allocated to Saline, TIL, FTS, or TIL + FTS to reflect a 2 × 2 factorial design. Individual health and performance outcomes were measured on Day 60 and closeout. From Day 0 through Day 60, in both strata, TIL resulted in significantly ($P \leq 0.05$) fewer BRD retreatment events, fewer 3rd BRD treatments, fewer steers that did not finish, and greater average daily gain when compared to steers that were not treated with TIL. From Day 0 through closeout, cattle with a WS ≥ 2, treated with TIL had fewer animals ($P \leq 0.05$) that did not finish compared to steers not treated with TIL. In this study, feedlot steers with clinical signs of BRD and rectal temperatures lower than traditional cutoffs displayed a positive response to antimicrobial therapy. A clear benefit of FTS was not observed in this study. Calves with a WS ≥ 2 were lighter at the time of first BRD treatment compared to calves with a WS = 1. However, standalone TIL therapy was the optimal BRD treatment modality across WS strata in this study.

Keywords: bovine respiratory disease complex, tildipirosin, flunixin transdermal solution, cattle, diagnosis, negative control

INTRODUCTION

The traditional case-definition for bovine respiratory disease (BRD) diagnosis in feedlot cattle reflects an animal exhibiting clinical signs of BRD such as anorexia, depression, nasal discharge, cough, respiratory difficulty; and, rectal temperature >104° F (1–6). This temperature threshold is also utilized in the BRD case-definition within the regulatory approval process for antibiotics in the United States (7–11). However, the diagnostic accuracy of that case-definition has previously been shown to be relatively poor (12, 13).

Antimicrobial therapy is indicated for an animal meeting those above criteria for a BRD diagnosis. Tildipirosin (TIL) is an antimicrobial medication indicated for treatment and control of bovine respiratory disease (BRD) associated with *M. haemolytica, P. multocida,* and *H. somni.* This drug has previously shown efficacy when applied to animals meeting the above BRD case-definition (14).

In practice, an animal that exhibits a sufficient clinical illness score (CIS) but fails to meet this specific threshold criterium for rectal temperature may be returned to its home-pen without treatment. Cattle that do not fit the case-definition, by not meeting the threshold for rectal temperature, may be misclassified or mistreated; thereby, jeopardizing animal well-being (not treating an animal that really is sick), misusing medication (wasting medication by treating an animal that won't benefit), subsequently impacting animal performance and profitability. Little data are available regarding "response to treatment" of cattle that have those clinical signs and rectal temperature ≤103.9° F. An additional question that has yet to be answered is if cattle that exhibit a sufficient clinical illness score but fail to meet the rectal temperature criteria of ≥104° F have the potential to respond to non-antimicrobial therapy. Flunixin meglumine Transdermal Solution (FTS) is indicated for control of pyrexia associated with bovine respiratory disease and the control of pain associated with foot rot. Using the conventional BRD case definition, utilizing FTS as an ancillary therapy (i.e., in addition to antimicrobial therapy) has not provided added value compared to the antimicrobial alone (15). However, to date, no data are available (to the authors' knowledge) that has assessed FTS as a standalone therapy among animals that exhibit clinical signs of BRD but fail to meet a traditional rectal temperature cutoff.

Given the perceived lack of accuracy afforded by current BRD diagnostic modalities, additional information (i.e., in addition to CIS and rectal temperature) may be necessary to improve overall accuracy while potentially improving the treatment decision-making process. Whisper® technology offers unique information that estimates the lung health of an individual calf at the time it has been identified with a tentative BRD diagnosis (16–19).

The objective of this study was to use a refined case-definition of BRD based on CIS, rectal temperature (≥102.5° F to ≤103.9° F) and results of computer-assisted lung auscultation (Whisper®) to compare clinical and performance outcomes of cattle treated because of BRD. The null hypothesis was that calves meeting the refined BRD case definition would not respond to antimicrobial, non-antimicrobial, or a combination of both therapies.

MATERIALS AND METHODS

The study protocol was submitted to the MVS Institution for Animal Care and Use Committee (IACUC) where the protocol received approval on 30 January 2018. The assigned IACUC number is AC17100B.

Animals

The same study protocol was followed at each of two study sites (Oakland, NE; Manhattan, KS). Beef or beef-cross feeder steers (N = 3,376) with moderate to high risk for developing BRD were procured through several livestock auctions in Nebraska, Iowa, South Dakota, and Missouri across 24 shipments from late February to late November of 2018. All steers were weaned at the time of procurement; and, the history of vaccination or treatments was not known. When the steers arrived at the study site, their health was evaluated; they were identified with an individual number; they were vaccinated (modified-live viral, multi-valent clostridial toxoid), dewormed, and implanted with a growth-promotant; and, weighed. No antimicrobials were administered to control BRD (metaphylaxis). Steers that were not healthy were not eligible for enrollment which occurred from March through December of 2018. Steers were housed in open-air, dirt-floor pens. Conditions and management of the pens were according to standard feedlot practices. All steers were fed a ration appropriate for the size, age, and stage of feeding. After a brief step up period (~1 week), cattle were fed once daily a finisher diet, which included (DM basis): 54.1% high moisture corn, 25.3% wet distillers grain, 12.6% sweat brand 60, 3.4% corn stalks, 2.6% liquid supplement, and 2.0 micromineral mix ingredients [including 400 mg of monensin/animal and 85 mg of tylosin/animal per day (Elanco Animal Health, Greenfield, IN)]. Fresh feed was delivered each morning. Fresh water was available *ad libitum*. Waterers were monitored daily and cleaned when necessary. Any health-related intervention not described in the study protocol was administered at the discretion of the attending veterinarian after consultation with the sponsor. The monitor of the study was notified when such treatments were administered or when any steer was euthanized. The attending veterinarian at each site performed a necropsy on any steer found dead or was euthanized. If BRD was diagnosed at necropsy during the first 60 days of the study (Day 0 to Day 60), real-time polymerase chain reaction (RT-PCR) was performed with samples of lung to identify the following specific pathogens: infectious bovine rhinotracheitis (IBR) virus, bovine viral diarrhea virus (BVDV), bovine parainfluenza virus type 3 (PI3), bovine respiratory syncytial virus (BRSV), bovine influenza virus (BIV), *Mannheimia haemolytica, Pasteurella multocida, Histophilus somni,* and *Mycoplasma bovis.*

Inclusion Criteria

Twenty-four hours after processing at arrival, steers were eligible for enrollment. The case-definition of BRD, refined for this study, was a clinical illness score (CIS) of 1, 2, or 3; rectal temperature >102.5° F and ≤103.9° F; and, a Whisper® score (WS) of 1 or ≥2. The CIS was assigned a number (0–4) based on the description in **Table 1**. Rectal temperatures were measured with digital GLA Agricultural Electronics thermometers that were calibrated prior to the study. The Whisper® Veterinary Stethoscope is a computerized stethoscope that measures and analyzes the sounds of the lungs and heart of individual animals using a machine-learning algorithm that assigns a score of 1 through 5 and estimates lung health at the time of clinical disease identification with increasing severity as scores rise (16–19). A

TABLE 1 | Clinical illness scoring system used for this study.

Score	Description
0 = Healthy	Normal, healthy behavior
1 = Mild	May stand isolated with its head down or ears drooping; but, will quickly respond to minimal stimulation
2 = Moderate	May remain recumbent or stand isolated with head down; may show signs of muscle weakness (standing cross-legged, knuckling, or swaying when walking), depression obvious when stimulated
3 = Severe	May be recumbent and reluctant to rise, or if standing isolated and reluctant to move; when moving, is ataxic, knuckling or swaying evident; head carried low with ears drooping; eyes dull, excess salivation/lacrimation possible, obviously gaunt
4 = Moribund	Unable to stand; approaching death; highly unlikely to respond to any antimicrobial treatment

lung health estimate of 1 indicates that the lung tissue of the respective calf is relatively healthy. Conversely, a lung health estimate of 5 reflects severely compromised lung tissue. Scores 2–4 reflect intermediary changes in lung health as the scale increases. The bell of the stethoscope was placed approximately two inches caudal and dorsal to the point of the right elbow of the calf. The area was cleaned if needed and sounds were recorded for 8 s. If the recording was not acceptable ("flagged" by the computer; <M60% of the entire recording present on the computer screen; or, the operator had reason to consider the recording to be inadequate), another recording was obtained.

Enrollment Procedure

A steer with CIS of 1, 2, or 3 was brought to a processing chute where its rectal temperature was measured. If that temperature met the criterion for the case-definition, a WS was obtained. Two levels of stratification were used based on the WS. Stratum 1 was comprised of steers with WS = 1; stratum 2 was comprised of steers with WS ≥ 2. These stratums were determined based upon the prevalence of each score category observed in field settings (data not shown). Within each stratum, steers were randomly assigned to one of 4 treatment groups in a 2 × 2 factorial design (see **Table 2**). On a given day (i.e., block), only full treatment blocks, per strata, were enrolled and commingled within pen. Steers that met one of the BRD case definitions but failed to fill all 4 treatments were no longer eligible for enrollment. When a steer met the inclusion criteria and was enrolled, it was weighed and treated as assigned (**Table 2**). Steers assigned to be negative controls (no treatment administered) were treated with sterile saline (1 mL 0.9% NaCl/cwt, SC). A steer was not eligible for enrollment in the study if it had an unacceptable health condition; had a CIS, a rectal temperature, or a WS outside the criteria stated; or if a full treatment block was not filled.

Post-enrollment Procedures

Daily throughout the study general health of the steers was observed by trained personnel who were blinded to treatments. All adverse events were reported by the same personnel. After

TABLE 2 | Two strata (WS = 1; or WS > 2) were created based on the Whisper Score (WS) at the time of enrollment.

			Flunixin transdermal solution[b]	
			Yes	**No**
WS = 1	Tildipirosin[a]	Yes	340	340
		No (PSS[c])	340	170
WS > 2	Tildipirosin[a]	Yes	340	340
		No (PSS[c])	340	170

Within the respective stratum, a 2 × 2 factorial (binomial) design was used for assignment to experimental treatment. Two thousand three hundred eighty (2,380) calves were randomly assigned to one of the treatments described below based upon their individual WS at the time of enrollment.

[a]Zuprevo® 18% (180 mg tildipirosin/mL) solution; 4 mg tildipirosin/kg (1 mL/cwt) BW, SC.

[b]Banamine Transdermal® (50 mg flunixin meglumine/mL); 3.33 flunixin meglumine/kg (1 mL/15 kg) BW, applied to dorsal midline of back between withers and tailhead.

[c]PSS, Physiologic Saline Solution; 0.9% NaCl; 1 mL/cwt, SC.

TABLE 3 | Protocol for 2nd and 3rd treatment of BRD if needed.

BRD event	Antimicrobial	Dose (mL/cwt)	PTI (days)
2	Nuflor®	6 [mg/kg]	3
3	Baytril® 100	5.5 [mg/kg]	Considered chronic BRD

The 1st treatment was that assigned when the steer was enrolled in the study. No more than 3 treatments were allowed.

enrollment a 2-day post-treatment interval (PTI) was imposed on all treatment groups (including negative controls). Steers were then eligible for additional diagnostic procedures and for retreatment (**Table 3**). The BRD retreatment case definition reflected a CIS of 1 or 2 and a rectal temperature ≥104° F, or a CIS = 3 regardless of rectal temperature across all treatment groups within both WS strata. Steers with a CIS = 4 were eligible for removal and/or euthanasia at the discretion of the Study Investigator. After the third treatment, a steer was retained in the pen of origin unless its well-being was in jeopardy, it required additional treatment, or it died in the pen. If any of those situations occurred, the steer was removed from the pen, weighed, and removed from the study. If a steer was found dead or was euthanized, a necropsy was performed by authorized personnel. Data pertaining to the individual, to the day of removal, were retained for analysis. Values for the response variables were recorded to Day 60. On Day 61, steers enrolled in the study were moved to larger pens where they were commingled with calves that were not in the study. At closeout (average: Day 274; range: Day 255–281) all steers enrolled in the study were transported to one of three facilities where they were commercially harvested and processed. No final body weights were captured; however, an "adjusted final live weight" was estimated using a carcass yield of 63%.

Design and Analysis

A stratified, randomized, 2 × 2 factorial design was used. Two (2) strata were determined *a priori* and were based on WS. Stratum 1 was comprised of steers with a WS = 1; and, Stratum 2 was comprised of steers with a WS ≥ 2 (**Table 2**). Within each stratum, a 2 × 2 factorial design was applied with two (2) levels of "tildipirosin; TIL" and two (2) levels of "Flunixin transdermal solution; FTS" comprising those factorials. Descriptive statistics were generated (SAS, version 9.4; Cary, NC) for CIS, rectal temperature, and incoming body weight. Inferential statistics were generated (SAS, version 9.4; Cary, NC) for the dependent/outcome variables which included the following: BRD retreatment risk, days on feed at BRD retreatment, BRD 3rd treatment risk, BRD case-fatality risk, removal risk, did not finish risk (DNF; a combination of both calves that died or were removed due to BRD), and average daily gain (ADG). Steers were randomly assigned to one of those experimental treatments. Statistical analyses were performed using generalized linear mixed models that were fitted using binomial (proportional outcomes; PROC GLIMMIX), multinomial (ordinal carcass grades; PROC GLIMMIX), or normal (continuous outcomes, PROC MIXED) distributions. Degrees of freedom were adjusted via Kenward-Roger estimation. A random intercept was included in all models to account for potential clustering effects within the design structure (lack of independence between the 2 study-sites, among pens within each site, and treatment groups within each pen). Random effects for all carcass metrics included an effect for the plant in which harvest occurred. Treatment group was included as the fixed effect. Enrollment body weight and rectal temperatures were evaluated for differences across treatments between both strata. If associations were observed, the respective independent variable was included in the model statement as a covariate.

TABLE 4 | Descriptive statistics of steers at time of enrollment.

Pool (hd)	3,376	
Enrolled by site (hd)	NE = 1,708	KS = 672
Enrolled total (hd)	2,380	
CIS 1 (hd)	2,149	
CIS 2 (hd)	230	
CIS 3 (hd)	1	
Average body weight (lb) [range]	658.1 lb [418–938]	
Average rectal temperature (°F) [range]	103.0 °F [102.5–103.9]	

RESULTS

No adverse events associated with the products used were observed during this study.

Three thousand, three hundred seventy-six (3,376) steers comprised the pool from which 2,380 steers (70.5% of the pool) were enrolled in this study at two sites (NE = 1,708 steers; KS = 672 steers). Descriptive statistics for those steers are presented in **Table 4**. Steers with a WS = 1 at the time of enrollment were heavier ($P < 0.05$) compared to steers possessing a WS ≥ 2 (**Figure 1**). Additionally, although minimal, steers with a WS = 1 at the time of enrollment displayed a reduced rectal temperature ($P < 0.05$; 103.03, 95% confidence interval [95% CI]; 103.01, 103.05) compared to steers possessing a WS ≥ 2 (103.07, 95% CI; 103.05, 103.09). Descriptive statistics for health-related outcomes from Day 0 to Day 60; and, from Day 0 to closeout are presented in **Figure 2**.

Fifteen (15) steers died due to BRD during Day 0 to Day 60. Samples of lungs from 11 of those 15 (73.3%) were submitted for detection of pathogens using rT-PCR. Of those 11 steers, nine

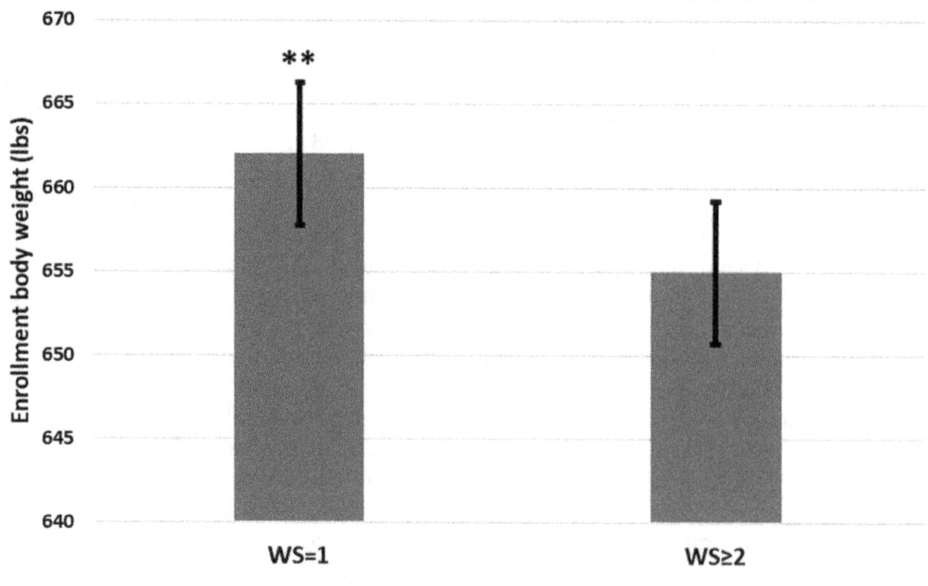

FIGURE 1 | Body weight at enrollment between mixed-breed beef feedlot steers meeting the case definition* of bovine respiratory disease (BRD) with a Whisper Score (WS) of 1 compared to steers with a WS ≥ 2. Error bars denote 95% confidence intervals. *The BRD case definition consisted of an animal displaying a clinical illness score of 1–3 and a rectal temperature of >102.5° F and <103.9° F. A WS was subsequently captured and calves were stratified by WS = 1 or >2. **A statistical difference of $P < 0.05$.

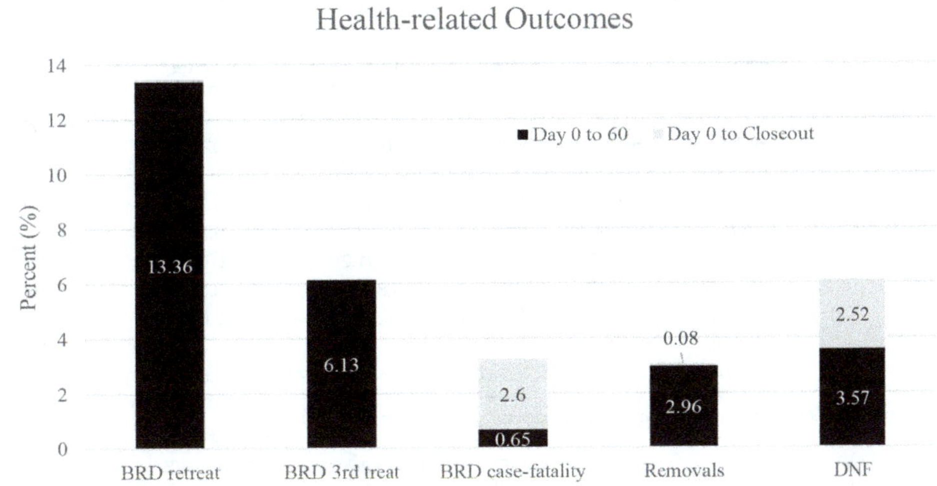

FIGURE 2 | Descriptive statistics for health-related outcomes for all steers from Day 0 to Day 60; and, from Day 0 to closeout. Values for BRD retreatments or for 3rd treatments were not retained after Day 60.

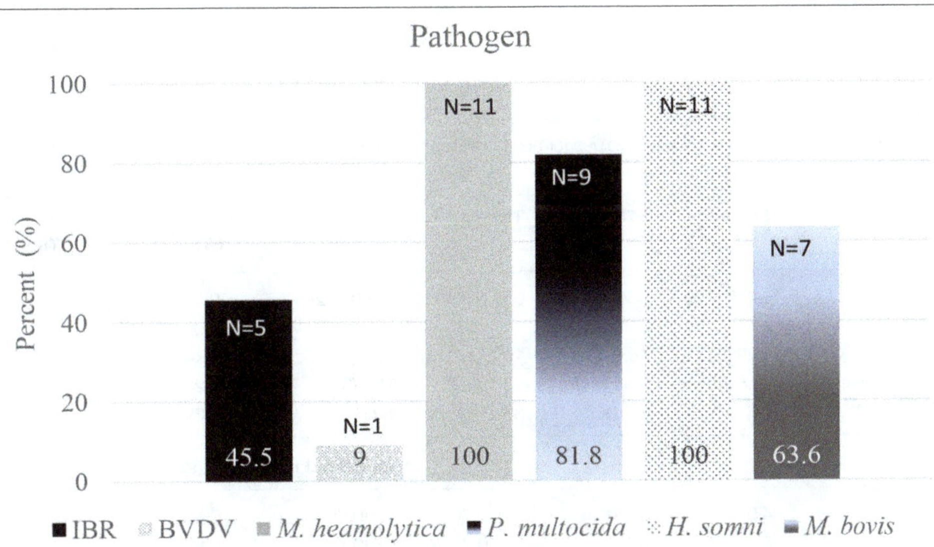

FIGURE 3 | Results of rT-PCR tests to identify pathogens in samples of lung from 11 of 15 steers that died during Day 0 to Day 60. Parainfluenza Type 3 (PI3), BRSV, or BIV were not identified in any sample.

were housed in one pen, and two were housed in one other pen. Results of rT-PCR tests to identify pathogens in samples of lung from those steers are shown in **Figure 3**. Parainfluenza Type 3 (PI3), BRSV, or BIV were not identified in any sample. Non-BRD conditions resulting in deaths or euthanasia were dietary acidosis ($N = 1$), fibrinous peritonitis (hardware; $N = 1$), severe lameness ($N = 2$), and injury ($N = 1$). Between Day 0 and Day 60 the average day of death due to BRD was Day 29; the average day of death from Day 0 to closeout was Day 135.

Model-adjusted estimates for health-related outcomes and for ADG at the end of the study on Day 60 are presented in **Tables 5A,B**. Within each stratum (WS = 1 vs. WS $\geq$ 2), tildipirosin resulted in fewer ($P \leq 0.05$) BRD retreatments, longer interval to BRD retreatment, fewer BRD 3rd treatments, fewer BRD removals (steers removed but did not die), fewer steers that did not finish (steers that died or were removed), and greater ADG than did steers that were not treated with tildipirosin.

Model-adjusted estimates for BRD case-fatality, removals, steers that did not finish, and adjusted-ADG from Day 0 to closeout were analyzed and results are presented in **Tables 6A,B**. Steers with a WS $\geq$ 2 that were treated with tildipirosin had fewer removals ($P < 0.05$), and fewer steers that did not finish ($P < 0.05$) compared to those that were not treated with tildipirosin. That was not observed for steers in stratum WS = 1. For steers in WS = 1, there was an interaction (tildipirosin x FTS; $P \leq 0.05$) for steers treated concurrently with tildipirosin and FTS; and, fewer

TABLE 5A | Model-adjusted means* (SEM) and corresponding *P*-values for health-related outcomes and ADG from Day 0 to Day 60 by treatment group for steers with a WS = 1.

Parameter	Saline[a]	FTS[a]	TIL[a]	TIL + FTS[a]	*P*-value FTS[α]	*P*-value TIL[β]	*P*-value TIL + FTS[δ]
Incoming body weight (lbs)	663.7 (5.5)	660.0 (4.0)	663.4 (4.0)	660.8 (4.0)	0.48	0.95	0.90
BRD retreatment (%)	15.0 (2.8)	18.5 (2.2)	10.4 (1.7)	8.2 (1.5)	0.95	<0.01	0.17
Day on Feed (DOF) at BRD retreatment (%)	21.6 (3.6)	23.1 (2.7)	31.6 (3.3)	34.1 (3.3)	0.32	<0.01	0.80
BRD 3rd treatment (%)	7.4 (2.1)	9.9 (1.7)	3.4 (1.0)	3.2 (1.0)	0.68	<0.01	0.48
BRD case-fatality (%)	0.57 (0.6)	1.2 (0.6)	0.49 (0.4)	0.85 (0.5)	0.39	0.76	0.91
Removals (%)	2.4 (1.2)	5.0 (1.2)	1.8 (0.7)	1.2 (0.5)	0.67	0.04	0.17
DNF (%)[b]	2.9 (1.3)	5.8 (1.3)	2.3 (0.8)	2.0 (0.8)	0.41	0.07	0.26
ADG (lbs/day)[c]	3.2 (0.1)	3.0 (0.1)	3.5 (0.1)	3.6 (0.1)	0.59	<0.01	0.06

Mixed models with a random effect to account for lack of independence among treatment groups within pens, and pens within 2 different sites. Mean and SEM listed above reflect the interactive means of the model.
[a]*Saline, negative control; FTS, Flunixin transdermal solution; TIL, tildipirosin; and TIL + FTS, concurrent administration of TIL and FTS.*
[b]*DNF, did not finish; a combination of both calves that died or were removed due to BRD from Day 0 to 60 of this study.*
[c]*ADG, Average Daily Gain.*
***P-values reflect the overall effect of FTS, TIL, and their interaction, respectively. P-values for each main effect reflect a model-adjusted average between treatments incorporating the product compared to those that do not. For example, the P-value for the FTS main effect reflects the comparison between treatments that implement FTS (i.e., FTS and TIL + FTS) vs. those that do not (i.e., Saline + TIL). Only when the P-value for the interaction is significant (P ≤ 0.05) are direct comparison made between the four treatment groups.*
[α]*P-value for main effect of Flunixin transdermal solution.*
[β]*P-value for main effect of tildipirosin.*
[δ]*P-value for interaction of tildipirosin and Flunixin transdermal solution.*

TABLE 5B | Model-adjusted means* (SEM) and corresponding *P*-values for health-related outcomes and ADG from Day 0 to Day 60 by treatment group for steers with a WS ≥ 2.

Parameter	Saline[a]	FTS[a]	TIL[a]	TIL + FTS[a]	*P*-value FTS[α]	*P*-value TIL[β]	*P*-value TIL + FTS[δ]
Incoming body weight (lbs)	649.5 (5.8)	654.4 (4.2)	653.5 (4.2)	660.0 (4.2)	0.21	0.30	0.86
BRD retreatment (%)	15.9 (3.0)	18.0 (2.2)	10.2 (1.7)	10.0 (1.7)	0.74	<0.01	0.66
Day on Feed (DOF) at BRD retreatment (%)	20.5 (3.5)	20.4 (3.0)	25.1 (3.2)	31.3 (3.1)	0.28	<0.01	0.25
BRD 3rd treatment (%)	6.6 (2.0)	9.8 (1.7)	3.7 (1.0)	3.9 (1.1)	0.39	<0.01	0.48
BRD case-fatality (%)				**Model did not converge**[†]			
Removals (%)	4.0 (1.5)	5.8 (1.3)	1.8 (0.7)	1.8 (0.7)	0.63	<0.01	0.60
DNF (%)[b]	5.2 (1.7)	6.1 (1.3)	2.3 (0.8)	1.8 (0.7)	0.86	<0.01	0.50
ADG (lbs/day)[c]	3.2 (0.1)	3.0 (0.1)	3.5 (0.1)	3.6 (0.1)	0.58	<0.01	0.10

Mixed models with a random effect to account for lack of independence among treatment groups within pens, and pens within 2 different sites.
[a]*Saline, negative control; FTS, Flunixin transdermal solution; TIL, tildipirosin; and TIL + FTS, concurrent administration of TIL and FTS.*
[b]*DNF, did not finish; a combination of both calves that died or were removed due to BRD from Day 0 to 60 of this study.*
[c]*ADG, Average Daily Gain.*
***P-values reflect the overall effect of FTS, TIL, and their interaction, respectively. P-values for each main effect reflect a model-adjusted average between treatments incorporating the product compared to those that do not. For example, the P-value for the FTS main effect reflects the comparison between treatments that implement FTS (i.e., FTS and TIL + FTS) vs. those that do not (i.e., Saline + TIL). Only when the P-value for the interaction is significant (P ≤ 0.05) are direct comparison made between the four treatment groups.*
[†]*Model did not converge: Lack of enough observations from Day 0 to 60 to generate a model-adjusted estimate.*
[α]*P-value for main effect of Flunixin transdermal solution.*
[β]*P-value for main effect of tildipirosin.*
[δ]*P-value for interaction of tildipirosin and Flunixin transdermal solution.*

removals ($P \leq 0.05$) and fewer steers that did not finish ($P \leq 0.05$) than did steers treated with only FTS.

Results of analyses of carcass characteristics are presented in **Tables 7A,B**. For yield and quality grades, data were available for approximately 75% of the steers across all treatment groups within each stratum (data not shown). In stratum WS = 1, tildipirosin resulted in higher marbling scores ($P \leq 0.05$) and thicker backfat ($P = 0.08$) than did steers not treated with tildipirosin. In stratum WS ≥ 2, steers treated with tildipirosin displayed higher ($P = 0.08$) hot carcass weight (HCW) than did steers that were not treated with tildipirosin.

TABLE 6A | Model-adjusted means* (SEM) and corresponding *P*-values for health-related outcomes and ADG from Day 0 to closeout by treatment group for steers with a WS = 1.

Parameter	Saline[1]	FTS[1]	TIL[1]	TIL + FTS[1]	*P*-value FTS[α]	*P*-value TIL[β]	*P*-value TIL + FTS[δ]
BRD case-fatality (%)	3.5 (1.4)	4.2 (1.1)	4.0 (1.1)	2.6 (0.9)	0.73	0.64	0.35
Removals (%)	2.4 (1.2)[a]	5.2 (1.2)[a,b]	3.7 (1.0)[a]	1.2 (0.6)[a,c]	0.66	0.19	0.02**
DNF (%)[2]	5.7 (1.8)[a]	8.7 (1.6)[a,b]	7.4 (1.5)[a]	3.8 (1.0)[a,c]	0.61	0.25	0.03
Adjusted-ADG (lbs/day)[3]	3.3 (0.04)	3.3 (0.03)	3.3 (0.03)	3.3 (0.03)	0.39	0.36	0.51

Mixed models with a random effect to account for lack of independence among treatment groups within pens, and pens within 2 different sites.
***Different superscripts denote significant differences ($P \leq 0.05$) between treatment groups; Pairwise comparisons were only evaluated if the interaction effect (TIL + FTS) was observed to be statistically significant ($P \leq 0.05$). All pairwise comparisons were adjusted for multiple comparisons (Tukey method).*
[1]*Saline, negative control; FTS, Flunixin transdermal solution; TIL, tildipirosin; and TIL + FTS, concurrent administration of TIL and FTS.*
[2]*DNF, did not finish; a combination of both calves that died or were removed due to BRD from Day 0-closeout of this study.*
[3]*Adjusted-ADG: adjusted Average Daily Gain based on a 63% carcass yield.*
***P-values reflect the overall effect of FTS, TIL, and their interaction, respectively. P-values for each main effect reflect a model-adjusted average between treatments incorporating the product compared to those that do not. For example, the P-value for the FTS main effect reflects the comparison between treatments that implement FTS (i.e., FTS and TIL+FTS) vs. those that do not (i.e., Saline + TIL). Only when the P-value for the interaction is significant ($P \leq 0.05$) are direct comparison made between the four treatment groups.*
[α]*P-value for main effect of Flunixin transdermal solution.*
[β]*P-value for main effect of tildipirosin.*
[δ]*P-value for interaction of tildipirosin and Flunixin transdermal solution.*

TABLE 6B | Model-adjusted means* (SEM) and corresponding *P*-values for health-related outcomes and ADG from Day 0 to closeout by treatment group for steers with a WS > 2.

Parameter	Saline[a]	FTS[a]	TIL[a]	TIL + FTS[a]	*P*-value FTS[α]	*P*-value TIL[β]	*P*-value TIL + FTS[δ]
BRD case-fatality (%)	3.1 (1.4)	3.4 (1.0)	3.3 (1.0)	1.5 (0.7)	0.54	0.50	0.44
Removals (%)	5.3 (1.8)	6.3 (1.4)	1.8 (0.7)	2.1 (0.8)	0.66	<0.01	0.95
DNF (%)[b]	8.8 (2.1)	9.4 (1.6)	5.0 (1.2)	3.5 (1.0)	0.68	<0.01	0.31
Adjusted-ADG (lbs/day)[c]	3.3 (0.05)	3.3 (0.03)	3.3 (0.03)	3.3 (0.03)	0.94	0.11	0.79

Mixed models with a random effect to account for lack of independence among treatment groups within pens, and pens within 2 different sites.
[a]*Saline, negative control; FTS, Flunixin transdermal solution; TIL, tildipirosin; and TIL + FTS, concurrent administration of TIL and FTS.*
[b]*DNF, did not finish; a combination of both calves that died or were removed due to BRD from Day 0-closeout of this study.*
[c]*Adjusted-ADG: adjusted Average Daily Gain based on a 63% carcass yield.*
***P-values reflect the overall effect of FTS, TIL, and their interaction, respectively. P-values for each main effect reflect a model-adjusted average between treatments incorporating the product compared to those that do not. For example, the P-value for the FTS main effect reflects the comparison between treatments that implement FTS (i.e., FTS and TIL+FTS) vs. those that do not (i.e., Saline + TIL). Only when the P-value for the interaction is significant ($P \leq 0.05$) are direct comparison made between the four treatment groups.*
[α]*P-value for main effect of Flunixin transdermal solution.*
[β]*P-value for main effect of tildipirosin.*
[δ]*P-value for interaction of tildipirosin and Flunixin transdermal solution.*

DISCUSSION

A traditional diagnosis of BRD is based on the presence of clinical signs of the disease, and a rectal temperature ≥104° F, before treatment is prescribed. Results of this study indicate that steers with clinical signs of BRD and rectal temperature <104° F also respond favorably to antimicrobial treatment. In this study tildipirosin resulted in beneficial outcomes that were measurable from Day 0 to Day 60, and from Day 0 to closeout. There were no statistical benefits (or detriments) for steers treated with FTS alone or concurrently with tildipirosin. In stratum WS = 1, a greater proportion of steers treated with FTS alone did not finish compared to steers treated with FTS + tildipirosin. However, no differences were observed among FTS, Saline, and Tildipirosin across these specific outcomes. Additionally, the use of FTS, alone or in conjunction with tildipirosin, did not augment the outcome among calves in either WS strata.

The normal body temperature of beef cattle ranges from 98 to 102.4° F (20). Therefore, given the diurnal variation in body temperature and the cross-sectional nature of rectal temperature data collection, it is likely that a subpopulation of calves presumptively identified with clinical signs of BRD will possess a rectal temperature <104° F. Response to therapy across both Whisper strata among calves with a rectal temperature <104° F may reflect the reality that current BRD diagnostic modalities involve a one point in time event and do not robustly describe the clinical severity of the individual animal. Theurer et al. observed no direct relationship between rectal temperature at the time of the first BRD treatment and the animal's probability of finishing the feedlot phase of production

TABLE 7A | Model-adjusted* means (SEM) and corresponding *P*-values for carcass characteristics by treatment group for steers with a WS = 1.

Parameter		Saline[1]	FTS[1]	TIL[1]	TIL + FTS[1]	*P*-value FTS[α]	*P*-value TIL[β]	*P*-value TIL + FTS[δ]
HCW[2], lbs		924.4 (6.8)	915.2 (4.9)	926.2 (4.9)	922.7 (4.9)	0.25	0.39	0.61
Ribeye area		15.1 (0.2)	15.3 (0.2)	15.3 (0.2)	15.3 (0.1)	0.45	0.58	0.86
Marbling		462.8 (11.1)	458.2 (8.0)	487.6 (8.0)	482.8 (7.8)	0.59	<0.01	0.99
Backfat		0.57 (0.02)	0.55 (0.01)	0.58 (0.01)	0.60 (0.01)	0.68	0.08	0.26
Calculated Yield Grade		2.9 (0.1)	2.6 (0.1)	3.0 (0.1)	2.9 (0.1)	0.09	0.12	0.29
[a]Yield Grade (*N* = 891)***	1	5.3% (7)	9.9% (25)	10.7% (27)	7.5% (19)		**Model did not converge	
	2	39.8% (53)	39.5% (100)	42.1% (106)	39.5% (100)			
	3	38.3% (51)	36.8% (93)	36.1% (91)	39.9% (101)			
	4	12.8% (17)	12.6% (32)	10.7% (27)	11.5% (29)			
	5	3.8% (5)	1.2% (3)	0.4% (1)	1.6% (4)			
	N	133	253	252	253			
[a]Quality Grade (*N* = 894)	Prime	2.3% (3)	2.4% (6)	1.6% (4)	2.7% (7)	0.73	0.81	0.66
	Choice	61.8% (81)	65.0% (165)	62.9% (158)	59.3% (153)			
	Select	32.8% (43)	30.3% (77)	31.5% (79)	32.2% (83)			
	Other	3.1% (4)	2.4% (6)	4.0% (10)	5.8% (15)			
	N	131	254	251	258			

*Mixed models with a random effect to account for lack of independence among treatment groups within pens, pens within 2 different sites, and sites within 3 different processing plants.
[a]Each cell within the Yield and Quality grade outcomes reflects the raw proportions and counts for each treatment group.
**Insufficient observations to generate a model-adjusted estimate within the hierarchical structure of the model. Due to non-convergence of the model, the effect of "processing plant" was removed from the random effect and was included as a covariate in the model for "yield grade". However, the model still did not converge within this WS stratum.
***Total number of steers in each treatment group for Yield and Quality Grade is specified. The proportion of missing data was the same for all treatment groups.
[1]Saline, negative control; FTS, Flunixin transdermal solution; TIL, tildipirosin; and TIL + FTS, concurrent administration of TIL and FTS.
[2]HCW, Hot Carcass Weight.
**P-values reflect the overall effect of FTS, TIL, and their interaction, respectively. P-values for each main effect reflect a model-adjusted average between treatments incorporating the product compared to those that do not. For example, the P-value for the FTS main effect reflects the comparison between treatments that implement FTS (i.e., FTS and TIL + FTS) vs. those that do not (i.e., Saline + TIL). Only when the P-value for the interaction is significant ($P \leq 0.05$) are direct comparison made between the four treatment groups.
[α]P-value for main effect of Flunixin transdermal solution.
[β]P-value for main effect of tildipirosin.
[δ]P-value for interaction of tildipirosin and Flunixin transdermal solution.

(21). Rather, this relationship was influenced by additional parameters including time of year, gender, and the days on feed prior to first BRD diagnosis (21). These variables likely contribute to the poor diagnostic performance of current BRD diagnostic methods (12, 13).

In this study, the Whisper technology was used in conjunction with traditional diagnostic modalities (clinical signs and rectal temperature) to delineate severity of BRD and to potentially aid in the BRD treatment decision. Since a WS cannot be randomly assigned to an animal, inferences cannot be made between treatments across WS strata; conversely, those decisions can only be made within the chosen strata analyzed in the present study. Although prior studies have shown an association between a rising Whisper Score and worsening lung health (18, 19) and calves enrolled with a WS ≥ 2 were lighter compared to calves with a WS = 1, the data generated in this study indicates that regardless of lung health status, calves in both WS strata require antimicrobial therapy to significantly reduce the risk of BRD relapse. This raises the question as to how to leverage the WS data. As an observation, the positive effects of tildipirosin observed at the 60-day mark within the WS = 1 stratum were not observed at closeout (**Table 6A**). Conversely, a significant tildipirosin effect was observed in the WS ≥ 2 strata for both the removal and DNF outcomes from Day 0 to closeout (**Table 6B**). This may suggest that calves identified with clinical signs of BRD, a rectal temperature <104° F and a WS = 1 are more likely to finish the feeding phase of production compared to calves with a WS ≥ 2 and a rectal temperature <104° F at the time of first BRD diagnosis. This observation among calves with a WS = 1 raises two potential opportunities to utilize these data: (1) Given that calves in both WS strata responded positively to antimicrobial therapy, perhaps a less potent (and cheaper) antimicrobial may be applicable in this subpopulation of cattle stricken with BRD; and (2) perhaps the value of the WS may be realized in the subsequent management of calves with more severe lung health issues at the time of first BRD diagnosis rather than impacting antimicrobial treatment decisions. More work is necessary to test these theories.

One potential limitation of this study is that the study population was not maintained within their original cohort from the time of enrollment until closeout. Rather, they were placed in a larger general population after 60 days post-BRD diagnosis. This occurrence may have led to an underestimation of overall BRD morbidity due to further reduction in BRD diagnostic accuracy within a larger group

TABLE 7B | Model-adjusted* means (SEM) and corresponding *P*-values for carcass characteristics by treatment group for steers with a WS ≥ 2.

Parameter		Saline[1]	FTS[1]	TIL[1]	TIL + FTS[1]	*P*-value FTS[α]	*P*-value TIL[β]	*P*-value TIL + FTS[δ]
HCW[2], lbs		912.6 (7.2)	914.5 (5.1)	920.4 (5.0)	926.5 (5.0)	0.48	0.08	0.72
Ribeye area		15.2 (0.2)	15.3 (0.1)	15.3 (0.1)	15.4 (0.1)	0.52	0.51	0.94
Marbling		475.7 (10.3)	481.6 (7.4)	470.2 (7.2)	472.3 (7.1)	0.62	0.36	0.82
Backfat		0.57 (0.02)	0.56 (0.01)	0.56 (0.01)	0.59 (0.01)	0.57	0.60	0.40
Calculated Yield Grade		2.9 (0.1)	2.9 (0.1)	2.8 (0.1)	3.0 (0.1)	0.44	0.87	0.26
[a]Yield Grade (*N* = 902)	1	9.4% (12)	9.7% (25)	11.8% (30)	10.3% (27)	0.69	0.83	0.42
	2	32.0% (41)	38.5% (99)	38.0% (97)	34.4% (90)			
	3	49.2% (63)	38.5% (99)	40.8% (104)	43.1% (113)			
	4	8.6% (11)	11.3% (29)	9.0% (23)	9.9% (26)			
	5	0.8% (1)	1.9% (5)	0.4% (1)	2.3% (6)			
	N	128	257	255	262			
[a]Quality** Grade (*N* = 902)	Prime	1.6% (2)	5.8% (15)	1.2% (3)	3.5% (9)	0.19	0.70	0.32
	Choice	64.1% (82)	62.0% (160)	67.2% (172)	65.4% (170)			
	Select	32.8% (42)	29.1% (75)	27.7% (71)	27.3% (71)			
	Other	1.6% (2)	3.1% (8)	3.9% (10)	3.8% (10)			
	N	128	258	256	260			

**Mixed models with a random effect to account for lack of independence among treatment groups within pens, pens within 2 different sites, and sites within 3 different processing plants.*
[a]Each cell within the Yield and Quality grade outcomes reflects the raw proportions and counts for each treatment group.
***Total number of steers in each treatment group for Yield and Quality Grade is specified. The proportion of missing data was the same for all treatment groups.*
[1]Saline, negative control; FTS, Flunixin transdermal solution; TIL, tildipirosin; and TIL + FTS, concurrent administration of TIL and FTS.
[2]HCW, Hot Carcass Weight.
***P-values reflect the overall effect of FTS, TIL, and their interaction, respectively. P-values for each main effect reflect a model-adjusted average between treatments incorporating the product compared to those that do not. For example, the P-value for the FTS main effect reflects the comparison between treatments that implement FTS (i.e., FTS and TIL + FTS) vs. those that do not (i.e., Saline + TIL). Only when the P-value for the interaction is significant (P ≤ 0.05) are direct comparison made between the four treatment groups.*
[α]P-value for main effect of Flunixin transdermal solution.
[β]P-value for main effect of tildipirosin.
[δ]P-value for interaction of tildipirosin and Flunixin transdermal solution.

size. Additionally, final body weights were not captured to avoid unnecessary stress on the finished animals which necessitated back calculation and estimation of final weights based on HCW and carcass yields (63%). This likely had an impact on the precision of the ADG estimates at closeout. However, these management decisions were applied universally across the study population and individual identification was accurately maintained through closeout.

In this study, calves exhibiting clinical signs of BRD but with rectal temperatures <104° F (regardless of WS) responded favorably to tildipirosin therapy at the time of first BRD diagnosis. Withholding antimicrobial medication from feedlot animals that have not reached the traditional threshold for rectal temperature may not be prudent for the best interest of the animal or the producer.

AUTHOR CONTRIBUTIONS

This study was designed and the protocol generated by JN and LB. This study was executed by CC and KL and monitored by JN and LB. Statistical analysis was performed by JN. Manuscript writing reflected a collaboration amongst all authors.

REFERENCES

1. Kilgore WR, Spensley MS, Sun F, Nutsch RG, Rooney KA, Skogerboe TL. Therapeutic efficacy of tulathromycin, a novel triamilide antimicrobial, against bovine respiratory disease in feeder calves. *Vet Ther.* (2005) 6:143–53.
2. Skogerboe TL, Rooney KA, Nutsch RG, Weigel DJ, Gajewski K, Kilgore WR. Comparative efficacy of tulathromycin versus florfenicol and tilmicosin against undifferentiated bovine respiratory disease in feedlot cattle. *Vet Ther.* (2005) 6:180–96.
3. Nutsch RG, Skogerboe TL, Rooney KA, Weigel DJ, Gajewski K, Lechtenberg KF. Comparative efficacy of tulathromycin, tilmicosin, and florfenicol in the treatment of bovine respiratory disease in stocker cattle. *Vet Ther.* (2005) 6:167–79.
4. Van Donkersgoed J, Berg J, Hendrick S. Comparison of florfenicol and tulathromycin for the treatment of undifferentiated fever in Alberta feedlot calves. *Vet Ther.* (2008) 9:275–81.
5. Robb EJ, Tucker CM, Corley L, Bryson WL, Rogers KC, Sturgess K, et al. Efficacy of tulathromycin or enrofloxacin for initial treatment of naturally occurring bovine respiratory disease in feeder calves. *Vet Ther.* (2007) 8:127–35.
6. Torres S, Thomson DU, Bello NM, Nosky BJ, Reinhardt CD. Field study of the comparative efficacy of gamithromycin and tulathromycin for the treatment

of undifferentiated bovine respiratory disease complex in beef feedlot calves at high risk of developing respiratory tract disease. *Am J Vet Res.* (2013) 74:847–53. doi: 10.2460/ajvr.74.6
7. FDA. *Freedom of Information Summary: Nuflor® Injectable Solution.* NADA 141-063 (1998).
8. FDA. *Freedom of Information Summary: Baytril 100 Injectable Solution.* NADA 141-068 (1998).
9. FDA. *Freedom of Information Summary: Naxcel XT Sterile Suspension.* NADA 141-209 (2003).
10. FDA. *Freedom of Information Summary: Draxxin Injectable Solution.* NADA 141-244 (2005).
11. FDA. *Freedom of Information Summary: Florfenicol and Flunixin Meglumine injectable Solution.* NADA 141-299 (2009).
12. White BJ, Renter DG. Bayesian estimation of the performance of using clinical observations and harvest lung lesions for diagnosing bovine respiratory disease in post-weaned beef calves. *J Vet Diagn Invest.* (2009) 21:446–53. doi: 10.1177/104063870902100405
13. Timsit E, Dendukuri N, Schiller I, Buczinski S. Diagnostic accuracy of clinical illness for bovine respiratory disease (BRD) diagnosis in beef cattle placed in feedlots: a systematic literature review and hierarchical Bayesian latent-class meta-analysis. *Prev Vet Med.* (2016) 135:67–73. doi: 10.1016/j.prevetmed.2016.11
14. Theurer MEF JT, Bryant LK, Nickell JS, Hutcheson, JP. Treatment efficacy of tildipirosin or tulathromycin for first treatment of naturally occurring bovine respiratory disease in a commercial feedlot. *Bovine Practitioner.* (2018) 52:154–9.
15. Wilson BK, Step DL, Maxwell CL, Wagner JJ, Richards CJ, Krehbiel CR. Evaluation of multiple ancillary therapies used in combination with an antimicrobial in newly received high-risk calves treated for bovine respiratory disease. *J Anim Sci.* (2015) 93:3661–74. doi: 10.2527/jas.2015-9023
16. Mang AV, Buczinski S, Booker CW, Timsit E. Evaluation of a computer-aided lung auscultation system for diagnosis of bovine respiratory disease in feedlot cattle. *J Vet Intern Med.* (2015) 29:11126. doi: 10.1111/jvim.12657
17. DeDonder KD, Thomson DU, Loneragan GH, Noffsinger T, Tayler W, Apley MD. Lung auscultation and rectal temperature as a predictor of lung lesions and bovine respiratory disease treatment outcome in feedyard cattle. *Bovine Pract.* (2010). 44:146–53.
18. Baruch J, Cernicchiaro N, Cull CA, Lechtenberg KF, Nickell JS, Renter DG. Performance of multiple diagnostic methods in assessing the progression of bovine respiratory disease in calves challenged with infectious bovine rhinotracheitis virus and Mannheimia haemolytica1. *J Anim Sci.* (2019) 97:2357–67 doi: 10.1093/jas/skz107
19. Zeineldin MM, Ghanem MM, Abd El-Raof YM, El-Attar HA. Lung ultrasonography and computer-aided scoring system as a diagnostic aid for bovine respiratory disease in feedlot cattle. *Glob Vet.* (2016). 17:588–94.
20. Cunningham JG. Thermoregulation. In: Cunningham JG, editor. *Textbook of Veterinary Physiology*. Philadelphia, PA: W.B. Saunders Company (1997). p. 634–45.
21. Theurer ME, White BJ, Larson RL, Holstein KK, Amrine DE. Relationship between rectal temperature at first treatment for bovine respiratory disease complex in feedlot calves and the probability of not finishing the production cycle. *J Am Vet Med Assoc.* (2014) 245:1279–85. doi: 10.2460/javma.245.11.1279

Comparison of Multiplex Real-Time PCR and PCR-Reverse Blot Hybridization Assays for the Direct and Rapid Detection of Porcine Circovirus Type 2 Genotypes

Hye-young Wang [1]***, Joong Ki Song*** [2]***, Seongho Shin*** [2] ***and Hyunil Kim*** [1*]

[1] *Optipharm, Inc., Cheongju-Si, South Korea,* [2] *Optipharm Animal Disease Diagnostic Center, Cheongju-Si, South Korea*

***Correspondence:**
Hyunil Kim
hikim@optipharm.co.kr

Porcine circovirus type 2 (PCV2), the causative agent of porcine circovirus-associated diseases (PCVAD), poses a serious economic threat for the swine industry. Currently, PCV2 is classified into five major genotypes: PCV2a, PCV2b, PCV2c, PCV2d, and PCV2e. The aim of this study is to evaluate the performance of two commercially available methods, multiplex real-time PCR assay and PCR-reverse blot hybridization assay (REBA), for the rapid detection of PCV2 and direct identification of PCV2 genotypes from clinical samples as well as to compare the results with that of sequence analysis. Molecular diagnostic methods were used to evaluate a total of 180 samples, including tissues and blood samples from pigs that were suspected of PCVAD infection. The results of this study showed that the detection rate for positive PCV2 was 48.3% ($n = 87$) in both multiplex real-time PCR and PCR-REBA methods. Using sequence analysis, which is the gold standard, and multiplex real time PCR assay, the sensitivity, specificity, positive predictive value, and negative predictive value of PCV2 genotyping were found to be 97.1% ($n = 67$, 95% CI 0.894–0.998, $p < 0.001$), 100% ($n = 93$, 95% CI 0.966–1.000, $p < 0.001$), 100% (95% CI 0.953–1.000, $p < 0.001$), 97.9% (95% CI 0.921–0.998, $p < 0.001$), respectively. The results of PCR-REBA were found to be consistent with those of sequence analysis for all the samples and showed good agreement ($\kappa = 1$). The most prevalent genotypes detected in this study were PCV2d ($n = 53$, 60.9%), followed by PCV2a ($n = 17$, 19.5%), PCV2b ($n = 14$, 16.1%), and PCV2a/b co-infection ($n = 3$, 3.5%). Both the methods required ~3 h for completion. Therefore, we conclude that two molecular methods are rapid and reliable for the characterization of the causative pathogen with PCV2 genotypes.

Keywords: porcine circovirus type 2, multiplex real-time PCR, PCR-REBA, ORF2, diagnosis

INTRODUCTION

Different from the non-pathogenic porcine circovirus (PCV) type 1 strain (1), PCV type 2 is considered to be an important emerging pathogen that causes porcine circovirus associated diseases (PCVAD) including postweaning multisystemic wasting syndrome (PMWS), porcine dermatitis nephropathy syndrome (PDNS), porcine respiratory disease complex (PRDC), enteritis, reproductive failure (2, 3), and one of the most economically important swine diseases worldwide (4). Whenever there are outbreaks of respiratory clinical signs, wasting, and granulomatous inflammation of lymphoid tissues in pigs, PMWS is clinically suspected (5). PCV2-associated systemic infection is clinically characterized by wasting, dyspnea, and lymphadenopathy, and in some cases, might be associated with diarrhea, pallor, and jaundice (6). PCV2, belonging to the genus *Circovirus* of the family *Circoviridae*, is a small non-enveloped virus with a circular single-stranded DNA genome (7). The PCV2 genome is ~1.7 kb nucleotide long and encodes for two open reading frames (ORFs) (8, 9). In the viral genome, ORF1 codes for the replicase (Rep) protein and ORF2 for the capsid (Cap) protein. Rep is a non-structural protein and is responsible for the viral replication, while the structural Cap protein controls the immunogenicity of the virus (10–13). With emerging viral strains, PCV2 has undergone much genetic variation in recent years and has been divided into five genotypes, namely PCV2a-e strains, which are classified based on the diversity level of the ORF2 nucleotide sequences (14, 15). Continuous mutations in the PCV2 genome have made the identification of PCV more difficult, especially by traditional molecular detection methods (16, 17). It has also been demonstrated experimentally that subclinical PCV2 infection might be associated with decreased vaccine efficacy (18). Therefore, PCV2 subclinical infection is not only the most common form of infection in pigs but is also resistant to the effect of vaccines. Hence, rapid and early identification of PCV2 subclinical infection is very important for the effective prophylaxis against PCVAD (19).

Until now, commercial diagnostic tests based on ELISA (9, 12) and PCR (19) have only been developed to confirm the presence or absence of PCV2. Although it has the advantage of being able to detect PCV2 in a short time, it is required expensive antibodies for diagnostic purposes, and the PCV2 genotypes cannot be distinguished simultaneously, so most PCV2 genotypes have been identified separately using PCR-based Restriction Fragment Length Polymorphism (RFLP) (20) or sequence analysis (13, 17, 20–22). In this study, a novel diagnostic assay based on multiplex real-time PCR (Opti PCV2-genotyping; Optipharm, Osong, Republic of Korea) was developed for the rapid and accurate identification of PCV2 as well as to discriminate between the PCV2 a/e, b, and d genotypes. The PCR-based reverse blot hybridization assay (PCR-REBA, REBA PCV2-genotyping; Optipharm) was to detect PCV2 and distinguish between PCV2a, PCV2b, PCV2c, PCV2d, and PCV2e genotypes. In this study, we evaluated the clinical applicability of multiplex real-time PCR and PCR-REBA methods and compared their efficiency to that of the sequence analysis method used for detecting PCV2 and differentiating the different PCV2a-e genotypes directly from the serum and tissue samples of pigs.

METHODS

Preparation of DNA Samples

To evaluate the diagnostic performance of the multiplex real-time PCR and PCR-REBA methods, a total of 180 samples suspected to be infected with PCVAD including 109 tissues and 71 bloods were provided by the Optipharm Animal Disease Diagnostic Center, which was commissioned from January to December, 2019. DNA was extracted from 200 μL of serum or 20 mg of organ tissue homogenate using a commercial automated system (Miracle-AutoXT Automated Nucleic Acid Extraction System, intronbio, Seongnam, Republic of Korea) according to the manufacturer's recommendations. To avoid cross contamination, all the samples were processed individually and stored at −20°C. The content and purity of the extracted DNA were assayed by measuring absorbance at 260 and 280 nm using an Infinite 200 NanoQuant (Tecan, Switzerland) spectrophotometer.

Multiplex Real-Time PCR Assay

Detection of PCV2 and identification of genotypes in clinical samples was performed with Opti PCV2-genotyping (Optipharm), a quantitative multiplex real-time PCR-based assay, using the CFX-96 real-time PCR system (Bio-Rad, Hercules, CA, USA) for thermocycling and fluorescence detection. Both the detection and genotype identification of PCV2 can be performed in a single tube using this assay [PCV2 (Cy5), PCV2a/e (FAM), PCV2b/d (CAL Flour Red 610), and PCV2d (HEX)] by incorporating specific TaqMan probes labeled with different fluorophores. Real-time PCR amplification was performed in a total reaction volume of 20 μL containing 10 μL of 2× Thunderbird probe qPCR mix (Toyobo, Osaka, Japan), 5 μL of a mixture of primer and TaqMan probe that were labeled with different fluorophores, and 5 μL template DNA. The real-time PCR kits consisted of an internal control (IC) DNA, which was used to indicate successful nucleic acid extraction, the quality of the sample and to check for the presence of PCR inhibitors in the reaction. The IC DNA is designed to have minimal sequence similarity with the target gene and also facilitates detection of false negatives. Therefore, it does not directly compete with the amplification of the species-specific target in multiplex real-time PCR. Positive (Plasmid DNA with mixed PCV2a, b, d genotypes) and negative controls consisting of molecular grade (DNAse/RNAse-free) water (Ultra pure water; Welgene, Gyeongsan, Republic of Korea) without template DNA were included in each assay and the assay was performed under the following conditions: 95°C for 3 min followed by 40 cycles of 95°C for 20 s and 55°C for 40 s. Each sample was tested in duplicate by running the PCR cycles twice. The viral load was quantified by determining the cycle threshold (C_T), and the number of PCR cycles required for the fluorescence to exceed a value significantly higher than the background fluorescence. Positive result was indicated when the C_T value was <38.

PCR-Reverse Blot Hybridization Assay (PCR-REBA)

Oligonucleotide primers corresponding to both strands of the ORF2 region of PCV2 (**Figure 1**) were designed by Primer3Plus (http://www.bioinformatics.nl/cgi-bin/primer3plus/primer3plus.cgi). The primers were made as probes corresponding to the complementary strand and were used exclusively thereafter. To validate the efficiency of the selected probes, target DNA samples amplified from the PCV2

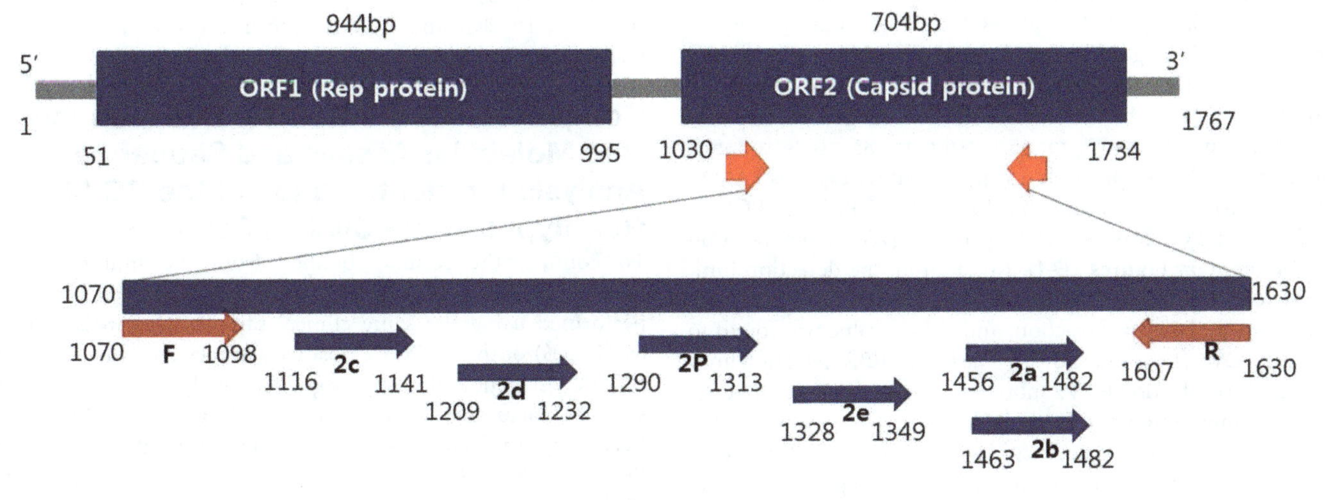

FIGURE 1 | Schematic representation of the ORF2 gene to distinguish PCV2 genotyping from positions of primer and probes used in this study.

strains were applied to the REBA membrane strips and spotted with the selected probes. Two types of DNA samples (PCV2c and PCV2e) were synthesized (Bioneer, Daejeon, Republic of Korea) and amplified with custom PCR primers (PCV2c, F-5′-TAAGTGGGGGGTCTTTAAGA-3′ and R-5′-TCCTCCGCC GCCGCCCCTGG-3′; PCV2e, F-5′-TAAGTGGGGGGTCTT TAA-3′ and R-5′-CTTGGCCATATCCTCCGCC-3′), resulting in amplicons of 630 and 640 bp, respectively. The resultant products were mutagenized after subcloning into the pBHA vector. Two plasmids were extracted from the transformants, and the mutated sequences were confirmed by sequence analysis (CosmoGenetech, Daejeon, Republic of Korea). PCR was performed using a 20 μL reaction mixture (GeNet Bio, Daejeon, Republic of Korea) containing 2× master mix (10 μL), 2 μL of primer mixture, 5 μL sample DNA, and 3 μL Ultra pure water (Welgene) to make up the final volume. The reactions were run on a Verity thermocycler (Applied Biosystems, CA, USA) under the following conditions: one cycle at 94°C for 5 min, followed by 35 cycles of 94°C for 30 s, annealing 60°C for 30 s, initial extension at 72°C for 30 s, and a final extension of 72°C for 10 min to complete the synthesis of all strands. The amplified target was visualized as a single band corresponding to a length of 620 bp using the ChemiDoc system (Vilber Lourmat, Eberhardzell, Germany).

For REBA PCV2 genotyping, the hybridization and washing processes were performed as follows; each sample was tested in duplicate and all PCR-REBA runs were performed twice. In brief, biotinylated PCR products were denatured at 25°C for 5 min in denaturation solution and then the denatured single-stranded PCR products suspended in hybridization solution were incubated with REBA PCV2-genotyping membrane strips at 55°C with shaking at 90 rpm in a blotting tray for 30 min. The strips were then washed twice with gentle shaking in 1 ml of washing solution for 10 min at 55°C, incubated at 25°C with 1:2,000 diluted streptavidin-alkaline phosphatase (AP) conjugate (Roche Diagnostics, Mannheim, Germany) in conjugate diluent solution (CDS) for 30 min, and finally washed twice with 1 ml CDS at room temperature for 1 min. The colorimetric hybridization signals were visualized by adding a 1:50 dilution of nitro blue tetrazolium chloride/5-bromo-4-chloro-3-indolyl (NBT/BCIP) AP-mediated staining solution (Roche Diagnostics), and then incubated until a color change was detected. Finally, the band pattern was read and interpreted visually.

Sequence Analysis

To confirm the results of the two molecular diagnostic methods, the PCR amplicons of all the clinical samples were sequenced using an ABI 3730 automated DNA sequencer (Applied Biosystems, Foster City, CA, USA) and the ABI Prism BigDye Terminator (Applied Biosystems) system (CosmoGenetech, Republic of Korea). The primer set used to amplify the target ORF2 gene was 5′-TCTGAATTGTACATACATRGTTAYACGG-3′ (1070F) and 5′- TACCGYTGGAGAAGGAAAAATGG-3′ (1630R), which resulted in a 560-bp PCR product. The obtained sequences were compared with sequences in the National Center for Biotechnology Information (NCBI) GenBank database for species identification.

RESULTS

Analytical Sensitivity and Specificity of the Multiplex Real-Time PCR and PCR-REBA Methods

Analytical sensitivity of the two molecular methods for the detection of PCV2 was determined by using 10-fold diluted (1 ng, 100 pg, 10 pg, 1 pg, 100 fg, 10 fg, and 1 fg) samples for obtaining the standard curve for the DNA extracted from PCV2 strains. The detection limit of the multiplex real-time PCR assay for PCV2-P (PCV2 species-specific probe), PCV2a/e-P (PCV2a/e genotype-specific probe), PCV2b/d-P (PCV2b/d genotype-specific probe),

PCV2c (PCV2c genotype-specific probe), PCV2d-P (PCV2d genotype-specific probe), and PCV2e-P (PCV2e genotype-specific probe) ranged from 100 to 10 fg DNA per reaction. The C_T values for PCV2-P, PCV2a/e, PCV2b/d, PCV2c, PCV2d, and PCV2e for each DNA concentration ranged from 17 to 36.8, 16.5 to 34.9, 16.7 to 35.1, 16.1 to 35, 16.8 to 35.3, and 15.5 to 33.1, respectively (**Supplementary Figures 1A–D**). The PCR-REBA detection limit for PCV2a, PCV2b, PCV2c, PCV2d, and PCV2e was ~100 fg to 10 fg DNA per reaction (**Supplementary Figures 1E–J**). In addition, the detection limit for mixed co-infection PCV2 subtypes in multiplex real-time PCR was 1 pg DNA per reaction, and the C_T value was found to be 17.97–32.86 (Data not shown). The PCR-REBA detection limit for mixed co-infection PCV2 subtypes detected ~100 fg DNA per reaction (**Supplementary Figure 1K**).

To determine the specificity of the two molecular assays, primers and probes for detecting PCV2 positive genotypes were used for testing 55 DNA samples, respectively, extracted from specific pathogen-free swine serum samples and used as negative controls. The multiplex real-time PCR and PCR-REBA assay for detecting PCV2 positive genotypes yielded negative results with all strains except PCV2 strains (including mixed co-infection PCV2 subtypes), hence, the cross reactivity was not detected (**Supplementary Table 1**).

Detection of PCV2 DNA Using Multiplex Real-Time PCR and PCR-REBA Methods in Clinical Samples

To evaluate the performance of the multiplex real-time PCR and PCR-REBA assay, a total of 180 clinical samples including tissue ($n = 109$, 60.6%) and whole blood ($n = 71$, 39.4%) were analyzed. Of 180 clinical samples, 87 (48.3%) samples were positive for PCV2, and 93 (51.7%) samples were negative as detected by both multiplex real-time PCR and PCR-REBA (**Table 1**).

Multiplex Real-Time PCR and PCR-REBA Methods for the Detection of PCV2 Genotyping in Clinical Samples

Of the 87 PCV2 positive samples, 53 (60.9%), 17 (19.5%), 12 (13.8%), and 3 (3.5%) samples showed positive fluorescence signals for PCV2d, PCV2a, PCV2b, and PCV2a/b co-infections, respectively, as evaluated using multiplex real-time PCR assay (**Figure 2A**) while no PCV2 genotypes were detected in 2 cases (2.3%). All the clinical samples showed positive IC signals and the C_T values of the 87 positive and 93 negative samples ranged from 23.62 to 32.7 (mean 24.89, SD ± 1) and 22.47 to 33.4 (mean 25.36, SD ± 0.47), respectively. The C_T values of the PCV2d, PCV2a, PCV2b, and PCV2a/b co-infections samples ranged from 15.75 to 35.08 (mean 23.43, SD ± 5.6), 20.97 to 33.85 (mean 26.5, SD ± 4.07), 22.89 to 34.37 (mean 28.81, SD ± 5.78), and 21.2 to 30.73 (SD ± 2.4), respectively. PCR-REBA, which is another method for performing the molecular identification of PCV2 genotypes, was performed with the same clinical samples (**Figure 2B**). Of the 87 positive samples, the following PCV2 genotypes were identified using PCR-REBA: PCV2d was the most prevalent at 60.9% ($n = 53$), followed by PCV2a ($n = 17$, 19.5%), PCV2b ($n = 14$, 16.1%), and PCV2a/b co-infections ($n = 3$, 3.5%), respectively (**Table 2**).

Comparison of the Results Between the Two Molecular Assays and Sequence Analysis for Identification of the PCV2 Genotypes in the Clinical Samples

To confirm the results obtained from the multiplex real-time PCR and PCR-REBA assay, sequence analysis was performed using the same clinical samples (**Figure 2C**). Only 69 (79.3%) of the 87 PCV2 positive samples could be identified for PCV2 genotyping by sequence analysis. Therefore, 18 samples including 11 PCV2d, 2 PCV2a, 4 PCV2b, and 1 PCV2a/b co-infected samples identified by multiplex real-time PCR and PCR-REBA were excluded from the comparative analysis. The results of the multiplex real-time PCR and sequence analysis methods were consistent except for two cases. In these two cases, while PCV2 genotypes were not detected using multiplex real-time PCR, the samples were identified as PCV2b-positive by sequence analysis. The results of the PCR-REBA for PCV2 genotyping of all 69 samples were consistent with the sequencing results (**Table 2**). The phylogenetic tree was constructed using Phylogeny.fr software (23) after alignment of the 69 sequenced results. Analysis of the phylogenetic tree indicated that the sequences could be divided into three genotypes (PCV2d, PCV2a, and PCV2b), which accounted for 60.9, 24.6, and 14.5%, respectively (**Figure 3**).

DISCUSSION

Although the severity of the economic losses caused by PCV2 infection has been mitigated by vaccination, PCVAD is still detected quite often and is an important porcine pathogen. It is important to distinguish between the PCV2 genotypes for the laboratory diagnosis of PCV2 as different PCV2 genotypes have been found in samples from pigs affected with other PCVAD (24). The currently used PCR-based methods for diagnosis, including nucleotide sequencing, PCR, nested PCR, and PCR-RFLP (25–28), are time consuming for general veterinary clinical applications; they can only be used in specialized diagnostic institutes as these methods require specialized equipment and reagents, and need to be inspected by professionals to differentiate the subtype virus. Therefore, there is an increasing requirement for diagnostic techniques that can be complemented with traditional methods in clinical diagnostic laboratories.

In the present study, two molecular assays were developed for detecting PCV2 genotypes. The purpose of the present study was to evaluate the clinical efficacy of the multiplex RT-PCR assay (Opti PCV2-genotyping) and PCR-REBA (REBA PCV2-genotyping) for rapid and accurate detection as well as identification of PCV2 genotypes based on the ORF2 regions. We also compared the results of these two molecular assays with those obtained from conventional methods such

TABLE 1 | Detection of porcine circovirus 2 DNA in 180 clinical samples suspected of PCVAD infection using the multiplex real-time PCR and PCR-REBA assay.

Sample	Total no. (%) of samples	Multiplex real-time PCR		PCR-REBA	
		Positive (%)	Negative (%)	Positive (%)	Negative (%)
Tissue	109 (60.6)	54 (49.5)	55 (50.5)	54 (49.5)	55 (50.5)
Blood	71 (39.4)	33 (46.5)	38 (53.5)	33 (46.5)	38 (53.5)
Total	180 (100)	87 (48.3)	93 (51.7)	87 (48.3)	93 (51.7)

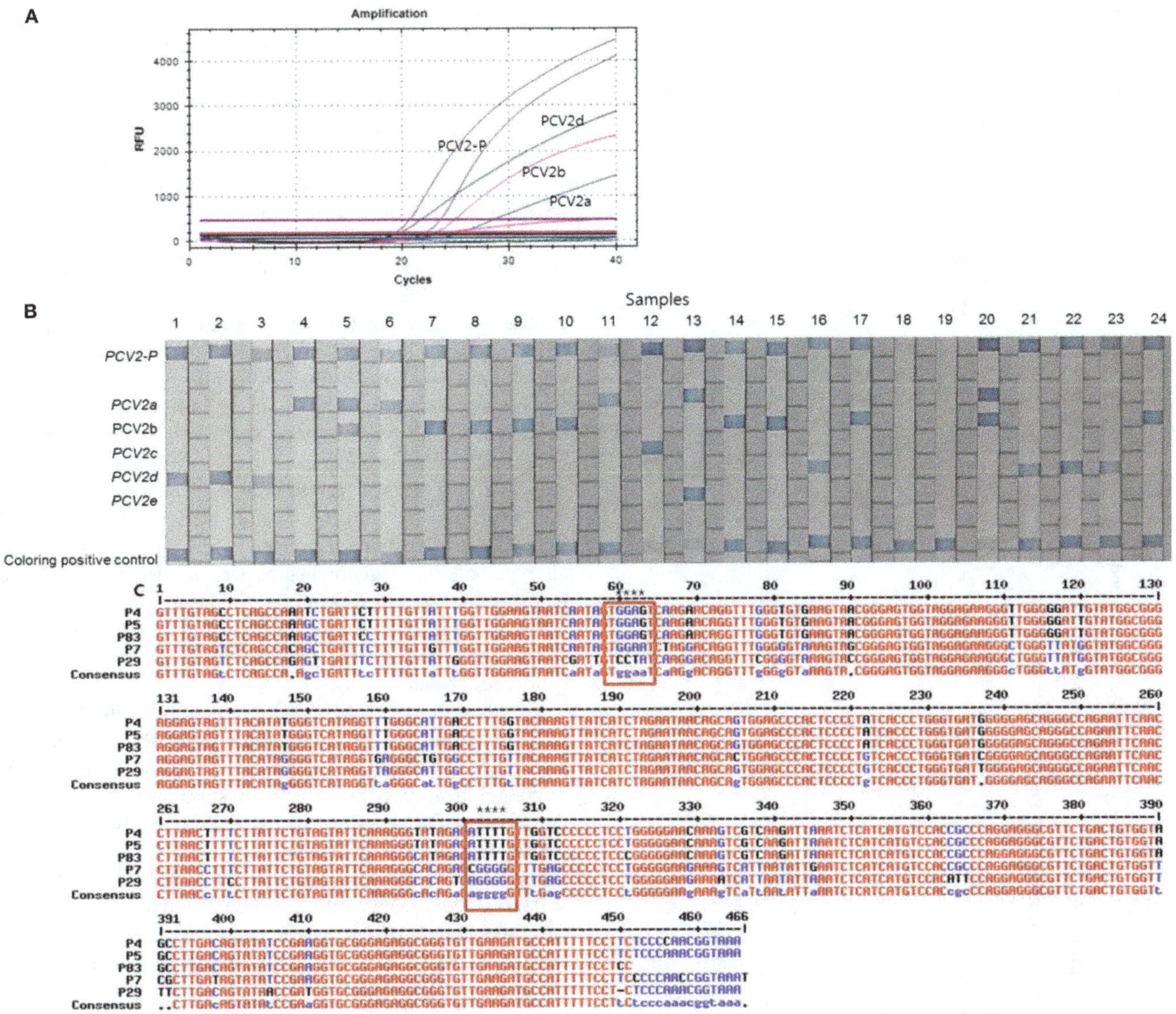

FIGURE 2 | Typical results of the multiplex real-time PCR, PCR-REBA, and sequence analysis with clinical samples. **(A)** Overall results for PCV2-positive, PCV2a, PCV2b, and PCV2d. Fluorescent dyes of specific TaqMan probes for multiplex real-time PCR were used PCV2 (Cy5), PCV2a/e (FAM), PCV2b/d (CAL Flour Red 610), and PCV2d (HEX), respectively. **(B)** Results of PCR-REBA; Lanes 1–3, 16, 21–23: PCV2d; lanes 4, 6, and 11: PCV2a; lanes 5 and 20: PCV2a and PCV2b co-infection; lane 7–10, 14–15, 17, and 24: PCV2b; lane 12: PCV2c; lane 13: PCV2e; lane 18 and 19: negative. PCV2c and PCV2e were used to synthesize the DNA as a control. **(C)** Sequence alignment results of a fragment of the genomic sequence of the clinical samples; P4, PCV2a; P7, PCV2b, P29, PCV2d, P5 and P83 showed that the two samples detected as PCV2a/b co-infection positive by the multiplex real-time PCR and PCR-REBA methods were shown as only PCV2a positive by sequence analysis; The red boxes indicate the position where three genotypes (PCV2a, 2b, and 2d) can be identified.

TABLE 2 | Comparison of multiplex real-time PCR, PCR-REBA, and sequence analysis results for the detection of PCV2 genotypes in 180 clinical samples suspected of PCVAD.

PCV2 genotyping	Molecular methods										
	PCR-REBA		Multiplex real-time PCR		Sequence analysis			Sensitivity (%)	95% CI	Specificity (%)	95% CI
	Positive (%)	Negative (%)	Positive (%)	Negative (%)	Positive (%)	N/A (%)	Consistent results				
PCV2 positive ($n = 87$)	**87 (48.3)**	**0 (0)**	**85 (97.7)**	**2 (2.3)**	**69 (79.3)***	**18 (20.7)**	**69 (100)**	100	0.954–1.000	100	0.979–1.000
Single infection ($n = 84$)	**84 (96.6)**	**0 (0)**	**82 (96.5)**	**2 (100)**	**67 (97.1)**	**17 (94.4)**	**67 (100)**	100	0.953–1.000	100	0.972–1.000
PCV2d	53 (63.1)	0 (0)	53 (63.1)	0 (0)	42 (79.2)	11 (20.8)	42 (100)	100	0.927–1.000	100	0.884–1.000
PCV2a	17 (20.2)	0 (0)	17 (20.2)	0 (0)	15 (88.2)	2 (11.8)	15 (100)	100	0.784–1.000	100	0.940–1.000
PCV2b	14 (16.7)	0 (0)	12 (14.3)	2 (2.4)	10 (71.4)	4 (28.6)	10 (100)	100	0.787–1.000	100	0.954–1.000
Multiple infection ($n = 3$)	**3 (3.4)**	**0 (0)**	**3 (3.5)**	**0 (0)**	**2 (2.9)**	**1 (5.6)**	**2 (100)**	100	0.425–1.000	100	0.961–1.000
PCV2a and PCV2b	3 (100)	0 (0)	3 (100)	0 (0)	2 (66.7)	1 (33.3)	2 (100)	100	0.369–1.000	100	0.953–1.000
PCV2 negative ($n = 93$)	**0 (0)**	**93 (100)**	**0 (0)**	**93 (100)**	–	–	–	–	–	–	–
Total ($n = 180$)	87 (48.3)	93 (51.7)	85 (47.2)	95 (52.8)	69 (79.3)	18 (20.7)	–	–	–	–	–

*N/A, not applicable; *A total of 18 samples including 11 PCV2d, 2 PCV2a, 4 PCV2b, and 1 PCV2a/b co-infection identified by multiplex real-time PCR and PCR-REBA were excluded because they were not sequenced; 95% CI, 95% confidence interval.*

as sequence analysis. The characteristics of the multiplex real-time PCR and PCR-REBA used in this study were similar as they were both rapid (turnaround time of 2–3 h), sensitive, specific, and comparatively easy to perform without requiring any specialized laboratory equipment, other than a PCR machine and water bath.

The Opti PCV2-genotyping assay is designed to simultaneously detect PCV2 and to distinguish PCV2a/e, PCV2b, and PCV2d genotypes. Multiplex real-time PCR, a recognized technique, is faster and more effective for the rapid detection of bacterial or viral infection compared to conventional PCR and other detection methods. Multiplex real-time PCR assay is a rapid method with a turnaround time of ~1.5–2 h, which includes 30 min for DNA preparation and 1.5 h for target DNA amplification. The combination of excellent sensitivity and specificity as well as ease of handling enable rapid and simultaneous detection of multiple species, and minimizes the possibility of contamination by eliminating the need for additional post-PCR processing of the samples, which has made this technology appealing for clinical microbiology laboratory applications (29). PCR-REBA is a highly sensitive and specific probe-based method in which multiple oligonucleotide probes are immobilized on nitrocellulose strips, hybridized with biotin-labeled PCR products, and can be used to derive rapid results within 4 h (30). In addition to the time required for target DNA amplification (1.5 h), PCR-REBA is a 3-step process with a hybridization step (30 min), a washing step (20 min), and a chromogenic detection and data interpretation step (40 min). It also requires a fully automated system for the washing, hybridization, and interpretation steps. The PCR-REBA molecular diagnostic assay can be used to isolate all types of PCV2 genotypes as well as detect PCV2 directly from serum or tissue samples. In addition, PCR-REBA has the advantage of the flexibility to add more specific-probes to the membrane strip for increasing the range of PCV2 genotypes detected.

In this study, the concordance rate of the multiplex real-time PCR assay and sequence analysis was 98.8% (95% confidence interval [CI] 0.953–0.999, $p < 0.001$). Using sequence analysis as the gold standard, the sensitivity, specificity, and positive and negative predictive values of the PCV2 genotyping results by multiplex real-time PCR assay were 97.1% ($n = 67$, 95% CI 0.894–0.998, $p < 0.001$), 100% ($n = 93$, 95% CI 0.966–1.000, $p < 0.001$), 100% (95% CI 0.953–1.000, $p < 0.001$), 97.9% (95% CI 0.921–0.998, $p < 0.001$), respectively. The results of PCR-REBA were found to be consistent with those of sequence analysis and showed good agreement ($\kappa = 1$).

Studies have shown that the most common PCV2 genotypes detected worldwide are PCV2b (53.1%) and PCV2a (34.4%) in Taiwan (24), PCV2b (87.5%) and PCV2a (12.5%) in Mexico (31), and PCV2d (45.3%) and PCV2b (41.1%) in China (13). In this study, the most prevalent genotypes detected were PCV2d ($n = 53$, 60.9%), followed by PCV2a ($n = 17$, 19.5%), PCV2b ($n = 14$, 16.1 %), and PCV2a/b co-infection ($n = 3$, 3.5%). Co-infection of PCV2a and PCV2b in clinical samples has been suggested to be the primary cause of other PCVAD while dual heterologous infection of

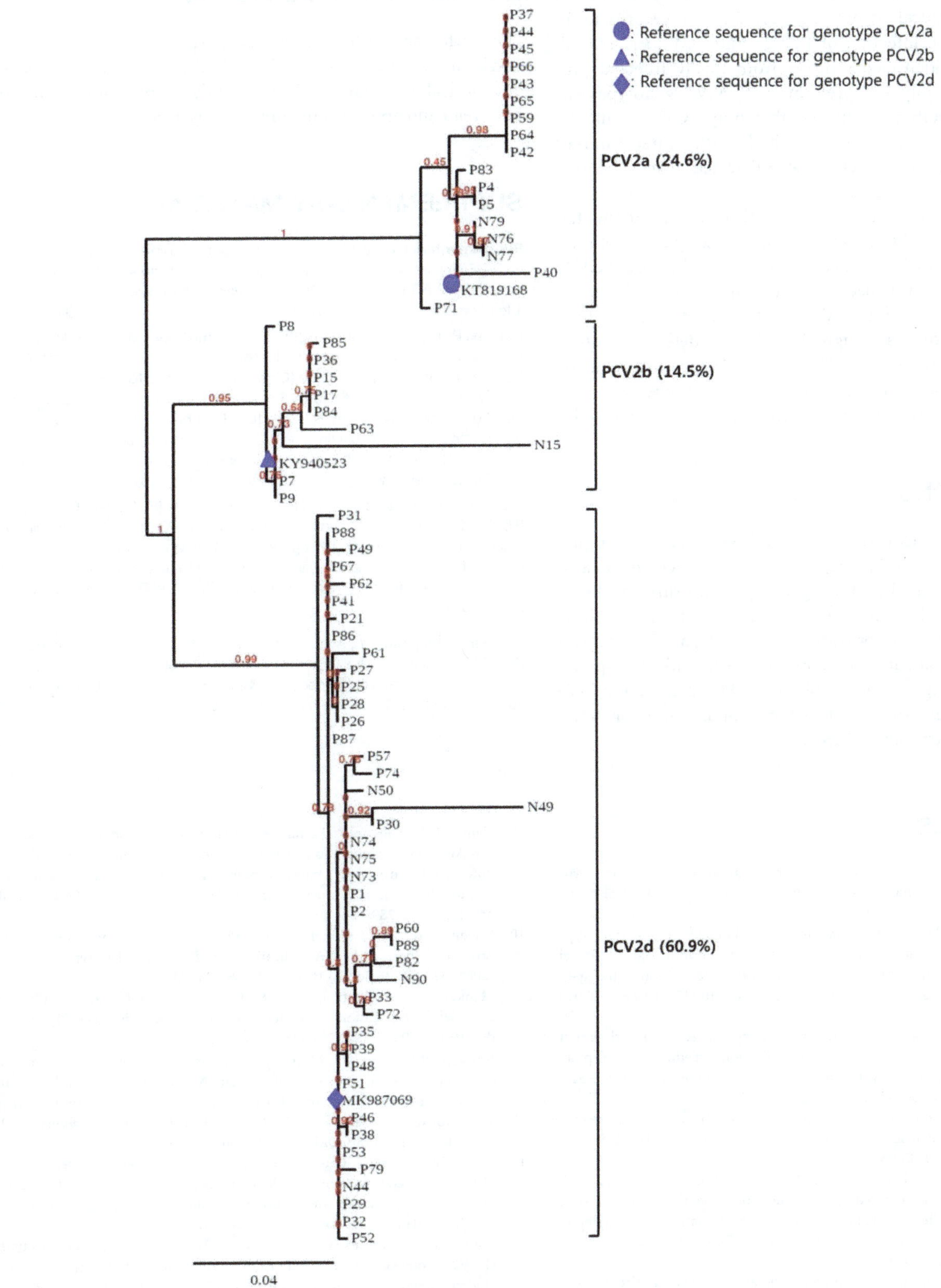

FIGURE 3 | Phylogenetic analysis of the 69 PCV2 isolates. The phylogenetic tree was constructed using Phylogeny.fr software after alignment of the 69 sequenced results. The PCV2genomes were mainly assigned to three genotypes (PCV2a, PCV2b, and PCV2d).

PCV2a and PCV2b in gnotobiotic pigs has been shown to induce severe clinical symptoms (24, 32). Therefore, rapid identification of co-infection of PCV2a and PCV2b is crucial. Generally, when identified samples from dually infected pigs were sequenced, only the predominant PCV2 genotype was detected. Our results also showed that only PCV2a could be identified by sequence analysis method in the three samples in which PCV2a/b co-infection was detected using the two molecular diagnostic methods.

There are potential limitations in this study. Firstly, the multiplex real-time PCR assay cannot distinguish between PCV2a type and PCV2e type, and does not include PCV2c type that has not yet been detected in Korea. Therefore, there should be an additional tube to include all of these genotypes. Secondly, although PCR-REBA detect all other genotypes in addition to PCV2, additional steps are required after PCR. Thirdly, the PCV2c and PCV2e genotypes were not detected in this study and further investigations of the samples are required.

CONCLUSIONS

The two recently developed molecular assays are accurate, rapid, and convenient tools for identifying PCV2. These assays can also discriminate between the PCV2 genotypes and directly detect PCV2 from clinical samples in only 2–3 h. Therefore, these two molecular assays can provide essential information that can help expedite therapeutic decisions for early and appropriate vaccinations during the acute phase of PCV2 infection. We believe that these assays can reduce the labor and time for PCV2 diagnosis in industrial animal area.

AUTHOR CONTRIBUTIONS

HW performed evaluation of the experiments, analyzed the data, and drafted the manuscript. JS and SS provide clinical samples and clinical information. HK revised the manuscript. All authors have read and approved the final manuscript.

SUPPLEMENTARY MATERIAL

Supplementary Figure 1 | Detection limits of the multiplex real-time PCR and PCR-REBA methods evaluated using 10-fold serial diluted samples. Serially diluted PCV2-P, PCV2a/e, PCV2b, and PCV2d DNA samples ranging from 1 ng to 1 fg per reaction were used to determine the detection limit of the multiplex real-time PCR and PCR-REBA methods. In the multiplex real-time PCR assay, the amplification curve of the specific probe **(A)** for detecting PCV2 ($R^2 = 0.997$), PCV2a/e probe **(B)**, PCV2b probe **(C)**, and PCV2d probe **(D)**, for detecting PCV2 genotypes ($R^2 = 0.999$) are shown. The overall detection limit of this assay for the PCV2 genotypes ranged from ~100 to 10 fg DNA per reaction. C_T was plotted against the input of the quantity of PCV2, 2a/e, 2b, 2c, 2d, and 2e DNA (repeated 40 times). The intensity of fluorescence is shown on the Y-axis (R^2 = reporter signal/passive reference signal). RFU, relative fluorescence unit and R^2, fluorescence units. Serially diluted PCV2-P **(E)**, PCV2a **(F)**, PCV2b **(G)**, PCV2c **(H)**, PCV2d **(I)**, PCV2e **(J)**, and 5 mixed co-infection PCV2 subtypes **(K)** with DNA amounts from 1 ng (lane 1), 100 pg (lane 2), 10 pg (lane 3), 1 pg (lane 4), 100 fg (lane 5), 10 fg (lane 6), and 1 fg (lane 7) were used to determine the detection limit of the PCR-REBA **(E–J)**. N, negative control. PCV2c and PCV2e used synthesized DNA as a control.

Supplementary Table 1 | Analytical specificity of the multiplex real-time PCR and PCR-REBA assay for detecting PCV2 and PCV2 genotypes with 25 strains and 30 normal serum samples, respectively, obtained from pigs. ATCC, American type culture collection, PCV2, Porcine circovirus type2.

REFERENCES

1. Olvera A, Cortey M, Segalés J. Molecular evolution of porcine circovirus type 2 genomes: phylogeny and clonality. *Virology.* (2007) 357:175–85. doi: 10.1016/j.virol.2006.07.047
2. Opriessnig T, Meng XJ, Halbur PG. Porcine circovirus type 2 associated disease: update on current terminology, clinical manifestations, pathogenesis, diagnosis, and intervention strategies. *J Vet Diagn Invest.* (2007) 19:591–615. doi: 10.1177/104063870701900601
3. Qiu X, Li T, Zhang G, Cao J, Jin Y, Xing G, et al. Development of a loop-mediated isothermal amplification method to rapidly detect porcine circovirus genotypes 2a and 2b. *Virol J.* (2012) 9:318. doi: 10.1186/1743-422X-9-318
4. Chae C. Postweaning multisystemic wasting syndrome: a review of aetiology, diagnosis and pathology. *Vet J.* (2004) 168:41–9. doi: 10.1016/S1090-0233(03)00182-5
5. Rosell C, Segales J, Plana-Duran J, Balasch M, Rodriguez-Arrioja GM, Kennedy S, et al. Pathological, immunohistochemical, and *in-situ* hybridization studies of natural cases of postweaning multisystemic wasting syndrome (PMWS) in pigs. *J Comp Pathol.* (1999) 120:59–78. doi: 10.1053/jcpa.1998.0258
6. Harding JC. The clinical expression and emergence of porcine circovirus 2. *Vet Microbiol.* (2004) 98:131–5. doi: 10.1016/j.vetmic.2003.10.013
7. Allan GM, Ellis JA. Porcine circoviruses: a review. *J Vet Diagn Invest.* (2000) 12:3–14. doi: 10.1177/104063870001200102
8. Hamel AL, Lin LL, Nayar GP. Nucleotide sequence of porcine circovirus associated with postweaning multisystemic wasting syndrome in pigs. *J Virol.* (1998) 72:5262–7. doi: 10.1128/JVI.72.6.5262-5267.1998
9. Nainys J, Lasickiene R, Petraityte-Burneikiene R, Dabrisius J, Lelesius R, Sereika V, et al. Generation in yeast of recombinant virus-like particles of porcine circovirus type 2 capsid protein and their use for a serologic assay and development of monoclonal antibodies. *BMC Biotechnol.* (2014) 14:100. doi: 10.1186/s12896-014-0100-1
10. Cheung AK. The essential and nonessential transcription units for viral protein synthesis and DNA replication of porcine circovirus type 2. *Virology.* (2004) 313:452–9. doi: 10.1016/S0042-6822(03)00373-8
11. Mankertz A, Mankertz J, Wolf K, Buhk HJ. Identification of a protein essential for replication of porcine circovirus. *J Gen Virol.* (1998) 79:381–4. doi: 10.1099/0022-1317-79-2-381
12. Nawagitgul P, Harms PA, Morozov I, Thacker BJ, Sorden SD, Lekcharoensuk C, et al. Modified indirect porcine circovirus (PCV) type 2-based and recombinant capsid protein (ORF2)-based enzyme-linked immunosorbent assays for detection of antibodies to PCV. *Clin Diagn Lab Immunol.* (2002) 9:33–40. doi: 10.1128/CDLI.9.1.33-40.2002
13. Yao J, Qin Y, Zeng Y, Ouyang K, Chen Y, Huang W, et al. Genetic analysis of porcine circovirus type 2 (PCV2) strains between 2002 and 2016 reveals PCV2 mutant predominating in porcine population in Guangxi, China. *BMC Vet Res.* (2019) 15:118. doi: 10.1186/s12917-019-1859-z
14. Franzo G, Tucciarone CM, Cecchinato M, Drigo M. Porcine circovirus type 2 (PCV2) evolution before and after the vaccination introduction: a large scale epidemiological study. *Sci Rep.* (2016) 6:39458. doi: 10.1038/srep39458
15. Xiao CT, Harmon KM, Halbur PG, Opriessnig T. PCV2d-2 is the predominant type of PCV2 DNA in pig samples collected in the U.S. During 2014-2016. *Vet Microbiol.* (2016) 197:72–7. doi: 10.1016/j.vetmic.2016.11.009
16. Eddicks M, Fux R, Szikora F, Eddicks L, Majzoub-Altweck M, Hermanns W, et al. Detection of a new cluster of porcine circovirus type 2b

strains in domestic pigs in Germany. *Vet Microbiol.* (2005) 176:337–43. doi: 10.1016/j.vetmic.2015.01.013

17. Yang S, Yin S, Shang Y, Liu B, Yuan L, Zafar Khan MU, et al. Phylogenetic and genetic variation analyses of porcine circovirus type 2 isolated from China. *Transbound Emerg Dis.* (2018) 65:e383–92. doi: 10.1111/tbed.12768
18. Opriessnig T, McKeown NE, Harmon KL, Meng XJ, Halbur PG. Porcine circovirus type 2 infection decreases the efficacy of a modified live porcine reproductive and respiratory syndrome virus vaccine. *Clin Vaccine Immunol.* (2006) 13:923–9. doi: 10.1128/CVI.00074-06
19. Huang Y, Zhang X, Du Q, Wang F, Zhao X, Zhang W, et al. Preclinical detection of porcine circovirus type 2 infection using an ultrasensitive nanoparticle DNA probe-based PCR assay. *PLoS ONE.* (2014) 9:e97869. doi: 10.1371/journal.pone.0097869
20. Guo LJ, Lu YH, Wei YW, Huang LP, Liu CM. Porcine circovirus type 2 (PCV2): genetic variation and newly emerging genotypes in China. *Virol J.* (2010) 7:273. doi: 10.1186/1743-422X-7-273
21. Rincón Monroy MA, Ramirez-Nieto GC, Vera VJ, Correa JJ, Mogollón-Galvis JD. Detection and molecular characterization of porcine circovirus type 2 from piglets with porcine circovirus associated diseases in Colombia. *Virol J.* (2014) 11:143. doi: 10.1186/1743-422X-11-143
22. Xiao CT, Halbur PG, Opriessnig T. Global molecular genetic analysis of porcine circovirus type 2 (PCV2) sequences confirms the presence of four main PCV2 genotypes and reveals a rapid increase of PCV2d. *J Gen Virol.* (2015) 96:1830–41. doi: 10.1099/vir.0.000100
23. Dereeper A, Guignon V, Blanc G, Audic S, Buffet S, Chevenet F, et al. Phylogeny.fr: robust phylogenetic analysis for the non-specialist. *Nucleic Acids Res.* (2008) 36:W465–9. doi: 10.1093/nar/gkn180
24. Wang C, Pang VF, Lee F, Liao PC, Huang YL, Lin YL, et al. Development and evaluation of a loop-mediated isothermal amplification method for rapid detection and differentiation of two genotypes of porcine circovirus type 2. *J Microbiol Immunol Infect.* (2014) 47:363–70. doi: 10.1016/j.jmii.2013.05.003
25. Wen LB, Guo X, Yang HC. Genotyping of porcine circovirus type 2 from a variety of clinical conditions in china. *Vet Microbiol.* (2005) 110:141–6. doi: 10.1016/j.vetmic.2005.07.003
26. Cheung AK, Lager KM, Kohutyuk OI, Vincent AL, Henry SC, Baker RB, et al. Detection of two porcine circovirus type 2 genotypic groups in United States swine herds. *Arch Virol.* (2007) 152:1035–44. doi: 10.1007/s00705-006-0909-6
27. Li W, Wang X, Ma T, Feng Z, Li Y, Jiang P. Genetic analysis of porcine circovirus type 2 (PCV2) strains isolated between 2001 and 2009: genotype PCV2b predominate in postweaning multisystemic wasting syndrome occurrences in eastern China. *Virus Genes.* (2010) 40:244–51. doi: 10.1007/s11262-009-0438-y
28. Lyoo KS, Kim HB, Joo HS. Evaluation of a nested polymerase chain reaction assay to differentiate between two genotypes of Porcine circovirus-2. *J Vet Diagn Invest.* (2008) 20:283–8. doi: 10.1177/104063870802000304
29. Wang HY, Kim H, Choi EH, Lee H. Performance of the Real Fungus-ID kit based on multiplex RT-PCR assay for the rapid detection and identification of *Trichophyton* spp. and *Microsporum* spp. in clinical specimens with suspected dermatophyte infection. *J Appl Microbiol.* (2016) 120:234–47. doi: 10.1111/jam.12993
30. Ajbani K, Shetty A, Mehta A, Rodrigues C. Rapid diagnosis of extensively drug-resistant tuberculosis by use of a reverse line blot hybridization assay. *J Clin Microbiol.* (2011) 49:2546–51. doi: 10.1128/JCM.02511-10
31. Bedolla López F, Trujillo Ortega ME, Mendoza Elvira S, Quintero Ramírez V, Alonso Morales R, Ramírez-Mendoza H, et al. Identification and genotyping of porcine circovirus type II (PCV2) in Mexico. *Virus Dis.* (2018) 29:385–9. doi: 10.1007/s13337-018-0460-6
32. Harding JC, Ellis JA, McIntosh KA, Krakowka S. Dual heterologous porcine circovirus genogroup 2a/2b infection induces severe disease in germ-free pigs. *Vet Microbiol.* (2010) 145:209e19. doi: 10.1016/j.vetmic.2010.03.026

Molecular Characterization of the Nsp2 and ORF5 (ORF5a) Genes of PRRSV Strains in Nine Provinces of China during 2016–2018

Baishuang Yin [1†], Shanshan Qi [2†], Wanli Sha [1], Hongyu Qin [1], Liming Liu [1], Jinyan Yun [1], Jinhai Zhu [2], Guojiang Li [1] and Dongbo Sun [1,2*]*

[1] College of Animal Science and Technology, Jilin Agricultural Science and Technology University, Jilin, China, [2] Laboratory for the Prevention and Control of Swine Infectious Diseases, College of Animal Science and Veterinary Medicine, Heilongjiang Bayi Agricultural University, Daqing, China

***Correspondence:**
Guojiang Li
jlliguojiang@126.com
Dongbo Sun
dongbosun@126.com

† These authors have contributed equally to this work*

Porcine reproductive and respiratory syndrome virus (PRRSV) causes a highly contagious disease and brings huge economic losses to commercial pork production worldwide. PRRSV causes severe reproductive failure in sows and respiratory distress in piglets. To trace the evolution of PRRSV in pigs with respiratory diseases in some regions of China, 112 samples were collected from nine provinces in China during 2016–2018. All samples were detected by RT-PCR and analyzed by the Nsp2/ORF5 (ORF5a)-genes-phylogeny. Sequence analysis and recombination analysis were conducted on the Nsp2/ORF5 (ORF5a) genes of the identified strain in the study. The RT-PCR result shown that the positive rate of PRRSV was 50.89% (57/112). Phylogenetic analysis showed that the identified PRRSV strains were all NA genotype and belonged to lineage 1, 3, and 8. The Nsp2 gene of identified PRRSV strains exhibited nucleotide homologies of 53.0 ∼ 99.8%, and amino acid homologies of 46.8 ∼ 99.7%. The ORF5 gene of identified PRRSV strains exhibited nucleotide homologies of 82.4 ∼ 100%, and amino acid homologies of 79.6 ∼ 100%. Sequence analysis revealed that a discontinuous 30-amino-acid deletion (positions 481 and 533–561) and a 131-amino-acid discontinuity deletion (positions 323–433, 481, and 533–551) in Nsp2 of PPRSV isolates; all identified strains in this study may be wild strains, and most identified strains may be highly virulent strains. Sequence analysis of ORF5 and ORF5a revealed that the mutation sites of GP5 were mainly concentrated in the signal peptide and epitopes region, while the mutation sites of ORF5a were mainly concentrated in the transmembrane and the intramembrane region. The recombination analysis indicated that there may be multiple recombination regions in identified strains, and the recombination pattern was more complex. This study showed that the prevalent PRRSV strain in some regions of China was still HP-PRRSV, while NADC30 strain also occupied a certain proportion; different types of PRRSV strains showed different patterns and variation in China. This study suggested that the monitoring of PRRSV prevalence and genetic variation should be further strengthened.

Keywords: porcine reproductive and respiratory syndrome virus, Nsp2 gene, ORF5 gene, ORF5a gene, genetic evolution

INTRODUCTION

Porcine reproductive and respiratory syndrome (PRRS) is a major threat to the global swine industry, causing significant economic losses each year. The causative agent is PRRS virus (PRRSV), a member of the *Arteriviridae* family, order *Nidoviridales*. PRRSV is a single positive-strand RNA virus with a genome length of ~15.4 kb (1, 2). The PRRSV contains at least 10 open reading frames (ORFs), which are ORF1a, ORF1b, ORF2a, ORF2b, ORF5a, and ORF3 ~ 7 from the 5' to the 3' untranslated regions (UTR) (3, 4). ORF1a and ORF1b are cleaved into at least 13–16 non-structural proteins (Nsps) by a complex proteolytic cascade (3).

PRRSV was first reported in commercial pigs by the United States in 1987 (5), and the disease quickly spread worldwide with frequent break outs. PRRSV is still considered a highly contagious disease in the pig industry and creates huge economic losses (1, 6, 7). PRRSV was divided into two genotypes: the European genotype (type I) and North American genotype (type II) (3). There are three main subtypes of PRRSV (type II) isolates in Chinese pig populations: classical PRRSV (type II) including CH-1a, S1, and BJ-4; highly pathogenic PRRSV (HP-PRRSV) including JXA1, HuN4, and TJ; and NADC30-like PRRSV including JL580, CHsx1401, and HNjz15 (8). The genetic characteristic of HP-PRRSV isolates have a discontinuous 30-amino-acid deletion in Nsp2, and NADC30-like PRRSV isolates have a discontinuous 131-amino-acid deletion in Nsp2 (9, 10). PRRSV has mutated in the epidemic process to produce new strains due to the high frequency of gene mutation and recombination, in which new strains often have stronger environmental adaptations. The above factors have made the PRRSV epidemic more complicated, and it also brings great difficulties to disease prevention (11, 12). Nsp2 and ORF5 (ORF5a) are highly variable and ORF5 is associated with the neutralizing epitope (13, 14). They are usually used as target genes for PRRSV molecular epidemiological surveillance.

This study intends to reveal the prevalence and genetic evolution of PRRSV during 2016–2018 in different regions of China. The current study used the Nsp2 and ORF5 (ORF5a) genes to analyze the genetic evolution of the identified PRRSV strains. Our aim is to provide a theoretical basis for further monitoring of genetic variations of PRRSV in China.

METHODS

Sampling

In total, 112 samples of the lung or lymph node tissues from pigs with respiratory diseases were collected between 2016 and 2018 in nine provinces or municipalities of China, including Heilongjiang, Jilin, Liaoning, Hubei, Jiangsu, Jiangxi, Zhejiang, Hebei, and the Inner Mongolia Autonomous Region. The lung or lymph node tissues were ground to powder with liquid nitrogen and diluted with three volumes of phosphate-buffered saline (PBS). The samples were centrifuged at 5,000 × g for 15 min at 4°C and the supernatants were transferred to a 1.5 mL tube. The genomic RNA was extracted from the supernatant using a commercial TIANamp Stool RNA Kit (Tiangen Biotech Co., Ltd, Beijing, China). The viral cDNA was synthesized using Moloney murine leukemia virus (RNaseH-) reverse transcriptase (Novoprotein Scientific Inc., Shanghai, China) in conjunction with six-random-nucleotide primers. The extracted genomic RNA and cDNA was stored at −80°C.

PCR Detection and Sequencing of PRRSV Strains

The primer of ORF5 full-length gene (including complete ORF5a gene) can be found in the report by Cao et al. (15). A pair of primers of Nsp2 gene were designed based on the alignment of published PRRSV genome sequences obtained from the NCBI GenBank database. Primer information is shown in **Table 1**. The amplification reactions were carried out in a 25 μL reaction volume containing 12.5 μl of EmeraldAmp® PCR Master Mix (2×Premix) (TaKaRa Biotechnology Co., Ltd., Dalian, China), 0.5 μM of the forward primer, 0.5 μM of the reverse primer, 1 μL of cDNA, and an appropriate volume of double-distilled (dd) H_2O. The cycling parameters of ORF5 gene were: 36 cycles of 94°C for 30 s, 55°C for 30 s, and 72°C for 1 min, followed by a final extension at 72°C for 10 min. The cycling parameters of Nsp2 gene were: 35 cycles of 95°C for 30 s, 57.6°C for 30 s, and 72°C for 3 min, followed by a final extension at 72°C for 10 min. The PCR products were analyzed by electrophoresis in a 1% agarose gel under UV light, and the samples with positive results were recorded. After the amplification, products were purified using the AxyPrep DNA Gel Extraction kit (A Corning Brand, Suzhou, China), and cloned into pGM-T Vector (TaKaRa Biotechnology Co., Ltd., Dalian, China). Each fragment was sequenced at least three times. All nucleotide

TABLE 1 | Primers specific for ORF5 and Nsp2 genes of PRRSV.

Target gene	Primer name	Primer sequence(5′-3′)	Amplified length(bp)
ORF5/ORF5a	ORF5-F	GTTTTAGCCTGTCTTTTTGCC	731
	ORF5-R	TATATCATCACTGGCGTGTAGG	
Nsp2	Nsp2-nF	GAAGGGAATTGTGGTTGGCA	2 175 ~ 2 568
	Nsp2-nR	AGACCCAGAAAACACACCCA	

TABLE 2 | The results of PRRSV sample positive rate in China between 2016 and 2018.

Region	Province	Positive rate	Total
Northeast China	Heilongjiang	60.46% (26/43)	52.3% (34/65)
	Jilin	0% (0/1)	
	Liaoning	36.36% (8/22)	
Central China	Hubei	11.11% (1/9)	11.11% (1/9)
East China	Jiangsu	100% (5/5)	85.7% (12/14)
	Jiangxi	100% (7/7)	
	Zhejiang	0% (0/2)	
North China	Inner Mongolia	44.44% (4/9)	43.5% (10/23)
	Hebei	42.86% (6/14)	
Total			50.89% (57/112)

sequences generated in this study have been submitted to the GenBank database.

Phylogenetic and Sequence Analysis of PRRSV Strains

For the phylogenetic analysis, the Nsp2 and ORF5 (ORF5a) genes of PRRSV reference strains were retrieved from the NCBI nucleotide database as reference sequences. Detailed information and the GenBank number of PRRSV reference strains is shown in **Supplementary Table 1**. To construct phylogenetic trees, nucleotide sequences of the target gene using the ClustalX alignment tool in the MEGA 6.06 software (16). Neighbor-joining phylogenetic trees were constructed with 1,000 bootstrap replicates and the remaining default parameters in the MEGA 6.06 software. The generated phylogenetic tree was annotated using the online software ITOL (https://itol.embl.de/) (17). The PRRSV-identified strains and reference strains were analyzed by MegAlign program in DNASTAR^{TM} 5.06 software. Nucleotide/amino acid homology of Nsp2 and ORF5 (ORF5a) genes of PRRSV-identified strains, and reference strains were gained using the Pairwise/Multiple Align function in Geneious Prime software.

Recombination Analysis

When RDP, GENECONV, BootScan, MaxChi, Chimera, SiScan, and 3eq methods were used to detect potential

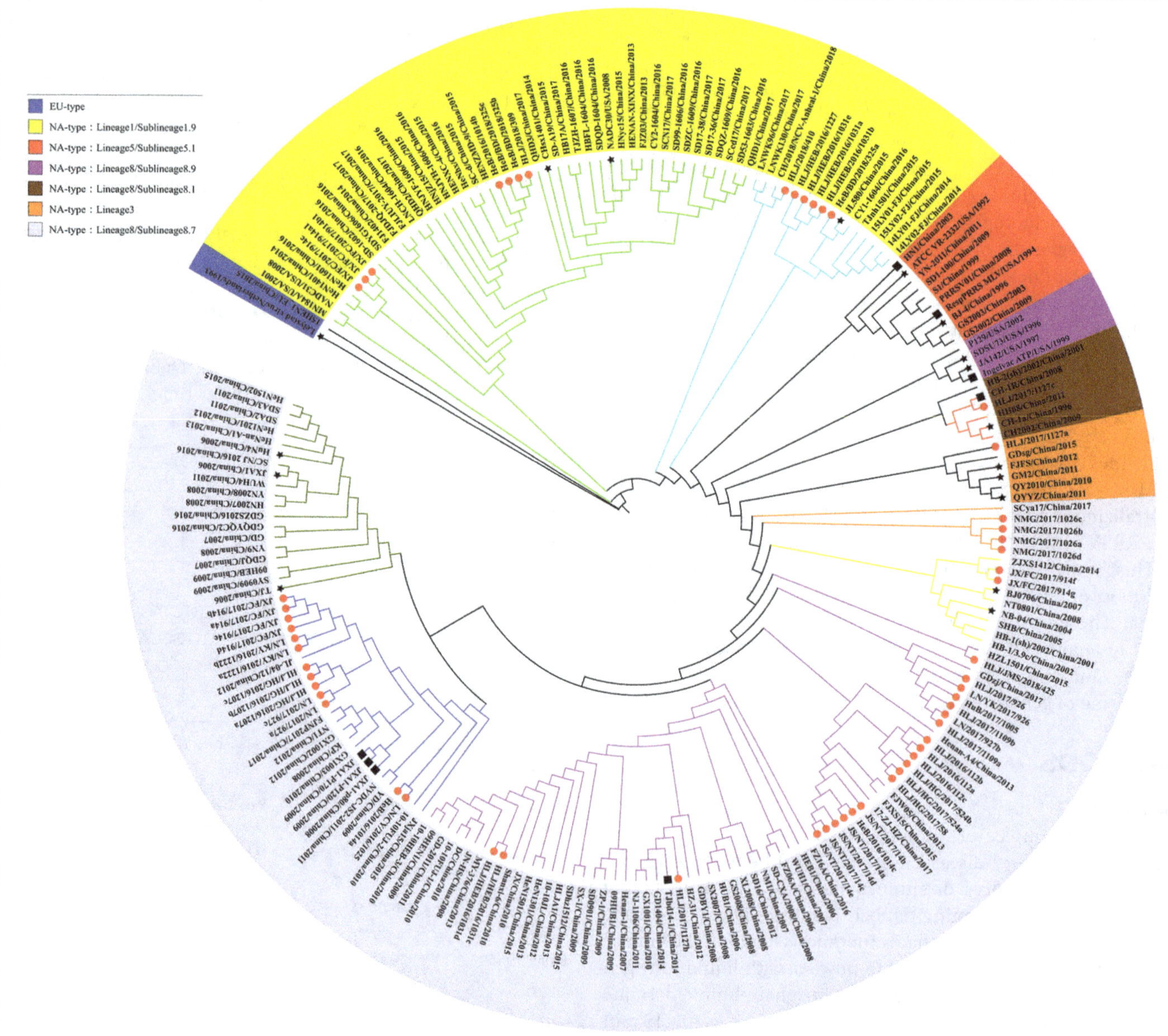

FIGURE 1 | Phylogenetic analysis based on Nsp2 gene. The red circle diagram represents PRRSV strains identified in our study, black star diagram represents PRRSV reference strains, and the black square diagram represents PRRSV vaccine strains.

recombinant events, five or more methods were identified as gene recombination and $P < 0.05$ in RDP4.0 software. The strains in this event were determined to be recombinant strains. In addition, the detected recombination events were further confirmed by SimPlot 3.5.1.

RESULTS

Detection and Analysis of PRRSV

In this study, 112 samples from nine provinces or municipalities of China were detected for PRRSV by RT-PCR. Of these tested samples, 50.89% (57/112) were positive for PRRSV. The infection rate of PRRSV was the highest in East China (85.71%, 12/14), including Jiangsu, Jiangxi, and Zhejiang province, and the lowest in Central China (11.11%, 1/9), including Hubei province. The infection rate of PRRSV in Northeast China was 52.3% (34/65), including Heilongjiang, Jilin, and Liaoning province, while the infection rate of PRRSV in North China was 43.5% (10/23), including Hebei province and the Inner Mongolia Autonomous Region (**Table 2**). Although the sources of the samples in different regions were non-uniform, the results showed that the presence of PRRSV was severe in some parts of China.

Phylogenetic Analysis of PRRSV

In 2010, Shi et al. conducted a systematic classification of type II PRRSVs based on ORF5 gene, and classified the

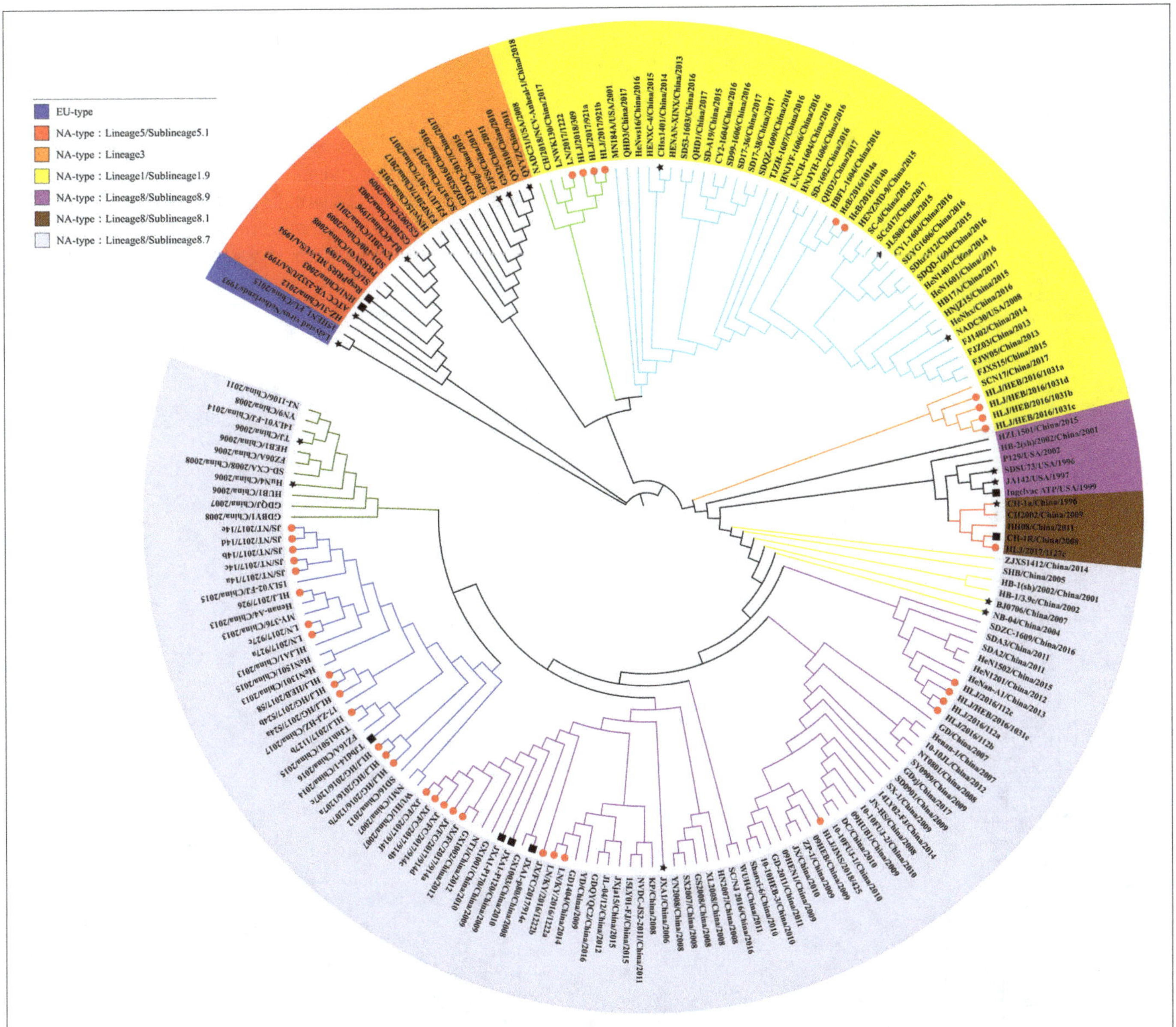

FIGURE 2 | Phylogenetic analysis based on ORF5 gene. The red circle diagram represents PRRSV strains identified in our study, the black star diagram represents PRRSV reference strains, and the black square diagram represents PRRSV vaccine strains.

PRRSVs into nine Lineage and 37 sublineage (18). Referring to the reported genotyping study by Shi et al., all the previously identified lineage reference sequences were also clustered in the same lineage in the phylogenetic tree of this study. The Nsp2 and ORF5-genes-based phylogenetic analysis revealed that all 56 PRRSV strains identified in this study belong to the North American genotype and were distributed in lineage 1, 3, and 8, among which the proportion of identified strains is the highest in sublineage 8.7 (73.2%, 41/56) and the lowest in lineage 3 (1.8%, 1/56) (**Figures 1, 2**). In addition, some identified strains were distributed differently in phylogenetic trees constructed with different genes. For instance, HeB/2016/1014a and HLJ/HEB/2016/1031(c, d) belong to the sublineage 8.7 while HLJ/HEB/2016/1031e and JX/FC/2017/914c belong to lineage 1 of the phylogenetic tree based on Nsp2 gene. However, the distribution of the identified strains was reversed in

TABLE 3 | Nucleotide and deduced amino acid homologies analysis based on Nsp2 gene (%).

		Identified strain				Reference strain					
		Sublineage 8.1	Lineage 3	Lineage 1	Sublineage 8.7	VR-2332	CH-1a	JXA1	NADC30	QYYZ	JA142
Sublineage 8.1	nt	100	82.5	62.3 ~ 69.7	76.6 ~ 88.5	85.9	98.8	89.0	65.2	81.9	92.6
	aa	100	78.0	55.3 ~ 63.7	73.1 ~ 84.3	81.7	98.4	85.1	59.7	76.2	89.0
Lineage 3	nt		100	61.9 ~ 67.1	77.3 ~ 88.4	76.1	82.6	88.5	63.9	74.7	79.6
	aa		100	55.9 ~ 62.0	73.8 ~ 84.7	70.6	77.8	85.7	58.7	70.5	74.3
Lineage 1	nt			72.5 ~ 99.6	**53.0**[a] ~ 73.5	63.4 ~ 68.3	62.2 ~ 69.7	63.5 ~ 73.4	76.5 ~ 93.9	56.1 ~ 62.5	62.2 ~ 67.7
	aa			66.0 ~ 99.5	**46.8**[a] ~ 69.3	56.8 ~ 62.9	55.3 ~ 63.7	57.3 ~ 69.3	72.0 ~ 92.0	49.1 ~ 55.6	55.9 ~ 61.7
Sublineage 8.7	nt				77.8 ~ **99.8**[b]	69.1 ~ 80.3	76.5 ~ 88.5	85.5 ~ 98.8	54.9 ~ 65.8	65.1 ~ 77.0	73.0 ~ 84.9
	aa				74.7 ~ **99.7**[b]	63.4 ~ 74.3	72.6 ~ 84.2	84.3 ~ 97.9	50.1 ~ 60.8	59.6 ~ 71.6	68.3 ~ 80.1
All strain	nt					63.4 ~ 85.9	62.2 ~ 98.8	63.5 ~ 98.8	54.9 ~ 93.9	56.1 ~ 81.9	62.2 ~ 92.6
	aa					56.8 ~ 81.7	55.3 ~ 98.4	57.3 ~ 97.9	50.1 ~ 92.0	49.1 ~ 76.2	55.9 ~ 89.0

Mark a at the top right for the lowest value, Mark b at the top right for the highest value.

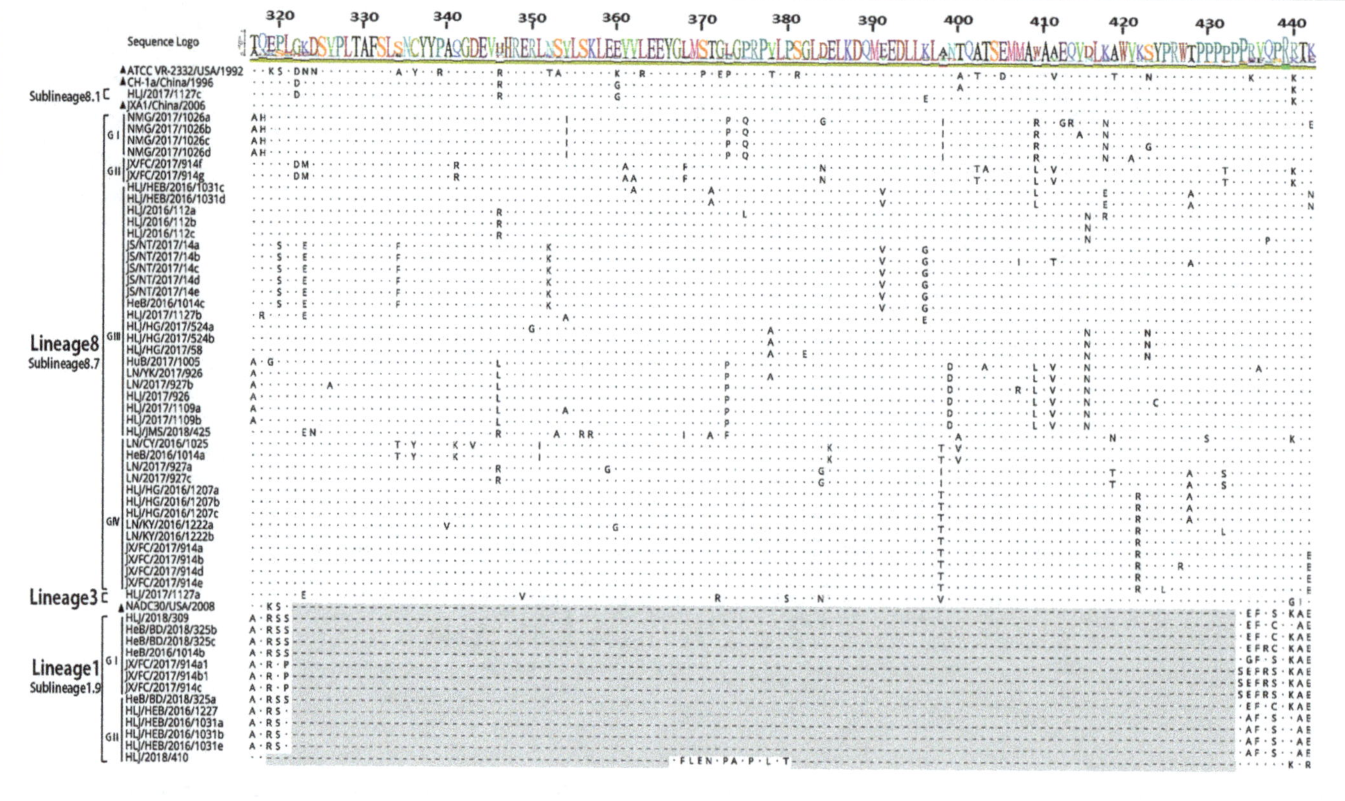

FIGURE 3 | Amino acid sequence alignment of Nsp2 protein.

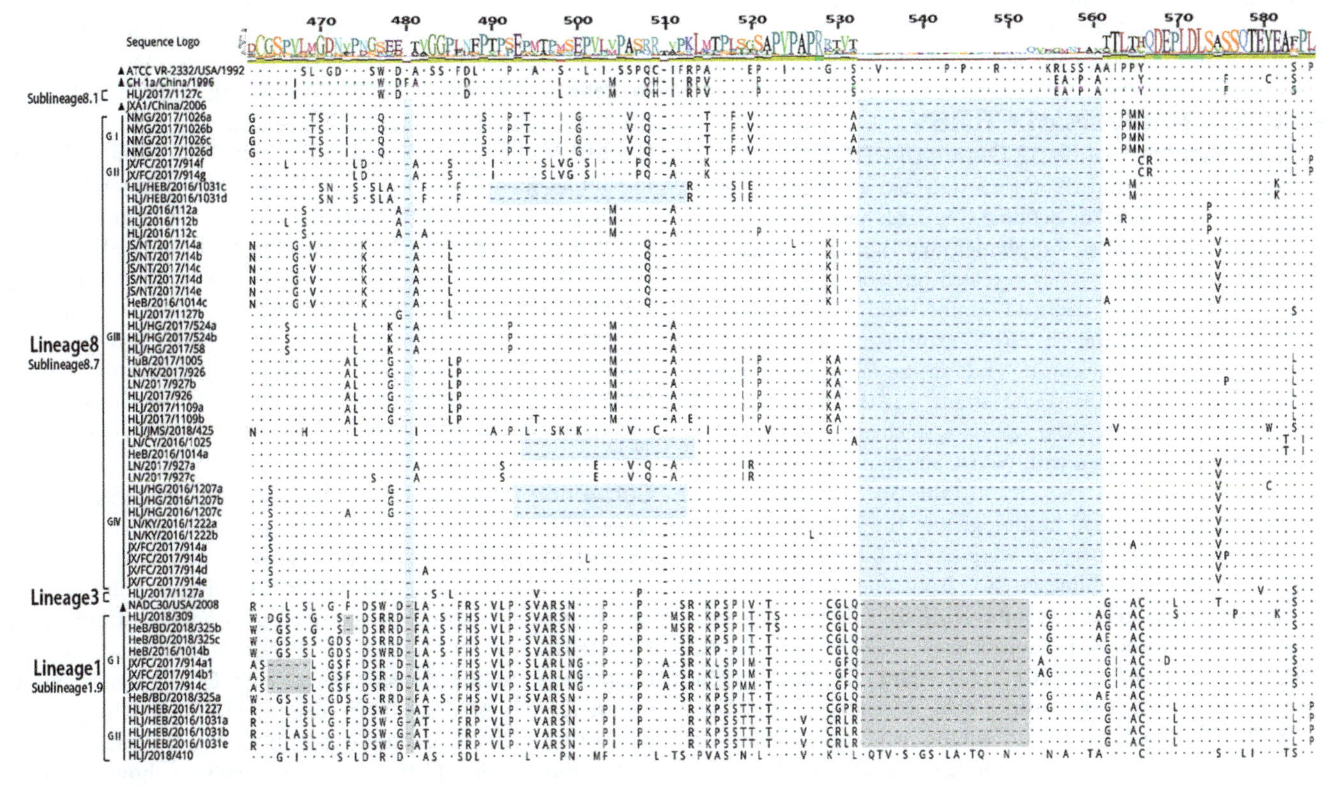

FIGURE 4 | Amino acid sequence alignment of Nsp2 protein.

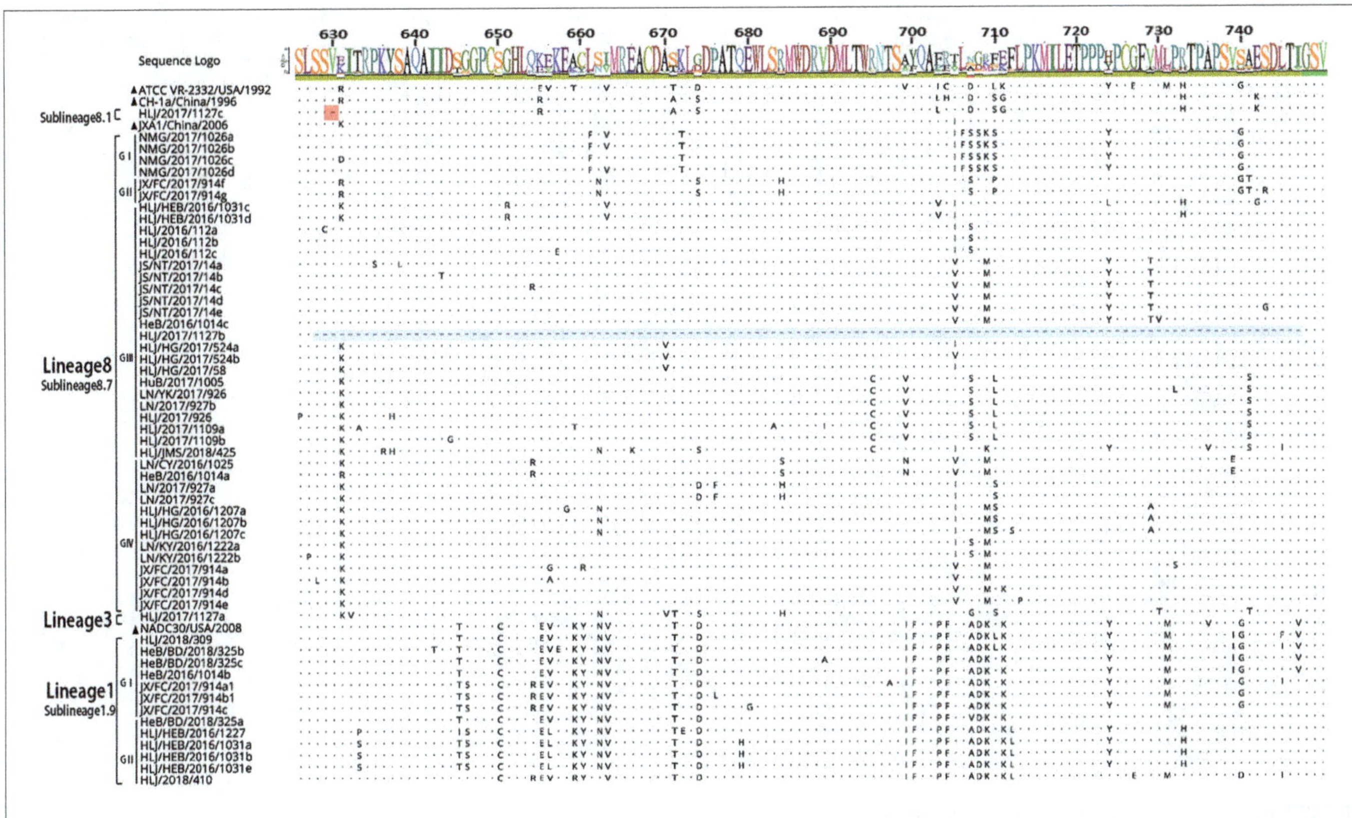

FIGURE 5 | Amino acid sequence alignment of Nsp2 protein.

the phylogenetic tree constructed with the ORF5 gene. With the rapid growth of sequence deposition into the databases, it would be complicated for the diversity of PRRSV sequences.

Sequence Analysis of PRRSV

Sequence Analysis of Nsp2 Genes of PRRSV

The 56 Nsp2 genes and 39 ORF5 (ORF5a) of PRRSV were successfully sequenced. The detailed GenBank number of the 56 PRRSV strains is shown in **Supplementary Table 2**. A sequence comparison of the Nsp2 genes revealed nucleotide homologies of 53.0 ~ 99.8% and deduced amino acid homologies of 46.8 ~ 99.7% among the 56 PRRSV strains. Along with the reference strain, its nucleotide and amino acid homologies compared with HP-PRRSV JXA1 strain was the highest (63.5 ~ 98.8% and 57.3 ~ 97.9%), and its nucleotide and amino acid homologies compared with NADC30 strain was the lowest (54.9 ~ 93.9% and 50.1 ~ 92.0%) (**Table 3**). In addition, the nucleotide and amino acid homologies of the identified strain in sublineage 8.1 and lineage 3 were higher than that of some identified strains in sublineage 8.7 from the same lineage. For example, HLJ/2017/1127c and HLJ/2017/1127b exhibited nucleotide and amino acid homologies of 76.6 and 73.1%, respectively. However, HLJ/2017/1127c and HLJ/2017/1127a exhibited nucleotide and amino acid homologies of 82.5 and 78.0%. The nucleotide and amino acid homologies of HLJ/2017/1127a and the representative strain QYYZ of lineage 3 was lower than the representative strain JXA1 of the 8.7 sublineage. This further suggests HLJ/2017/1127a is likely to be generated by recombinant strains in lineage 3 and sublineage 8.7. The classical PRRSV (type II) ATCC VR-2332 was used as the reference standard; the identified strain HLJ/2017/1127c had the same mutation pattern with vaccine strain CH-1R, which lacked a V at position 630 aa in the Nsp2. The identified strains of sublineage 8.7 and lineage 3 all showed a discontinuous 30-amino-acid deletion (positions 481 and 533–561) that conforms to the classical deletion mutation pattern of the HP-PRRSV-like strain. Excluding HLJ/2018/410, all strains identified in lineage 1 showed 131-amino-acid discontinuity deletion (positions 323–433, 481, and 533–551), that conforms to the classical deletion mutation pattern of the NADC30-like strain (**Figures 3–6**). The prevalent PRRSV strain in some regions of China was still HP-PRRSV, while NADC30 strain also occupied a certain proportion.

Sequence Analysis of ORF5 Genes of PRRSV

A sequence comparison of the ORF5 genes revealed nucleotide homologies of 82.4 ~ 100% and deduced amino acid homologies of 79.6 ~ 100% among the 39 PRRSV strains. The nucleotide and amino acid homologies compared with JXA1 strain was the highest (84.9 ~ 99.7%, 84.1 ~ 99.0%), and its nucleotide and amino acid homologies compared with QYYZ strain was the lowest (81.9 ~ 84.6%, 80.1 ~ 86.6%) (**Table 4**). The mutation sites of ORF5 were mainly concentrated in the signal peptide and epitopes region. GP5 virulence-related sites showed that nine of the 39 identified strains had mutated at the position 13th aa

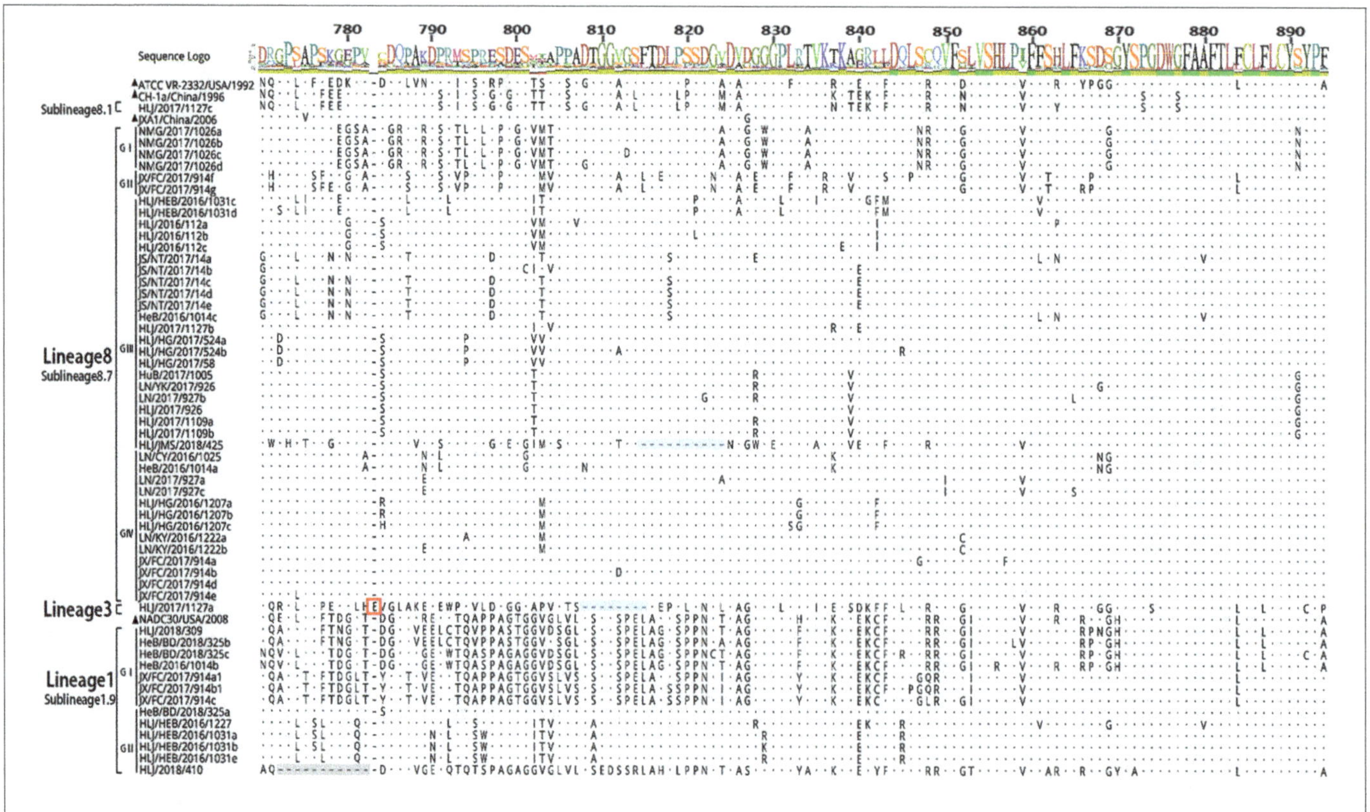

FIGURE 6 | Amino acid sequence alignment of Nsp2 protein.

(R→ Q). A total of 12 identified strains of sublineage 8.7 and lineage 1 had mutated at position 151 aa (R→ K), The 137th aa of all identified strains was conservative and was S (**Figure 7**). It is observed that all identified strains may be wild strains, and most identified strains may be highly virulent strains in the study.

Sequence Analysis of ORF5a Genes of PRRSV

A sequence analysis of the ORF5a genes among the 39 PRRSV strains exhibited nucleotide homologies of 84.0 ~ 100% and deduced amino acid homologies of 80.8 ~ 100%. The nucleotide and amino acid homologies compared with JXA1 strain was the highest (87.2 ~ 99.4%, 84.6 ~ 100%), and its nucleotide and amino acid homologies compared with QYYZ strain was the lowest (70.5 ~ 79.5%, 67.3 ~ 78.8%) (**Table 5**). All the ORF5a proteins of the identified strains encoded 46 aa, and HLJ/2017/1127c exhibited high sequence similarity compared with CH-1a strain, with only a few point mutations, such as $M^8 \rightarrow I^8$, $F^{20} \rightarrow L^{20}$, and $S^{42}/F^{42} \rightarrow I^{42}$; A part of identified strains had two amino acid mutations in the transmembrane region, $G^{12}/V^{12} \rightarrow A^{12}$, $R^{24} \rightarrow C^{24}$, and two amino acid mutations in the intramembrane region, $Q^{36} \rightarrow R^{36}$, $Q^{38} \rightarrow R^{38}/P^{38}$. Compared with NADC30, some of the strains identified had one amino acid mutation in the transmembrane region, $V^{26}/I^{26} \rightarrow T^{26}$, and one amino acid conformity mutation in the intramembrane region, $S^{42} \rightarrow I^{42}/L^{42}$ (**Figure 8**). This shows that the mutation sites of ORF5a were mainly concentrated in the transmembrane region and the intramembrane region.

Recombination Analysis

The recombination analysis of Nsp2 gene showed that there were five potential recombination events (**Table 6**). The recombination analysis of Nsp2 gene showed that the recombinant strains in event 1 and 2 were produced by recombination of lineage 1 and sublineage 8.7 (**Supplementary Figure 1**). The high frequency mutation and recombination make the virus gain more genetically diverse (19). This recombination pattern is the most common in PRRSV recombinant strains in China, and animal tests have confirmed that the virulence of some recombinant strains is higher than the prototype strain NADC30 (9). The identified strain HLJ/2017/1127a in recombinant event 3 was produced by recombination of lineage 3 and sublineage 8.7 wild strain. The main parental strain was FZ06A, while the minor parental strain was QYYZ. Previous studies have shown that the low virulence prototype strain QYYZ even became highly virulent after recombination with the vaccine strain derived from HP-PRRSV (20). The identified strain JS/NT/2017/14b in recombinant event four showed that the main parental strain HLJ/2017/1127b belongs to subline 8.7, while the minor parental strain JS/NT/2017/14a belongs to subline 8.7. Three recombinant strains in recombinant event five were from the same origin as JS/NT/2017/14b, but the recombinant sites are different. The recombination analysis of ORF5 genes showed that the recombinant event included four recombinant strains of lineage 1 (**Table 7**). The main parental strain CY1-1604 belongs to lineage 1, while the minor parental strain GS2008 belongs to sublineage 8.7 (**Supplementary Figure 2**). Combined with the recombination analysis of Nsp2 gene, the identified strain HLJ/HEB/2016/1031 (a, b) was also recombined in ORF5 gene, which indicated that there may be multiple recombination regions in identified strains, and the recombination pattern was more complex.

DISCUSSION

Since the outbreak of HP-PRRSV in 2006, PRRSV has been widely spread across the world. In previous studies, the positive rate of PRRSV was shown to be 55.21% (7,490/11,3567) in 29 provinces of China in 2012–2015 (21). In Central and Southern China, there was a positive rate of 50.62% (530/1,047) of PRRSV among 257 pig farms (22). In our study, the total positive rate of PRRSV was 50.89% (57/112) in nine provinces of China from 2016 to 2018, which was in accordance with the above scholars. PRRS is one of the most prevalent and threatening infectious diseases in Chinese pig farms.

Nsp2 and ORF5 (ORF5a) genes have the highest variability in PRRSV genome and are used as main target genes for PRRSV genetic variation. Phylogenetic tree analysis showed that all the 56 PRRSV strains identified in this study belong to the North American genotype and were distributed in lineage 1, 3, and 8 according to Shi et al. (18). In this study, the HP-PRRSV strain accounted for the highest proportion of epidemic strains in China; the NADC30-like strain had increased gradually, which was in accordance with the results of Gao et al. (23). However, some studies have shown that the NADC30-like strain in some regions of China have replaced the HP-PRRSV strain, and has become a new dominant strain (22). The rising infection rate of HP-PRRSV and NADC30-like strains may lead to a significant decrease in the effective protection rate of vaccines on pig farms.

The sequence alignments of Nsp2 gene revealed that the identified strain HLJ/2017/1127c in subline 8.1 had a high similarity with vaccine strain CH-1R, and existed a V deletion in the 630aa, suggesting that the identified strain may be a vaccine strain or a recombinant strain of a vaccine strain. Sequence alignments identified a discontinuous 30-amino-acid deletion (positions 481 and 533–561) and a 131-amino-acid discontinuity deletion (positions 323–433, 481, and 533–551) in Nsp2 of PPRSV isolates. JX/FC/2017/914(c, a1, b1) had the same deletion pattern as PRRSV strains HeN1401 and HeN1601, isolated by Zhang et al. (24). The recombinant analysis of the two epidemic strains revealed that HeN1401 and HeN1601 strains were generated by the recombinant weak vaccine strains TJbd14-1 and NADC30 (24). This further suggests that the identified strain JX/FC/2017/914(c, a1, b1) may also be a recombinant strain.

The GP5 protein sequences of different subline strains showed high similarity with the representative strains of the subline. The mutation sites of GP5 were mainly concentrated in the signal peptide and epitopes region. But some identified strains also have some amino acid consistent mutations in immune-related regions. Allende et al. found that nine amino acid site mutations may be closely related to the virulence of the PRRSV and that two sites (13 and 151 aa) were located in GP5 protein. The

TABLE 4 | Nucleotide and deduced amino acid homologies analysis based on ORF5 gene (%).

		Identified strain			Reference strain						
		Sublineage 8.1	**Sublineage 8.7**	**Lineage 1**	**VR-2332**	**CH-1a**	**JXA1**	**NADC30**	**QYYZ**	**JA142**
Sublineage 8.1	nt	100	90.9 ~ 94.0	84.9 ~ 91.0	91.0	98.7	94.4	87.1	84.4	93.4
	aa	100	87.1 ~ 89.6	81.1 ~ 88.6	89.1	97.5	90.5	85.1	81.6	94.0
Sublineage 8.7	nt		91.4 ~ **100**[b]	**82.4**[a] ~ 92.2	86.4 ~ 89.2	91.9 ~ 95.0	94.9 ~ 99.7	83.1 ~ 86.1	81.9 ~ 84.4	88.1 ~ 91.0
	aa		91.0 ~ **100**[b]	**79.6**[a] ~ 91.5	84.6 ~ 89.1	89.6 ~ 92.0	93.5 ~ 99.0	83.6 ~ 87.1	80.1 ~ 83.1	88.1 ~ 90.5
Lineage 1	nt			85.9 ~ **100**[b]	84.7 ~ 87.7	85.6 ~ 91.9	84.9 ~ 92.5	88.2 ~ 94.0	83.6 ~ 84.6	85.4 ~ 90.2
	aa			85.1 ~ **100**[b]	83.1 ~ 87.1	83.6 ~ 91.0	84.1 ~ 90.5	89.6 ~ 94.0	81.6 ~ 86.6	85.1 ~ 91.0
All strain	nt				84.7 ~ 91.0	85.6 ~ 98.7	84.9 ~ 99.7	83.1 ~ 94.0	81.9 ~ 84.6	85.4 ~ 93.4
	aa				83.1 ~ 89.1	83.6 ~ 97.5	84.1 ~ 99.0	83.6 ~ 94.0	80.1 ~ 86.6	85.1 ~ 94.0

Mark a at the top right for the lowest value, Mark b at the top right for the highest value.

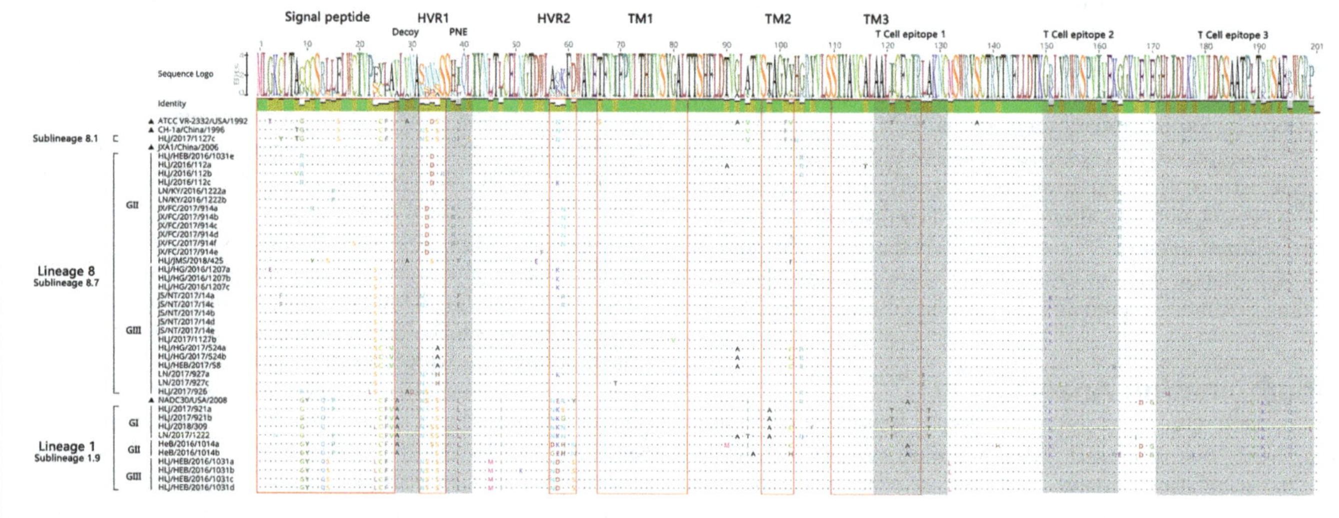

FIGURE 7 | Amino acid sequence alignment of GP5 protein.

TABLE 5 | Nucleotide and deduced amino acid homologies analysis based on ORF5a gene (%).

		Identified strain			Reference strain						
		Sublineage 8.1	**Sublineage 8.7**	**Lineage 1**	**VR-2332**	**CH-1a**	**JXA1**	**NADC30**	**QYYZ**	**JA142**
Sublineage 8.1	nt	100	87.8 ~ 90.4	87.2 ~ 90.4	80.1	97.4	91.0	88.5	74.4	83.3
	aa	100	82.7 ~ 88.5	84.6 ~ 86.5	75.0	94.2	88.5	84.6	69.2	80.8
Sublineage 8.7	nt		89.7 ~ **100**[b]	**84.0**[a] ~ 91.0	76.9 ~ 81.4	89.7 ~ 92.9	93.6 ~ 99.4	83.3 ~ 88.5	70.5 ~ 74.4	76.9 ~ 80.8
	aa		86.5 ~ **100**[b]	**80.8**[a] ~ 86.5	71.2 ~ 76.9	84.6 ~ 90.4	92.3 ~ 100	80.8 ~ 84.6	67.3 ~ 71.2	75.0 ~ 80.8
Lineage 1.9	nt			88.5 ~ **100**[b]	77.6 ~ 81.4	89.7 ~ 92.0	87.2 ~ 90.4	91.0 ~ 97.4	75.0 ~ 79.5	78.2 ~ 81.4
	aa			92.3 ~ **100**[b]	80.8 ~ 84.6	88.5 ~ 92.3	84.6 ~ 86.5	94.2 ~ 98.1	73.1 ~ 78.8	78.8 ~ 86.5
All strain	nt				76.9 ~ 81.4	89.7 ~ 97.4	87.2 ~ 99.4	83.3 ~ 97.4	70.5 ~ 79.5	76.9 ~ 83.3
	aa				71.2 ~ 84.6	84.6 ~ 94.2	84.6 ~ 100	80.8 ~ 98.1	67.3 ~ 78.8	75.0 ~ 86.5

Mark a at the top right for the lowest value, Mark b at the top right for the highest value.

GP5 protein of high virulence strains generally were shown as R^{13} and R^{151} (25). Wesley et al. showed that the 137aa of GP5 protein can distinguish the attenuated vaccine strain (A^{137}) and the wild strain (S^{137}) (26). Therefore, the above three amino acid sites are often used to predict the virulence of PRRSV strains. The sequence analysis of GP5 protein showed that only one mutation pattern ($R^{13} \rightarrow Q^{13}$ and $R^{151} \rightarrow K^{151}$) existed in this study. Nine identified strains had mutated at position 13 aa,

TABLE 6 | Recombination analysis of Nsp2 gene.

Recombination event	Recombinant strains	Main parental strain	Minor parental strain	Recombinant breakpoint	Recombination analysis method
1	HeB/2018/325a HLJ/2016/1031a HLJ/2016/1031b HLJ/2016/1031e HLJ/HEB/1227	HENZMD-9	10-10FUJ-2/China	18-2043 (18–1591)	RDP ($P = 1.22 \times 10^{-18}$) GENECONV ($P = 9.49 \times 10^{-28}$) BootScan ($P = 1.78 \times 10^{-28}$) MaxChi ($P = 4.14 \times 10^{-26}$) Chimaera ($P = 6.68 \times 10^{-8}$) SiScan ($P = 9.44 \times 10^{-27}$) 3seq ($P = 3.61 \times 10^{-8}$)
2	JX/2017/914c JX/2017/914a1 JX/2017/914b1	HENZMD-9	10-10FUJ-1/China	654–2600 (654–2015)	RDP ($P = 6.81 \times 10^{-40}$) GENECONV ($P = 3.43 \times 10^{-34}$) BootScan ($P = 6.79 \times 10^{-28}$) MaxChi ($P = 7.71 \times 10^{-20}$) Chimaera ($P = 4.31 \times 10^{-22}$) SiScan ($P = 2.28 \times 10^{-25}$) 3seq ($P = 2.27 \times 10^{-14}$)
3	HLJ/2017/1127a	FZ06A	QYYZ	1892–2730 (1742–2442)	RDP ($P = 2.08 \times 10^{-5}$) GENECONV (NS) BootScan ($P = 6.97 \times 10^{-5}$) MaxChi ($P = 6.41 \times 10^{-18}$) Chimaera ($P = 9.90 \times 10^{-16}$) SiScan ($P = 1.48 \times 10^{-8}$) 3seq ($P = 7.66 \times 10^{-15}$)
4	JS/NT/2017/14b	HLJ/2017/1127b	JS/NT/2017/14a	732–2227 (732–2077)	RDP ($P = 4.54 \times 10^{-7}$) GENECONV ($P = 4.83 \times 10^{-6}$) BootScan ($P = 7.00 \times 10^{-8}$) MaxChi ($P = 2.44 \times 10^{-11}$) Chimaera (NS) SiScan ($P = 7.43 \times 10^{-12}$) 3seq ($P = 3.88 \times 10^{-12}$)
5	JS/NT/2017/14d JS/NT/2017/14c JS/NT/2017/14e	HLJ/2017/1127b	JS/NT/2017/14a	561–2534 (561–2267)	RDP ($P = 1.75 \times 10^{-5}$) GENECONV ($P = 2.27 \times 10^{-4}$) BootScan($P = 1.16 \times 10^{-5}$) MaxChi ($P = 6.46 \times 10^{-8}$) Chimaera (NS) SiScan ($P = 7.01 \times 10^{-17}$) 3seq ($P = 8.06 \times 10^{-9}$)

NS, No significant P-value.

TABLE 7 | Recombination analysis of ORF5 gene.

Recombination event	Recombinant strains	Main parental strain	Minor parental strain	Recombinant breakpoint	Recombination analysis method
1	HLJ/HEB/2016/1031a HLJ/HEB/2016/1031b HLJ/HEB/2016/1031c HLJ/HEB/2016/1031d	CY1-1604	GS2008	249–580 (249–580)	RDP ($P = 1.92 \times 10^{-7}$) GENECONV ($P = 2.51 \times 10^{-6}$) BootScan ($P = 1.72 \times 10^{-6}$) MaxChi ($P = 2.60 \times 10^{-10}$) Chimaera ($P = 3.00 \times 10^{-9}$) SiScan ($P = 6.72 \times 10^{-12}$) 3seq ($P = 2.29 \times 10^{-12}$)

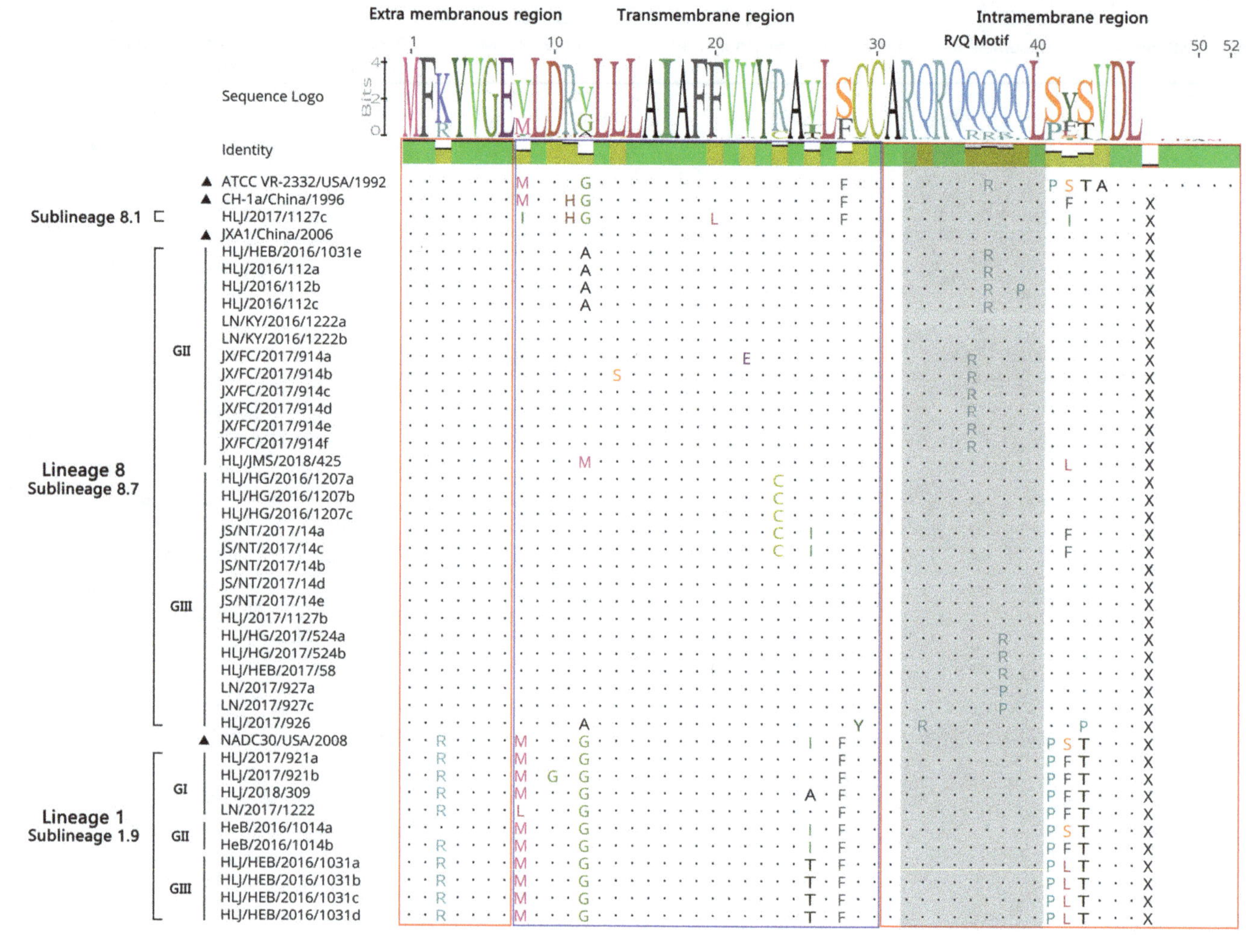

FIGURE 8 | Amino acid sequence alignment of GP5a protein.

and 12 identified strains mutated at position 151 aa. In addition, the 137 aa of all identified strains is S. The results suggest that all identified strains may be wild strains, and most identified strains may be highly virulent strains in nine provinces of China during 2016–2018.

Studies have shown that ORF5a protein is essential for viral viability and infectivity (27, 28). There is fairly limited information available on current genetic variations of PRRSV ORF5a gene (29). Therefore, this study explored the genetic variation of ORF5a gene of PRRSV epidemic strains in China by molecular biological methods. The ORF5a protein generally encoded 46–51 amino acids of which ORF5a protein of PRRSV strains encoded 46 amino acids in lineage 1 and 8, and 51 amino acids in lineage 3 and 5 (30). All the ORF5a proteins identified in this study encoded 46 amino acids. Compared with the reference strain, the identified strains also showed high sequence similarity, and the mutation sites of ORF5a were mainly concentrated in the transmembrane region and the intramembrane region, while the other region was highly conserved. Our study demonstrated the existence of multiple different strains in the same region and extensive genetic mutation of PRRSV in China from 2016 to 2018.

The recombination analysis indicated that there may be multiple recombination regions in identified strains, and the recombination pattern was more complex. At present, many studies have shown that PRRSV strain in lineage 1 is prone to recombinant mutation, and some of the recombinant strains are more virulent than others (10, 19). Although the recombination pattern of the virus identified in this study is in accordance with that reported by some previous scholars, the change of pathogenicity of PRRSV by gene recombination is not absolute. This study only carried out partial gene (Nsp2 and ORF5) recombination analysis without the virus isolation and whole genome sequences of PRRSV, so the recombination of whole genome sequences is more complicated and different.

CONCLUSION

This study showed that PRRSV infection was prevalent in nine provinces of China from 2016 to 2018, and thc prcvalcnt PRRSV strain in most regions was still HP-PRRSV, while the NADC30 strain also occupied a certain proportion. There was a discontinuous 30-amino-acid deletion (positions 481 and 533–561) and a 131-amino-acid discontinuity deletion (positions 323–433, 481, and 533–551) in Nsp2 of PPRSV isolates. All identified strains in this study may be wild strains, and most identified strains may be highly virulent strains. This study identified highly homologous HP-PRRSV variants with distinct genetic mutation, which contributes to further analyzing the epidemics and evolution of PRRSV in the field.

AUTHOR CONTRIBUTIONS

DS and GL conceived the study. BY, SQ, and JZ analyzed the data. BY and SQ wrote the manuscript for submission. WS, HQ, LL, and JY participated in the design of the study, performed the data collection and analysis, and commented on the manuscript. All authors approved the final manuscript.

REFERENCES

1. Baron T, Albina E, Leforban Y, Madec F, Guilmoto H, Plana Duran J, et al. Report on the first outbreaks of the porcine reproductive and respiratory syndrome (PRRS) in France. Diagnosis and viral isolation. *Ann Rech Vet.* (1992) 23:161–6.
2. Li Y, Treffers EE, Napthine S, Tas A, Zhu L, Sun Z, et al. Transactivation of programmed ribosomal frameshifting by a viral protein. *Proc Natl Acad Sci USA.* (2014) 111:E2172–81. doi: 10.1073/pnas.1321930111
3. Fang Y, Treffers EE, Li Y, Tas A, Sun Z, van der Meer Y, et al. Efficient−2 frameshifting by mammalian ribosomes to synthesize an additional arterivirus protein. *Proc Natl Acad Sci USA.* (2012) 109:E2920–8. doi: 10.1073/pnas.1211145109
4. Lunney JK, Fang Y, Ladinig A, Chen N, Li Y, Rowland B, et al. Porcine Reproductive and Respiratory Syndrome Virus (PRRSV): pathogenesis and interaction with the immune system. *Annu Rev Anim Biosci.* (2016) 4:129–54. doi: 10.1146/annurev-animal-022114-111025
5. Keffaber KK. Reproductive failure of unknown etiology. *Am Assoc Swine Pract Newsl.* (1989) 2:1–9.
6. Neumann EJ, Kliebenstein JB, Johnson CD, Mabry JW, Bush EJ, Seitzinger AH, et al. Assessment of the economic impact of porcine reproductive and respiratory syndrome on swine production in the United States. *J Am Vet Med Assoc.* (2005) 227:385–92. doi: 10.2460/javma.2005.227.385
7. Kuwahara H, Nunoya T, Tajima M, Kato A, Samejima T. An outbreak of porcine reproductive and respiratory syndrome in Japan. *J Vet Med Sci.* (1994) 56:901–9. doi: 10.1292/jvms.56.901
8. Chen N, Ye M, Huang Y, Li S, Xiao YZ, Li XS, et al. Identification of two porcine reproductive and respiratory syndrome virus variants sharing high genomic homology but with distinct virulence. *Viruses.* (2019) 11:875. doi: 10.3390/v11090875
9. Zhao K, Ye C, Chang XB, Jiang CG, Wang SJ, Cai XH, et al. Importation and recombination are responsible for the latest emergence of highly pathogenic porcine reproductive and respiratory syndrome virus in China. *J Virol.* (2015) 89:10712–6. doi: 10.1128/JVI.01446-15
10. Zhou L, Wang Z, Ding Y, Ge X, Guo X, Yang H. NADC30-like strain of porcine reproductive and respiratory syndrome virus, China. *Emerg Infect Dis.* (2015) 21:2256–7. doi: 10.3201/eid2112.150360
11. Lu WH, Tun HM, Sun BL, Mo J, Zhou QF, Deng YX, et al. Re-emerging of porcine respiratory and reproductive syndrome virus (lineage 3) and increased pathogenicity after genomic recombination with vaccine variant. *Vet Microbiol.* (2015) 175:332–40. doi: 10.1016/j.vetmic.2014.11.016
12. Lu WH, Wei ZY, Zhang GQ, Li ZL, Ma JY, Xie QM, et al. Complete genome sequence of a novel variant porcine reproductive and respiratory syndrome virus (PRRSV) strain: evidence for recombination between vaccine and wild-type PRRSV strains. *J Virol.* (2012) 86:9543. doi: 10.1128/JVI.01341-12
13. Wang PP, Dong JG, Zhang LY, Liang PS, Liu YL, Wang L, et al. Sequence and phylogenetic analyses of the Nsp2 and ORF5 genes of porcine reproductive and respiratory syndrome virus in Boars from South China in 2015. *Transbound Emerg Dis.* (2017) 64:1953–64. doi: 10.1111/tbed.12594
14. Nilubol D, Tripipat T, Hoonsuwan T, Tipsombatboon P, Piriyapongsa J. Genetic diversity of the ORF5 gene of porcine reproductive and respiratory syndrome virus (PRRSV) genotypes I and II in Thailand. *Arch Virol.* (2013) 158:943–53. doi: 10.1007/s00705-012-1573-7
15. Cao ZX, Jiao PR, Huang YM, Qin HY, Kong LW, Pan QH, et al. Genetic diversity analysis of the ORF5 gene in porcine reproductive and respiratory syndrome virus samples from South China. *Acta Vet Hung.* (2012) 60:157–64. doi: 10.1556/avet.2012.013
16. Tamura K, Stecher G, Peterson D, Filipski A, Kumar S. MEGA6: molecular evolutionary genetics analysis version 6.0. *Mol Biol Evol.* (2013) 30:2725–9. doi: 10.1093/molbev/mst197
17. Letunic I, Bork P. Interactive Tree Of Life (iTOL): an online tool for phylogenetic tree display and annotation. *Bioinformatics.* (2007) 23:127–8. doi: 10.1093/bioinformatics/btl529
18. Shi M, Lam TT, Hon CC, Murtaugh MP, Davies PR, Hui RK, et al. Phylogeny-based evolutionary, demographical, and geographical dissection of North American type 2 porcine reproductive and respiratory syndrome viruses. *J Virol.* (2010) 84:8700–11. doi: 10.1128/JVI.02551-09
19. Murtaugh MP, Stadejek T, Abrahante JE, Tommy TL, Frederick CL. The ever-expanding diversity of porcine reproductive and respiratory syndrome virus. *Virus Research.* (2010) 154:18–30. doi: 10.1016/j.virusres.2010.08.015
20. Dong J, Wang Y, Yu L, Zhang P, Liu X, Zhang L, et al. Pathogenicity of a newly emerged recombined porcine reproductive and respiratory syndrome virus strain (subgenotype III) in China. *Vet Microbiol.* (2017) 210:162–6. doi: 10.1016/j.vetmic.2017.09.018
21. Peng Z, Zhao T, Liang W, Song W, Gao Z, Tang X, et al. RT-PCR detection of porcine reproductive and respiratory syndrome virus based on the ORF5 gene in mainland China, 2012–2015. *Acta Virol.* (2017) 61:336–40. doi: 10.4149/av_2017_312
22. Liang W, Zhao T, Peng Z, Sun Y, Stratton CW, Zhou D, et al. Epidemiological and genetic characteristics of porcine reproductive and respiratory syndrome virus circulating in central and South China in 2016. *Acta Trop.* (2019) 190:83–91. doi: 10.1016/j.actatropica.2018.11.004
23. Gao JC, Xiong JY, Ye C, Chang XB, Guo JC, Jiang CG, et al. Genotypic and geographical distribution of porcine reproductive and respiratory syndrome viruses in mainland China in 1996–2016. *Vet Microbiol.* (2017) 208:164–72. doi: 10.1016/j.vetmic.2017.08.003
24. Zhang Z, Zhou L, Ge X, Guo X, Han J, Yang H. Evolutionary analysis of six isolates of porcine reproductive and respiratory syndrome virus from a single pig farm: MLV-evolved and recombinant viruses. *Infect Genet Evol.* (2018) 66:111–9. doi: 10.1016/j.meegid.2018.09.024
25. Allende R, Kutish GF, Laegreid W, Lu Z, Lewis TL, Rock DL, et al. Mutations in the genome of porcine reproductive and respiratory syndrome virus responsible for the attenuation phenotype. *Arch Virol.* (2000) 145:1149–61. doi: 10.1007/s007050070115
26. Wesley RD, Mengeling WL, Lager KM, Clouser DF, Landgraf JG, et al. Differentiation of a porcine reproductive and respiratory syndrome virus vaccine strain from North American field strains by restriction fragment length polymorphism analysis of ORF5. *J Vet Diagn Invest.* (1998) 10:140–4. doi: 10.1177/104063879801000204
27. van Dinten LC, den Boon JA, Wassenaar AL, Spaan WJ, Snijder EJ. An infectious arterivirus cDNA clone: identification of a replicase point mutation

that abolishes discontinuous mRNA transcription. *Proc Natl Acad Sci USA.* (1997) 94:991–6. doi: 10.1073/pnas.94.3.991

28. Firth AE, Brown CM. Detecting overlapping coding sequences in virus genomes. *BMC Bioinformatics.* (2006) 7:75. doi: 10.1186/1471-2105-7-75
29. Firth AE, Zevenhoven-Dobbe JC, Wills NM, Go YY, Balasuriya UB, Atkins JF, et al. Discovery of a small arterivirus gene that overlaps the GP5 coding sequence and is important for virus production. *J Gen Virol.* (2011) 92:1097–106. doi: 10.1099/vir.0.029264-0
30. Zhang Q, Bai J, Hou H, Song Z, Zhao Y, Jiang P. A novel recombinant porcine reproductive and respiratory syndrome virus with significant variation in cell adaption and pathogenicity. *Vet Microbiol.* (2017) 208:150–8. doi: 10.1016/j.vetmic.2017.07.028

22

Socially vs. Privately Optimal Control of Livestock Diseases: A Case for Integration of Epidemiology and Economics

Ângelo J. Mendes[1], Daniel T. Haydon[1], Emma McIntosh[2], Nick Hanley[1] and Jo E. B. Halliday[1]*

[1] *College of Medical, Veterinary and Life Sciences, Institute of Biodiversity, Animal Health and Comparative Medicine, University of Glasgow, Glasgow, United Kingdom,* [2] *College of Medical, Veterinary and Life Sciences, Institute of Health and Wellbeing, University of Glasgow, Glasgow, United Kingdom*

***Correspondence:**
Ângelo J. Mendes
a.mendes.1@research.gla.ac.uk

This paper aims to illustrate the interdependencies between key epidemiological and economic factors that influence the control of many livestock infectious diseases. The factors considered here are (i) farmer heterogeneity (i.e., differences in how farmers respond to a perceived disease risk), (ii) off-farm effects of farmers' actions to control a disease (i.e., costs and benefits borne by agents that are external to the farm), and (iii) misalignment between privately and socially optimal control efforts (i.e., privately optimal behavior not conducive to a socially optimal outcome). Endemic chronic diseases cause a wide range of adverse social and economic impacts, particularly in low-income countries. The actions taken by farmers to control livestock diseases minimize some of these impacts, and heterogeneity in those actions leads to variation in prevalence at the farm level. While some farmers respond to perceived disease risks, others free-ride on the actions of these individuals, thereby compromising the potential benefits of collective, coordinated behavior. When evaluating a plausible range of disease cost to price of control ratios and assuming that farmers choose their privately optimal control effort, we demonstrate that achievement of a socially optimal disease control target is unlikely, occurring in <25% of all price-cost combinations. To achieve a socially optimal disease control outcome (reliant on farmers' voluntary actions), control policies must consider farmer heterogeneity, off-farm effects, and the predicted uptake of control measures under the assumption of optimized behavior.

Keywords: livestock, infection, disease control, model, epidemiology, economics

INTRODUCTION

Livestock production is vital to economic development in many low-income countries, contributing to poverty alleviation, investment in children's education, and food security (1, 2). Infectious diseases jeopardize these societal functions, yet their control has become increasingly reliant upon privately funded actions (3–8). This "voluntary approach" to disease control distributes costs and responsibility between private agents (farmers that invest in control measures) and the government (animal health authorities that promote and often regulate farmers' actions) (9). The problem of the voluntary approach is that self-interested behavior can fail to produce a socially optimal level of disease control (i.e., the level of disease control that maximizes the sum of all agents' payoffs in society, the social optimum) (8, 10). The market thus "fails" to achieve the social optimum.

One reason for such "market failure" in disease control is the presence of externalities: costs and benefits borne by agents who are not parties to a market transaction (8). Externalities can be positive (e.g., a farmer enjoys a lower risk of disease incursion into his herd when neighboring farmers vaccinate their animals) or negative (e.g., a farmer has a higher risk of disease incursion into his herd when other farmers sell sick animals into a livestock market). One farmer's investment in animal health can thus influence other farmers' levels of disease risk. The way individual farmers perceive and act upon their level of risk may fail to produce a social optimum: some farmers free-ride on the control efforts of others, and the potential benefits of one farmer's actions can be limited by others' inaction (9, 11). Achieving the socially optimal level of disease control often requires governments to intervene (e.g., through financial incentives and regulation) in a way that accounts for the nature of farmers' decision-making processes and the interdependencies between farmers' choices and disease dynamics (3, 8, 9, 12–19).

The way farmers perceive and respond to disease risks is not only affected by disease spread but also impacts upon it. There are feedback processes between how a disease spreads and the responses of farmers to changing risks (20–22). When the inter-dependent dynamics of economic, behavioral, and epidemiological factors are not understood or well-represented in models of disease transmission, then policies aimed at promoting farmers' action may have perverse effects (23–26).

Our objective in this paper is to illustrate interdependencies between key epidemiological and economic factors that are not consistently taken into account in models of livestock diseases: (i) farmer heterogeneity (i.e., differences between farmers in how they respond to perceived risks); (ii) associated externalities; and (iii) misalignment between privately and socially optimal control efforts. We demonstrate the impact of farmer heterogeneity on disease prevalence over time. We quantify the externalities associated with farmer heterogeneity and show how the outcome of any individual farmer's control effort depends on the behavior of others. Finally, we examine a farmer's decision in trading-off *ex ante* disease prevention expenditure and *ex post* treatment expenditure and output loss, to estimate the probability that adoption of privately optimal behavior will achieve a socially optimal disease control target. The consequences of a socially sub-optimal control level depend on, among other factors, the population at risk. Here, for simplicity and to illustrate the general case, groups of farmers represent society.

METHODS

We explore the relationships between epidemiological and economic factors using a deterministic compartmental model (27). The model assumes a chronic infectious disease of livestock with a low basic reproduction number ($R_0 = 1.11$), a livestock species with an average lifespan of five time units, and a constant herd size over time (250 animals on farm). We apply the model in three scenarios that explore farmer heterogeneity, quantify externalities, and examine differences between privately and socially optimal control efforts. In all scenarios, the animal-level prevalence in each farm starts at 10% (the endemic equilibrium, i.e., when prevalence remains steady and the effective reproductive number, R_e, is 1.00). We simulate the time required to achieve a prevalence of <2% following a hypothetical awareness-raising event (e.g., information provision at time zero) and a time horizon of 25 time units. This target prevalence of <2% represents an economic optimum from society's perspective (i.e., the socially optimal level of disease control). A 2% threshold can also be considered a prevalence level below which costly government-led strategies aimed at eliminating the disease (e.g., test-and-slaughter) are required (28). In our simulations, for simplicity and without loss of generality, we assume infected animals show chronic symptoms and lose productivity, but there is no disease-associated mortality or infertility. Individuals can be either susceptible or infected; once infected, they remain infected and infectious for the remainder of their lives. Complete recovery from the disease is not possible.

The model set-up is as simple as possible for demonstration purposes. The basic features are (i) two states (susceptible—S; and infected—I), (ii) continuous time steps, (iii) equal birth and death rates ($\alpha = \mu = 0.20$), and (iv) an initial transmission rate (β) of approximately 8.89×10^{-4}, reflecting the endemic equilibrium. The model can be run with one or more farms, and disease transmission can occur within farm only or both within and between farms. The proportion of the initial overall β attributable to between-farm transmission (q) is 0.0 when there is no transmission between farms, and 0.1 when between-farm transmission is included. The amount of control effort applied on farm is represented by a proportionate reducer on β (r_i^{β}). The model's differential equations are as follows:

$$\frac{dS_i}{dt} = \alpha\,(S_i + I_i) - (1 - q)\left(1 - r_i^{\beta}\right)\beta S_i I_i - q\beta S_i \sum_{\substack{j=1 \\ j \neq i}}^{n} I_j - \mu S_i \quad (1)$$

$$\frac{dI_i}{dt} = (1 - q)\left(1 - r_i^{\beta}\right)\beta S_i I_i + q\beta S_i \sum_{\substack{j=1 \\ j \neq i}}^{n} I_j - \mu I_i \quad (2)$$

The differential equations were solved in *R* (29) (version 3.6.2) with the package *deSolve* (30) (version 1.27.1). All plots were generated using the *ggplot2* package (version 3.3.0) (31).

We demonstrate the effect of farmer heterogeneity on the predicted prevalence of disease over time by simulating transmission-reducing measures in three farms following a hypothetical awareness-raising event. As farmers continually assess the benefits and costs of their actions over time, the amount of control effort in each farm is set to be a function of disease prevalence (p_i). We assume that (i) disease transmission occurs within each farm only, and (ii) as the prevalence (and disease impact) at the farm declines, the control effort applied (r_i^{β}) also falls (32), as follows:

$$r_i^{\beta} = \frac{1}{1 + e^{-100(p_i - \gamma_i)}} \quad (3)$$

where γ_i represents the farmer responsiveness. γ was set at 0.025, 0.100, and 0.175 for the farmer that is "highly responsive," "moderately responsive," and "slightly responsive," respectively. Note that, as the prevalence decreases in any farm due to the control effort applied, the farmer responsiveness does not change—it is a characteristic of each individual farmer.

We then estimate the off-farm effects (externalities) of livestock disease control in two of the above farms: one in which the farmer is highly responsive and the other in which the farmer is slightly responsive. Firstly, we quantify the *ex post* cost of disease over time at the farm level by assigning a monetary value (δ) to the cost of each infected animal per time step. We assume that the *ex post* cost of the disease varies linearly with prevalence (i.e., the cost per time step is the product of the number of infected animals and the cost per infected animal). We then compare the *ex post* cost of disease over time in each farm when the transmission rate between farms (bβ) is 0% (q is 0.0) and 10% (q is 0.1) of the initial within-farm transmission rate (wβ). Actions taken by each farmer to reduce transmission in their farms only reduce the wβ and do not influence bβ, which is kept constant over time. By holding the bβ constant over time and at a common value for the two farms, we demonstrate the off-farm effects of on-farm actions only—this assumes that (i) the contact rate between farms is kept constant, and (ii) the force of infection is proportional to the number of infected animals on each farm. Variation in farm number and density is unlikely to affect the qualitative inferences from this simulation.

We define "cost of disease" as the sum of disease-related output loss (production potential that is not realized over time) and expenditure on treatment of infected animals, plus the cost of control. Treating infected animals does not affect their infectiousness. Cost of control refers to money spent on reducing the wβ to prevent new cases, for instance, through improvements in hygiene and biosecurity. The cost of disease can thus be split into *ex ante* cost (cost of control) and *ex post* cost (disease-related output loss and treatment-related expenditure).

We demonstrate the market failure in livestock disease control by comparing the private net profit of farmer i (Π_i) with the social net profit (Π_s), the sum of the private net profits of n farmers ($\Pi_s = \sum_{i=1}^{n} \Pi_i$). Π_i denotes the private net profit of farmer i for the whole simulation period of 25 time units ($\Pi_i = \sum_{t=1}^{25} \Pi_{it}$). The example has only two farmers for simplicity, so $\Pi_s = \Pi_R + \Pi_r$; the social net profit is the net profit of the highly responsive farmer (R) plus the net profit of the slightly responsive farmer (r). Considering that the benefit (b_i, the number of animal infections averted) enjoyed by the highly responsive farmer as a result of disease control effort is a function of control effort applied in their farm (r_R^{β}) as well as in the other farm (r_r^{β}) (i.e., $b_R = f\left(r_R^{\beta}, r_r^{\beta}\right)$), the net profit Π_{Rt} (in time step t) is given by $\delta b_R - \theta r_R^{\beta}$, where δ is the *ex post* cost per infected animal (treatment expenditure and output loss), and θ is the unit price of control action (the price of reducing the transmission rate by 1%). For this simulation, we assume that δ and θ are fixed at 50 and 0.10 monetary units, respectively.

We examine the effect of optimizing behavior on disease prevalence by assuming that the farmer reduces the wβ so that the total cost of the disease (the sum of *ex ante* and *ex post* costs) at each time step is minimized (32). This process is repeated iteratively for each level of the unit price of control (θ, ranging from 0.00 to 1.25 monetary units per time step) and *ex post* cost per infected animal (δ, ranging from 10 to 85 monetary units per time step). We assume (conservatively) that (i) the farmer has perfect information of both the *ex ante* and *ex post* costs of disease, and (ii) their behavior is no longer determined by a pre-specified logistic function. Instead, at each time step, the farmer reviews and optimizes their control effort given the prevalence. The short planning horizon (one time step, equivalent to one-fifth of the animals' average lifespan) reflects the generally high time-preference rates in low-income countries (33).

The qualitative inferences drawn from the model outputs are observed under a range of alternative scenarios and assumed parameter values. Readers can explore different scenarios and assumptions in the interactive web application, which is available here: http://boydorr.gla.ac.uk/eemodel/epiecon. This application was developed with *shiny* (34) (version 1.4.0) and *shinydashboard* (35) (version 0.7.1) packages in R (29). The R script for all the simulations is available at: https://doi.org/10.5281/zenodo.4108335.

RESULTS

The Impact of Farmer Heterogeneity

The prevalence of the disease is estimated over time within three model farms managed by three different "types" of farmers who vary in their responsiveness to an awareness-raising event. The responsiveness level of each farmer type is given by a behavioral parameter (γ_i). The model uses this parameter in a logistic function that determines the reduction in transmission rate caused by each farmer's different actions at any given level of prevalence (**Figure 1A**). For instance, at the initial prevalence of 10%, (i) the highly responsive farmer reduces transmission by 100% (red solid line), (ii) the moderately responsive farmer reduces transmission by 50% (green dotted line), and (iii) the slightly responsive farmer does not reduce transmission at all (blue dashed line). The impacts of these three levels of responsiveness on disease prevalence over time are shown in **Figure 1B**. The heterogeneity in farmer responsiveness has an impact on the level of control effort applied and thus on the reduction in prevalence achieved. Among the three farmer types, only the highly responsive type achieves the target prevalence (i.e., <2%) within 25 time units.

Externalities: The Off-Farm Effects of Farmers' Control Actions

Now we model disease prevalence in two neighboring farms (managed by highly and slightly responsive farmers, respectively), allowing for between-farm transmission, to explore the off-farm effects of farmers' control actions upon within-farm and societal costs of disease, represented by the sum of costs over the two neighboring farms.

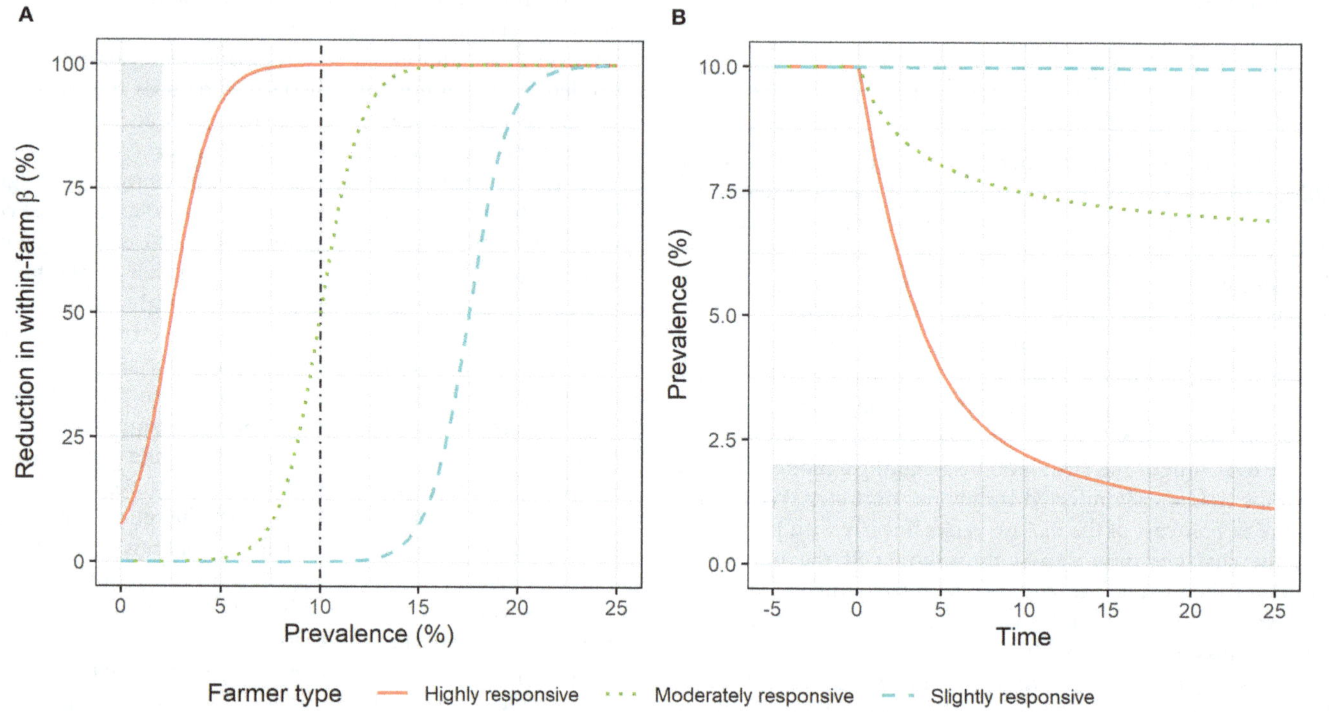

FIGURE 1 | Effect of farmer type on disease prevalence following a common starting prevalence and a hypothetical awareness-raising event (at time zero). **(A)** Control effort applied (percentage reduction in transmission rate—β—within the farm in relation to the initial β in endemic equilibrium) as a function of disease prevalence for three different farmer types. The vertical dash-dotted line indicates initial prevalence. **(B)** Disease prevalence over time within the three farms. In both panels, the gray shaded area indicates the target prevalence level from society's perspective (<2%).

For each farm, we estimate the *ex post* cost of disease over time following an awareness-raising event. **Figure 2** shows the estimated *ex post* cost in two farms with and without between-farm transmission. With no off-farm effects (i.e., $b\beta = 0$, and thus no effects of neighbor's actions on costs), a highly responsive farmer (solid red line) reduces prevalence and *ex post* cost. In contrast, for a slightly responsive farmer (dotted blue line), the prevalence and the *ex post* cost are unchanged over time. When the off-farm effects or externalities are included (i.e., $b\beta > 0$, transmission between farms is possible), the highly responsive farmer sees a reduced benefit of their actions, and the slightly responsive farmer benefits from their neighbor's actions (compared to the equivalent costs when $b\beta = 0$). The extent by which the first farmer (highly responsive) reduces the prevalence of disease (and its associated cost) is limited by the force of infection originating from the second farm, where the farmer is only slightly responsive. Also, despite the lack of control action, the prevalence and *ex post* cost of disease at the second farm drops over time as a result of a decreasing force of infection originating from the first farm, where the prevalence is decreasing due to the control measures applied. Using a discount rate of 5%[1], the extent of market failure[2] is the difference between the Π^s (849 monetary units) and Π^R (695 monetary units). This difference is due to the benefits enjoyed by the slightly responsive farmer, who does not incur any costs of control.

Privately Optimal Behavior and Reductions in Prevalence

Here we model disease prevalence (with a single farm and $b\beta = 0$) to establish if privately optimal actions of a farmer will achieve the socially optimal target prevalence (i.e., <2%). The prevalence over time assuming privately optimal behavior for different unit prices of control (from "free" to "high") is shown in **Figure 3**. Following an awareness-raising event (at time zero) and assuming a fixed *ex post* cost per infected animal ($\delta = 50$ monetary units), the extent by which the within-farm prevalence is reduced varies inversely with the unit price of control (θ). Achieving the socially optimal target prevalence is possible if the unit price of control is very low. Disease elimination (prevalence below 0.4% or <1 infected animal in a herd of 250; note that the predicted prevalence is strictly continuous) only occurs when the unit price of control is equal or <0.05 monetary units (first line above "free" in **Figure 3**). When the unit price of control is above 0.05 monetary units, the farmer's optimal control effort either reduces the prevalence until it reaches a new endemic equilibrium or does not reduce it at all (shown as the uppermost flat line in **Figure 3**; the prevalence remains at the initial endemic equilibrium level). This model of optimizing behavior shows that self-interested farmers, who optimize their

[1]The discount rate accounts for the decreasing value of benefits and costs over time in "real terms," as viewed from the present.

[2]More details available here: http://boydorr.gla.ac.uk/eemodel/epiecon.

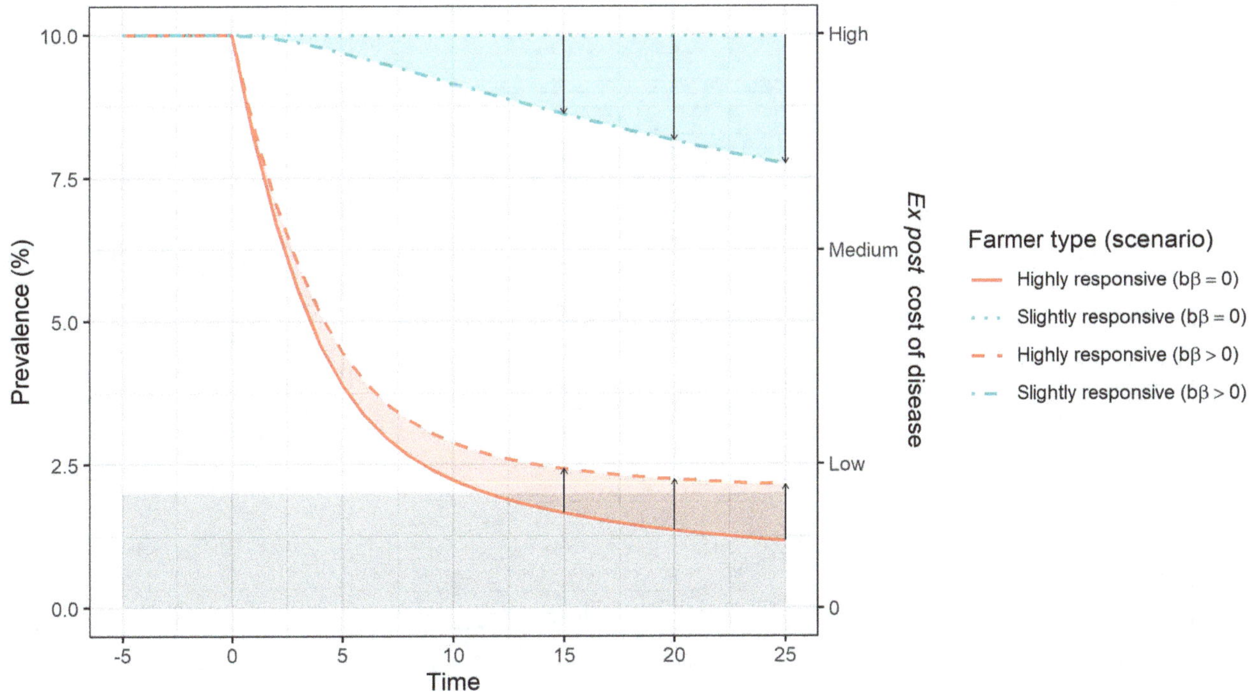

FIGURE 2 | Externalities occurring as a result of different effort to achieve disease control in two neighboring farms. Arrows indicate a simulation scenario shift, from absence of transmission between farms ($b\beta = 0$) to a situation in which between-farm transmission is possible ($b\beta > 0$). Assuming an *ex post* cost per infected animal per time step (δ) of 50 monetary units, the labels "Low," "Medium," and "High" on the right vertical axis correspond to 313, 781, and 1,250 monetary units. Blue and red shaded areas correspond to the positive and negative externalities, respectively. The gray shaded area indicates the target prevalence level from society's perspective (<2%).

private investment in disease control, as assumed here, may not achieve the target prevalence from society's perspective in the absence of an intervention by, for example, the government.

In our simulations, under the assumption of optimizing farmer behavior, as prevalence drops, the marginal cost of control actions (i.e., the cost of reducing the prevalence by an additional unit, 1%), increases sharply. It is more expensive to reduce the prevalence from 3 to 2% than from 10 to 9% because the number of cases prevented per time step by reducing the transmission rate depends on the number of currently infected individuals. If the number of currently infected individuals is high (e.g., 10% prevalence), the prevention of new cases yields a quick reduction in prevalence. If the number of currently infected individuals is low (e.g., 3% prevalence), further reductions of the prevalence rely to a greater extent on the elimination of currently infected individuals. Under the assumption of optimizing behavior, as the marginal costs of control increase, the farmer's investment in control therefore gradually declines until an equilibrium is reached in both epidemiological and economic terms (shown as the plateau for each line in **Figure 3**). This equilibrium prevalence level is reached when the *ex ante* expenditure in one time step equals the averted *ex post* cost of disease.

The achievement of a socially optimal outcome prevalence depends on the specific values of the unit price of control and cost per infected animal selected. The results shown in **Figure 3** considered a fixed *ex post* cost of one infected animal (δ = 50 monetary units). However, for the same disease and animal species, this value could in practice vary with the price of livestock, cost of production inputs, type of production system, etc. **Figure 4** shows the predicted prevalence after 25 time units for a range of values of price per control unit and a range of values of *ex post* cost per infected animal. When we allow the cost per infected animal to vary in plausible ranges in relation to the price of control unit (e.g., eliminating disease transmission by 100% would cost a maximum of 125 monetary units per time step, which is <1.5 times the highest *ex post* cost of one infected animal, i.e., 85 monetary units), the previously observed pattern holds: farmers who optimize their control effort may not achieve the target prevalence from society's perspective.

DISCUSSION

Analytical frameworks introducing human behavioral dynamics in the field of livestock infectious disease modeling have emerged in the last two decades. From the pioneering works of Bicknell et al. (24) and McInerney et al. (32) to the most recent individual-based, network-based, and game-theoretic models (9, 36–38), many significant contributions have improved our understanding of the interplay between human behavior and livestock disease spread (and the likelihood of disease control). However, this study is unique and contributes to that body of knowledge for two reasons. Firstly, it provides a simple but robust

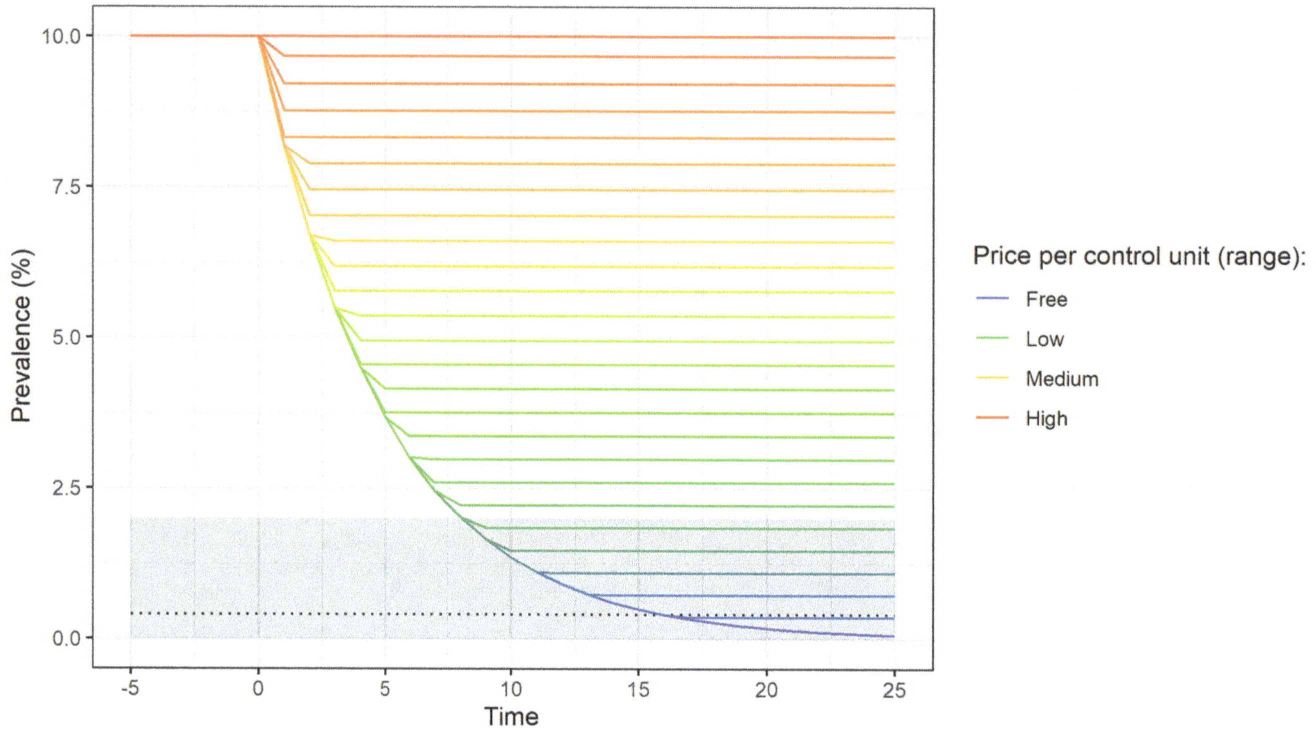

FIGURE 3 | Disease prevalence over time, assuming privately optimal behavior in a single farm for a range of prices per control unit. This simulation assumes a cost of one infected animal per time step (δ) of 50 monetary units. The price of reducing the transmission rate by 1% (θ) ranges from "Free" (0.00 monetary units) to "High" (1.25 monetary units). "Low" and "Medium" correspond to 0.40 and 0.85 monetary units, respectively. Colored lines represent increases by 0.05 monetary units. The gray shaded area indicates the target prevalence level from society's perspective (<2%). The black dotted horizontal line indicates a prevalence consistent with disease elimination (0.4%; <1 infected animal in a herd of 250 animals).

framework for exploring key factors in the control livestock diseases: farmer heterogeneity, externalities, and private-social misalignment of control optima. Secondly, we apply this framework to the control of endemic chronic diseases through privately funded actions in a low-resource setting.

Despite the growing literature on livestock infectious disease modeling, very little attention has been given to the assumption of homogeneous human behavior, the validity of which we evaluate here. Models of livestock disease typically assume that the farmers' perception of risk and the way they respond to that level of perceived risk remain unchanged over time (22). In addition, many epidemiological models entirely ignore the effects of changing prevalence on privately optimal spending on disease control (22, 23). However, several empirical studies have shown that a farmer's likelihood to take control actions is the result of a dynamic and complex interplay between epidemiological, economic, environmental, cultural, and social factors (39–43). Models of disease transmission that ignore such heterogeneity are likely to be misleading, resulting in reduced value for informing control efforts. Like many decision-makers, farmers make decisions based on conscious and unconscious, cognitive and affective shortcuts or rules of thumb (42, 44, 45). We model the implications of this type of individual decision-making process by simulating the effects on prevalence and costs of different levels of farmer responsiveness. These simulations quantify the consequences of heterogeneous behavior, the occurrence of externalities, and the consequent disparities between privately and socially optimal control efforts.

The simulations of our theoretical scenario of optimizing behavior assumed perfect information and rational behavior by the individual farmer. In this scenario, the farmer was able to accurately choose the optimal control effort at any point in time by trading-off the marginal benefits of reducing the prevalence against the marginal costs of their actions. These models assume a conservative range of values for the unit price of control action (from 0.00 to 1.25 monetary units to reduce the transmission rate by 1% per time step) and cost of one infected animal (from 10 to 85 monetary units per time step). For example, without administration and overhead charges, the annual cost of vaccinating a herd of 250 cattle for brucellosis in India (167.50 USD; 0.67 USD times 250) would be over twice as much the average loss caused by brucellosis per infected animal (73.44 USD) (46). The values that we used are considered appropriate and conservative for this evaluation because the highest possible cost of eliminating disease transmission completely would be equivalent to <1.5 times the highest *ex post* cost of one infected animal per time step. Despite these conservative assumptions, the societal disease control target was only achieved for high disease cost to price of control ratios (<25% of all price-cost combinations; **Figure 4**). Given these findings, we can infer that

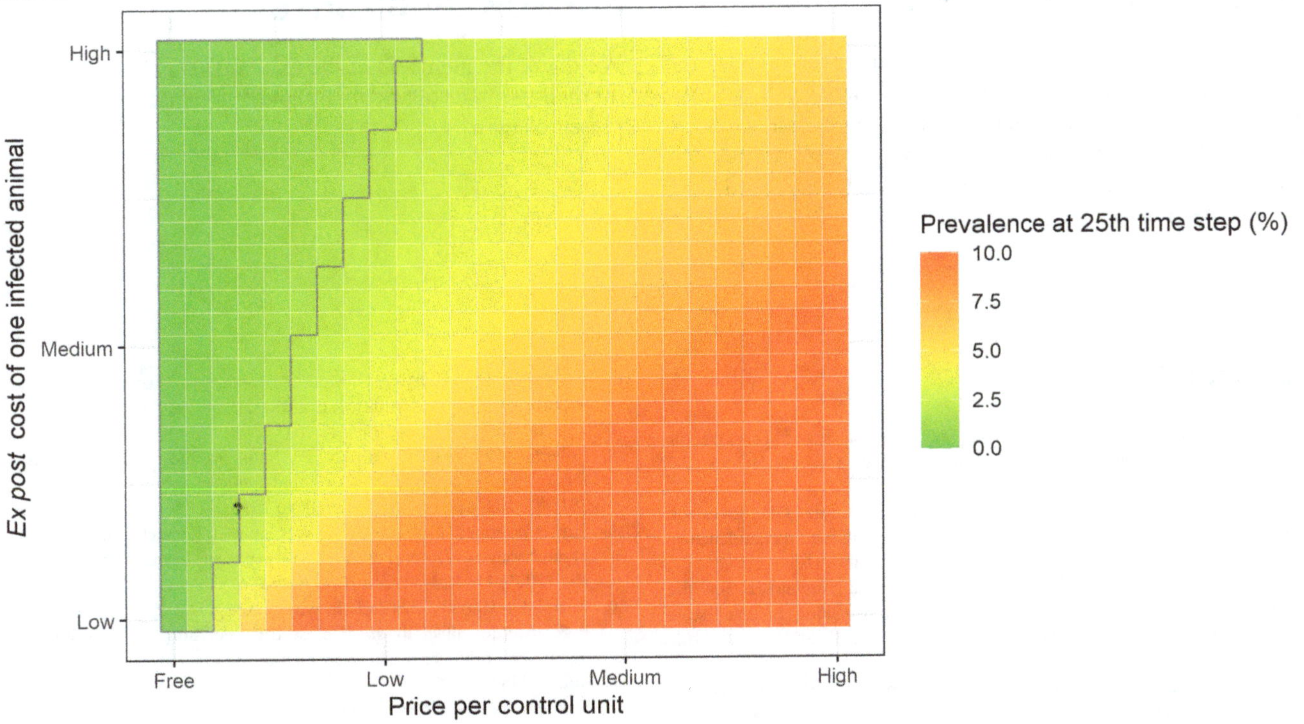

FIGURE 4 | Predicted prevalence at 25th time step for different values of price per control unit ("Free" = 0.00; "Low" = 0.40; "Medium" = 0.85; and, "High" = 1.25 monetary units) and *ex post* cost per infected animal ("Low" = 10; "Medium" = 46; and, "High" = 85 monetary units), assuming privately optimal behavior in a single farm. The polygon with gray border indicates the target prevalence level from society's perspective (<2%).

effective disease control through voluntary actions is unlikely to be privately optimal in many real-world cases. Additionally, as prevalence decreases, there is a sharp increase in the marginal costs of control action, which leads to a fall in optimal control effort. This result is consistent with the economic principle of diminishing returns and has also been reported by other theoretical (32) and empirical studies, namely those that analyzed control actions against tuberculosis (24, 47) and brucellosis (48, 49) in cattle.

Our model illustrates the misalignment of private and social optima for livestock disease control through a basic trade-off between the benefits of reductions in herd prevalence and the costs of transmission-reducing actions. Essentially, farmers "buy reductions in disease transmission," which is a simple and logical representation of many disease control actions. However, this approach is likely to underestimate the gap between private and social optima in many cases: the model does not capture many of the benefits of farmers' actions such as (i) the control of multiple pathogens through improved biosecurity, and (ii) the human health benefits in the cases of zoonoses. For instance, brucellosis is a bacterial zoonosis that causes abortion in livestock and debilitating symptoms (e.g., fever, joint pain, myalgia) in humans (50, 51). Given this burden on human health, in addition to animal health, voluntary actions taken by farmers to control the disease in their livestock (e.g., through vaccination) generate positive externalities, as society benefits from farmers' actions whilst not bearing the costs of these actions. This is a market failure that requires coordinated action to achieve socially optimal outcomes in terms of both human and animal health and productivity (48). Hence, the benefits enjoyed and the costs born by both public and private sectors must be considered throughout the planning phase of control interventions, which can include, among others, the provision of subsidized goods and services (e.g., vaccination), creating and enforcing regulations (e.g., movement restrictions) and setting compensation schemes (e.g., for culled seropositive animals) (8, 48).

To enable private farmers' actions to achieve a socially optimal disease control target, policy design and development must consider the heterogeneity of farmer behavior, the associated off-farm effects or externalities, and the predicted uptake of control measures under optimized farmer behavior. Failure to acknowledge these factors may result in potentially misleading predictions about disease transmission and the associated economic costs. This, in turn, perpetuates conditions in which private investments by farmers are inadequate to achieve disease control from society's perspective. For multi-host diseases that can impact multiple sectors (e.g., multi-host livestock diseases and zoonoses), inadequate disease control can have profound repercussions on international trade and, indeed, threaten human health.

AUTHOR CONTRIBUTIONS

ÂM, DH, EM, NH, and JH contributed to conception and design of the study and writing of the manuscript. ÂM and DH wrote the code in R. ÂM developed the interactive web application. All authors contributed to the article and approved the submitted version.

ACKNOWLEDGMENTS

We thank the members of the OHRBID lab (Univ. of Glasgow) for their useful feedback on the epidemiological-economic model presented here.

REFERENCES

1. FAO. *World Livestock: Transforming the Livestock Sector Through the Sustainable Development Goals*. Rome. Licence: CC BY-NC-SA 3.0 IGO (2018).
2. Marsh TL, Yoder J, Deboch T, McElwain TF, Palmer GH. Livestock vaccinations translate into increased human capital and school attendance by girls. *Sci Adv.* (2016) 2:e1601410. doi: 10.1126/sciadv.1601410
3. Chilonda P, Van Huylenbroeck G. A conceptual framework for the economic analysis of factors influencing decision-making of small-scale farmers in animal health management. *Rev Sci Tech.* (2001) 20:687–700. doi: 10.20506/rst.20.3.1302
4. Ilukor J. Improving the delivery of veterinary services in Africa: insights from the empirical application of transaction costs theory in Uganda and Kenya. *Rev Sci Tech.* (2017) 36:279–89. doi: 10.20506/rst.36.1.2628
5. Leonard DK, Koma LM, Ly C, Woods PS. The new institutional economics of privatising veterinary services in Africa. *Rev Sci Tech.* (1999) 18:544–61. doi: 10.20506/rst.18.2.1178
6. van Veen TWS, de Haan C. Trends in the organization and financing of livestock and animal health services. *Prev Vet Med.* (1995) 25:225–40. doi: 10.1016/0167-5877(95)00540-4
7. Perry BD. Disease control programmes in developing countries: prospects and constraints. In: Dijkhuizen AA, Morris RS, editors. *Animal Health Economics: Principles and Applications*. Sydney, NSW: Post Graduate Foundation Publication (1997). p. 209–32.
8. Rushton J, Leonard DK. The New institutional economics and the assessment of animal disease control. In: Rushton J, editor. *The Economics of Animal Health and Production*. Wallingford: CABI (2009). p. 144–8. doi: 10.1079/9781845931940.0144
9. Sok J, Fischer EAJ. Farmers' heterogeneous motives, voluntary vaccination and disease spread: an agent-based model. *Europ Rev Agr Econ.* (2019) 47:1201–22. doi: 10.1093/erae/jbz041
10. Hanley N, Shogren J, White B. (eds.). Market failure. In: *Environmental Economics: In Theory and Practice*. 2nd ed. Basingstoke: Palgrave Macmillan (2007). p. 42–81.
11. Kristensen E, Jakobsen EB. Danish dairy farmers' perception of biosecurity. *Prev Vet Med.* (2011) 99:122–9. doi: 10.1016/j.prevetmed.2011.01.010
12. Fournie G, Rushton J, Pfeiffer D. Disease modelling and the human factor. *Vet Rec.* (2012) 170:157–8. doi: 10.1136/vr.e588
13. Gilbert W, Rushton J. Incentive perception in livestock disease control. *J Agr Econ.* (2018) 69:243–61. doi: 10.1111/1477-9552.12168
14. Horan RD, Wolf CA, Fenichel EP. Dynamic perspectives on the control of animal disease: merging epidemiology and economics. In: Zilberman D, Otte J, Roland-Holst D, Pfeiffer D, editors. *Health and Animal Agriculture in Developing Countries: Food and Agriculture Organization of the United Nations*. New York, NY: Springer Science+Business Media, LLC (2012). p. 101–18. doi: 10.1007/978-1-4419-7077-0_6
15. Mongoh MN, Hearne R, Khaitsa ML. Private and public economic incentives for the control of animal diseases: the case of anthrax in livestock. *Transbound Emerg Dis.* (2008) 55:319–28. doi: 10.1111/j.1865-1682.2008.01050.x
16. Morin BR, Kinzig AP, Levin SA, Perrings CA. Economic incentives in the socially optimal management of infectious disease: when R_0 is not enough. *EcoHealth.* (2018) 15:274–89. doi: 10.1007/s10393-017-1270-9
17. Rat-Aspert O, Fourichon C. Modelling collective effectiveness of voluntary vaccination with and without incentives. *Prev Vet Med.* (2010) 93:265–75. doi: 10.1016/j.prevetmed.2009.11.004
18. Roberts TW, Peck DE, Ritten JP. Cattle producers' economic incentives for preventing bovine brucellosis under uncertainty. *Prev Vet Med.* (2012) 107:187–203. doi: 10.1016/j.prevetmed.2012.06.008
19. Stott AW, Jones GM, Humphry RW, Gunn GJ. Financial incentive to control paratuberculosis (Johne's disease) on dairy farms in the United Kingdom. *Vet Rec.* (2005) 156:825–31. doi: 10.1136/vr.156.26.825
20. Bucini G, Merrill SC, Clark E, Moegenburg SM, Zia A, Koliba CJ, et al. Risk attitudes affect livestock biosecurity decisions with ramifications for disease control in a simulated production system. *Front Vet Sci.* (2019) 6:196. doi: 10.3389/fvets.2019.00196
21. Delabouglise A, Thanh NTL, Xuyen HTA, Nguyen-Van-Yen B, Tuyet PN, Lam HM, et al. Poultry farmer response to disease outbreaks in smallholder farming systems in southern Vietnam. *Elife.* (2020) 9:e59212. doi: 10.7554/eLife.59212
22. Hidano A, Enticott G, Christley RM, Gates MC. Modeling dynamic human behavioral changes in animal disease models: challenges and opportunities for addressing bias. *Front Vet Sci.* (2018) 5:137. doi: 10.3389/fvets.2018.00137
23. Barnes AP, Moxey AP, Vosough Ahmadi B, Borthwick FA. The effect of animal health compensation on 'positive' behaviours towards exotic disease reporting and implementing biosecurity: a review, a synthesis and a research agenda. *Prev Vet Med.* (2015) 122:42–52. doi: 10.1016/j.prevetmed.2015.09.003
24. Bicknell KB, Wilen JE, Howitt RE. Public policy and private incentives for livestock disease control. *Aust J Agric Resour Econ.* (1999) 43:501–21. doi: 10.1111/1467-8489.00092
25. Gramig BM, Horan RD. Jointly determined livestock disease dynamics and decentralised economic behaviour. *Aust J Agric Resour Econ.* (2011) 55:393–410. doi: 10.1111/j.1467-8489.2011.00543.x
26. Wolf CA. Using institutional and behavioural economics to examine animal health systems. *Rev Sci Tech.* (2017) 36:67–76. doi: 10.20506/rst.36.1.2610
27. Mancy R, Brock PM, Kao RR. An integrated framework for process-driven model construction in disease ecology and animal health. *Front Vet Sci.* (2017) 4:155. doi: 10.3389/fvets.2017.00155
28. European Comission. *Brucellosis in Sheep and Goats (Brucella melitensis)*. Adopted 12 July 2001. Report of the Scientific Committee on Animal Health and Animal Welfare. Health & Consumer Protection Directorate-General. Directorate C - Scientific Health Opinions. C2 - Management of scientific committees; scientific co-operation and networks. SANCO.C.2/AH/R23/2001 (2001).
29. R Core Team. *R: A Language and Environment for Statistical Computing*. Vienna: R Foundation for Statistical Computing (2018).
30. Soetaert K, Petzoldt T, Setzer RW. Solving differential equations in R: Package deSolve. *J Stat Softw.* (2010) 33:25. doi: 10.18637/jss.v033.i09
31. Wickham H. *ggplot2: Elegant Graphics for Data Analysis*. New York, NY: Springer-Verlag (2016).
32. McInerney JP, Howe KS, Schepers JA. A framework for the economic analysis of disease in farm livestock. *Prev Vet Med.* (1992) 13:137–54. doi: 10.1016/0167-5877(92)90098-Z
33. Anderson CL, Gugerty MK. Intertemporal choice and development policy: new evidence on time-varying discount rates from Vietnam and Russia. *Dev Econ.* (2009) 47:123–46. doi: 10.1111/j.1746-1049.2009.00080.x

34. Chang W, Cheng J, Allaire JJ, Xie Y, McPherson J. *shiny: Web Application Framework for R*. R package version 1.4.0. 2019. Available online at: https://CRAN.R-project.org/package=shiny
35. Chang W, Ribeiro BB. *shinydashboard: Create Dashboards with 'Shiny'*. R package version 0.7.1. 2018. Available online at: https://CRAN.R-project.org/package=shinydashboard
36. Delabouglise A, Boni MF. Game theory of vaccination and depopulation for managing livestock diseases and zoonoses on small-scale farms. *Epidemics*. (2020) 30:100370. doi: 10.1016/j.epidem.2019.100370
37. Hennessy DA. Biosecurity and spread of an infectious animal disease. *Am J Agric Econ*. (2007) 89:1226–31. doi: 10.1111/j.1467-8276.2007.01088.x
38. Tago D, Hammitt JK, Thomas A, Raboisson D. the impact of farmers' strategic behavior on the spread of animal infectious diseases. *PLoS ONE*. (2016) 11:e0157450. doi: 10.1371/journal.pone.0157450
39. Ahmed H, Call DR, Quinlan RJ, Yoder JK. Relationships between livestock grazing practices, disease risk, and antimicrobial use among East African Agropastoralists. *Environ Devel Econ*. (2017) 23:80–97. doi: 10.1017/S1355770X17000341
40. Chaters GL, Johnson PCD, Cleaveland S, Crispell J, de Glanville WA, Doherty T, et al. Analysing livestock network data for infectious disease control: an argument for routine data collection in emerging economies. *Philos Trans R Soc Lond B Biol Sci*. (2019) 374:20180264. doi: 10.1098/rstb.2018.0264
41. Ifft J, Roland-Holst D, Zilberman D. Production and risk prevention response of free range chicken producers in Viet Nam to highly pathogenic avian influenza outbreaks. *Am J Agric Econ*. (2011) 93:490–7. doi: 10.1093/ajae/aaq135
42. Manyweathers J, Field H, Longnecker N, Agho K, Smith C, Taylor M. "Why won't they just vaccinate?" Horse owner risk perception and uptake of the Hendra virus vaccine. *BMC Vet Res*. (2017) 13. doi: 10.1186/s12917-017-1006-7
43. Oparinde A, Birol E. Farm households' preferences for cash-based compensation versus livelihood-enhancing programmes: a choice experiment to inform avian flu (hpai h5n1) compensation policy in Nigeria. *J Afr Econ*. (2012) 21:637–68. doi: 10.1093/jae/ejs004
44. Findlater KM, Satterfield T, Kandlikar M. Farmers' risk-based decision making under pervasive uncertainty: cognitive thresholds and hazy hedging. *Risk Anal*. (2019) 39:1755–70. doi: 10.1111/risa.13290
45. Gigerenzer G, Gaissmaier W. Heuristic decision making. *Annu Rev Psychol*. (2011) 62:451–82. doi: 10.1146/annurev-psych-120709-145346
46. Singh BB, Kostoulas P, Gill JPS, Dhand NK. Cost-benefit analysis of intervention policies for prevention and control of brucellosis in India. *PLoS Negl Trop Dis*. (2018) 12:e0006488-e. doi: 10.1371/journal.pntd.0006488
47. Hone J. Diminishing returns in bovine tuberculosis control. *Epidemiol Infect*. (2013) 141:1382–9. doi: 10.1017/S0950268813000927
48. Peck D, Bruce M. The economic efficiency and equity of government policies on brucellosis: comparative insights from Albania and the United States of America. *Rev Sci Tech*. (2017) 36:291–302. doi: 10.20506/rst.36.1.2629
49. Peck DE. Bovine brucellosis in the greater yellowstone area: an economic diagnosis. *West Econ Forum*. (2010) 9:27–41. doi: 10.22004/ag.econ.176167
50. Corbel MJ. *Food and Agriculture Organization of the United Nations, World Organisation for Animal Health, World Health Organization*. Brucellosis in Humans and Animals. WHO/CDS/EPR/2006.7. Geneva: WHO Press (2006). p. 4–10.
51. Dean AS, Crump L, Greter H, Hattendorf J, Schelling E, Zinsstag J. Clinical manifestations of human brucellosis: a systematic review and meta-analysis. *PLoS Negl Trop Dis*. (2012) 6:e1929. doi: 10.1371/journal.pntd.0001929

PERMISSIONS

All chapters in this book were first published by Frontiers; hereby published with permission under the Creative Commons Attribution License or equivalent. Every chapter published in this book has been scrutinized by our experts. Their significance has been extensively debated. The topics covered herein carry significant findings which will fuel the growth of the discipline. They may even be implemented as practical applications or may be referred to as a beginning point for another development.

The contributors of this book come from diverse backgrounds, making this book a truly international effort. This book will bring forth new frontiers with its revolutionizing research information and detailed analysis of the nascent developments around the world.

We would like to thank all the contributing authors for lending their expertise to make the book truly unique. They have played a crucial role in the development of this book. Without their invaluable contributions this book wouldn't have been possible. They have made vital efforts to compile up to date information on the varied aspects of this subject to make this book a valuable addition to the collection of many professionals and students.

This book was conceptualized with the vision of imparting up-to-date information and advanced data in this field. To ensure the same, a matchless editorial board was set up. Every individual on the board went through rigorous rounds of assessment to prove their worth. After which they invested a large part of their time researching and compiling the most relevant data for our readers.

The editorial board has been involved in producing this book since its inception. They have spent rigorous hours researching and exploring the diverse topics which have resulted in the successful publishing of this book. They have passed on their knowledge of decades through this book. To expedite this challenging task, the publisher supported the team at every step. A small team of assistant editors was also appointed to further simplify the editing procedure and attain best results for the readers.

Apart from the editorial board, the designing team has also invested a significant amount of their time in understanding the subject and creating the most relevant covers. They scrutinized every image to scout for the most suitable representation of the subject and create an appropriate cover for the book.

The publishing team has been an ardent support to the editorial, designing and production team. Their endless efforts to recruit the best for this project, has resulted in the accomplishment of this book. They are a veteran in the field of academics and their pool of knowledge is as vast as their experience in printing. Their expertise and guidance has proved useful at every step. Their uncompromising quality standards have made this book an exceptional effort. Their encouragement from time to time has been an inspiration for everyone.

The publisher and the editorial board hope that this book will prove to be a valuable piece of knowledge for researchers, students, practitioners and scholars across the globe.

LIST OF CONTRIBUTORS

Rania Hamada
Photonics Control Technology Team, RIKEN Center for Advanced Photonics, Saitama, Japan
Department of Animal Medicine, Faculty of Veterinary Medicine, South Valley University, Qena, Egypt

Samy Metwally
Photonics Control Technology Team, RIKEN Center for Advanced Photonics, Saitama, Japan
Laboratory of Global Animal Resource Science, Graduate School of Agricultural and Life Sciences, The University of Tokyo, Tokyo, Japan
Department of Animal Medicine, Faculty of Veterinary Medicine, Damanhour University, Damanhour, Egypt

Meripet Polat and Liushiqi Borjigin
Nakamura Laboratory, Baton Zone Program, RIKEN Cluster for Science, Technology and Innovation Hub, Saitama, Japan

Alsagher O. Ali and Adel E. A. Mohamed
Department of Animal Medicine, Faculty of Veterinary Medicine, South Valley University, Qena, Egypt

A. A. A. Abdel-Hady
Department of Surgery, Anaesthesiology and Radiology, Faculty of Veterinary Medicine, South Valley University, Qena, Egypt

Satoshi Wada
Photonics Control Technology Team, RIKEN Center for Advanced Photonics, Saitama, Japan

Yoko Aida
Laboratory of Global Animal Resource Science, Graduate School of Agricultural and Life Sciences, The University of Tokyo, Tokyo, Japan
Nakamura Laboratory, Baton Zone Program, RIKEN Cluster for Science, Technology and Innovation Hub, Saitama, Japan

Raquel Álvarez-Alonso, Ion I. Zendoia, Jesús F. Barandika, Ana Hurtado and Ana L. García-Pérez
Animal Health Department, NEIKER-Instituto Vasco de Investigación y Desarrollo Agrario, Derio, Spain

Isabel Jado
Laboratory of Special Pathogens, Instituto de Salud Carlos III, Centro Nacional de Microbiología, Madrid, Spain

Ceferino M. López
Department of Animal Pathology, Veterinary Faculty, University of Santiago de Compostela, Lugo, Spain

Han Chang, Shengyong Feng, Qianqian Su, Bo Wang and Juan Du
National Research Center for Wildlife-Borne Diseases, Institute of Zoology, Chinese Academy of Sciences, Beijing, China
College of Life Sciences, University of Chinese Academy of Sciences, Beijing, China

Yutian Wang and Fuhuang Li
Department of Microbiology, Beijing General Station of Animal Husbandry, Beijing, China

Hongxuan He
National Research Center for Wildlife-Borne Diseases, Institute of Zoology, Chinese Academy of Sciences, Beijing, China

Qing-Long Gong
College of Chinese Medicine Materials, Jilin Agricultural University, Changchun, China
College of Animal Science and Technology, Jilin Agricultural University, Changchun, China

Yu-Han Sun, Yang Yang, Jian-Ming Li, Kun Shi, Xue Leng and Ying Zong
College of Chinese Medicine Materials, Jilin Agricultural University, Changchun, China

Bo Zhao, Qi Wang, Gui-Yang Ge and Zi-Yang Chen
College of Animal Science and Technology, Jilin Agricultural University, Changchun, China

Rui Du
College of Chinese Medicine Materials, Jilin Agricultural University, Changchun, China
Laboratory of Production and Product Application of Sika Deer of Jilin Province, Jilin Agricultural University, Changchun, China
Key Lab of Animal Production, Product Quality and Security, Ministry of Education, Jilin Agricultural University, Changchun, China

Ki Myung Choi
Optipharm, Inc., Cheongju, South Korea

Seongho Shin
Optipharm Animal Disease Diagnostic Center, Cheongju, South Korea

Thi Ngan Mai
Graduate School of Medicine and Veterinary Medicine, University of Miyazaki, Miyazaki, Japan
Faculty of Veterinary Medicine, Vietnam National University of Agriculture, Hanoi, Vietnam

Thanh Phong Bui
Branch of Cargill Vietnam Co., Ltd, Dong Van II Industrial Zone, Ha Nam, Vietnam

Thi My Le Huynh
Faculty of Veterinary Medicine, Vietnam National University of Agriculture, Hanoi, Vietnam

Yosuke Sasaki
Department of Animal and Grassland Sciences, Faculty of Agriculture, University of Miyazaki, Miyazaki, Japan
Center for Animal Disease Control, University of Miyazaki, Miyazaki, Japan

Shuya Mitoma
Graduate School of Medicine and Veterinary Medicine, University of Miyazaki, Miyazaki, Japan

Hala El Daous
Graduate School of Medicine and Veterinary Medicine, University of Miyazaki, Miyazaki, Japan
Faculty of Veterinary Medicine, Benha University, Toukh, Egypt

Watcharapong Fahkrajang
Department of Livestock Development, Ministry of Agriculture and Cooperatives, Bangkok, Thailand

Junzo Norimine and Satoshi Sekiguchi
Center for Animal Disease Control, University of Miyazaki, Miyazaki, Japan
Department of Veterinary Science, Faculty of Agriculture, University of Miyazaki, Miyazaki, Japan

Fenja Winter, Clara Schoneberg and Amely Campe
Department of Biometry, Epidemiology and Information Processing, WHO Collaborating Centre for Research and Training for Health at the Human-Animal-Environment Interface, University of Veterinary Medicine Hannover Foundation, Hanover, Germany

Annika Wolf, Benjamin U. Bauer and Martin Ganter
Clinic for Swine, Small Ruminants and Forensic Medicine, University of Veterinary Medicine Hannover Foundation, Hanover, Germany

T. Louise Prüfer and Martin Runge
Lower Saxony State Office for Consumer Protection and Food Safety - Food and Veterinary Institute Braunschweig/Hannover, Hanover, Germany

Silke F. Fischer
National Consulting Laboratory for Coxiella burnetii, State Health Office Baden-Württemberg, Stuttgart, Germany

Ursula Gerdes
Animal Disease Fund of Lower Saxony, Public Law Institution, Hanover, Germany

Lin Zheng
School of Food and Engineering, Jilin Agricultural University, Changchun, China
The Key Laboratory of Jilin Province for Zoonosis Prevention and Control, Changchun, China

Ling-Wei Zhu, Jie Jing, Jia-yao Guan, Ge-Jin Lu, Xue Ji, Yang Sun and Xue-Jun Guo
The Key Laboratory of Jilin Province for Zoonosis Prevention and Control, Changchun, China

Lin-Hong Xie and Dong Chu
Wild Animal Sources and Diseases Inspection Station, National Forestry and Grassl and Bureau, Beijing, China

Ping Chen
School of Food and Engineering, Jilin Agricultural University, Changchun, China

Kohei Makita, Lisa Haruta, Yuki Nakahara, Yuto Tamura, Takuto Watanabe, Hazumu Kadowaki and Shingo Asakura
Veterinary Epidemiology Unit, School of Veterinary Medicine, Rakuno Gakuen University, Ebetsu, Japan

Elly Steenbergen
Veterinary Epidemiology Unit, School of Veterinary Medicine, Rakuno Gakuen University, Ebetsu, Japan
Quantitative Veterinary Epidemiology Group, Wageningen University & Research, Wageningen, Netherlands

Saddam Hossain
Veterinary Epidemiology Unit, School of Veterinary Medicine, Rakuno Gakuen University, Ebetsu, Japan
Department of Medicine and Surgery, Faculty of Veterinary Medicine, Chittagong Veterinary and Animal Sciences University, Chittagong, Bangladesh

Peng Li, Dingxiu Zhang, Hongmei Li, Jinying Pang, Huijun Guo and Jianhua Qiu
College of Animal Science and Veterinary Medicine, Shandong Agricultural University, Tai'an, China
Shandong Provincial Key Laboratory of Animal Biotechnology and Disease Control and Prevention, Shandong Provincial Engineering Technology Research Center of Animal Disease Control and Prevention, Shandong Agricultural University, Tai'an, China

Linyang Yu, Yanling Liu, Shuangyun Wang, Leyi Zhang, Pengshuai Liang, Lei Wang and Changxu Song
College of Animal Science & National Engineering Center for Swine Breeding Industry, South China Agriculture University, Guangzhou, China

Jianguo Dong
School of Animal Husbandry and Medical Engineering, Xinyang Agriculture and Forestry University, Xinyang, China

Shan Wen Stacy Khaw, Joanne Meers and Joerg Henning
School of Veterinary Science, The University of Queensland, Gatton, QLD, Australia

Le Tri Vu
Regional Animal Health Centre VI, Ho Chi Minh City, Vietnam

Didik Yulianto
Disease Investigation Centre, Wates, Indonesia

Yu Pang, Defang Zhou, Jing Zhou, Jingwen Xue and Ziqiang Cheng
College of Veterinary Medicine, Shandong Agricultural University, Tai'an, China

Yiya Wang
School of Life Sciences, Qilu Normal University, Jinan, China

Katharina Giebel
School of Life Sciences, University of Warwick, Coventry, United Kingdom
School of Agriculture, Food and the Environment, Royal Agricultural University, Gloucestershire, United Kingdom

Laura E. Green
College of Life and Environmental Sciences, Institute for Microbiology and Infection, University of Birmingham, Birmingham, United Kingdom

Kevin J. Purdy
School of Life Sciences, University of Warwick, Coventry, United Kingdom

Lee V. Wisener and Jan M. Sargeant
Department of Population Medicine, Ontario Veterinary College, University of Guelph, Guelph, ON, Canada
Centre for Public Health and Zoonoses, University of Guelph, Guelph, ON, Canada

Terri L. O'Sullivan, Scott A. McEwen, Mark Reist and Katheryn J. Churchill
Department of Population Medicine, Ontario Veterinary College, University of Guelph, Guelph, ON, Canada

Annette M. O'Connor
Department of Large Animal Clinical Sciences, College of Veterinary Medicine, Michigan State University, East Lansing, MI, United States

Velma Kivali
International Livestock Research Institute, Nairobi, Kenya
Biomedical Sciences, Edinburgh Medical School, University of Edinburgh, Edinburgh, United Kingdom

Alice N. Kiyong'a and Philip Toye
International Livestock Research Institute, Nairobi, Kenya

Jenna Fyfe
Biomedical Sciences, Edinburgh Medical School, University of Edinburgh, Edinburgh, United Kingdom

Eric M. Fèvre and Elizabeth A. J. Cook
International Livestock Research Institute, Nairobi, Kenya
Institute of Infection, Veterinary and Ecological Sciences, University of Liverpool, Liverpool, United Kingdom

Jin-Yong Noh, Kyu-Jik Kim and Jun-Beom Kim
Konkuk Ctc bio Animal Vaccine KCAV Co. Ltd, Seoul, South Korea

Sun-Hak Lee, Deok-Hwan Kim and Sungsu Youk
Department of Avian Disease, College of Veterinary Medicine, Konkuk University, Seoul, South Korea

Chang-Seon Song
Konkuk Ctc bio Animal Vaccine KCAV Co. Ltd, Seoul, South Korea
Department of Avian Disease, College of Veterinary Medicine, Konkuk University, Seoul, South Korea

Sang-Soep Nahm
Department of Anatomy, College of Veterinary Medicine, Konkuk University, Seoul, South Korea

Jason Nickell
Allflex Livestock Intelligence, Madison, WI, United States

Lonty Bryant
Merck Animal Health, De Soto, KS, United States

Kelly F. Lechtenberg and Charley Cull
Midwest Veterinary Services, Oakland, NE, United States
Veterinary and Biomedical Research Center, Manhattan, KS, United States

Hye-young Wang and Hyunil Kim
Optipharm, Inc., Cheongju-Si, South Korea,

Joong Ki Song and Seongho Shin
Optipharm Animal Disease Diagnostic Center, Cheongju-Si, South Korea

Baishuang Yin, Wanli Sha, Hongyu Qin, Liming Liu, Jinyan Yun and Guojiang Li
College of Animal Science and Technology, Jilin Agricultural Science and Technology University, Jilin, China

Shanshan Qi and Jinhai Zhu
Laboratory for the Prevention and Control of Swine Infectious Diseases, College of Animal Science and Veterinary Medicine, Heilongjiang Bayi Agricultural University, Daqing, China

Dongbo Sun
College of Animal Science and Technology, Jilin Agricultural Science and Technology University, Jilin, China
Laboratory for the Prevention and Control of Swine Infectious Diseases, College of Animal Science and Veterinary Medicine, Heilongjiang Bayi Agricultural University, Daqing, China

Ângelo J. Mendes, Daniel T. Haydon, Nick Hanley and Jo E. B. Halliday
College of Medical, Veterinary and Life Sciences, Institute of Biodiversity, Animal Health and Comparative Medicine, University of Glasgow, Glasgow, United Kingdom

Emma McIntosh
College of Medical, Veterinary and Life Sciences, Institute of Health and Wellbeing, University of Glasgow, Glasgow, United Kingdom

Index

www.ingramcontent.com/pod-product-compliance
Lightning Source LLC
LaVergne TN
LVHW060521210926
848485LV00005B/1119
9781647404413